P9-DTF-282

American
Medical
Association

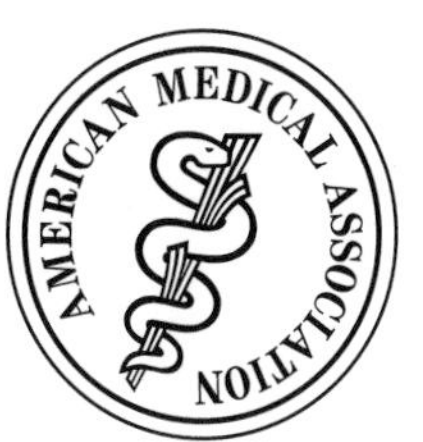

Complete Guide to Your Children's Health

Other books by the
American Medical Association

American Medical Association
Complete Guide to Women's Health

American Medical Association
Family Medical Guide

American Medical Association
Encyclopedia of Medicine

American Medical Association
Guide to Your Family's Symptoms

American Medical Association
Handbook of First Aid and Emergency Care

American Medical Association
Pocket Guide to Back Pain

American Medical Association
Pocket Guide to First Aid and Emergency Care

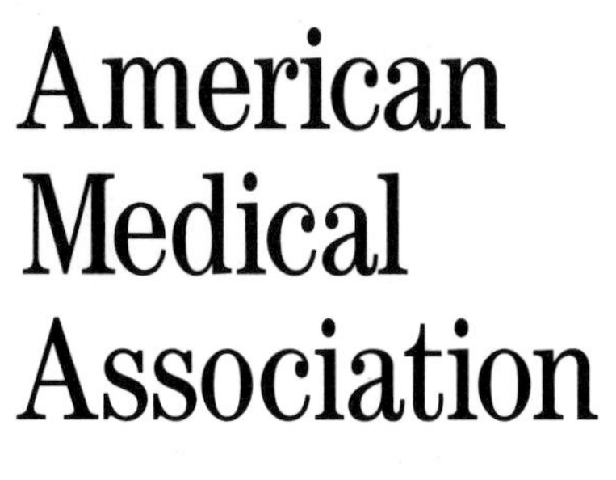

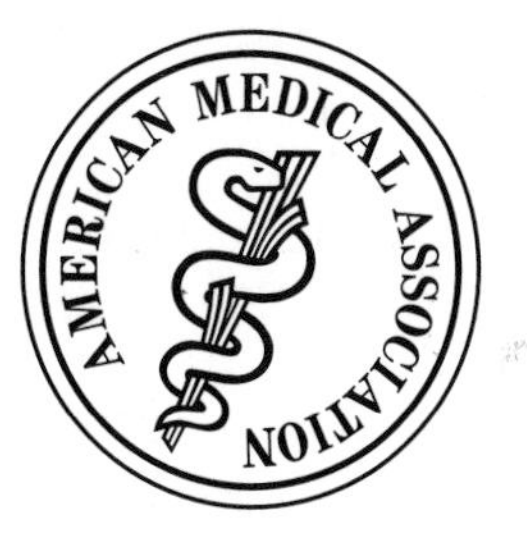

Complete Guide to Your Children's Health

Edward S. Traisman, MD
Pediatrician
Medical Editor

Karen Judy, MD
Pediatrician
Assistant Medical Editor

Mary Jane Staba, MD
Pediatrician
Assistant Medical Editor

Written by
Donna Kotulak
Dennis Connaughton

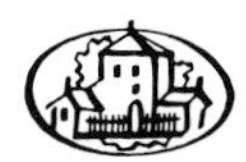

Random House New York

tions and information in this book are appropriate in most cases; however,
ostitute for medical diagnosis. For specific information concerning your child's
ı, the AMA suggests that you consult a physician. The names of organizations,
native therapies appearing in the book are given for informational purposes
only. Their inclusion does not imply AMA endorsement, nor does the omission of any organization, product, or alternative therapy indicate AMA disapproval.

Photograph of seborrheic dermatitis on page 23, copyright SPL Custom Medical Stock Photo

Photograph of poison ivy on page 23, copyright Custom Medical Stock Photo

Photograph of diaper rash on page 23, copyright Custom Medical Stock Photo

Photograph of cradle cap on page 23, copyright NMSB Custom Medical Stock Photo

Photograph of impetigo on page 23, copyright SPL Custom Medical Stock Photo

Photograph of cold sores on page 23, copyright Science Source/Photo Researchers

Photograph of chickenpox on page 24, copyright Martin/Custom Medical Stock Photo

Photograph of roseola on page 24, copyright Keith/Custom Medical Stock Photo

Photograph of hand-foot-and-mouth disease on page 24, copyright SPL Custom Medical Stock Photo

Photograph of fifth disease on page 24, copyright SPL Custom Medical Stock Photo

Photograph of measles on page 24, copyright NMSB Custom Medical Stock Photo

Photograph of German measles on page 24, copyright NMSB Custom Medical Stock Photo

Photograph of scarlet fever on page 24, copyright Custom Medical Stock Photo

Chart, page 113, adapted from the US Department of Agriculture Handbook No. 8

Chart, page 190, adapted from data provided by Procter & Gamble

Chart, page 196, adapted from the 1997 Monitoring the Future Study, University of Michigan/National Institute on Drug Abuse

Charts, pages 239-243, adapted with permission from Ross Laboratories

Vision chart, page 248, reprinted with permission from National Society to Prevent Blindness

Chart, page 444, adapted from data provided by American Cancer Association

Library of Congress Cataloging-in-Publication Data
American medical association complete guide to children's health
p. cm.
Includes index.
ISBN 0-679-45776-3 (alk. paper)
1. Children–Diseases–Popular works. 2. Children–Health and hygiene–Popular works. 3. Pediatrics–Popular works. 4. Child rearing–Health aspects–Popular works. I. American Medical Association.
RJ61.A535 1999 98-6970
618.92–dc21

Random House website address: www.atrandom.com

Printed in the United States of America
98765432
First Edition

American Medical Association

Physicians dedicated to the health of America

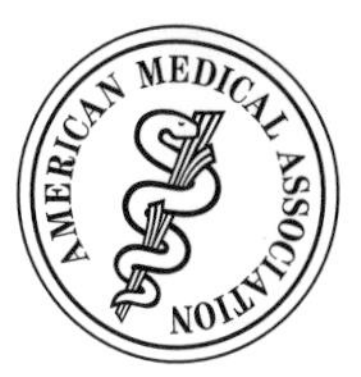

Foreword

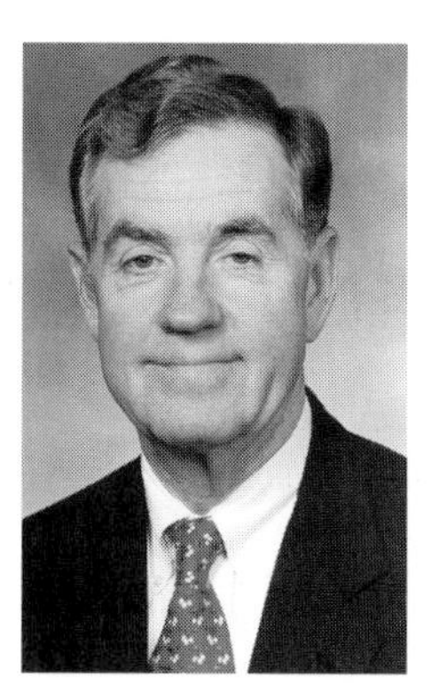

Nothing is more important to our future than the health and well-being of our children. The *American Medical Association Complete Guide to Your Children's Health* gives you, as parents, the information you need to keep your children healthy and safe, and to help them reach their full physical, intellectual, and emotional potential.

The first half of the book is devoted to your child's healthy development from birth through adolescence, including important issues such as preventive health, safety, emotional health, and finding quality child care. Highlighting new knowledge about brain development, several chapters explain what you can do during the critical first 3 years of your child's life to lay a strong foundation for his or her future health, happiness, and achievement. Simple measures such as talking and reading to a child can significantly enhance his or her development.

The second half of the book is an encyclopedia of the most common childhood diseases and disorders, providing current information about how these illnesses are diagnosed and treated. Today, we can successfully treat, cure, or control more childhood diseases than ever before, including some cancers, and we have discovered new ways to prevent many others.

You can look for additional information about children's health on the AMA website at **http://www.ama-assn.org.** You can also use this website to access Physician Select: Online Doctor Finder–a directory of licensed doctors nationwide.

The joy of seeing a child grow into a mature, happy adult is a parent's greatest pleasure and proudest achievement. We want the *American Medical Association Complete Guide to Your Children's Health* to be an indispensable, trusted reference for you and your family.

E. Ratcliffe Anderson, Jr, MD
Executive Vice President,
Chief Executive Officer

The American Medical Association

	E. Ratcliffe Anderson, Jr, MD	*Executive Vice President, Chief Executive Officer*
	Robert L. Kennett	*Senior Vice President, Publishing and Business Services*
	M. Frances Dyra	*Director, Product Line Development*
Editorial Staff	Edward S. Traisman, MD	*Medical Editor*
	Karen Judy, MD	*Assistant Medical Editor*
	Mary Jane Staba, MD	*Assistant Medical Editor*
	Dorothea Guthrie	*Managing Editor*
	Pam Brick	*Senior Editor*
	Donna Kotulak	*Writer*
	Dennis Connaughton	*Writer*
	Robin Fitzpatrick Husayko	*Editor*
	Anne White Michalski	*Medical Researcher*
	Erin Henke	*Medical Researcher*
	Laura Barnes	*Editorial Assistant*
	Mary Mortensen	*Indexer*
Illustration	Scott Thorn Barrows	*Medical Illustrator*
	Rolin Graphics Inc.	*General Illustrators*
Alison Brown Cerier Book Development, Inc.	Alison Brown Cerier	*Book Developer*
	Michaelis/Carpelis Design Associates, Inc.	*Designer*
	David Lynch	*Proofreader*
Medical Consultants	Eugene Anandappa, MD	*Nuclear Medicine*
	Ellen Chadwick, MD	*Infectious Diseases*
	Paul J. Chaiken, DDS	*Dentistry*
	Charles Czerpak, DDS	*Pediatric Dentistry*
	Mindy Hermann, MBA, RD	*Nutrition*
	Sheila Hickey, MSW	*Social Services*
	Andrew Lazar, MD	*Dermatology*
	Peg Maher	*Audiology*
	Amy Paller, MD	*Dermatology*
	Humphrey Roberts, DVM	*Veterinary Medicine*
	Ramona I. Slupik, MD	*Obstetrics and Gynecology*
	Nicky Ward, BSN, IBCLC	*Lactation*

Contents

PART 2: CARING FOR YOUR CHILD'S HEALTH 205

Quick reference lists

A parent's guides

These illustrated, two-page features give you the facts you need to take action on important health and safety concerns.

First aid and emergencies

This handy first-aid guide gives you concise instructions about how to handle common childhood emergencies.

Symptom charts

These charts lead you through a question-and-answer format to help you find the possible causes of many common childhood symptoms, either directing you to other parts of the book for more detailed information, advising you about care you can give at home, or recommending medical attention for your child.

Infants

Children

About this book

The *American Medical Association Complete Guide to Your Children's Health* gives you up-to-date information that enables you to help your children achieve their full physical, emotional, and intellectual potential. The book emphasizes healthy development, safety, the basics of a healthy lifestyle (such as nutritious eating and regular exercise), and helping children acquire self-esteem, self-discipline, and sound judgment.

The first part of the book, Your Healthy Child From Birth Through Adolescence, includes six chapters devoted to specific age groups from birth to age 21. In addition to describing the developmental advances that parents can expect at each stage, these chapters highlight what you as parents can do to stimulate your children's development and enhance their health. Each chapter provides helpful information about fundamentals such as nutrition, exercise, sleep, and discipline. It's a good idea to read ahead to the next stage of your child's development so you'll know what to expect.

The second part of the book, Caring for Your Child's Health, includes information about a variety of topics. Subjects include preventive health care (such as routine screening tests, vaccinations, and well-child visits to the doctor), dental hygiene, and at-home care for children with common illnesses such as a cold or sore throat. Other chapters explore such important concerns as finding quality child care, preventing injuries, and nurturing your children's emotional health. A chapter that speaks to parents of children with special health needs offers encouragement and helpful suggestions about how to be advocates for your children to get the help and services they need.

The third, largest part of the book, Childhood Diseases and Disorders, is an illustrated encyclopedia of the most common illnesses of childhood. The entries about specific illnesses include descriptions of their symptoms and current knowledge about how they are diagnosed and treated. Boxed features throughout this section provide additional information about particular disorders, such as ways to prevent or manage them, or detailed explanations of relevant medical terms, concepts, tests, or procedures.

At the front of the book, you'll find an anatomical atlas with colorful, detailed illustrations of the major systems and organs of the body and brief explanations of how they function. Throughout the book are two-page features, or parent guides, that give you practical facts about common health and safety concerns–from ear infections to how to childproof your home. For a list of these features and their location in the book, see page 13. Symptom charts, which are listed on page 357 and found on pages 358 to 400, suggest the possible causes and significance of many common symptoms, such as fever or vomiting, and help you determine what measures to take. A section at the back of the book, First Aid and Emergencies, provides instructions for giving first aid or taking other action in the event of an injury or emergency.

Atlas of the body

When it comes to anatomy, children are not just little adults. Their bones are softer, their head is proportionally larger, and they breathe faster because they have less lung volume than adults. These differences affect the way children respond to illness and injury. For example, children under age 5 have a shorter, narrower windpipe than do adults, making them more susceptible to airway obstruction.

This atlas illustrates the major systems and organs of a child's body. In most cases the drawings show the body systems of a 6-year-old child, unless otherwise noted. Use this atlas to learn how your child's body looks on the inside. Show your child the illustrations on these pages so he or she can learn about the body too. To find out more about your child's body systems, consult the index at the back of this book.

THE TORSO

The upper part of a child's torso, the chest, contains the heart and lungs. The lower part of the torso, the abdomen, holds the digestive, urinary, and reproductive systems. See page 22 for the position and function of the kidneys and bladder (not shown here).

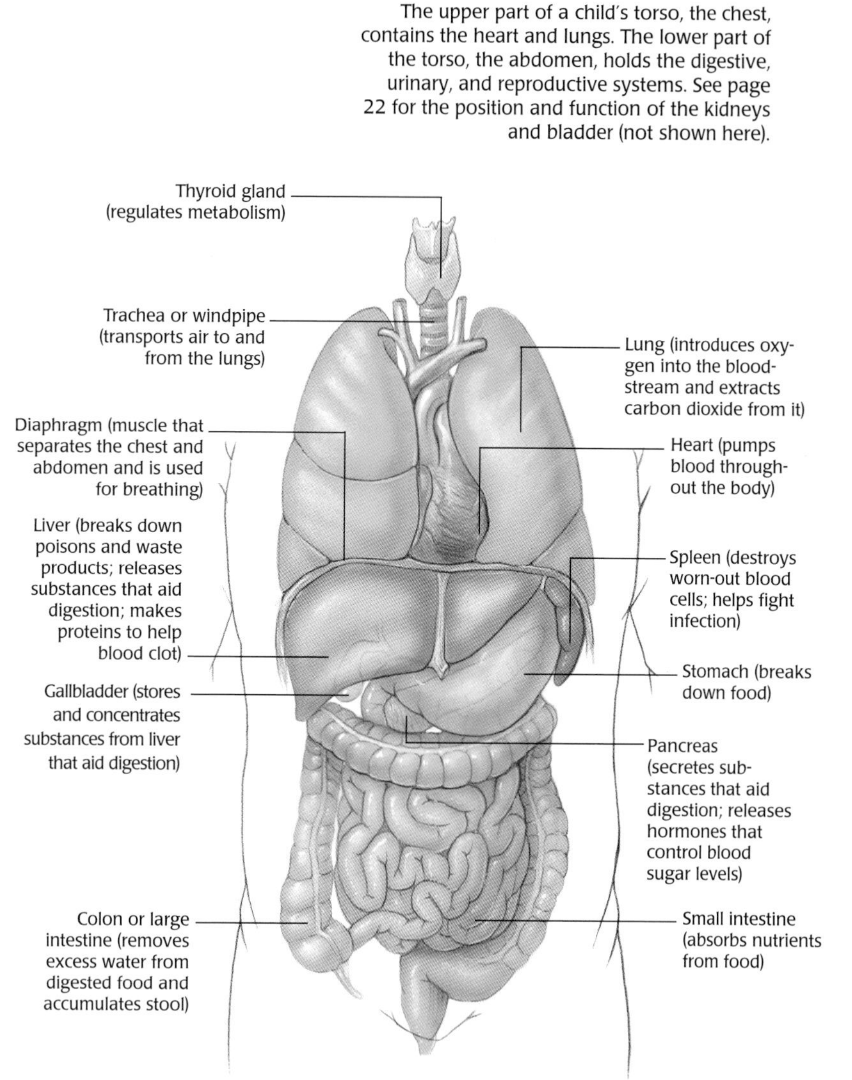

BONES AND MUSCLES

The 206 bones and more than 600 muscles in a child's body work together to support the body and help it move. They also protect the child's internal organs. Bones grow to their peak strength and density by about age 18, so now is the best time to help your child build strong bones. Provide your child with a calcium- and vitamin D-rich diet and encourage him or her to get plenty of exercise, which helps build strong bones and muscles.

BONES

An infant's skeleton is quite a bit different from that of an older child or adult. For example, the skull makes up about one fourth of an infant's body compared with only about one eighth in an older child. An infant's neck is shorter, the jaw smaller, and the forehead less prominent. The trunk of an infant is longer in proportion to the rest of the body, and the arms and legs are shorter. A child grows as much as 17 inches in the first 2 years of life and then 1 to 2 inches a year until the growth spurt of puberty. As a child grows, his or her bones become harder, thicker, longer, and stronger. In long bones such as the femur, the most active areas of growth lie near the ends of the bones, in areas called growth plates (see shaded area).

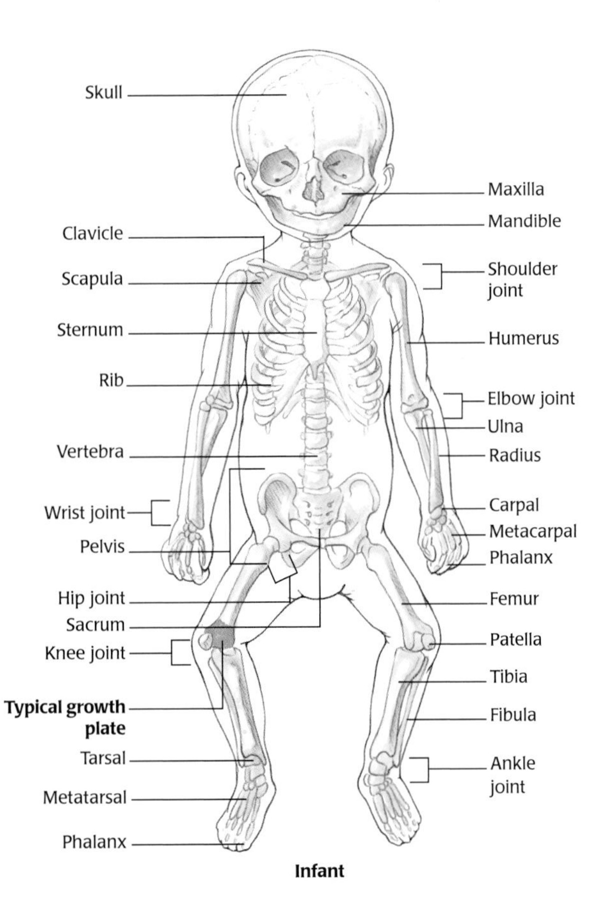

Infant

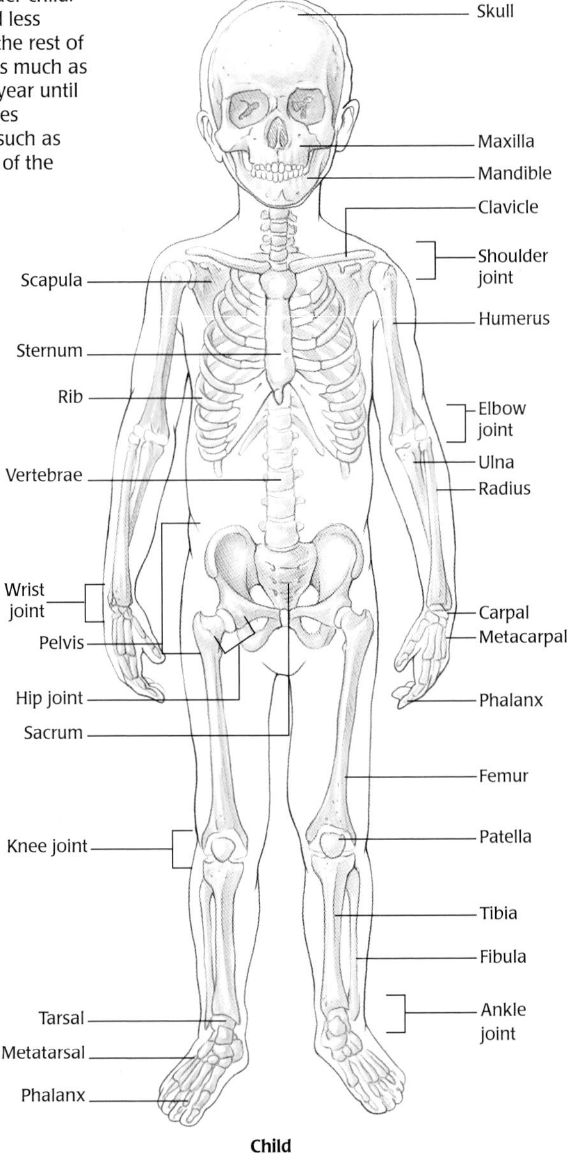

Child

MUSCLES

Muscles are composed of bundles of interlocking fibers that contract and relax. Skeletal muscles like those shown here are attached (directly or with a tendon) to two or more bones. When a muscle contracts, the attached bones move. Muscles often work together as a group—one contracts, another relaxes, and nearby muscles provide stability. In addition to skeletal muscles that can be moved voluntarily, a child's body has involuntary muscles in organs such as the heart and stomach.

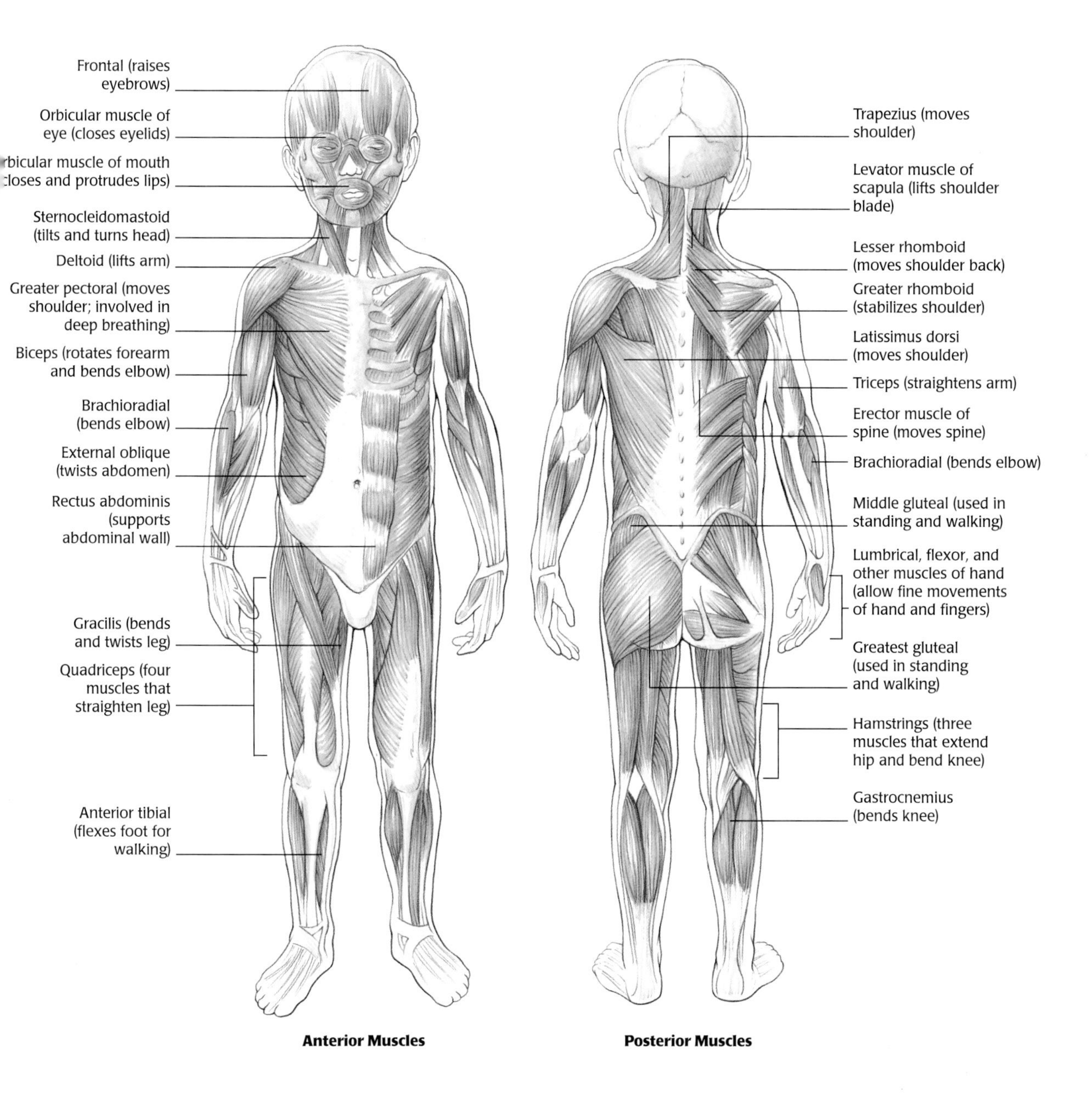

Anterior Muscles **Posterior Muscles**

THE HEART AND CIRCULATORY SYSTEM

The heart and blood vessels make up a child's circulatory system. The heart is a muscular organ made up of two side-by-side pumps. The right side receives oxygen-depleted blood from the body and sends it to the lungs, which remove carbon dioxide from the blood and nourish it with oxygen. The oxygen-rich blood then enters the left side of the heart. From there, the blood is pumped into the aorta and out via the arteries to the entire body. Arteries (red) carry oxygen-rich blood away from the heart to tissues throughout the body; veins (blue) return oxygen-depleted blood to the heart. The blood vessels also carry waste products through the body for eventual removal in urine or stool.

THE HEART

The heart pumps life-sustaining blood to the organs of your child's body. A child's heart muscle fibers are not fully developed until about age 5, when his or her heart function becomes similar to that of a healthy adult.

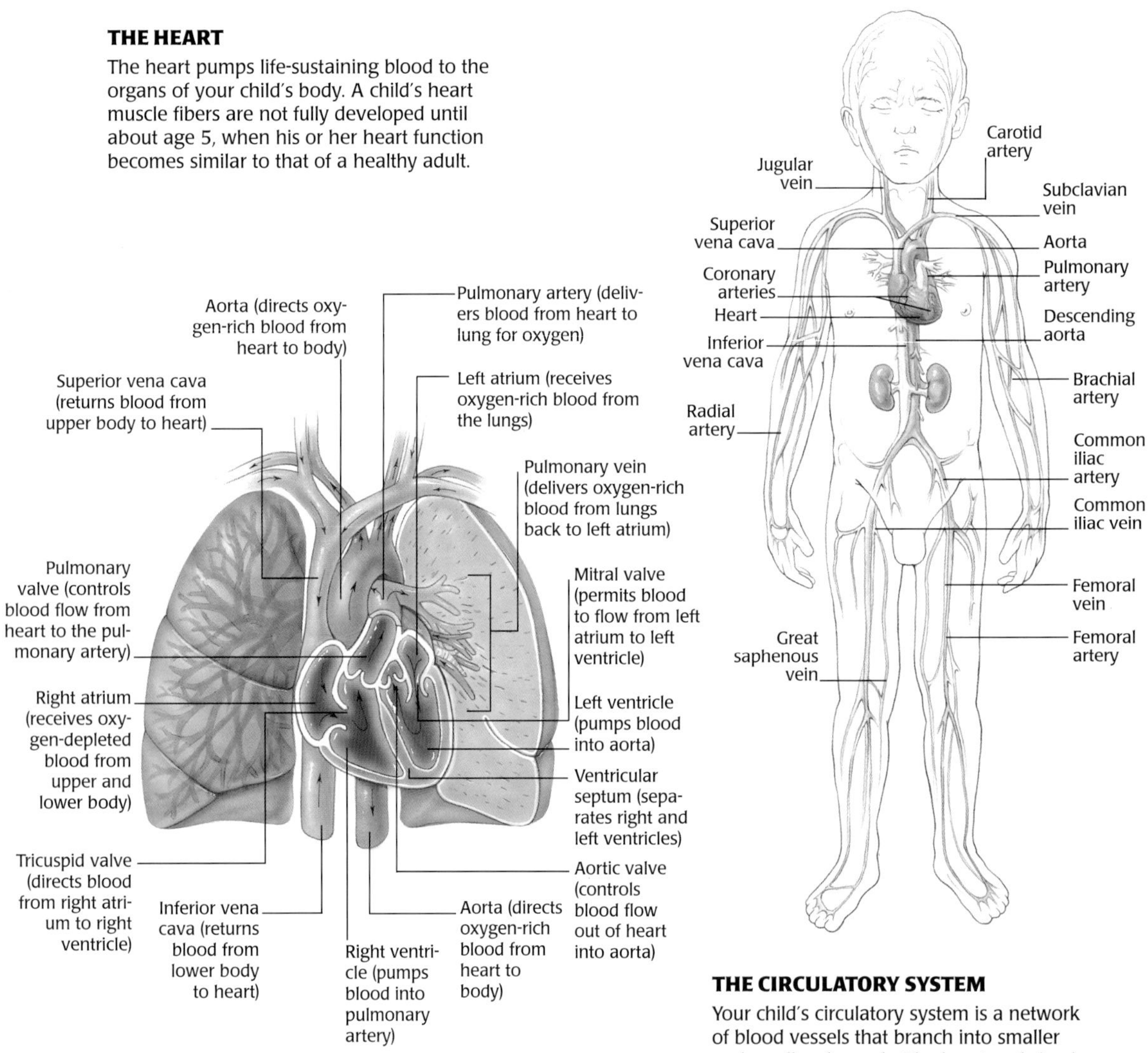

THE CIRCULATORY SYSTEM

Your child's circulatory system is a network of blood vessels that branch into smaller and smaller channels. The heart and circulatory system work as a single system to transport blood to all the cells of the body.

THE BRAIN AND NERVOUS SYSTEM

The brain and nervous system work like an intricate communications network that controls the inner workings of your child's body and helps him or her respond to the outside world. The nerves pass messages from the brain to every part of your child's body and back, enabling him or her to learn and develop new skills.

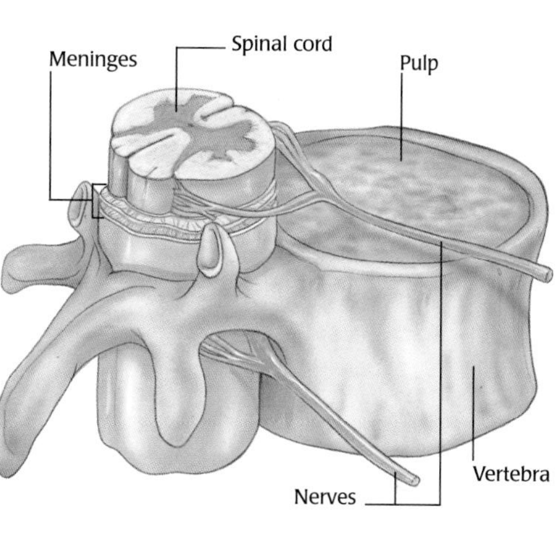

CROSS SECTION OF THE SPINAL CORD

The spinal cord is covered by three layers of protective membranes called the meninges. It has a central canal containing cerebrospinal fluid. Bones called vertebrae surround and protect the spinal cord. Spinal nerves send and receive messages about body sensation and movement to and from the brain by way of the spinal cord.

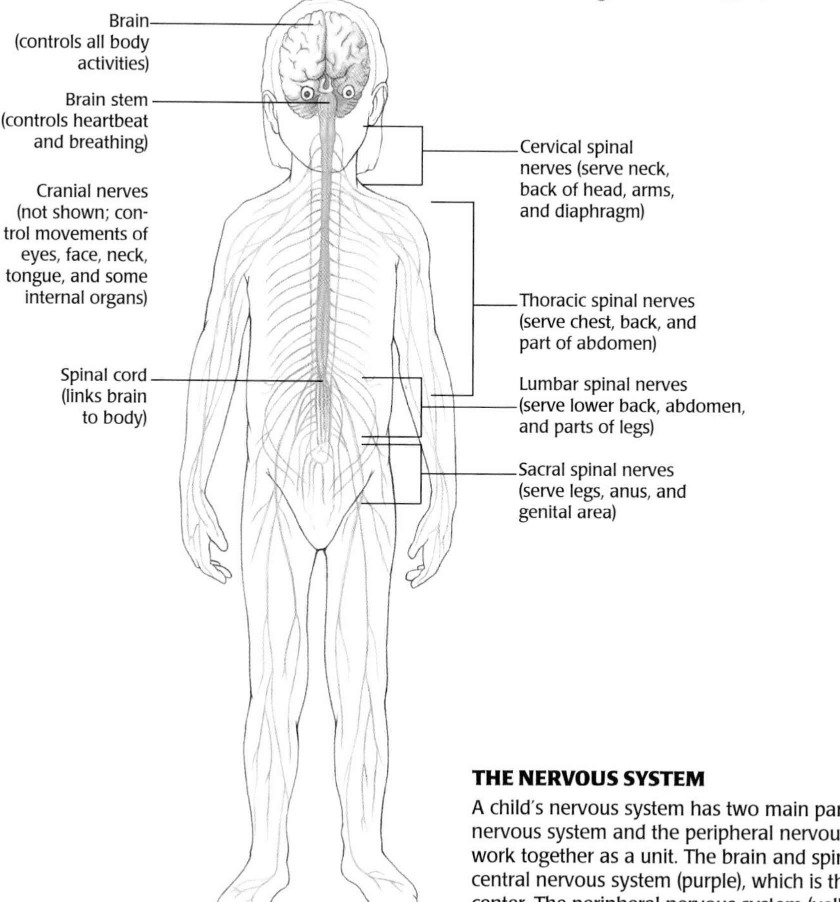

THE NERVOUS SYSTEM

A child's nervous system has two main parts—the central nervous system and the peripheral nervous system—that work together as a unit. The brain and spinal cord form the central nervous system (purple), which is the body's control center. The peripheral nervous system (yellow), a network of nerves that emanate from the spinal cord, connects the central nervous system to the child's skin, muscles, bones, and joints.

THE URINARY TRACT AND REPRODUCTIVE SYSTEM

A child's urinary tract filters and removes excess water and waste products from the body. The reproductive system serves the child's sexual and future reproductive needs. In both boys and girls, the lower urinary tract and reproductive organs are closely related.

THE URINARY AND REPRODUCTIVE TRACTS

The reproductive and urinary systems differ in boys and girls. A boy's urethra is longer than a girl's. A girl's urethra is short and lies just above the external genitals. A girl's bladder sits lower in the pelvis than does a boy's. A girl's reproductive organs reside inside the pelvis; a boy's reproductive organs are located outside the body in the scrotum. Girls are born with several hundred thousand eggs in their ovaries. In boys, sperm are continuously produced in the testicles beginning at puberty.

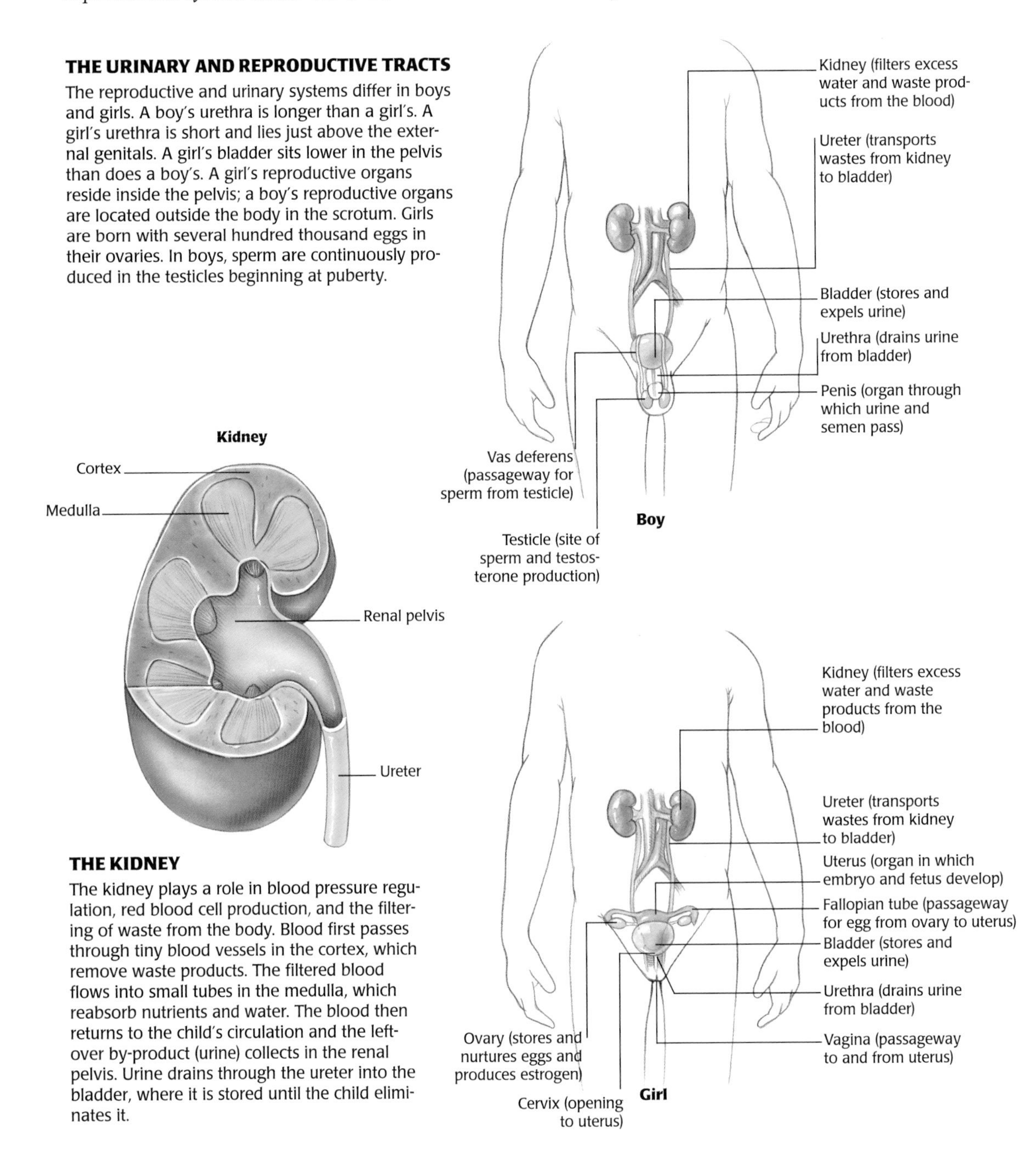

THE KIDNEY

The kidney plays a role in blood pressure regulation, red blood cell production, and the filtering of waste from the body. Blood first passes through tiny blood vessels in the cortex, which remove waste products. The filtered blood flows into small tubes in the medulla, which reabsorb nutrients and water. The blood then returns to the child's circulation and the leftover by-product (urine) collects in the renal pelvis. Urine drains through the ureter into the bladder, where it is stored until the child eliminates it.

Common childhood skin problems

A child's sensitive skin is especially vulnerable to irritation and infection. Most childhood skin conditions are minor and respond quickly to treatment or just go away on their own. Use this section to help you identify some common skin problems your child may develop.

INFANT RASHES

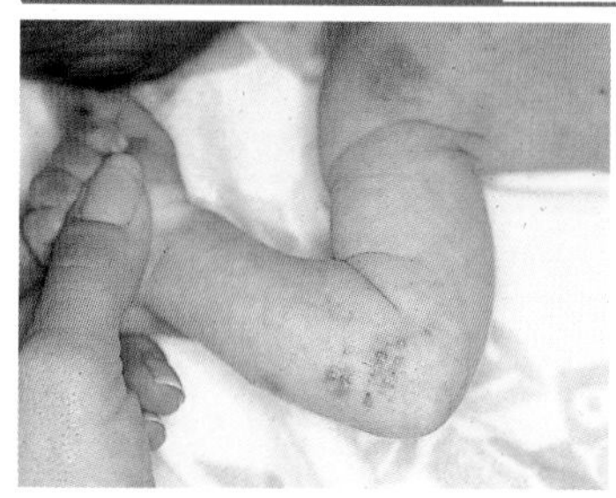

Erythema toxicum
A rash that occurs during the first 3 to 5 days of life. Small red spots turn into pimples with clear, whitish heads.

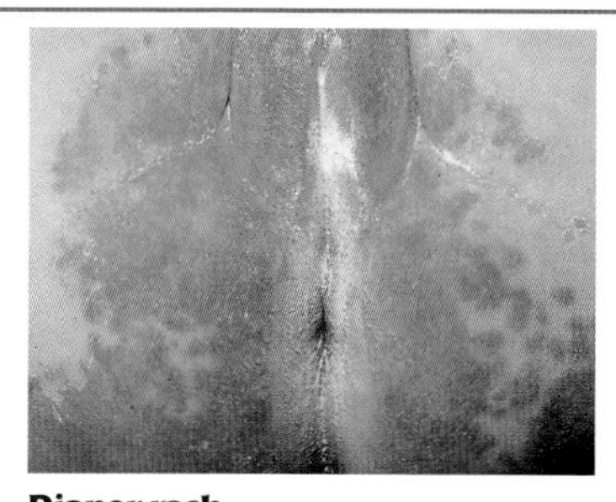

Diaper rash
A mild to severe skin irritation in the diaper area caused by urine, stool, baby wipes, or detergents.

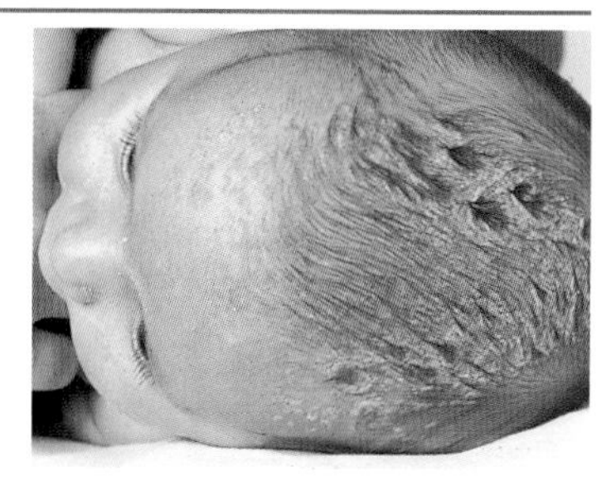

Cradle cap
Patches of thick yellow scales occurring on the scalp. Most common between 3 and 9 months of age.

ALLERGIC RASHES

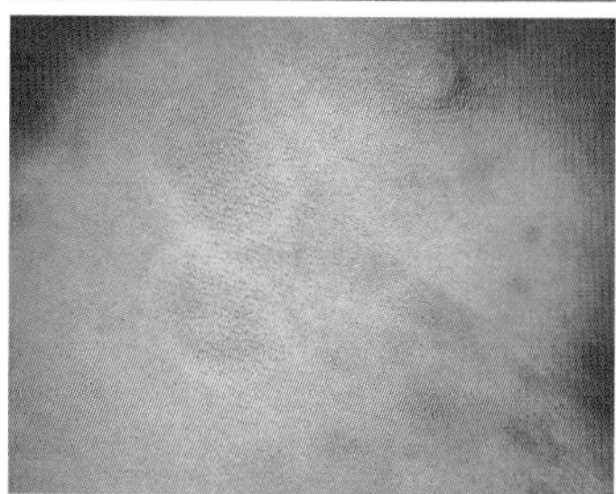

Hives
An allergic reaction that quickly produces an itchy, raised rash consisting of light-red patches with white centers.

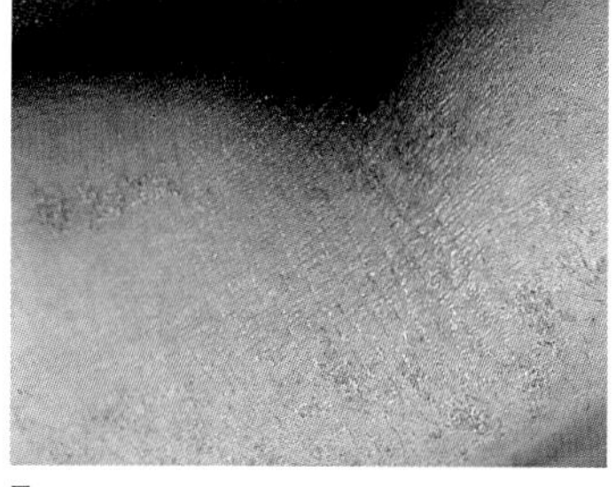

Eczema
An allergy that produces a red, itchy rash, sometimes with oozing blisters and scaling, most often on the cheeks.

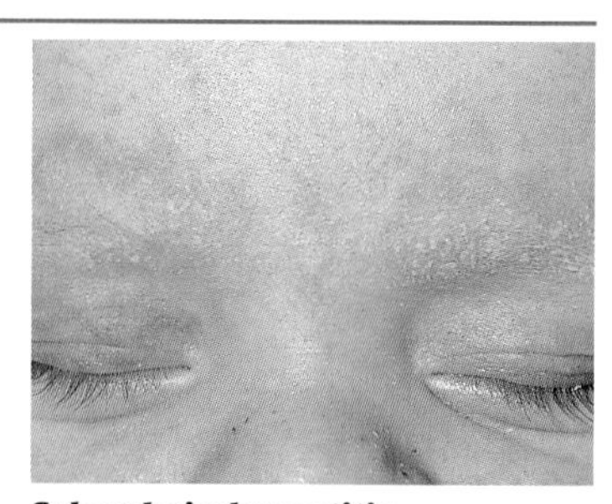

Seborrheic dermatitis
An allergic condition that produces a red, flaky, itchy rash on the face, scalp, upper chest, back, and armpits.

ALLERGIC RASHES

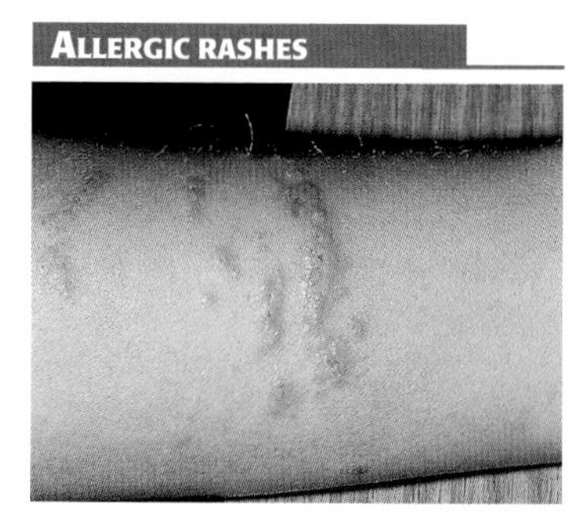

Poison ivy
An allergic reaction to contact with the poison ivy plant. Exposed areas burn and are red, itchy, and blistery.

RASHES FROM INFECTIONS

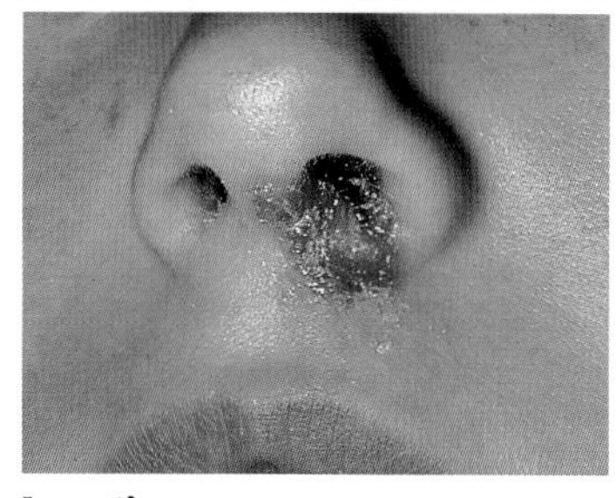

Impetigo
A bacterial infection; groups of blisters form on the face or limbs. The blisters burst and form crusty sores.

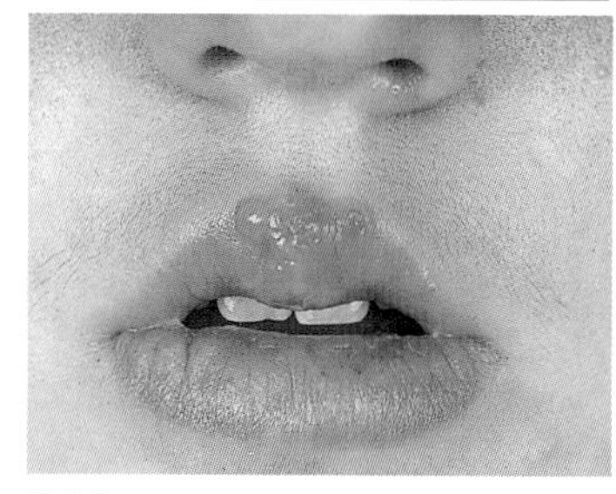

Cold sores
Infection by a virus that produces small blisters surrounded by inflamed skin on the lips or around the mouth.

RASHES FROM INFECTIONS

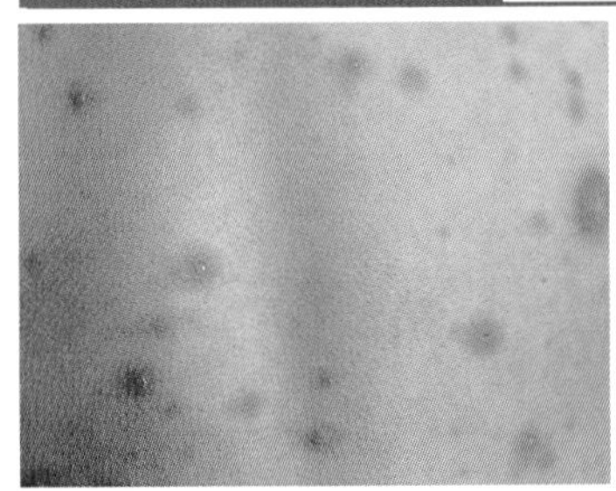

Chickenpox

Infection by a virus, producing small, red pimples that turn into itchy, fluid-filled blisters that rupture and scab. The rash mainly covers the limbs, trunk, and face, but may form in the mouth or nose.

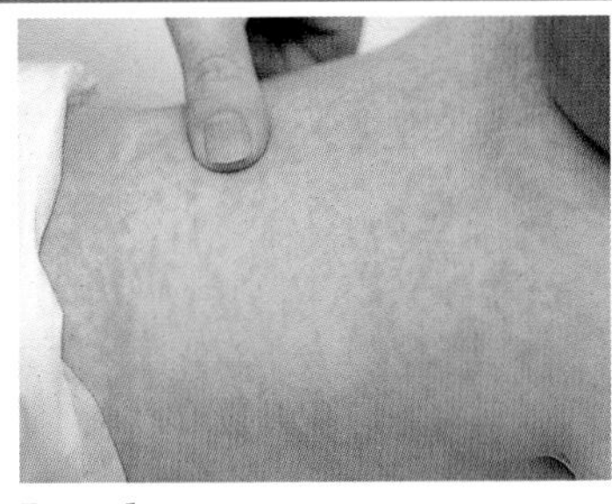

Roseola

Infection by a virus that occurs mainly in children under the age of 2. A faint rash appears on the child's face, neck, and trunk after a high fever that has lasted 3 to 4 days and then suddenly breaks.

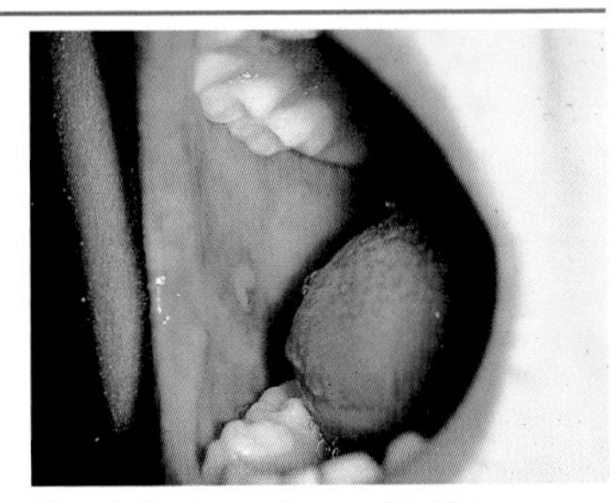

Hand-foot-and-mouth disease

Infection by a virus that produces a blistery rash on the palms of the hands, between the fingers, and on the soles of the feet. Shallow, painful ulcers also form in the mouth and on the tongue.

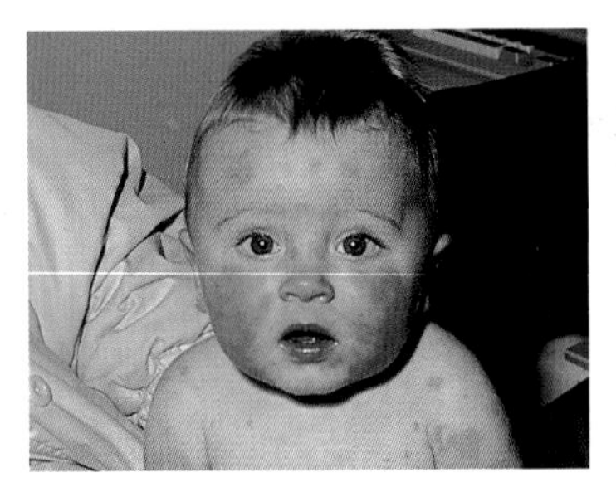

Fifth disease

Infection by a virus that first produces a bright red rash on the cheeks, giving the appearance that the cheeks have been slapped. The rash then spreads in a lacy pattern to the child's trunk, arms, and legs.

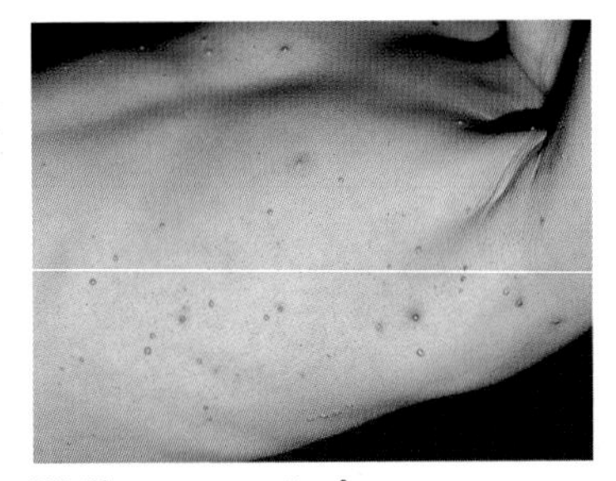

Molluscum contagiosum

Infection by a virus characterized by small, smooth, flesh-colored bumps, each with a tiny hole in the center. The bumps (which do not hurt or itch) are filled with a cheesy material and can appear almost anywhere on the body.

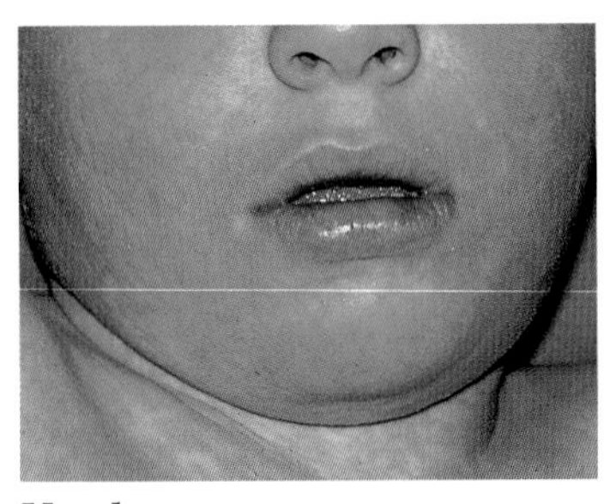

Measles

Infection by a virus producing flat or raised reddish spots that form blotches. The rash usually starts on the forehead and then spreads to the trunk. Tiny white spots may appear inside the mouth before the rash appears.

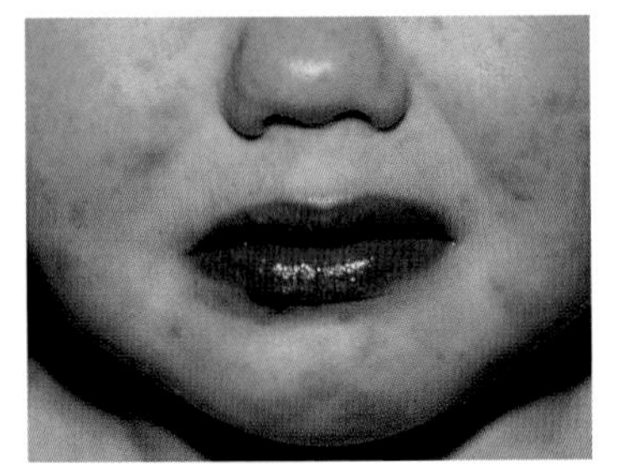

German measles (rubella)

Infection by a virus producing a rash similar to but less severe than that of measles (above right). Tiny, light-red spots merge to form evenly colored patches that appear mainly on the face, neck, trunk, and limbs.

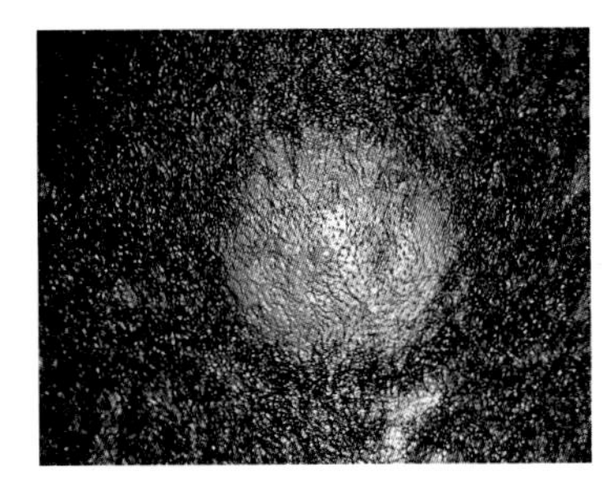

Ringworm

Infection by a fungus producing red, itchy, ring-shaped patches with bumpy edges and a pale center. Patches can appear on the scalp, trunk, groin, or buttocks. On the scalp, ringworm can cause bald patches.

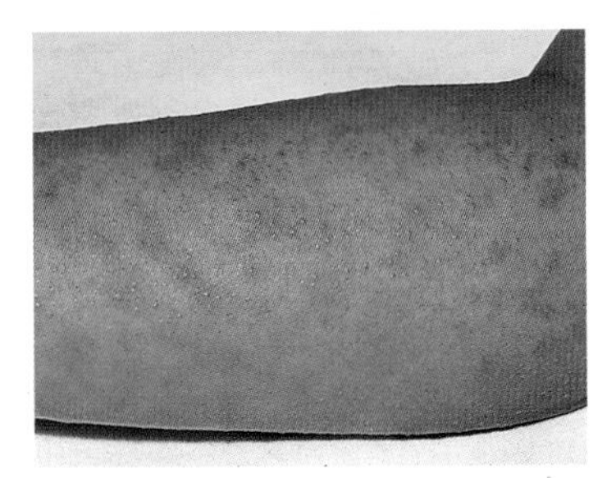

Scarlet fever

Infection by a bacterium that causes an inflammation known as strep throat. The child may get a bright red rash on the face and, later, the rest of the body. The skin on the fingertips and in the groin area may peel.

Your healthy child from birth through adolescence

CHAPTER • 1

Your newborn (birth to 3 months)

Having a newborn will delight and exhaust you. Caring for a baby demands attention and responsiveness during a time when you will be sleep-deprived. But taking care of a newborn will also be immensely gratifying. If you feel unprepared for parenthood, be assured that most new parents feel the same way. Try to be flexible, share the responsibilities with your partner, and enjoy this special time together with your new baby.

WHAT YOU CAN DO FOR YOUR CHILD NOW

The first 3 months of life set the stage for your baby's future development. To make sure that he or she gets the best start possible, follow these guidelines to help your newborn grow and thrive:

- **BREAST-FEED YOUR NEWBORN** (see page 44). Breast milk is the best nutrition available.
- **GIVE YOUR BABY LOTS OF LOVE AND ATTENTION**–touch, cuddle, and talk to him or her often. You can't "spoil" a baby of this age.
- **ALWAYS PUT YOUR BABY TO SLEEP ON HIS OR HER BACK** to reduce the risk of sudden infant death syndrome (see page 626).
- **WHENEVER YOUR BABY IS IN A CAR, PUT HIM OR HER IN A SAFETY SEAT** installed in the back seat and facing the back (see page 294).
- **CREATE A SAFE ENVIRONMENT FOR YOUR NEWBORN** (see page 76).
- **TAKE YOUR BABY FOR ALL THE RECOMMENDED CHECKUPS AND VACCINATIONS** (see page 226).
- **DON'T ALLOW SMOKING AROUND YOUR BABY.**
- **KEEP YOUR BABY OUT OF THE SUN** (sunscreen shouldn't be applied to infants under 6 months) and dress him or her appropriately for the weather.

Planning ahead for the birth of your baby

You need to plan ahead for the birth of your baby. You'll have to find a doctor (see page 221), set up the nursery (see page 30), make arrangements for child care if you and your partner both work, and decide whether or not your child should be breast-fed or circumcised if you have a boy. Once your baby is born, you won't have much free time, so try to finalize your decisions beforehand.

Prenatal care is extremely important to ensure a healthy pregnancy. A woman should see her doctor or state-licensed nurse-midwife (practicing under a doctor's supervision) as soon as she thinks she may be pregnant. She should have regular checkups throughout her pregnancy as her doctor recommends. Good prenatal care reduces the risk of complications, including premature delivery.

Mothers: Give your baby a healthy start

You can give your baby a healthy start long before you get pregnant by making sure your body is in the best condition to nurture a pregnancy and making sure you don't expose your baby before it is born to toxic substances or harmful conditions. Take these important steps:

- Eat a balanced, nutritious diet (see page 111).
- Exercise regularly.
- Take a daily multivitamin-mineral supplement that contains 400 micrograms (0.4 milligrams) of the B vitamin folic acid, which reduces the risk of serious neural tube defects (defects in the spine and brain) that can arise during the first 3 months of pregnancy. You should start taking folic acid 2 months before you try to become pregnant.
- Stop drinking alcohol now and abstain from alcohol throughout your entire pregnancy. Drinking during pregnancy, especially in the first 3 months, can cause fetal alcohol syndrome (see page 486)—a combination of serious birth defects including facial and limb deformities, heart defects, slow growth, and mental retardation. Even moderate drinking during pregnancy—an average of less than one drink a day—has been linked to developmental problems.
- Don't smoke. Smoking during pregnancy can reduce the amount of oxygen to the fetus, increasing the risk of miscarriage, stillbirth, or premature delivery. Mothers who smoke deliver babies that are smaller, have more medical problems, and have a higher risk of sudden infant death syndrome (see page 626) than babies of nonsmokers. Avoid secondhand smoke as much as possible.
- Avoid all street or recreational drugs. Many drugs pass through the placenta and can severely, even fatally, injure a growing fetus.
- If you have cats, ask a partner or friend to change the litterbox. Cat feces can transmit toxoplasmosis, a disease that can cause birth defects.
- Avoid raw or very rare meat or fish and unpasteurized cheeses. They can transmit germs that can harm you or the fetus.
- If you have never had chickenpox, avoid contact with those who have active disease.
- Check with your doctor before you take any prescription or over-the-counter medications, even aspirin or a cold remedy. If you regularly take a medication for a chronic condition, ask your doctor if he or she needs to change the medication or the dose during your pregnancy.
- Limit the stress in your life. You will often feel tired and your emotions may fluctuate greatly during pregnancy. Find time to rest or take a nap every day to restore your energy. Limit your commitments so you won't feel overextended.
- If you have never had German measles or chickenpox as a child, get immunized against these diseases before you get pregnant. German measles can cause severe birth defects and chickenpox can also harm the fetus. After getting these vaccinations, wait the period of time your doctor recommends (usually 4 months) before trying to become pregnant.

Although women physically carry the child, men can influence a child's health as well. Studies show that a father's behavior or work conditions—smoking, drinking alcohol, or exposure to chemicals or radiation on the job—can affect the growth of a fetus. A baby's father also needs to be in good shape to cope with the demands of raising a child. Eating a nutritious diet, exercising, avoiding alcohol and other drugs, and not smoking are smart choices for a prospective father. They also reinforce the mother's decision to lead a healthy lifestyle.

How will you feed your baby?

Pregnancy is the time to decide whether to breast-feed or bottle-feed your baby. Doctors recommend breast-feeding for 1 year because breast milk provides the best nutrition for your infant and immunity against disease. Breast-feeding has health benefits for a nursing woman as well. The more you know about breast-feeding, the easier it will be to start nursing your baby. While you are pregnant, read all you can about breast-feeding, take a childbirth class that covers it, choose a doctor who strongly supports it, and get acquainted with other women who have breast-fed their children so they can give you tips and answer your questions. Contact the local chapter of La Leche League, a volunteer organization that provides information and encouragement to women who are breast-feeding. For more information about breast-feeding, see page 44.

Some mothers feel uncomfortable with breast-feeding and a few women can't nurse because they or their baby have a health problem. If you decide to bottle-feed your baby, don't have misgivings about your decision. You can give your baby just as much love and affection as a mother who breast-feeds. Bottle-feeding has some advantages too: it allows both parents to feed the baby and frees the mother from the constant demands of nursing. Give your baby only specially prepared infant formula–not cow's milk–until he or she is 1 year old. See page 53 for more information on bottle-feeding.

Where do you want to deliver your baby?

Do you want to deliver your baby in the hospital, in a birthing center, or at home? Should you choose natural childbirth, which seeks to limit the use of pain medication, or do you plan to make use of medication as needed? These are some of the decisions you and your partner will face as you prepare for the birth of your child. A pregnant woman needs to talk to her doctor about whether she can deliver vaginally or if she may need to have a cesarean section. The doctor can also recommend a local childbirth education class, which will teach both partners what to expect during labor and delivery.

A woman and her partner will also want to make a decision about the type of hospital arrangement they would prefer after the baby is born. Your hospital or birthing center probably has an option called rooming-in, which permits you to stay with your infant constantly from birth to the end of your stay. Rooming-in allows you to become familiar with your baby and his or her sleep and feeding patterns while you have help from an experienced nursing staff. Another option is to keep the baby with you most of the time but to send him or her to the hospital nursery when you need to get some sleep. Don't feel you're being a bad parent if you want some moments to yourself during this time. You need to regain your strength as fully as possible after giving birth and the hospital is the ideal place to do it. You'll be at home with your baby soon enough tending to his or her needs full time.

BABY EQUIPMENT AND SUPPLIES

Be wary of the many claims by advertisers and well-meaning friends, relatives, and neighbors about items you and your baby "can't live without." Stick to the real necessities. Here are some of the things you will need for your baby and a list of other items that might be helpful. For supplies to keep in your medicine cabinet, see page 274. For infant clothing, see page 64.

Basic supplies

You'll spend a lot of time feeding, diapering, bathing, and playing with your baby. Here are some supplies you'll need:

Feeding If you are breast-feeding, you'll need a breast pump (hand, battery-operated, or electric) and two or three nursing bras. You may want to get absorbent breast pads to put inside your bra to soak up leaking milk. If you are bottle-feeding, you'll need about ten 8-ounce bottles with nipples (plastic bottles are safer than glass and can be used for breast milk), a few 4-ounce bottles, and a supply of the type of formula your doctor recommends. You may have to try a couple of different kinds of baby bottles and nipples to find out the type your baby prefers.

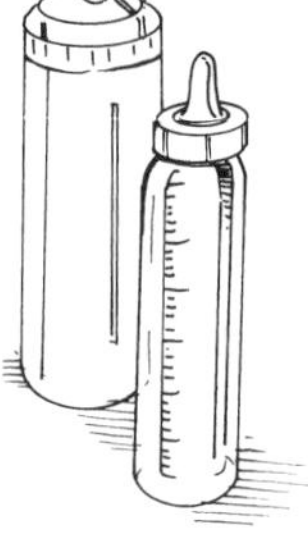
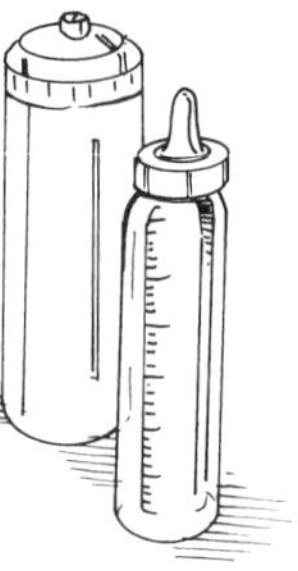

Playing Soft, cuddly toys such as teddy bears are comforting for young babies. Blocks help them learn to pick up and manipulate objects.

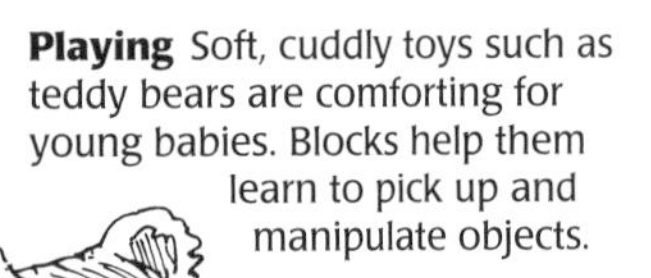

Sleeping In addition to a safe crib and mattress (see page 300), you'll need two felt-backed waterproof mattress pads, three or four fitted crib sheets, a crib blanket, and two cotton receiving blankets. Don't use bumper pads because they can pose a suffocation danger; they also prevent a baby from seeing out the sides of the crib.

Bathing Although a plastic washtub or the kitchen sink will do for a baby's bath, you'll find it easier and safer to bathe your baby in a portable infant tub that has a sponge lining to prevent slipping (see page 63). Get two or three terrycloth baby towels, preferably with hoods, or regular bath-size towels. Have three or four soft washcloths, with some in a different color to use only for cleaning baby's bottom.

Diapering Infants go through 10 to 13 diapers a day. If you are using disposable diapers, start with six to eight dozen—about a week's supply. If you are using cloth diapers, three to five dozen should be enough, because you'll be washing them every few days. With cloth diapers, you'll also need pins, several pairs of plastic pants, and a diaper pail. Diaper wraps, which are made of cotton or wool in the shape of disposable diapers, eliminate the need for pins and rubber pants (reducing the risk of diaper rash). Get baby wipes; even if you prefer not to use wipes at home, they're convenient on outings. Buy petroleum jelly and zinc oxide ointment in case your baby gets a diaper rash.

Many parents find the high surface of changing tables convenient for dressing and diapering their baby. Make sure the table is sturdy, has a guardrail or strap to prevent the baby from falling, and has room to store everything you need. Don't put the changing table near a window and always keep one hand on your baby even when he or she is strapped in.

Look for a diaper bag with several compartments (one of which is waterproof for wet clothes or soiled diapers), a zipper closing for the main compartment, and a padded shoulder strap for easy carrying. Some diaper bags come with a changing pad.

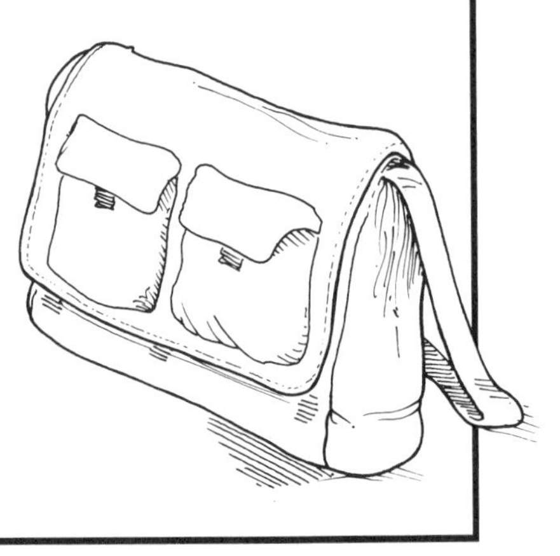

Baby equipment

Infant seat Infant seats are useful for very young babies who cannot yet sit on their own. Putting your baby in the infant seat for short periods during the day provides a different perspective of the world. But you need to take extra care when buying an infant seat because they are not covered by federal safety regulations. Get one with a wide, sturdy base to prevent tipping and a frame that allows the baby to sit deep inside. Always use the strap and harness and, when you carry the seat with your infant in it, hold it with both arms under the frame. Using carrying handles isn't as safe because the seat can more easily get bumped or overturned. Never put the seat on a high surface; your child could flip it over and fall. Check the manufacturer's weight guidelines and stop using the seat after your baby has outgrown it. Never use an infant seat as a car safety seat.

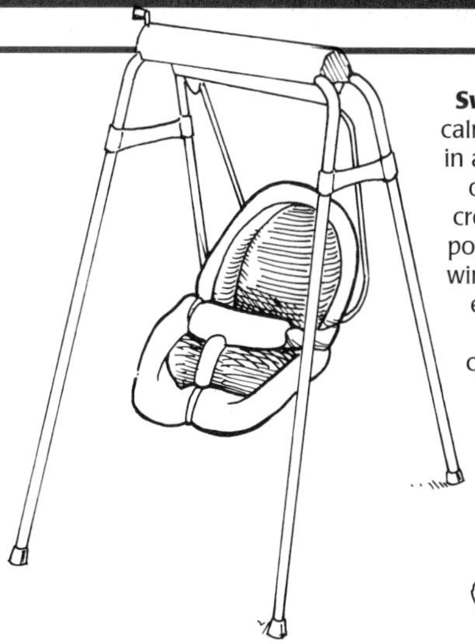

Swinging for comfort Many babies calm down instantly when they're put in an automatic swing. Make sure the one you buy has a sturdy base and crossbars. The battery- or pendulum-powered models are quieter than the windup ones; some babies are awakened by the winding action. Before putting your baby in the swing, check the manufacturer's minimum weight guidelines and safety instructions. Stop using the swing after your baby has outgrown it, usually at about 20 pounds.

No walkers A walker is one item that should not be on your list of things to buy. Children can get seriously injured while in a walker, especially if they fall down stairs. Also, because they keep children up on their toes, walkers and exercise saucers can hinder development of some of a child's muscles and the child's spine and can interfere with learning to walk. Crawling on the floor is healthier for your baby's development.

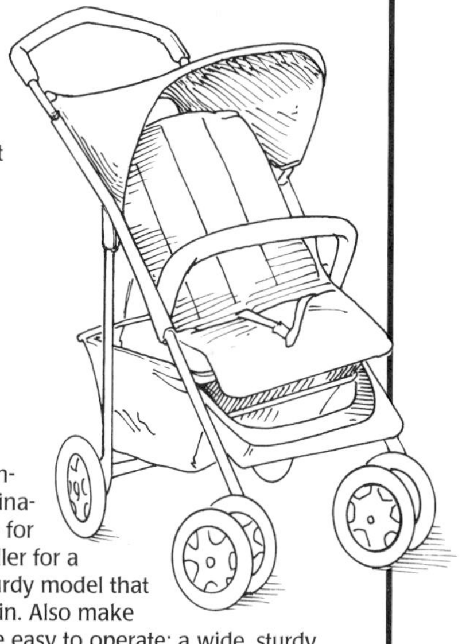

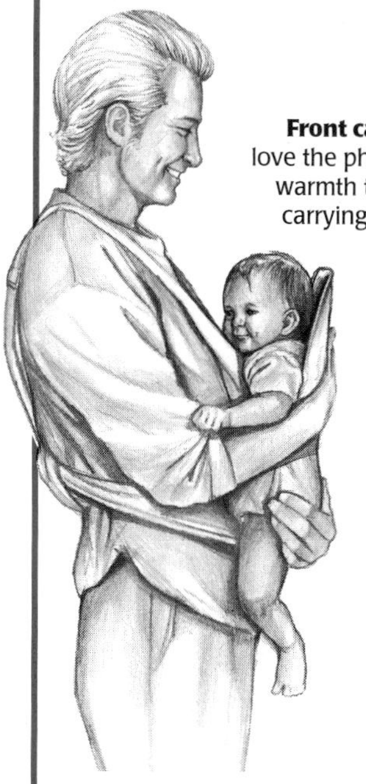

Front carriers Newborns love the physical contact and warmth they get in a front-carrying pack and you still have your hands free. Buy a front pack that has a support for the infant's head. By about 5 or 6 months of age, your baby will be too heavy to carry in front. For older babies, packs in which you can carry your baby on your back are available.

Carriages and strollers A convertible carriage-stroller combination can be used as a carriage for a newborn and then as a stroller for a baby who can sit up. Get a sturdy model that your baby can lie down or sit in. Also make sure that it has brakes that are easy to operate; a wide, sturdy base; a seat belt and harness; and a large sunshade. If the stroller is collapsible, make sure the release mechanism is out of your child's reach. Hanging bags or other items from the handles could tip the stroller backward. Umbrella strollers are good second strollers because they are lightweight, compact, inexpensive, and easy to store.

Nursery monitors Some parents use nursery monitors or intercoms to keep tabs on their baby when he or she is asleep in another room. Keep in mind that young babies normally have restless, noisy periods during sleep, so you don't have to respond to every movement or sound your baby makes. On the other hand, you shouldn't let a monitor function as a baby-sitter.

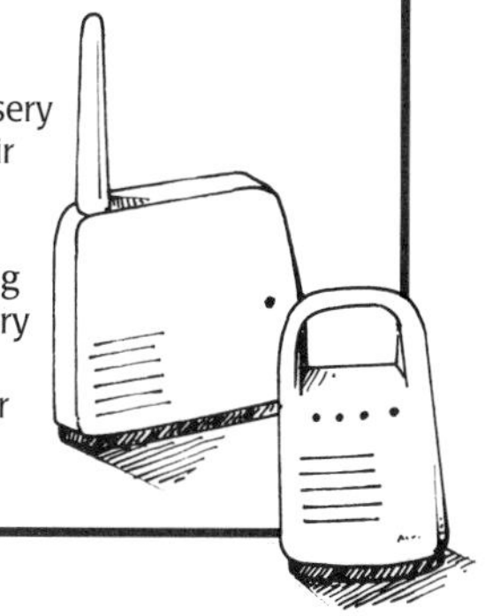

Finding quality child care

If you and your partner will both be working outside the home after the birth of your child, arrange for quality child care before the baby is born. It is essential for your child's healthy development—and for your peace of mind—to find a situation in which he or she will receive nurturing, loving, and stimulating care in your absence. Infants need to feel secure and loved, so it is ideal if one person (or a few consistent caregivers) provides all of your baby's care. For information about how to find quality day care, see chapter 7.

Before you leave the hospital, make sure you're ready; ask the maternity ward nurses for lessons on bathing, changing, feeding, and burping your baby. Do you feel comfortable being on your own with your baby? Have you made arrangements for someone to be there to help until you gain confidence? Home health care agencies can provide nurses who will visit you at home to make sure things are going well. Take advantage of this service, especially if you and your baby are discharged from the hospital early. Find out if the hospital or your health plan has a help line you can call with questions and concerns.

Some couples want to have their babies at home, in familiar and comfortable surroundings. If you choose a home birth, you will have to arrange to have a home birth practitioner, such as a state-licensed nurse-midwife under a doctor's supervision, at your side to help with your labor and delivery. Interview the practitioner before your due date so you can find out what kind of training, experience, and license he or she has and how he or she handles problems that could arise during delivery. Make sure that the practitioner can perform all the necessary newborn medical examinations and tests. See your pediatrician within 24 hours of birth for a thorough medical examination, administration of the hepatitis B vaccine, and state metabolic screening tests for disorders such as PKU (see page 595). Serious conditions can go undetected or untreated in babies who are born at home. Women who have a high-risk pregnancy—for example, women with medical conditions such as diabetes or those expecting multiple births—are probably not candidates for a home birth because their risk for complications may be high.

HOW DO YOU FEEL ABOUT CIRCUMCISION?

If you have a baby boy, you will have to decide whether or not to have him circumcised. Most boys are born with a fold of skin called the foreskin that covers the tip of the penis. Circumcision is a surgical procedure that removes the foreskin. An obstetrician-gynecologist or a pediatrician usually performs the procedure in the first day or two after birth.

Most Americans choose to have their sons circumcised for social or religious reasons. Men who are circumcised want their sons to look like them and like most of the other boys in school. Some religious groups have practiced circumcision for thousands of years and continue to circumcise their boys today.

Some doctors believe that routine circumcision is unnecessary. However, scientific evidence shows that circumcision decreases the risk of urinary tract infections early in life and cancer of the penis later in life. Like any surgery, circumcision carries a risk of infection and bleeding. In rare cases, the foreskin may be cut too short or too long, or the circumcision may heal improperly. The procedure is painful, and circumcised babies are often irritable for 24 to 48 hours afterward. If you choose circumcision, ask your child's doctor to use a local anesthetic to ease the pain. If you decide against circumcision at birth but later change your mind, your son will need general anesthesia, which carries more risks.

Circumcision is a personal decision but you should consult your child's doctor about it so that you understand the possible health benefits and risks.

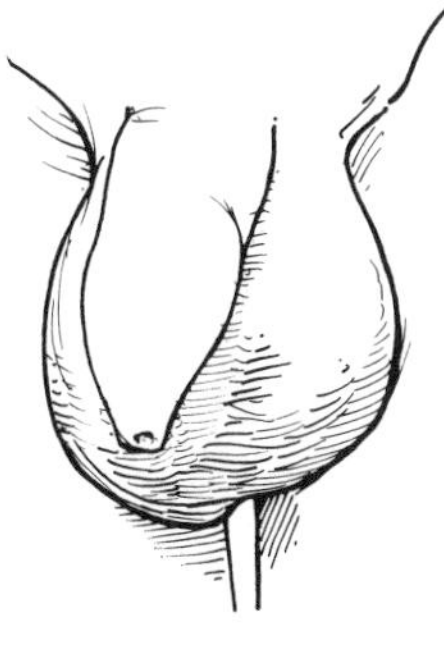

Uncircumcised penis
A loose fold of skin called the foreskin covers the tip of an uncircumcised penis. The foreskin gradually separates from the tip naturally during the first months or years of a boy's life.

Circumcised penis
The foreskin of a circumcised penis has been removed from the tip, leaving the tip permanently exposed. Healing can take up to 10 days after a circumcision.

Getting to know your baby

You and your partner will probably be able to hold your baby right after delivery. Some mothers make their first attempt at breast-feeding. But don't worry if you can't hold your baby immediately—for example, because the delivery was a cesarean, your baby needs immediate medical attention, or childbirth was simply too exhausting. The first few minutes after delivery are not critical; you'll have plenty of time to get to know and bond with your child.

THE FIRST MOMENTS

Immediately after delivery, the delivery team goes into action. Using a suction device, they remove any mucus that may be inside your baby's nose and mouth and place an antibiotic solution into his or her eyes to protect against infection. Your baby will receive an injection of vitamin K, which helps blood to clot. The nurses will examine your baby's entire body to check for any abnormalities. The doctor will check the baby's heart rate, make sure he or she is breathing normally, and measure his or her length, weight, and head circumference. Like all newborns, your baby will be given an evaluation, which will result in a rating called the Apgar score (see below). For more about newborn screening tests, see page 223.

Within minutes of birth, your newborn will begin exploring the world with his or her senses. Your baby can focus on objects that are 8 to 10 inches away and has a natural attraction to the human face, especially yours. Newborns can hear well, and recognize sounds they heard frequently during pregnancy, such as their parents' voices. This is the time to begin learning how to communicate with your baby by touching, holding, rocking, talking, singing, and playing. Infants thrive on contact with a loving person.

Although your newborn will sleep for much of the first few days, watch for the times when your baby is awake and alert. At these times, he or she is very receptive to interaction with you. Babies just a few days old produce facial expressions, such as yawning, grimacing, and smiling. It's never too early to start talking to your infant—talking to a baby is the single most important factor in shaping his or her future ability to think. Have fun getting to know your baby and trying out different ways of communicating.

What is an Apgar score?

The delivery team examines all newborns and gives them a score, called an Apgar score, at 1 and 5 minutes after birth. The score, conceived by American anesthesiologist Virginia Apgar, is the sum total of numbers that reflect the condition of a newborn's heart rate, breathing, muscle tone, reflexes, and color as the baby adjusts to life outside the uterus. Each response is given a rating from 0 to 2; the total score can range from 0 to 10. Most healthy babies score between 7 and 10. An Apgar score does not predict a baby's long-term health status or development. A newborn who has gone through a long labor or a difficult delivery may receive a low Apgar score, but is still likely to develop normally.

	Apgar score		
SIGN	**0**	**1**	**2**
Heart rate	None	Less than 100 beats per minute	More than 100 beats per minute
Breathing and crying	None	Weak cry, irregular breathing	Strong cry, regular breathing
Skin color*	Blue or pale	Pink body, blue hands and feet	All pink
Muscle tone	Limp	Some bending of arms and legs	Active bending of arms and legs
Reflex response	None	Grimaces	Cries

*For nonwhite infants, doctors assess skin color by examining the inside of the child's mouth and lips, palms, and soles of the feet.

IF YOUR BABY IS PREMATURE

A baby born before the 37th week of pregnancy is considered premature, or preterm. Preterm birth can result from a pregnancy-related condition, such as high blood pressure; from a maternal infection or chronic illness, such as diabetes; from the mother's use of recreational drugs; or from other causes. In most cases, the cause of preterm birth is unknown. Babies born as early as the 25th week of pregnancy have a chance of surviving. The longer the pregnancy continues, the better the child's chances of survival.

If you are at risk of having a preterm delivery, your doctor will arrange for you to deliver at a hospital that can provide the right kind of care for you and has an intensive care unit for at-risk newborns. Depending on the complications your preterm baby has, he or she may be sent to either the regular nursery or the neonatal intensive care unit.

Many premature infants have breathing problems that require ventilation (artificial breathing) or oxygen. Other complications of prematurity include

The Ohio bed

A premature infant is usually placed in an open bed with transparent sides, called an Ohio bed. Tubes and sensors may be attached to the baby to provide essential life support and help the nurses and doctors monitor his or her condition. Ohio beds are also used for infants who are born with serious infections, respiratory problems, or birth defects. Once the baby has grown sufficiently and his or her condition stabilizes, he or she will be transferred to an incubator.

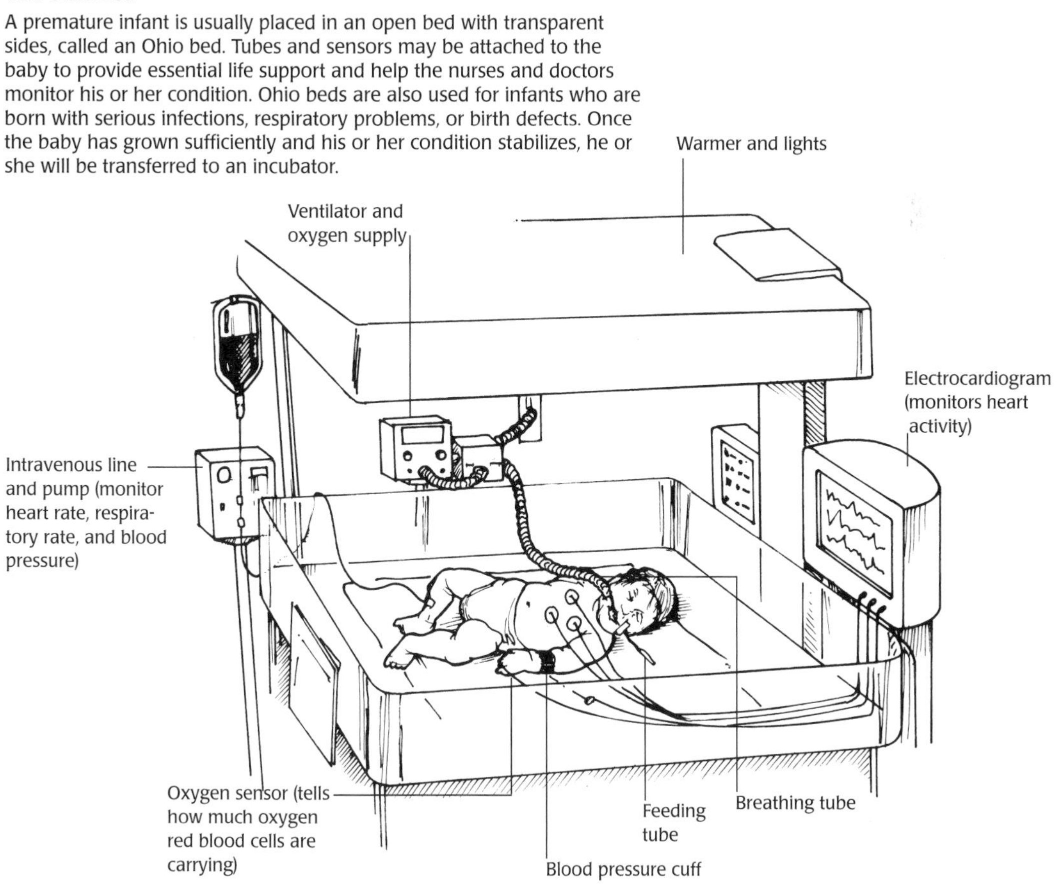

Premature infants in car seats

Most states require you to transport your baby in an approved car safety seat—starting with that first trip home from the hospital. The majority of car safety seats are designed to hold babies weighing more than 7 pounds. Babies who weigh less, especially preterm and low-birthweight infants, can sometimes have difficulty breathing when sitting semiupright in a safety seat. The hospital staff may evaluate your infant for these problems and recommend an alternate type of seat. If not, place a small rolled blanket or towel on each side of your child's head or purchase a neckroll to support his or her head and neck and to make breathing easier. If the baby's head flops forward, wedge a rolled towel or newspaper under the safety seat at the baby's feet so he or she lies in a more reclining position. Make sure the safety seat remains firmly attached to the seat of the car.

newborn infection (see page 575), retinopathy of prematurity (see page 608), intraventricular hemorrhage (see page 538), necrotizing enterocolitis (see page 575), jaundice (see page 540), and apnea (see page 416).

Your preterm baby will lie in a special bed called an Ohio bed (see page 35) or in an incubator. The nursing staff may attach several monitors and intravenous lines to your baby. He or she may also have a breathing tube in place that is hooked up to a ventilator (an artificial breathing machine). Because many premature infants have difficulty feeding (the sucking reflex starts during the 37th week of pregnancy) and are ill, they need to be fed intravenously at first. They require extra vitamins and additional calories to keep up with their rapid growth and development. When they become healthier, preterm infants can receive breast milk or formula through a feeding tube until they begin to suck.

One of the hardest parts of having a preterm baby is not being able to hold and cuddle him or her. Spend as much time as you can touching, stroking, and talking to your baby while he or she is in the Ohio bed or incubator. This kind of stimulation can dramatically improve your baby's breathing and physical growth. The contact will also help you and your baby bond.

Before you bring your baby home from the hospital, you will be given special instructions for caring for him or her. Your baby may temporarily need supplemental oxygen or may need to remain attached to a monitor that checks his or her breathing for signs of apnea (see page 416). Many hospitals encourage new parents of premature infants to spend at least one night in the hospital in a special unit. The overnight stay gives the parents a chance to practice taking care of their infant, while the hospital staff is still close by to guide them and answer questions.

Your child can go home when he or she can feed on his or her own and is gaining weight and when his or her condition has stabilized. Frequent follow-up visits will allow the doctor to monitor your baby's growth. Developmentally, most premature infants catch up to full-term babies by 18 to 24 months of age.

THE FIRST WEEKS AT HOME

You and your baby will probably leave the hospital within 24 to 48 hours after delivery. Most infants do well during their first few days of life, but a few develop problems, such as excessive weight loss, dehydration (see page 283), and jaundice (see page 540). Breast-fed babies are most at risk because the mother's milk may not yet have come in. That's why it's important for your baby to have a

YOUR NEWBORN'S APPEARANCE

Your baby may not look the way you expected—you might not even consider him or her to be very cute. But don't be alarmed. Most newborn characteristics will disappear in the first few days or weeks of your baby's life and he or she will look more like the cuddly baby you hoped for.

Skin may be covered with a white, creamy, protective coating called vernix and may look blotchy and be red, blue, or gray. Bruises and birthmarks are common from pressure during birth. A dark-skinned baby may have patches of lighter skin. Upper body may be covered with fine hair called lanugo.

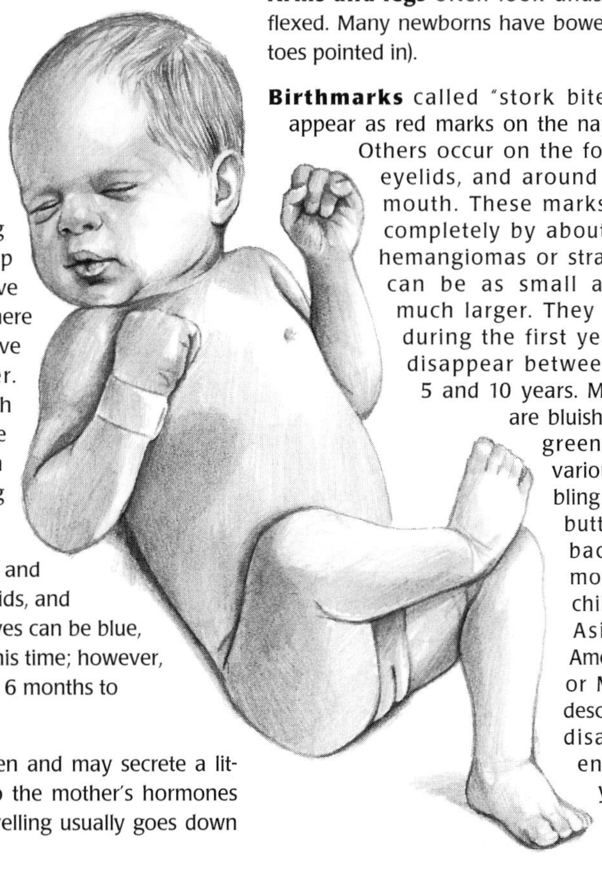

Head may be cone-shaped and is large in relation to the rest of the body. Scalp may be swollen from passing through birth canal. Top and back of the head have a soft spot (fontanelle) where the bones of the skull have not yet grown together. Some babies are born with no hair, while others have a full head of hair, which they usually start shedding at about 1 month.

Face may have a flat nose and ears, puffy or swollen eyelids, and wrinkled facial features. Eyes can be blue, green, gray, or brown at this time; however, true eye color takes about 6 months to develop.

Breasts are usually swollen and may secrete a little milk from exposure to the mother's hormones during pregnancy. The swelling usually goes down within a few weeks.

Genitals may look disproportionately large. Girls may have a clear or white discharge or bleeding from the vagina from exposure to the mother's hormones. Ask your doctor about these discharges if they concern you. In boys, the testicles usually lie in the scrotum. However, in a small number of boys one or both testicles may still be in the groin. In most of these boys, the testicles will descend into the scrotum within a few months.

Arms and legs often look unusually thin and flexed. Many newborns have bowed legs (with the toes pointed in).

Birthmarks called "stork bites" frequently appear as red marks on the nape of the neck. Others occur on the forehead, upper eyelids, and around the nose and mouth. These marks usually fade completely by about age 2. Some hemangiomas or strawberry marks can be as small as freckles or much larger. They often enlarge during the first year but usually disappear between the ages of 5 and 10 years. Mongolian spots are bluish-gray or bluish-green flat marks of various sizes resembling bruises on the buttocks or lower back. They are most common in children of black, Asian, Native American, Hispanic, or Mediterranean descent and usually disappear by the end of the first year.

First bowel movements consist of a dark, sticky substance called meconium, which fills the intestines before delivery. The stool changes color and consistency once a baby starts to take breast milk or formula during the first week of life.

Newborn reflexes

For the first 3 to 4 months, a newborn's reflexes may include sucking, grasping, and startling. They will disappear as your baby develops conscious control over his or her muscles.

The rooting reflex

Stroking your newborn's cheek will stimulate the rooting reflex. Your newborn will turn his or her head toward your finger and open his or her mouth, searching for a breast or bottle on which to feed. Stimulating this reflex is a helpful way to start your baby's first feedings at the breast or bottle. The reflex lasts about 3 or 4 months.

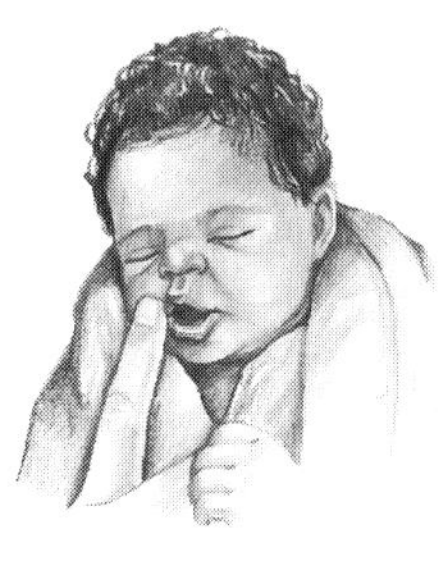

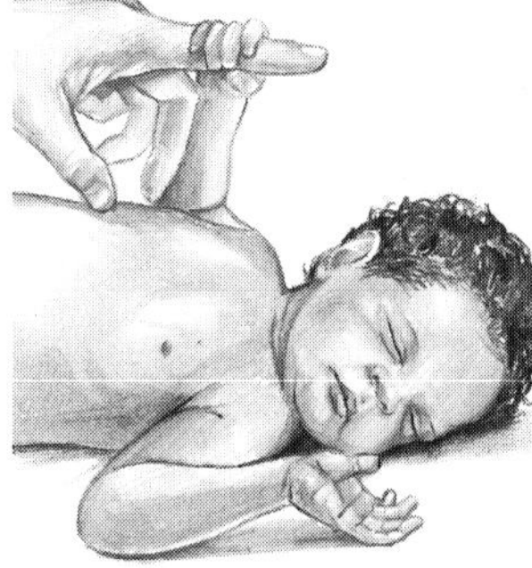

The grasping reflex

Your baby's fingers will automatically tighten around your finger or anything else that is pressed into his or her palm. This reflexive grasp is so strong that it can support the baby's entire weight. It usually lasts until about 5 or 6 months of age.

The startle reflex

A young baby will react to a loud noise or the sensation of falling by extending his or her arms, legs, fingers, and neck and by arching his or her back. The baby then quickly brings his or her arms together into the chest with fists clenched. This reflex, called the Moro reflex, lasts about 3 months.

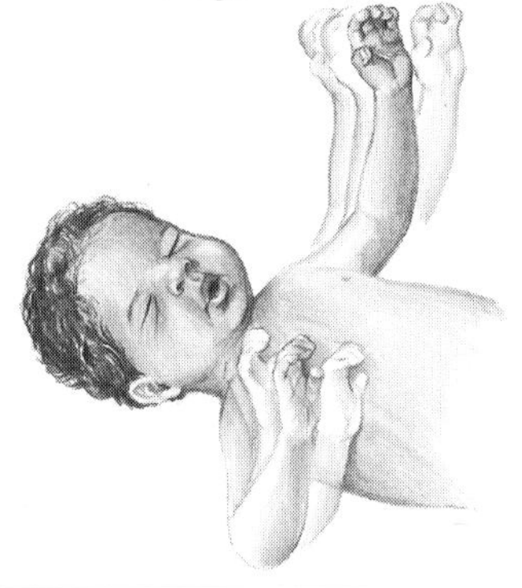

medical follow-up examination within 2 to 4 days after leaving the hospital. Don't wait for the first recommended well-baby visit (see page 237) at 1 or 2 weeks. Make an appointment with the doctor before you leave the hospital. You will either have to bring the baby in for a checkup or arrange for a nurse to visit your home to evaluate your baby's progress. The doctor or nurse will check your child's weight, make sure he or she is feeding well, look for signs of jaundice or heart or breathing problems, and draw blood for any laboratory tests your child might need. If you are having trouble breast-feeding, the nurse or doctor may recommend a lactation specialist.

Any illness during the first month of life can be serious, so report all symptoms to your doctor, including poor color, fever, or coughing. Keep track of your baby's eating, sleeping, and crying patterns so that you can recognize changes. Call your doctor immediately if you notice any of the following problems:

- **Breathing difficulty** Your baby's breathing rate is more than 60 breaths a minute and you notice labored chest movements, flaring of the nostrils, grunting while breathing, or bluish skin. Breathing difficulty is the most common problem in newborns.
- **Excessive sleepiness** Your infant is rarely alert, doesn't wake up regularly for feedings, or seems too tired to eat.
- **Excessive crying** Your baby's usual pattern of crying changes or lasts unusually long.
- **Lack of appetite** Your infant isn't eating as much as usual or sucks poorly.
- **Blue skin** Your baby's skin looks bluish, even when he or she is warm. Blue skin could indicate a lack of oxygen in the blood, which requires immediate medical attention.
- **Vomiting** Your baby vomits for more than 4 hours, vomits forcefully, vomits and has a fever or diarrhea, or vomits after more than two consecutive feedings.

- **High or low temperature** Your baby's temperature is either over 100°F taken rectally (99°F taken under the arm) or below 96.5°F. See page 267 for how to take a temperature.
- **Swollen abdomen** Your baby's abdomen feels swollen and hard and he or she has not had a bowel movement for more than 1 or 2 days or is vomiting. (Your baby's abdomen should feel soft between feedings.)
- **Excessive coughing** Your baby coughs persistently, or frequently chokes during feedings.
- **Diarrhea** Your baby has more than six to eight loose, watery bowel movements a day.
- **Dehydration** Your baby is fussy or too quiet, feeds poorly, and requires fewer than four to six diaper changes in 24 hours.
- **Constipation** Your baby does not have a bowel movement in 5 to 7 days.

If your baby has jaundice More than half of all newborns become jaundiced–a yellowing of the skin and whites of the eyes–by the second or third day after birth. Jaundice is caused by the buildup in the blood of bilirubin, which is produced by the normal breakdown of red blood cells. Before birth, your child needs more oxygen-carrying red blood cells than he or she does after birth. The excess blood cells break down after birth and form bilirubin, which is mostly processed by the liver and eliminated from the body in the stool. But sometimes a newborn's immature liver and kidneys can't handle the amount of bilirubin. It can then build up in the blood and cause jaundice.

Most newborn jaundice clears up without treatment when the baby is about a week to 10 days old. An abnormally high level of bilirubin requires phototherapy (light therapy) treatment. Phototherapy delivers ultraviolet light

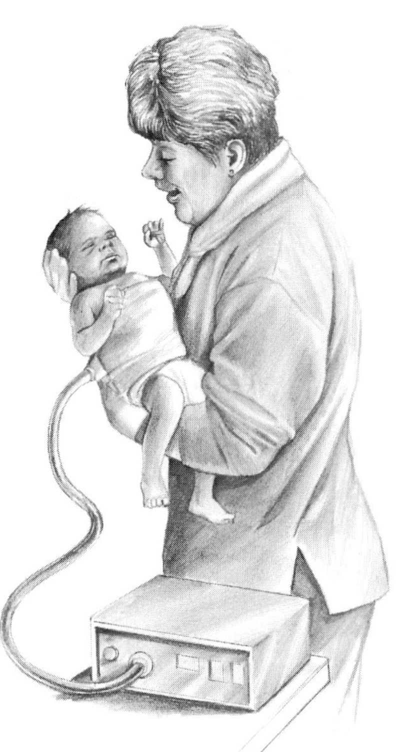

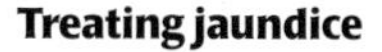

Treating jaundice

If your baby needs phototherapy for jaundice, you may be able to give him or her the treatment yourself at home. Your doctor will arrange for a visiting nurse to teach you how to use the phototherapy equipment. The nurse will also monitor your baby's progress during daily visits to your home. The ultraviolet light is delivered through a fiberoptic panel that wraps around the baby like a wide belt. The panel fits into a cotton flannel sleeve that feels soft against the baby's skin. You can hold, feed, and change your baby while the belt is on. The longer the infant wears the belt each day, the faster the treatment works. Each day, the visiting nurse will check your baby's condition and take a blood sample to measure his or her bilirubin level, which usually comes down to a safe level within 3 to 4 days. Health insurance sometimes covers the cost of the nursing care and phototherapy equipment.

that helps the infant excrete bilirubin in his or her urine. It also helps induce bowel movements, so the child can excrete bilirubin in the stool. Phototherapy can be done in the hospital or at home. In severe cases, the doctor will hospitalize the child so he or she can be closely monitored and to find out if an underlying medical condition, such as biliary atresia (see page 430) or hemolytic anemia (see page 411), might be causing the excessively high bilirubin buildup. In the hospital, the infant will receive phototherapy and may need intravenous fluids. He or she may need an exchange blood transfusion, in which the baby's entire blood supply is replaced by donated blood. Untreated bilirubin levels that stay high for a long period can cause brain damage.

RESPONDING TO YOUR BABY'S CRIES

Babies cry when they need something; they cry less when their needs are met quickly. You will soon learn to identify your newborn's different cries–whether they signal hunger, pain, fear, discomfort, fatigue, boredom, overstimulation, or the need for comforting. Through trial and error, you will learn the calming techniques that your baby likes best.

Most babies eventually develop their own way of calming themselves, by sucking a thumb, finger, or pacifier, or snuggling up to a favorite blanket. Watch your baby to see if he or she develops a self-comforting method. Your doctor can give you helpful tips for calming your child. Some proven techniques include:

- **Motion** Gentle movement (especially if it is repetitive) is a calming influence on many babies. Rock your baby, carry him or her in a front carrier while you do chores, put him or her in an automatic infant swing (but make sure the baby's head is supported), or take him or her for a ride in the stroller or car.
- **A calm environment** Play soft, soothing music, sing, or hum. Turn off the television. Avoid sudden, loud noises and harsh lighting.
- **White noise** Some babies are soothed by monotonous humming; shaking of rattles; or even the sound of a dishwasher, washing machine, or vacuum cleaner.
- **Touch** Give the baby a warm bath (if your baby enjoys the water). Rhythmically stroke or massage his or her back, arms, or legs. Help him or her find a finger or thumb to suck on or offer a pacifier.
- **Distraction** Point out and describe bright, colorful drawings, toys, or other objects.
- **A change in feeding technique** When feeding your baby (either breast milk or formula), burp him or her more frequently. If you are feeding your baby formula, use a bottle with a collapsible bag to help reduce the amount of air he or she sucks in; hold the baby upright for half an hour after a feeding to minimize the amount he or she spits up.

Thumbs and pacifiers Some babies seem to need to suck more than others and are not satisfied by only the breast or bottle. This need is most intense between 2 and 4 months of age. A thumb or finger is a convenient self-comforting device—and it's always available. But if your baby has not discovered his or her thumb or finger and wants to suck between feedings, try offering a pacifier, which babies also find comforting.

Choose a sturdy, one-piece pacifier that has ventilation holes in the shield. If you can't find a one-piece pacifier, choose one that has a securely attached nipple that won't come loose and be swallowed by your baby. The pacifier should be dishwasher safe so you can thoroughly clean it, especially for the first 6 months when your child is most at risk of getting infections. Nipples come in a variety of shapes; buy a few different types and see which one your child prefers. Many doctors recommend orthodontic-type pacifiers to minimize possible tooth-alignment problems in the future.

Keep several pacifiers on hand so you always have a clean one available when your baby loses or drops one outdoors. Never attach a pacifier to the crib, stroller, or playpen and never hang one from a ribbon, string, or cord around your baby's neck or wrist. It's OK to clip one attached to a ribbon onto your baby's shirt when he or she is up and about and you are watching him or her closely.

Most children give up sucking on thumbs, fingers, and pacifiers between the ages of 2 and 4, with no harm done to their teeth (see page 266). Children who suck their thumb usually do so only when they're tired or upset and want comfort. Some doctors think that constant use of a pacifier can affect a child's ability to make sounds and talk. Try to limit the use of the pacifier after 4 months of age—before it becomes more of a habit than a means of comfort. Remember that, whether your child sucks on a finger or a pacifier, he or she would probably prefer to be comforted by you. Close physical contact with you or another loving person is more beneficial for your child's development than anything else.

When your baby has colic Colic is a common condition in children younger than 3 months old. It is characterized by fierce crying—distinct from the baby's usual way of crying—usually in the late afternoon or early evening. Episodes usually occur at least three times a week. An attack begins suddenly, the baby cries loudly and continuously for 3 hours or more, and his or her face may be flushed. The skin around the infant's mouth can turn pale, his or her abdomen may be swollen and tight, and the baby may draw his or her knees up toward the abdomen and clench his or her hands. Nothing comforts the child for more than a few minutes and the attack may end only after the baby is completely exhausted and falls asleep, or when he or she has a bowel movement or passes gas. The cause of colic is unknown and occurs in both breast-fed and bottle-fed babies. Some doctors believe that colic may be the result of an immature digestive system.

Colic usually goes away when the child is about 3 to 4 months old. Until then, you may feel exhausted and frustrated that you can't comfort your crying infant. Remember that you are not to blame for your child's colic and take

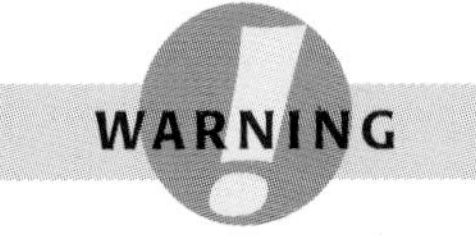

Is it more than just colic?

If your baby is vomiting or you notice anything unusual in his or her bowel movements, such as blood or mucus, talk to your doctor. These are not symptoms of colic. A medical examination is necessary to rule out a more serious condition, such as an intestinal obstruction.

a break whenever you can. Ask someone else to take over or put your baby in a safe place such as the crib or a swing, go into another room, and do something else while your baby cries for a while. Try to schedule your day so that you have fewer other demands during your child's fussy time. Ask your doctor for suggestions. He or she might recommend giving your baby an over-the-counter antigas medication (in drops), which relieves discomfort in some children. If you are breast-feeding your baby, reducing the amount of dairy products and caffeine in your diet may help; if you are bottle-feeding, try using a soy or lactose-free formula. If the frustration of dealing with your child ever makes you feel that you want to hurt your child, get help immediately. For information about how to deal with anger, see page 327. To find out how to comfort a crying baby, see page 40.

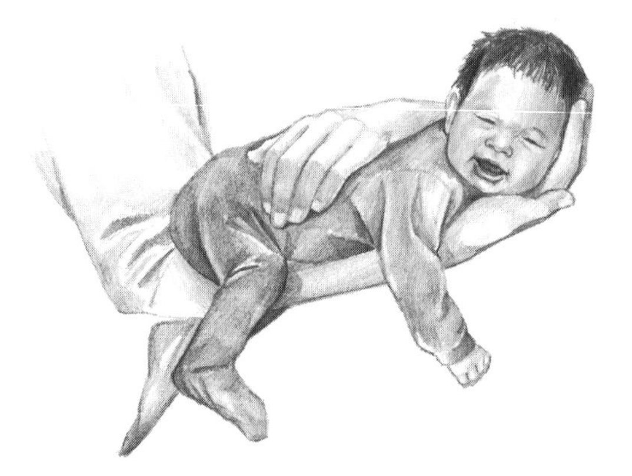

Calming the colicky baby

If your baby has colic, you have probably already tried countless measures to soothe him or her. Many parents find that holding their baby in the "football" position shown here, which puts pressure on the baby's abdomen, often provides some relief. Place your baby facedown on your arm, supporting his or her head and neck with your hand. You could also try lying your child facedown across your lap and massaging his or her back. Make sure your baby can breathe freely while on your lap.

Making adjustments

The first weeks at home with your new baby will be the most demanding and difficult. This period also marks a transition in your relationship with your partner and in your lives, which will never be the same again. You are both likely to be exhausted much of the time and will need to make an extra effort to catch up on sleep whenever you can—for example, when your baby is napping. You'll be better able to take care of your baby when you are rested.

For the mother, the first few weeks will involve some major adjustments in her body. The hard work that your body is doing to recover from childbirth can contribute to your fatigue. You will likely have a menstrual period for several weeks after the birth, with the flow being heavy at first. Your abdomen will be loose and saggy, gradually tightening up over the next month or two.

Try to have some fun too. Plan a date night or another special time to be together as a couple and make an effort to stick with it. If one of you feels overwhelmed by all the new responsibilities involved in caring for the baby, share more of the tasks. For example, if the mother is breast-feeding, her partner can tend to the baby's cries in the middle of the night by changing the baby's diaper and bringing him or her in for nursing. Don't hesitate to ask friends and relatives for help with daily tasks such as meals, housework, and child care—they will probably be happy to help.

The "after baby" blues

Most women feel a bit moody and depressed in the first few days after giving birth. You may feel lonely, overwhelmed by your new responsibilities, anxious, or angry. These feelings usually go away within several days or weeks.

But some women develop a longer-lasting condition called postpartum depression. They feel intense anxiety or despair that makes even the smallest task seem difficult. The cause of postpartum depression is not fully understood but may result from a sudden reduction in a woman's hormone levels after childbirth. Other contributing factors include a lack of sleep, pain from childbirth, or breast engorgement. You might also be having a hard time adjusting to caring for a new infant.

Getting emotional support to help you cope with these new circumstances is essential—both for yourself and your baby, who tunes into your moods and emotions and can be profoundly affected. Share your feelings with your partner and other relatives and friends who have children. Talk with your doctor about the need for counseling if you experience any of the following symptoms:

- Anxiety or hopelessness that lasts for more than 2 weeks
- Inability to sleep even when you feel tired
- Sleeping too much, even when your baby is awake
- Anxiety or panic attacks
- Lack of interest in your baby or other family members
- Fear of harming the baby or yourself (see page 327)

Feeding your baby

Whether you choose to breast-feed or bottle-feed your baby, the time you spend feeding your child is a valuable opportunity to learn about and bond with him or her. It's also a chance for you to watch, touch, talk to, play with, and sing to your infant. While many doctors encourage mothers to breast-feed, the feeding process should take into account the mother's health and the family's lifestyle. If you are having trouble deciding whether to breast- or bottle-feed, talk to your doctor.

BREAST-FEEDING

If you decide to breast-feed, you are giving your baby the best nutrition possible–whether you nurse for just a few weeks or for several months or more. Breast-feeding also provides a unique opportunity for mother and child to form a special bond. Breast-feeding benefits the mother in many ways:

- Helps your uterus return to its normal size more rapidly.
- Helps you lose weight faster.
- Helps reduce your risk of breast cancer by causing potentially protective changes in breast cells if you nurse for at least 3 months. The risk of breast cancer is further reduced each time you nurse another baby for at least 3 months.
- Eliminates the inconvenience and expense of preparing formula and washing bottles; breast milk is sterile, always available, and at just the right temperature.
- Each breast-feeding session gives you a much-needed chance to relax.

Breast-feeding is good for your baby because it:

- Provides a unique mixture of nutrients, hormones, and proteins essential for digestion, brain development, and growth.
- Provides infection-fighting proteins (antibodies) that reduce the risk of infections of the middle ear, digestive system, and respiratory tract.
- Reduces the risk of food allergies.
- Causes fewer digestive problems, such as constipation or diarrhea, than formula.
- Reduces the risk of some chronic diseases later in life.

Your breasts were made for nursing a baby–you don't need to do anything to prepare them. In fact, experts now say that the less a woman does, the better. Ask your obstetrician to examine your breasts during pregnancy for any anatomical features, such as inverted nipples, that might interfere with breast-feeding. If you have inverted nipples, your doctor or the lactation nurse (a specialist trained to help new mothers learn how to breast-feed) may recommend wearing a special nipple shield along with performing certain exercises in the last 3 months of pregnancy to draw out the nipple.

Women with some rare health conditions, such as infection with HIV, the virus that causes AIDS (see page 404), should not breast-feed (HIV can be passed to a nursing baby in breast milk). If you are concerned about any condition you have, ask your doctor about it. Medications taken by a nursing mother–for treating cancer, high blood pressure, or mental disorders–can harm a nursing baby. Inform your doctor if you are taking any medications regularly; he or she can tell you if it's OK for you to breast-feed or if you should take the medication just after a nursing session or before your baby goes to bed at night. If the doctor prescribes any new medication, be sure to tell him or her that you are breast-feeding.

Some diseases, such as galactosemia (see page 493) or PKU (see page 595), prevent a baby from breast-feeding because the child cannot tolerate the nutrients in breast milk. In such cases, your child's doctor will prescribe special formula.

Starting to breast-feed Even though breast-feeding may seem awkward at first, you will eventually succeed. But most mothers and infants need to learn how to breast-feed—although some are more proficient than others from the start. Be patient, persistent, and confident, and don't let anyone try to discourage you from nursing. It can take a few weeks for you and your infant to become skilled breast-feeding partners. As you and your baby begin, problems may arise and you will undoubtedly have questions. If you feel you are having a problem breast-feeding, get help immediately. Ask your doctor or the hospital for a referral to a lactation nurse, one who specializes in breast-feeding.

The first few days after delivery, your breasts produce a small amount of colostrum, a thin, creamy substance that supplies your baby with essential nutrients and antibodies (infection-fighting proteins) until your milk begins to flow. This first food is completely adequate for your baby's first few days of life. Your milk will come in between the second and fifth day after delivery. Also, you may experience some breast and nipple discomfort from engorgement and the baby's sucking efforts. This resolves with time.

If this is your first time breast-feeding, be patient with yourself and your baby. Both of you need time to adjust to a new routine. Here are some tips to

QUESTIONS MOTHERS ASK

Breast-feeding

Q Will I have to stop eating some of my favorite foods when I'm breast-feeding?

A You should be able to continue eating the same foods you always have. Some breast-feeding women say that when they eat caffeine-containing, spicy, or gas-producing foods—such as chocolate or onions—their baby seems to be fussy. Other women don't notice any effects. Excessive amounts of dairy products can cause gas in some infants. If you wonder about a specific food, eat a small amount and see if your baby is affected. Look for a reaction 6 to 8 hours afterward.

Q My breasts are small. Will I be able to breast-feed?

A Breast size has nothing to do with the ability to breast-feed successfully. Expect your breasts to increase in size during pregnancy and breast-feeding. They will return to the same pre-pregnancy size when you stop breast-feeding.

Q Will breast-feeding make my breasts sag?

A The appearance of your breasts depends more on how large your breasts become during pregnancy than on breast-feeding. Wear a good support bra during both pregnancy and breast-feeding.

help make your breast-feeding experience pleasant, satisfying, and successful:

- Feed your baby whenever he or she is hungry; you will eventually establish a pattern. For the first several weeks, breast-fed babies may want to nurse every 1½ to 2 hours. As your baby grows, he or she will be able to go longer between feedings and eventually will sleep through the night (see page 57).
- If your newborn does not wake at least every 3 to 3½ hours demanding to be fed, try awakening him or her, even during the night; infrequent feedings will prevent you from building up an adequate milk supply for your baby and put him or her at risk of being underfed.
- Sit or lie down in a comfortable position. Position pillows under your supporting arm as needed, so that your arm won't get sore.
- Use both breasts at every feeding and alternate the breast you start with, emptying one breast completely before starting on the other. (You can move a safety pin from one bra strap to the other to help you remember which side to start on.) Alternating breasts helps prevent nipple soreness and ensures that both breasts produce a similar amount of milk. Also, the composition of the milk changes during the nursing session.
- Let the baby nurse for up to 20 minutes on the first side before changing sides. (After 20 minutes, the milk supply is usually exhausted from the breast, and soreness can occur from prolonged sucking.)
- Position your baby so that his or her whole body faces you.
- Use your thumb and index finger to point your nipple outward and brush it against the baby's cheek to stimulate the rooting reflex (see page 38). Your baby will turn toward the nipple and suck. Quickly draw your infant to your breast when he or she opens his or her mouth wide.
- Be sure your whole nipple and part of the areola (the dark, circular area around it) are in the baby's mouth—otherwise, your nipple will become sore.
- Although it may seem impossible, try to get plenty of rest. Being relaxed will help stimulate your let-down reflex.
- Drink lots of fluids while you're nursing. Aim for six to eight glasses of water a day; you might try sipping a glass while nursing. Avoid carbonated beverages and excessive amounts of dairy products, which may give your baby gas, and caffeinated beverages, which can be dehydrating to you and overstimulating to your infant. Avoid alcohol, which passes into breast milk.

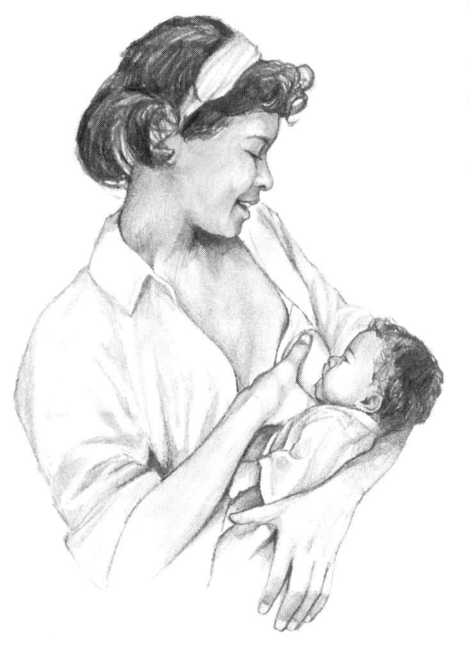

Latching on

To be in the right position for breast-feeding, your baby's entire body should be facing you. Make sure the whole nipple and part of the areola (the darker, circular area around the nipple) are in the baby's mouth. Your baby's mouth will be flared outward on your breast. If your nipples hurt throughout the feeding, your baby has not latched on properly.

Nature designed breast-feeding as a wonderfully efficient system of supply and demand: the more a baby nurses on your breast, the more milk your breast will produce. As a baby nurses less—for example, when you eventually add solid foods to your child's diet or begin weaning him or her—your breasts will produce less and less milk. Minimize giving supplemental bottles of formula during the first 6 weeks because they can interfere with the quantity of your milk production. Also, babies who get bottles frequently early on may reject breast-feeding because it is easier for them to get formula from a bottle. Giving the baby a bottle periodically after the first 6 weeks to allow yourself a rest or to feed the baby will not interfere with milk production. However, many infants who are solely breast-fed reject an artificial nipple. Breast milk contains all the fluid a baby needs, so you don't need to give your baby water or other fluids.

If breast milk is your baby's sole source of nourishment, your child's doctor may recommend giving him or her a daily supplement containing vitamins A, D, and E, which are not always present in sufficient amounts in breast milk. Because breast milk provides iron, which helps prevent anemia (see page 412),

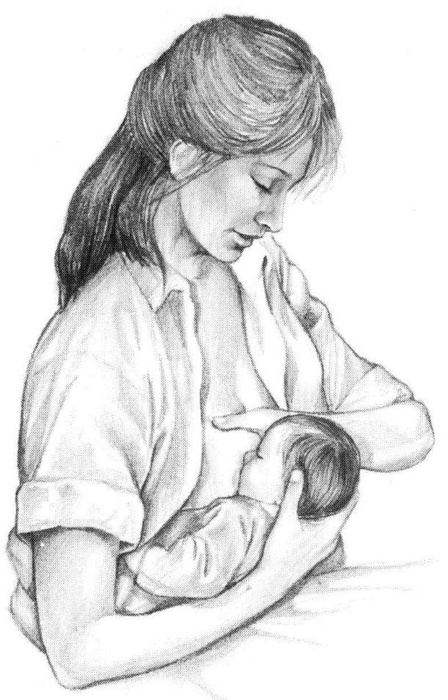

Football hold

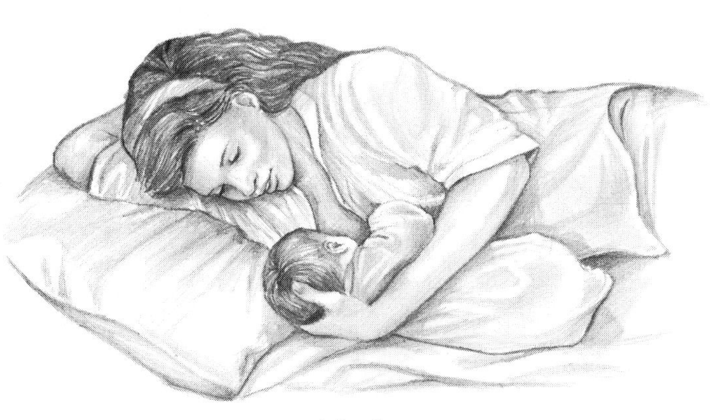

Lying down

Alternate breast-feeding positions

The best way to prevent breast pain and soreness is to vary your nursing position from feeding to feeding, especially at first. If your baby is very small, try the so-called football hold (left), in which you hold your baby at your side. In addition to the most common, child-on-lap position, try breast-feeding lying down (right), which makes for especially restful sessions.

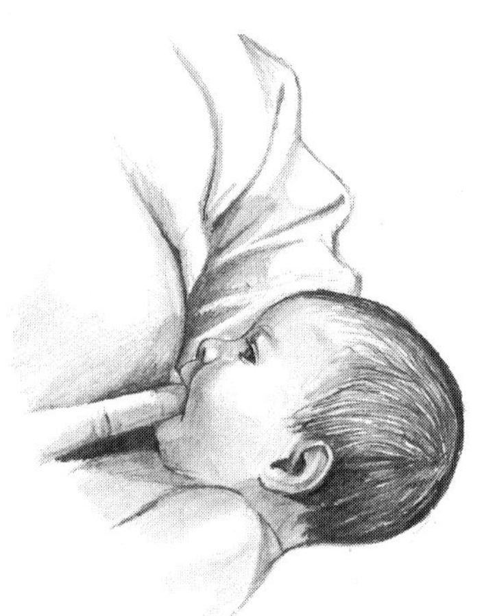

you won't need to give your child a supplement containing iron until your child begins eating solid foods. Fluoride is not present in breast milk, so, if your child is not drinking fluorinated water after 6 months of age, the doctor may also recommend a fluoride supplement.

You may notice a brief tingling, pins-and-needles, or tightening sensation, and milk may drip or spray from your breasts before or during a nursing session. This response, called the let-down or milk-ejection reflex, is your body's way of making your milk flow easily for your baby. This reflex may also be triggered when you hear your baby cry, think about nursing your baby, or take a shower. Apply pressure to the nipple with your finger to stop the flow. You can wear disposable or washable cotton nursing pads inside your bra to prevent leakage.

Remove your baby from the breast gently

When your baby is finished nursing, break the suction of the baby's mouth by putting your finger between your baby's upper and lower gums. You can also gently press your fingers into your breast near the baby's mouth or gently push down on the baby's chin. This technique will help prevent nipple soreness.

Common breast-feeding problems Remember that, even though breast-feeding is a natural process, you and your baby need to learn how to breast-feed together, so expect some minor difficulty and uncertainty. Here are some of the most common problems women encounter when starting to breast-feed:

• Your breasts may become engorged with milk and swell painfully, especially when your milk first comes in. Hot showers can help. Ask your doctor if it's OK to take acetaminophen or ibuprofen for the discomfort. A properly fitting support bra will help relieve some of the discomfort, but the best prevention for engorged breasts is to put your baby to the breast and let him or her nurse. The swelling will go away in a few days. If your breasts are so engorged that your baby cannot latch on properly, hand pump a little milk from each breast before bringing the baby to your nipple.

• Your nipples may become sore, especially during the first week or two. Proper positioning of your infant can prevent some of the soreness. Alternate your nursing position so that the baby does not always suck hardest on the same side of the nipple. Avoid using soap because it can dry out your nipples; wash your breasts with water only. After each feeding, coat your nipples with breast milk, which is a natural moisturizer. (Don't apply lotions or lubricants around your nipples; your baby may taste or ingest them while nursing.) To keep your nipples dry, expose them to the air as much as possible (try keeping the flaps of your nursing bra down for a while after each feeding), change a wet nursing bra right away, and don't keep milk-soaked nursing pads in your bra. If your nipples continue to hurt after the first week or so or become cracked, talk to a lactation specialist recommended by your child's doctor or by the local La Leche League. Sore nipples are the most common reason for breast-feeding failure.

• During the first few days, you may have some uterine cramps (like menstrual cramps) at the beginning of each nursing session. These cramps are caused by contractions that help your uterus return to its original size. They will disappear after the first week.

Don't rely on breast-feeding alone for contraception

Although you may not have a period (after the initial postpartum flow) for as long as you nurse your baby, you cannot assume that breast-feeding is a reliable form of contraception. Your ovaries may be releasing eggs so you can still become pregnant. Check with your doctor about when it's OK to resume having intercourse. You'll need to use some form of contraception whenever you have sex. Don't use combined birth-control pills while you are breast-feeding because the hormones they contain can reduce the amount of breast milk you produce. Instead, use a low-dose, progestin-only pill (the minipill) or a barrier method such as a condom, diaphragm, or spermicide during this time.

Taking care of yourself Breast-feeding burns a lot of calories. While you are breast-feeding, you will need to consume about 500 calories more per day than you did before you got pregnant or about 200 more than you ate during pregnancy. Eat a well-balanced, nutritious diet with plenty of fruits, vegetables, and whole grains. Get at least 1,000 milligrams of calcium each day to keep your bones strong. Good sources of calcium include skim milk and other low-fat dairy products. If you are not getting enough nutrients in your diet, your doctor will probably recommend that you continue taking the prenatal supplement you took during pregnancy, as well as a calcium supplement. You will notice how much more thirsty you are while breast-feeding. Drinking at least six to eight glasses of fluids a day, including water, juice, and milk, will satisfy your and your baby's fluid needs. Avoid tobacco, alcohol, and other drugs, which can pass to your baby in breast milk.

Regular aerobic exercise keeps you strong and doesn't affect the quality of your milk. You may find it more comfortable to nurse before exercising so your breasts will be less heavy with milk.

Is my baby getting enough breast milk? When you first start breast-feeding, you might worry that your baby is not getting enough milk. You won't know exactly how many ounces he or she is taking at each feeding, as you would with bottle-feeding. All babies normally lose some weight during the first few days after birth. Most breast-fed babies regain their birthweight by about 2 weeks of age.

One clue that your baby is not getting enough is if he or she acts hungry after nursing, such as frequently sucking on his or her hands or displaying the rooting reflex (see page 38). If you are unsure about your baby's weight gain, take him or her to the doctor's office for a weight check. You can be assured that your baby is getting enough milk if you notice several of the following signs during the first few weeks:

- Your baby's sucking is strong, steady, and rhythmic for at least 10 minutes at every feeding.
- You can hear your baby swallowing while feeding.
- Your baby wakes up every 2 to 3 hours and wants to nurse; he or she nurses at least 8 to 12 times every 24 hours.

- Your baby has at least six to eight wet diapers and two yellowish bowel movements every 24 hours.
- Your breasts feel full before feedings and softer afterward.
- Your baby regains his or her birthweight by 2 weeks of age.

Your baby's bowel movements By the fourth or fifth day of life, a breast-fed baby's bowel movements will be yellowish and loose (even watery for the first 3 to 4 weeks), have a seedy consistency, and have an odor of yogurt. Between about 4 days and 4 weeks of age, your baby will have at least four bowel movements a day, usually one during or after each nursing session. Don't be alarmed if the bowel movements are noisy; this is normal. The bowel

Burping your baby

Burping helps to relieve your baby's stomach distention and may reduce spitting up. You generally don't need to burp your baby more than twice during a feeding, for about 1 minute each time. These are the burping methods that many parents have found effective. Try them all; you may have more success with one than another.

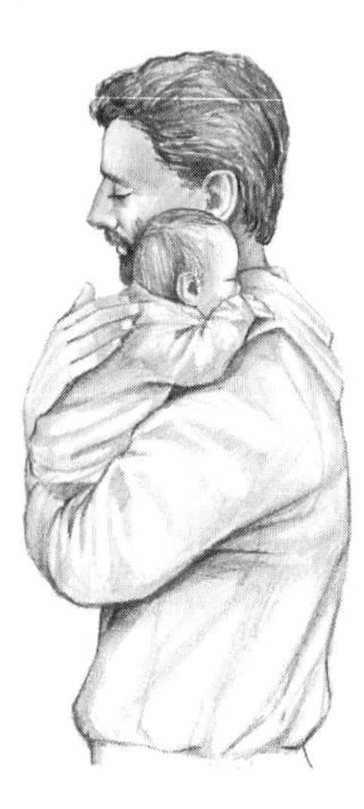

Over your shoulder
Drape a towel or cloth diaper over your shoulder. Hold your baby so that his or her head rests on your shoulder and gently pat or rub his or her back.

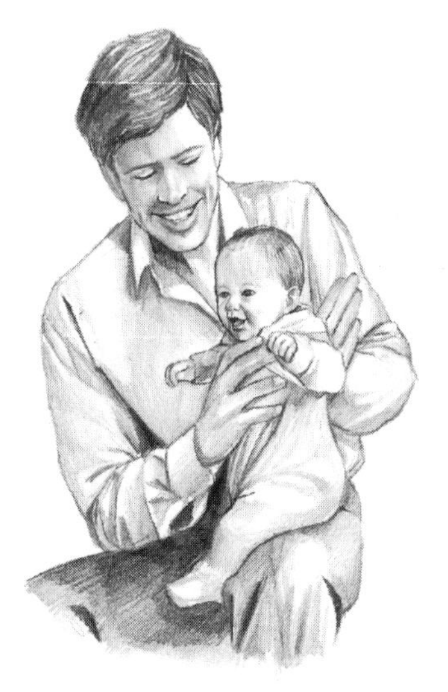

Sitting up
Place a towel or cloth diaper on one leg. Sit your baby sideways on your other leg, leaning him or her forward over your covered leg as you support the chest and chin with one hand and gently pat his or her back with your other hand.

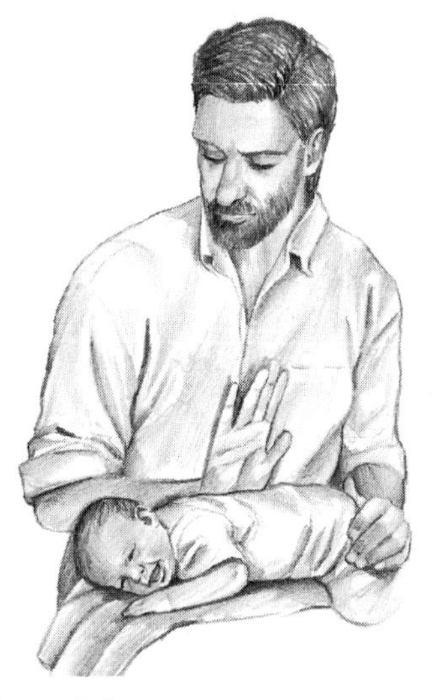

Stomach down
Place a towel or cloth diaper on your lap. Lay your baby stomach-down across your lap with his or her stomach on one of your legs and his or her head on the other. Position your legs so that the baby's head is slightly higher than his or her chest. Turn the baby's head to the side and gently pat or rub his or her back with your hand.

movements will become less frequent as the baby's digestive system matures. By the time your breast-fed baby is 2 to 3 months old, he or she may have one bowel movement every 5 to 7 days. Don't worry about your baby being constipated as long as the stool is soft when it does come. If your baby seems uncomfortable and is crying as if in pain, or if his or her bowel movements smell bad or are persistently runny or hard, call your child's doctor.

Supplemental bottles Try to wait until your milk supply is firmly established (about 6 weeks) before giving your infant a supplemental bottle of breast milk or formula. If you're going to be away at feeding time, express your milk beforehand and refrigerate it in a bottle so someone else can give it to the baby while you're out. That way, you'll avoid giving the baby formula and can maintain your supply of breast milk. If you do use formula, express milk from your breasts anyway to keep your milk supply from diminishing.

Several kinds of breast pumps are available for expressing milk. If you are seldom away from your baby, expressing milk by hand or with a hand pump should be sufficient. But, if you are returning to work or need to be away for long periods, consider buying a battery-operated pump, or rent or buy an electric pump from your local hospital. Both are faster and more efficient and comfortable than a hand pump. Ask your doctor about these options. Whichever type you choose, you will probably need some help at first to learn how to use it.

You can store breast milk in the refrigerator for 24 hours and in the freezer for up to 6 months. Use clean plastic containers or disposable baby bottle bags (some of the infection-fighting substances in breast milk can stick to glass). To thaw frozen milk, place it in the refrigerator overnight or in a bowl or pan of warm water. Never microwave breast milk or heat it in boiling water because you could destroy some of the protective substances in the milk or make the milk too hot. After thawing breast milk in the refrigerator, use it within 24 hours. Never reuse leftover milk; throw it away.

Breast problems You can develop breast problems while you are nursing. Call your doctor if you have any of the symptoms described below. The following conditions are the most common and are usually easy to treat:

BLOCKED MILK DUCT After your milk comes in and you are nursing regularly, you may develop a blocked milk duct. The duct may back up because of a missed feeding, or simply because of the way the duct curves or bends. You may experience tenderness or redness in one relatively small area of the breast. It may be hard and feel like a bruise. Try starting feedings on that breast and point the baby's nose toward the affected area. After nursing, apply moist heat (a warm washcloth) for 10 to 15 minutes at a time. If left untreated, a blocked duct can develop into mastitis.

MASTITIS Mastitis is an infection of the milk ducts in the breast that can occur when bacteria enter through the nipple, usually from a nursing baby's mouth. The breast becomes extremely sore, hard, red, and swollen. You may also have chills and a fever. Your doctor will prescribe an antibiotic along with a pain reliever—if you need one—that is safe to take while breast-feeding. Expressing breast milk helps relieve the symptoms. Some doctors recommend nursing on the infected breast while others do not. Ask your child's doctor what he or she recommends. Some women have recurrent episodes of mastitis.

BREAST ABSCESS A breast abscess is a collection of pus that forms a red, hot, firm, extremely tender lump in the breast. It occurs when bacteria from the baby's mouth enter the breast through a cracked or sore nipple; it usually clears up with antibiotics. Your doctor may recommend draining the abscess with a needle or through a tiny incision. This procedure is performed in the doctor's office using a local anesthetic. You may be able to continue to nurse during treatment. Talk to your doctor.

THRUSH Some breast-feeding women develop a yeast infection called thrush, which causes the nipples to become sore and cracked. The nursing baby also contracts the infection, which produces white patches on the baby's tongue (see page 648). Your doctor will prescribe medicated cream that you can apply to your nipples several times a day and medicated mouth drops to give to your baby. Thrush can recur and persist and often requires several weeks of treatment. Continue to breast-feed during treatment and expose your nipples to the air as much as possible to help promote healing.

Nursing when you go back to work You can give your baby the benefits of breast milk even after you return to work. You can express milk from your breasts once or twice a day at work using a breast pump, refrigerate the milk, and bring it home for the baby's caregiver to feed to the baby the next day. The nutritional benefits to your baby are worth the inconvenience. Some employers set aside a private area where nursing mothers can pump milk from their breasts. Find out what options your employer offers.

On the other hand, you may decide to breast-feed for as long as you are on maternity leave and then start bottle-feeding before returning to work. You can still breast-feed when you're at home in the morning, evening, and at bedtime, but your milk supply will naturally begin to decrease as your baby nurses less. You will be most comfortable and your baby more accepting if you wean him or her gradually, eliminating one breast feeding at a time. If you stop abruptly, your breasts may become swollen and sore.

If your baby refuses to suck on a bottle nipple, be patient. Try different kinds of nipples or have someone else feed him or her while you leave the room. (Nursing babies often refuse to accept a bottle from their mothers.) Some babies can be weaned directly to a capped cup. Once you have begun weaning, stop expressing milk from your breasts so you can naturally reduce your milk supply. As your baby adjusts to the withdrawal of one feeding at the breast, eliminate another. During the transition from breast to bottle, spend more time cuddling and playing with your baby to make you both feel better as you adjust to the change in feeding patterns. For information about weaning an older baby, see page 90.

BOTTLE-FEEDING

Breast-feeding is not for everyone. If you can't breast-feed or choose not to (for example, if you take certain medications or develop a severe breast infection), a variety of nutritious formulas are available. Infant formulas are designed to resemble the nutritional content of breast milk as closely as possible. Ask your pediatrician which formula he or she recommends.

Bottle-feeding has several advantages. It frees the mother from her baby; other family members, especially dad, get a chance to be more involved with feeding. With a bottle, you know exactly how much your baby is taking at each feeding. A bottle-fed baby still gets the needed cuddling and closeness at mealtime. But avoid propping the bottle up so you won't have to hold your baby during a feeding. You will deny yourself and your baby important opportunities for closeness and bonding. Propping a bottle can also increase a baby's risk of choking and make him or her more susceptible to ear infections.

Giving formula Your doctor will probably recommend a formula based on cow's milk, fortified with iron, and that comes in a powder or liquid concentrate that you mix with water or in a ready-to-feed form. Babies under 1 year of age should not get regular cow's milk because the unprocessed protein it contains is hard to digest and the high protein and salt content can strain immature kidneys. All types of formula are basically the same in nutritional content; they differ only in price. The most convenient, ready-to-feed formula costs the most. Never try to make your own formula at home—your baby might not get the nutrients needed for growth, development, and good health.

Whatever type of formula you use, follow these preparation and refrigeration guidelines:

- Always check the expiration date before you buy or use any formula. Don't buy or use leaky, dented, or otherwise damaged containers.
- Always wash your hands before preparing formula.
- Wash bottles, nipples, and caps in hot, soapy water, rinse them carefully, and let them air dry. Running them through the dishwasher will kill even more germs. Rinsing out bottles and nipples right after feedings will make them easier to clean. Sterilizing is unnecessary.
- Refrigerate all opened cans of ready-to-feed and liquid concentrate and use them within the time specified on the can.
- Immediately refrigerate any unused formula you have prepared from powder or liquid concentrate.
- Don't use formula that has been frozen.
- When making formula from powder or liquid concentrate, use the exact amounts of water recommended on the label.

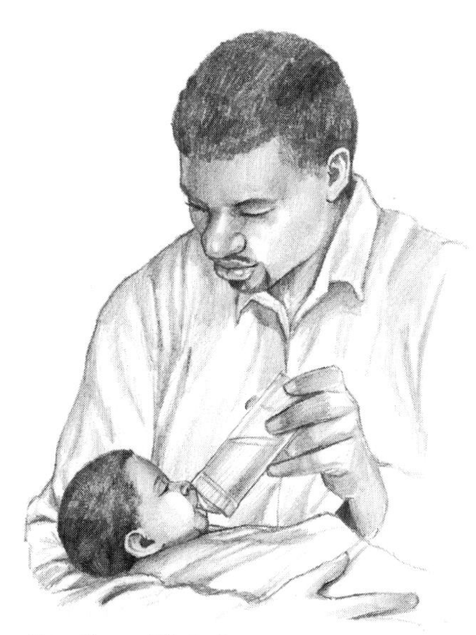

Bonding with dad
The major advantage that bottle-feeding has over breast-feeding is that dad doesn't get left out. Make each feeding session a chance to bond and get close to your baby.

Don't overfeed your baby

Overfeeding a baby in the first few months of life can lead to excessive weight gain, vomiting, and spitting up. Don't use the breast or bottle as a pacifier. All babies have a strong need to suck and it doesn't always mean that they are hungry. If you think your child is full but he or she continues to suck, try giving a pacifier or finger to help satisfy the need without overfeeding.

Too little water can cause problems for the infant's digestive system; too much will provide inadequate nutrition. Using incorrect amounts of water can also cause salt imbalances in the baby.

- When using water from the tap, always use cold water. Let it run for about 2 minutes to clear stale water out of the pipes and reduce the risk of lead contamination from older pipes.
- If you think your tap water might be impure, use undistilled bottled water (the process of distilling removes valuable minerals), boil the water for 5 minutes, or use a water filter system.
- Never reuse leftover formula; it can easily become contaminated with bacteria.

Getting started The nurses at the hospital will probably offer your baby some formula as soon as he or she wakes up from his or her first sleep about 3 to 6 hours after delivery. The baby will probably take only about half an ounce at the first feeding; a newborn's need for nutrition is minimal. By the third day, most babies take about 2 ounces every 3 to 4 hours. The younger and smaller an infant is, the more frequently he or she will want to eat.

Feeding time should be relaxing for you and your baby. Get comfortable and hold your baby in a semiupright position in the crook of your arm. Support your arm with a pillow. Try these suggestions for an easy feeding session:

- Stroke your baby's cheek with your finger or the tip of the nipple to trigger the rooting reflex (see page 38). Then gently place the nipple between your baby's lips.
- Hold the bottle tilted so that formula always fills the neck of the bottle and the nipple. Otherwise, your baby could swallow air and develop intestinal gas. You don't have to tilt the bottle if you're using disposable bottle liners, which automatically deflate as they're emptied.
- To make sure the formula is coming through the nipple at the right speed, turn the bottle upside down and give it a few quick shakes. If the formula

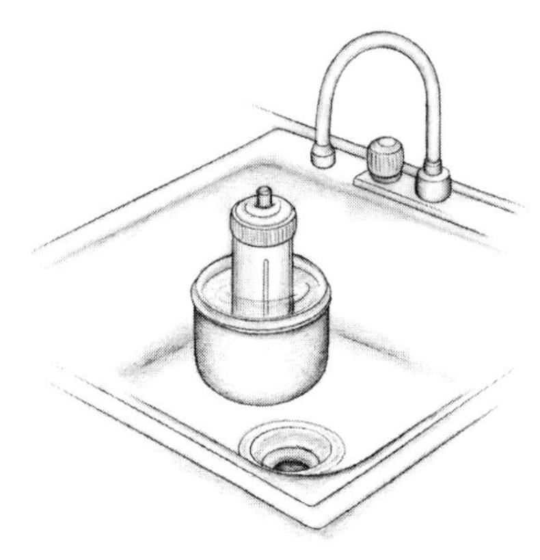

Warming formula

To warm formula, hold the filled bottle under warm running tap water or put the bottle in a pan or bowl of warm water and let it stand for a few minutes (left). Test the temperature by shaking a drop of formula onto your wrist before giving it to your baby (right). It should be lukewarm, not hot. Many babies will accept formula that's a little cool. Never warm formula in the microwave because it can destroy vital nutrients and heat unevenly, creating hot spots that can burn the baby.

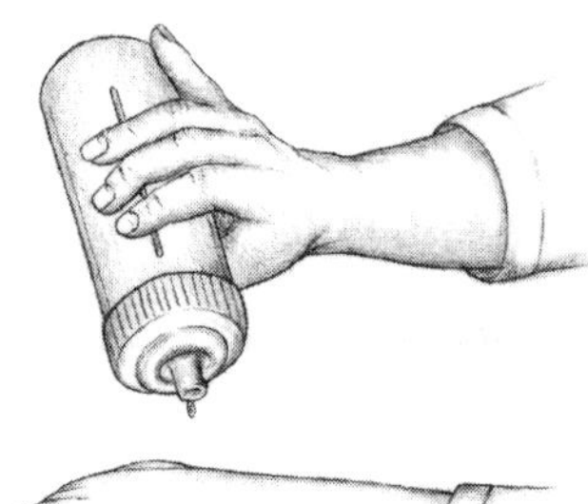

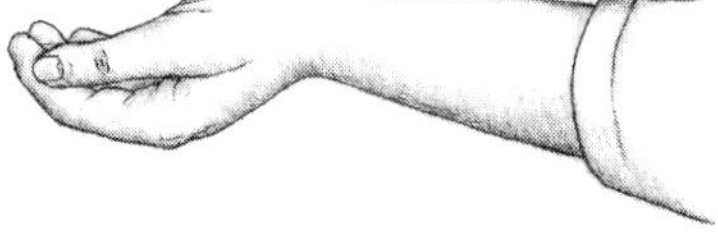

Allergies to formula

Some babies are allergic to the protein in cow's milk formula or have lactose intolerance (see page 549). Symptoms of an allergic reaction to cow's milk protein include vomiting, diarrhea (sometimes with blood), abdominal pain, and a rash. Lactose intolerance produces excessive gas, abdominal swelling and pain, and diarrhea. If your baby can't tolerate cow's milk formula, your doctor will probably recommend a lactose-free and/or soy-based formula. Some doctors recommend hydrolyzed-protein (predigested) formula, in which the cow's milk protein has already been broken down, making it less likely to cause an allergic reaction.

spurts out, it's flowing too fast for your baby. If just a few drops come out, it's not flowing fast enough. You should get a little spray and then some drops, so your baby does not have to gulp or have milk leaking out of his or her mouth.

- Feed your baby on demand. Babies usually take 3 to 4 ounces of formula per feeding, every 2 to 3 hours, by the end of the first month. The baby will take larger amounts less frequently as he or she gets older.
- Feedings shouldn't take more than 10 to 20 minutes. If they do, you might be overfeeding your baby, the nipple might be clogged, your child might be ill (and you should call the doctor), or your baby may be sucking for comfort.

Your baby's bowel movements Your baby's bowel movements should be soft but somewhat formed. Babies getting soy formula may have firm stools. The color may be pale yellow, yellowish brown, light brown, or brown-green, depending on his or her formula. If your baby is taking formula fortified with iron, or vitamin drops containing iron, the stool may be greenish, dark brown, or black. Bottle-fed babies sometimes get constipated. If your baby goes 3 or 4 days without a bowel movement and then has a movement that is hard or dry, he or she may need extra fluid. (If the movement is soft, your baby is not constipated.)

Make sure you are mixing the formula correctly; too little water can cause constipation as well as other, more serious problems. If the constipation persists longer than a few days, talk to your doctor. If your baby suddenly has frequent, liquid bowel movements, he or she may be allergic to the formula. Call your doctor right away. Prompt treatment is needed to avoid dehydration (see page 283), which is excessive loss of fluid.

Sleep

Good sleep is essential for good health, and most of a child's growth occurs during sleep. For the first several weeks, your baby's behavior will be very unpredictable and you'll be up for feedings at least twice a night. A newborn sleeps most of the time and wakes up for feedings. Most infants are more wakeful at night at first, but will gradually sleep longer during the night and stay awake longer during the day.

REDUCING THE RISK OF SIDS

SIDS (sudden infant death syndrome) (see page 626) is the death of an apparently healthy infant under 1 year of age (usually 6 months or younger) for which no cause can be found. Although there is no way to predict or prevent SIDS, you can substantially reduce your child's risk by always placing him or her to sleep on his or her back instead of the stomach. It's OK to place your child on his or her back even after a feeding. This will not increase the risk of the baby breathing in spit-up food. Placing your baby on his or her side to sleep is also safer than sleeping on the stomach. Bring the baby's arm that is on the mattress forward so he or she won't roll over onto the stomach.

Until your child is about 6 months old, alternate between placing him or her on the back or on either side, because lying in one position can temporarily flatten part of your child's head. When awake, your baby can lie tummy-down frequently, which helps him or her strengthen the arms and learn how to raise the head. When your baby learns how to roll over, put him or her to sleep on the back or side, but don't worry if he or she changes position. The risk of SIDS decreases at this stage.

Other measures that can help reduce the risk of SIDS include breast-feeding your baby, providing a firm mattress, keeping pillows and soft toys out of the crib, and keeping him or her away from secondhand smoke. Don't put your baby to bed on a beanbag chair or waterbed and never use plastic top sheets. Babies can't regulate their body temperature as efficiently as adults and get overheated when they are dressed too warmly or swaddled in a blanket. Overheating may be another risk factor for SIDS, so avoid swaddling your baby in a blanket when you put him or her to bed; put on clothing that is appropriate for the temperature and cover him or her loosely.

Exceptions to the rule on sleep positions

Some babies, such as those who have gastroesophageal reflux (see page 494) or an upper respiratory condition that raises the risk of airway obstruction, should be put to sleep on their side. You should elevate the head of the bed by placing a pillow under the mattress; this helps to decrease reflux and helps a baby with an upper respiratory condition to handle his or her secretions. If your child has a medical condition, ask your doctor which sleep position you should use.

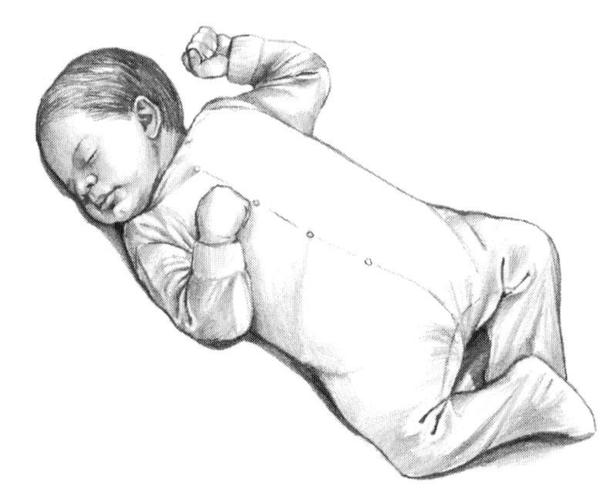

Safest sleeping position for your baby

Sleeping on the back can significantly reduce your child's risk of dying of SIDS (sudden infant death syndrome). The second safest position is on the side and the least safe is on the stomach. But give your baby plenty of "tummy time" on a blanket on the floor during the day, when you can watch him or her closely. (He or she can learn to push with the arms from this position.)

HELPING YOUR BABY SLEEP THROUGH THE NIGHT

By about 1 month of age you can start to influence your child's sleep schedule, but don't expect your baby to give up middle-of-the-night feedings until some time between the third and fifth month. There are no hard-and-fast rules for getting a child to sleep through the night. Some experts recommend putting a fussy baby to bed, leaving the room, and letting him or her cry until he or she falls asleep–no matter how long it takes. They promise that this technique works in 3 nights or less. Others say to put the child to bed, give a reassuring pat, leave the room, and let the child cry for increasing intervals before returning to the room and calmly reassuring him or her. This method promises to train a child to fall asleep on his or her own within 1 week. Most parents try these and other techniques and find a way that works for them.

Most experts discourage parents from letting their children sleep in bed with them. The restless sleep of an infant can prevent parents from getting enough sleep and can interfere with their need for intimacy. The baby can also fall out of bed or the parent can roll over onto the baby. Letting your child sleep with you can also make training the child to fall asleep independently even more difficult. Try some of the following tips to help your child sleep through the night:

- If you have just fed your baby and he or she is crying, check his or her diaper to make sure it is dry. If not, change the diaper.
- Try cuddling, rocking, or stroking your baby.
- If it has been 1 to 2 hours since the baby's last feeding, he or she may be hungry, especially during early infancy. Work toward five feedings every 24 hours by the time your baby is about 4 months old.
- Establish a regular sleep schedule. Small children thrive on routine. To help your child develop a regular sleep pattern, put him or her down for naps at about the same time each day and schedule your child's bedtime for the same time each night.
- Develop a bedtime routine. Before putting your infant to bed at night, engage in relaxing and enjoyable activities–a warm bath or a soothing massage, singing, soft music, or reading.
- Help your child distinguish between night and day. Spend lots of time during the day cuddling, socializing, and playing. Make middle-of-the-night feedings and diaper changes more brief and less fun, done only by the light of a nightlight.
- Put your baby in the crib when he or she is quiet, but not yet asleep. Gently rub or pat his or her stomach as you talk or sing softly to help him or her find ways to fall asleep.
- Minimize putting your young baby to bed with a pacifier. A pacifier may interfere with your child's ability to develop his or her own self-comforting techniques and the child could wake up when the pacifier falls out of his or her mouth.

Changing diapers

There are many different brands and types of disposable and cloth diapers. No matter which type you use, change them as soon as they are wet or soiled to avoid diaper rash (see page 59). If you use cloth diapers, you might want to try diaper wraps, which are pieces of fabric shaped like disposable diapers that fit over a cloth diaper. Diaper wraps fasten with plastic hook and loop closures, eliminating the need for pins and rubber pants. Although most cloth diapers are prefolded, you may need to fold them more to fit your newborn. Put the extra fabric in front for a boy, in back for a girl.

You can hire a diaper service to launder your baby's soiled cloth diapers. If you wash them yourself, launder them separately from your other laundry in hot water with a mild detergent and rinse them twice. Add half a cup of white vinegar to the last rinse cycle to help neutralize the ammonia in the baby's urine. Don't use fabric softeners or antistatic products because they can cause rashes.

The time you spend changing diapers can be a chance to play with your baby. Talk to him or her, sing, play peek-a-boo, and exercise his or her arms and legs (see page 67). While you are diapering your baby, keep one hand on him or her at all times and never turn your back on your baby—even for a second. A newborn can roll over and fall off a bed or changing table and be seriously injured. Use a changing table with a restraining strap, or simply change your baby on the floor.

How to change a diaper

Get in the habit of washing your hands before and after changing diapers. Assemble everything you need before you start. You'll need a clean diaper; a soft, wet washcloth or a container of baby wipes; petroleum jelly or a zinc oxide cream; a dry towel; and, possibly, a change of clothing. Some babies are sensitive to baby wipes; if they produce any irritation on your baby's skin, stop using them. (Don't use talcum or baby powder that contains talc because your baby could breathe in particles of powder and develop upper respiratory problems. If you wish to use cornstarch or baby powder without talc, use a small amount and apply by hand to minimize inhalation). You'll quickly develop your own diapering techniques but here are some basic steps:

1. If you're changing your baby on a surface other than a changing table, put down a protective towel, cloth diaper, or changing mat. Unfasten the diaper and, holding the baby's feet together with a finger in between the feet to keep the ankles from chafing, lift up the feet as you fold the soiled part of the diaper in on itself with your other hand. Set the soiled diaper aside.
2. Still holding the baby's feet, use a wet washcloth or baby wipe to gently clean your baby's bottom, around the genitals, in the skin folds on his or her thighs, and between the buttocks. Always wipe from front to back for girls to

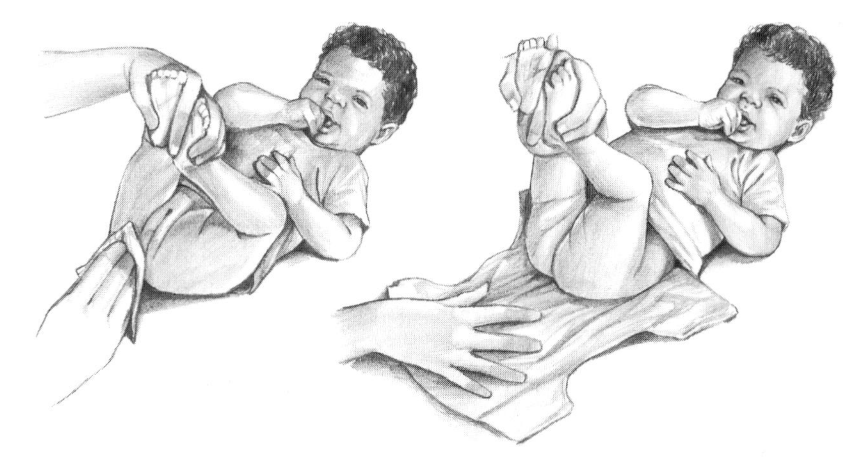

Cleaning your baby's bottom
Use a wet washcloth or baby wipe to clean your baby's diaper area every time you change a diaper.

Positioning the diaper
Holding the baby's feet together, place a clean diaper under your baby.

keep bacteria away from the urethra. Baby girls may get stool in and around the labia and vagina, so clean this area gently. If your son is not circumcised (see page 32), don't try to pull the foreskin back to clean under it.

3. Gently pat the diaper area dry with a small towel and let it air dry completely. If your baby has a rash, expose the rash to the air as long as possible, then apply petroleum jelly or a zinc oxide cream to the area. Some doctors recommend using these ointments to prevent rashes.
4. Hold your baby's feet together again and pull his or her bottom up as you place the diaper underneath. Bring the bottom half of the diaper up between the baby's legs and fasten it in front. If you're using a cloth diaper with pins, hold your hand between the baby's skin and the pin. (Stick the pin in a bar of soap first to make it go through the fabric more easily.) If you're using a disposable diaper, tape the back end of the fresh diaper onto the front end.
5. Gently shake out any stool into the toilet. Tightly retape a soiled disposable diaper and throw it away or rinse a soiled cloth diaper and put it in a tightly covered diaper pail until wash day. If you're out of the house, put the cloth diaper in a tightly sealed plastic bag until you get home.

DIAPER RASH

Diaper rash is a rash that develops in the diaper area–on the abdomen and genitals, in the skin folds of the thighs and buttocks, or in the rectal area. The rash can be mild or severe and occurs when your baby's sensitive skin is exposed to excessive moisture from prolonged contact with urine, feces, or both. Diaper rashes can also be caused by chafing or rubbing against the diaper, a yeast infection (see page

646), a bacterial infection, or an allergic reaction to the disposable diaper material or a detergent used to wash cloth diapers. Most babies develop a diaper rash between 4 and 15 months of age. See page 605 for prevention.

Call your child's doctor if you think the rash might be caused by diarrhea, a yeast infection, or a bacterial infection; these conditions should be treated first. You should also call the doctor if the rash has blisters or pus-filled sores, doesn't go away within 48 to 72 hours, spreads to other areas, or gets worse.

CARING FOR THE UMBILICAL CORD

At birth your baby's umbilical cord was cut off and clamped. The stump will become hard and dark, shrivel up, and fall off within 1 to 4 weeks. (Don't try to pull it off.) In the meantime, you will need to keep it clean and dry to prevent infection. Each time you change your baby's diapers, use a sterile cotton ball or gauze square soaked in rubbing alcohol or an alcohol pad to clean the cord and stump. Expose it to air as much as possible by folding the diaper below the cord or cutting a wedge in the front of the diaper and keeping the baby's T-shirt up. Don't give your baby a tub bath until the cord falls off and dries at the base; sponge bathe him or her only. If the cord gets wet, gently dry it off.

A small amount of oozing from the cord is normal, but it shouldn't soak through clothing. A few days before and after the cord falls off, you may notice some bleeding or discharge. Wipe away the discharge with a cotton ball dipped in alcohol. If you notice any redness around the cord or an unpleasant odor, or if the oozing or bleeding continues for longer than a few days after the cord has come off, your baby may have an infection. Call the doctor immediately. If the cord doesn't fall off in 1 to 2 months, the doctor may need to burn or tie it off.

CIRCUMCISION CARE

Circumcision is the removal of the layer of skin (foreskin) that covers the tip of the penis (see page 32). After a circumcision, the penis will appear red and swollen and it may bleed a little during the first 24 hours. After the procedure, the doctor will wrap the penis in gauze coated with petroleum jelly or an antibiotic ointment. Sometimes doctors use a clear piece of plastic resembling a bell. The nurses at the hospital will teach you how to clean the penis at home and change the gauze dressing over the next 3 days. The plastic bell does not require any special care; it stays intact and then falls off in 5 to 10 days.

Change your baby's diapers as soon as they are wet or soiled and gently cleanse the area with water. Reapply petroleum jelly or an antibacterial ointment to the penis for the first 3 to 4 days after the circumcision. Avoid soaps, powders, lotions, and baby wipes in the diaper area until the penis has healed because they can irritate a newly circumcised penis. Don't give your son a tub bath until the circumcision heals and the umbilical cord stump falls off.

Call the doctor right away if you notice increased bleeding or drainage from the penis, if urine comes out in dribbles or in a weak stream, if the head of the penis is blue or black, or if your son has signs of infection, such as a temperature above 100°F, an unpleasant smelling, yellowish-green discharge from the penis, increased redness, or swelling.

CARE OF AN UNCIRCUMCISED PENIS

No special care is needed for an uncircumcised penis. In fact, when bathing your child, the less you do the better. Soap and water are all that you need. Don't try to forcibly retract the foreskin or manipulate it in any way for cleaning. Retraction could cause bleeding, swelling, and pain. The foreskin could also get caught around the penis and obstruct the flow of urine.

At birth, the foreskin is firmly attached to the head of the penis (the glans). Over time, the foreskin and head of the penis begin to separate as cells continually shed from the inner lining of the foreskin and the surface of the glans. Some babies are born with the foreskin and glans already separated, but this is rare. Separation can occur a few days after birth, or days, weeks, months, or years later. In some boys, the foreskin doesn't fully separate, or retract, until adolescence. When your son is old enough to bathe himself and the foreskin is retractable, teach him to retract the foreskin, rinse the head of the penis and the inside fold of the foreskin with warm water, and slip the foreskin back into place over the head of the penis.

Bathing your baby

Infants do not need to be bathed frequently—every other day is usually sufficient, although you may want to bathe your baby daily in hot weather. Never turn your back on your baby when you are giving a bath, even for a few seconds. An infant can easily slip under the water and drown very quickly. If you need to answer the door or the phone, wrap your baby in a towel and take him or her with you.

GIVING A SPONGE BATH

Here are some suggestions for giving your baby a sponge bath during the first few weeks of life, or until his or her umbilical cord has fallen off.

1. Prepare the area where you'll be giving the bath—the counter next to the sink, a bed, a table, the floor, or a changing table. Pad hard surfaces with a blanket or fluffy towel and a bed or crib with a waterproof pad. If the surface is above the floor, always keep your eyes and at least one hand on your baby to prevent a fall.
2. Gather all the supplies before you begin: a basin of warm water, one or two small, soft washcloths, mild baby soap, baby shampoo (if you use it), and a towel (preferably a baby towel with a hood). If you will be diapering and

dressing your baby in the same place, assemble the supplies—a clean diaper, clean clothing, rubbing alcohol and cotton balls or alcohol pads for the umbilical cord, and ointment for diaper rash if needed.

3. Keep your baby wrapped in a towel and expose only the parts of the body you are washing.
4. Work from the face to the diaper area. You don't need to use soap on the baby's face. Gently clean both upper eyelids with a washcloth soaked in warm water, wiping from the nose outward. Clean only the outer part of the ears, including the creases behind the ears. Make sure you get into all the creases on the neck, arms, and elbows. In the diaper area, wash from front to back, getting all the creases and crevices. Spread a girl's labia apart and gently clean between them; carefully clean a boy's penis and scrotum. You can use soap or baby shampoo on your baby's hair once a week; the easiest way to rinse off shampoo is to hold your baby with the football hold (see page 42) over the sink as you squeeze clean water from a wet washcloth.
5. Diaper and dress your baby.

Cleaning the ears The old advice still applies: Don't put anything smaller than your elbow in your child's ear. That means you should not clean inside your child's ears—with cotton swabs, your fingers, or anything else. The ears produce wax to help keep them clean and earwax naturally moves outward. If you try to remove earwax, you could push it farther in or risk injuring the eardrum. Use a damp washcloth or cotton ball to clean the outer part of the ear. If your child's ears seem to have a lot of wax inside, talk to your doctor. Only he or she should clean inside your child's ears.

Trimming baby's nails A baby's fingernails grow quickly and you need to trim them to a safe level, but be very careful not to cut into the skin on the fingertip. Use special baby nail clippers or scissors, or file the nails with a worn emery board so you don't scrape the skin. Rounding off the corners of the nails can help prevent scratches. The best time to trim your baby's nails is right after a bath, when the nails are soft, or when he or she is asleep. The task is usually easier if you have someone hold the baby's hands while you trim. Biting your baby's nails off can cause infection.

GIVING A TUB BATH

As soon as your baby's umbilical cord and circumcision have healed, he or she is ready for a tub bath. Some babies love being in water; others hate it. If your baby strongly protests, keep on giving sponge baths for a few days and try again. Young babies have an innate fear of falling and feel vulnerable when they are naked, so always hold your baby firmly throughout the bath. Never take your eyes off your baby or leave him or her in the tub to get something you forgot or to answer the telephone—wrap the baby in a towel and bring him or her with you.

You'll find it easier to maneuver your baby in a small, portable tub designed for infants. Special sponge tub inserts are available that make the tub less slippery. Wash the tub regularly with disinfectant to keep it free of bacteria. You could also use a simple plastic basin or the kitchen sink, lining either one with a clean towel to make it less slippery. Avoid soap for the first few baths–it makes a wiggly baby slippery and even harder to handle. Just use plenty of warm water until you are accustomed to handling your baby in the tub.

Put the tub in a sink, on a counter, or on another area where there's plenty of room for the tub and all the bath supplies. Fill the tub with about 2 inches of warm water and, before putting the baby in the water, test the temperature with a bath thermometer–it should be between 98°F and 100°F. If you don't have a thermometer, test the water with your elbow–it should feel lukewarm, not hot. Don't put liquid soap or bubble bath in the water because they can dry your baby's skin.

Hold your baby securely, supporting his or her shoulder, neck, and head with one hand and the legs and buttocks with the other. Speak in comforting, reassuring tones as you gradually lower him or her into the tub, keeping his or her head and neck out of the water. While supporting the baby's head and neck with one hand (unless the tub has built-in support or your baby has good control of his or her head), wash him or her with your other hand, starting with the face and ending with the diaper area. To wash your baby's back and

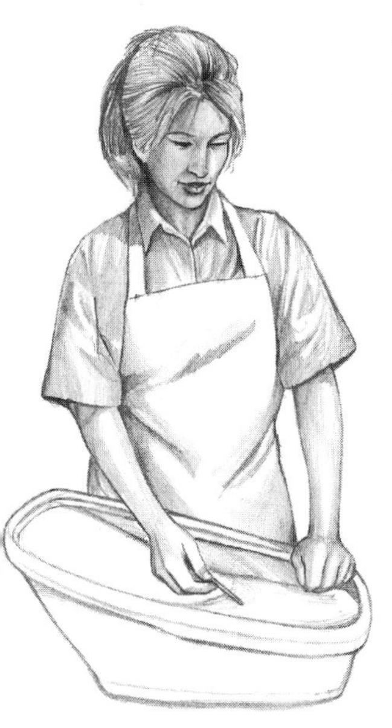

Testing the bath water
The most accurate way to test your baby's bath water is with a bath thermometer. The water should be between 98°F and 100°F.

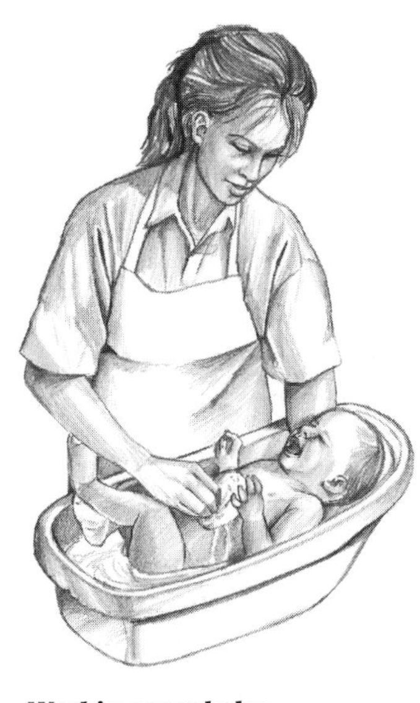

Washing your baby
Support your baby's head with one hand while you wash him or her with your other hand.

Drying your baby
When drying your baby, it's best to use a hooded towel so your baby doesn't feel cold.

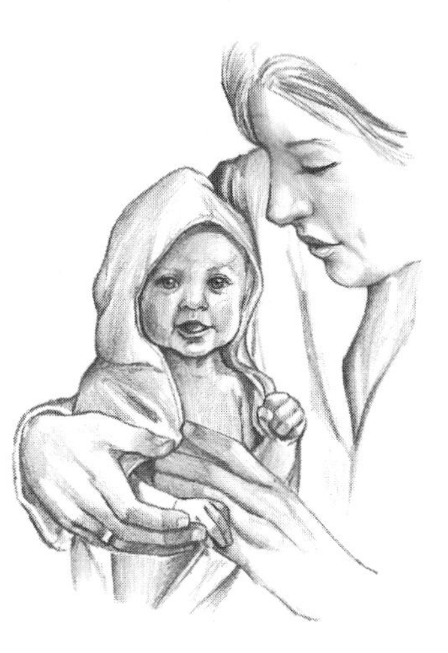

buttocks, turn him or her over on your arm and wash with the other hand. Rinse the baby thoroughly with a clean washcloth. Shampoo his or her hair once or twice a week, using mild baby soap or baby shampoo. Rinse by squeezing a wet washcloth over the infant's head, taking care not to get any water in the baby's eyes.

After the bath, wrap your baby in a towel, dry him or her thoroughly, put on a clean diaper, and dress your baby.

DRESSING YOUR BABY

To help make dressing a squirming baby easier, choose clothes that have easy-on, easy-off features, such as wide neck openings or snap closings, loose sleeves, snaps or zippers down the front instead of the back, and snaps or zippers down both legs to make diaper changes easier. Stretch or knit fabrics are easier to put on and take off. Don't buy clothing that has ribbons or string that

Infant clothing to grow into

Infants can outgrow clothing in newborn and 3-month sizes within a month. You may want to have a few small-sized T-shirts and sleepers, but buy the rest of your baby's clothes in size 6 months or larger. As your baby grows, buy clothing in sizes bigger than your child's age. (For example, buy size 9-, 12-, or 18-month clothes for a 6-month-old.) Here are the basics:

- One-piece sleepers (three to four)
- One-piece front-opening outfits (four or five)
- Front-snapping, cotton T-shirts (two in 3-month size, four in 6-month size)
- Sweaters (two)
- Bibs or cloth diapers for burping (four)
- Socks, booties, or some type of baby slipper boots (two pairs)
- Warm hat (one)
- Wide-brimmed sunbonnet (one)

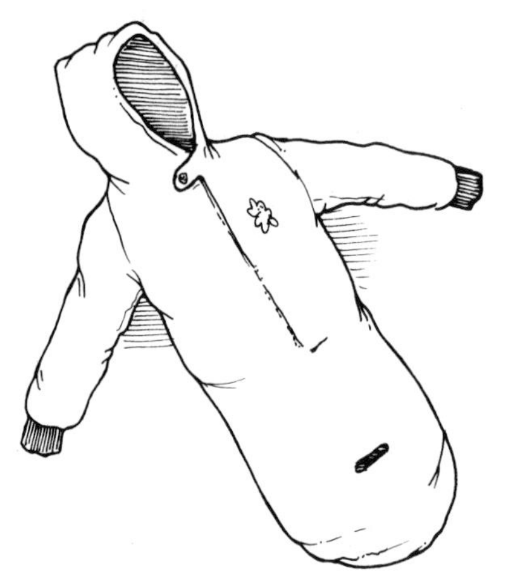

Cold weather clothing

A bunting (a one-piece blanketlike coat with a hood) will keep your baby warm and cozy in cold weather and is especially easy to put on and take off. Make sure you get one that has an opening between the legs so the car safety seat harness can be pulled through.

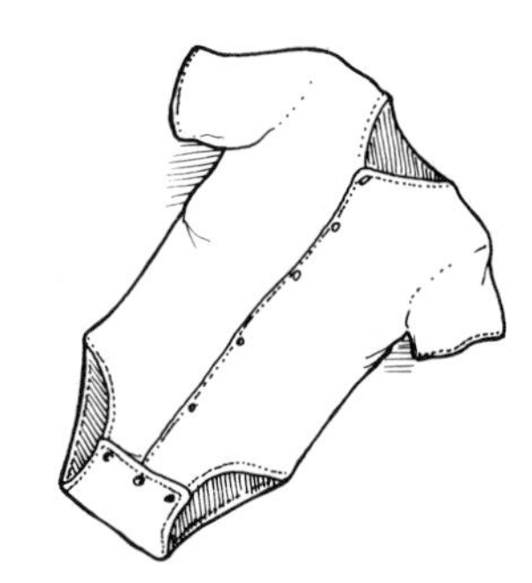

T-shirts

Few things are more difficult for new parents than pulling clothes over their newborn's head. It's not much fun for babies either. You'll find dressing a newborn much easier with clothes, including T-shirts, that open in the front.

can knot up, unravel, or wrap around your baby's neck and possibly cause choking. Here are some tips for making dressing your baby simple and enjoyable for you both:

- Dress your baby on a flat surface such as a bed, crib mattress, or changing table. When your baby can sit up, you can dress him or her on your lap.
- Before you pull a garment over your baby's head, stretch the neck opening as you ease it over his or her head, avoiding catching the nose or ears. Play peek-a-boo as you slip the garment over the baby's head.
- To put on a sleeve, reach through it from the outside with your hand, grasp the baby's hand, and pull the sleeve over the baby's arm.
- When closing a zipper, pull the garment away from your baby's body to avoid pinching the skin.
- When undressing your baby, take the sleeves off first, one at a time, as you support his or her back and head with one hand. Stretch the neckline as you gently slip the garment off, holding it away from the baby's face.
- Entertain your baby with constant, animated talk about anything you can think of–what you're doing, which item of clothing you're putting on, its color, parts of your baby's body, or a nursery rhyme–to stimulate learning.

Your baby's skin

A baby's skin is more sensitive than that of an adult so it is more susceptible to irritation. Your baby's skin usually doesn't need lotions, oils, or powders. If your baby's skin is very dry, use a mild moisturizing soap and apply some nonperfumed baby lotion to the dry areas after every bath and diaper change. If the dryness persists, bathe your baby less frequently. If lotion doesn't help, try baby oil or petroleum jelly.

INFANT ACNE

When your baby is about 3 or 4 weeks old, you may notice fleshy or red pimples on his or her cheeks, forehead, or chin. Whiteheads may also be present. Many babies develop this skin condition, called infant acne, which tends to come and go for a few months. The pimples are caused by exposure to the mother's hormones just before birth.

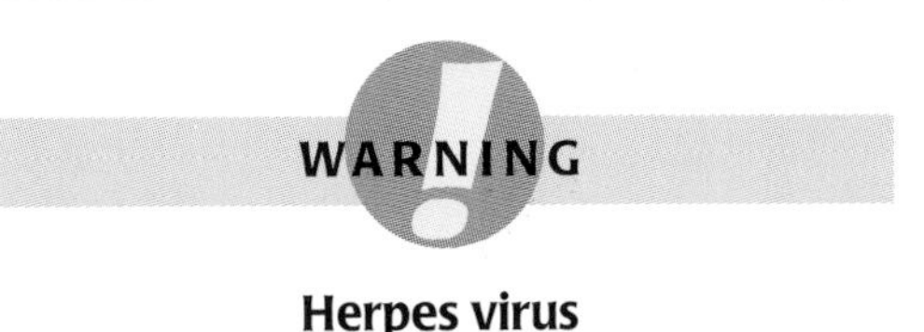

Herpes virus

If you notice that your child has developed blisters with pimples (especially on his or her scalp) during the first month of life, call the doctor. If the blisters are caused by exposure to the herpes virus (see page 499) during birth, your child will need treatment.

The condition clears up on its own. Just wash your baby's face with a washcloth and water two or three times a day. (Baby oil and ointments can make the problem worse.) During your baby's first week of life, a similar-looking rash called erythema toxicum may occur. This condition will disappear on its own.

Milia

Many infants develop tiny white bumps that resemble whiteheads on their nose and cheeks and sometimes on the chin and forehead. These bumps, called milia, are caused by clogged oil glands and will disappear by 1 to 2 months of age. Wash the bumps with a washcloth and water. Don't squeeze or scrub the bumps or apply ointments or creams.

Thrush

An infant's immune system is not fully developed. That is why babies are more susceptible to infections caused by common germs, such as Candida albicans, a yeast that normally lives in the mouth and other areas of the body. During the first few months of life, many babies develop a yeast infection called thrush on the tongue and inside the cheeks (see page 648). It looks like a thick coating of milk, but you won't be able to wipe it off. Call your child's doctor. If he or she diagnoses thrush, your child will need an antifungal medication, taken by mouth, to eliminate the infection. Sometimes the infection spreads through the baby's digestive system and causes a red, pimplelike rash around the anus, genitals, and inner thighs. The rash is treated by applying an antifungal cream to the affected area. Some nursing women develop thrush, and the nursing baby eventually develops the infection as well (see page 648).

Cradle cap

Cradle cap is a form of seborrheic dermatitis (see page 618) in which yellowish, crusty scales develop on an infant's scalp. The condition is not serious and usually clears up on its own. To help remove the scales, try shampooing more frequently with a mild baby shampoo. Leave the shampoo on for a few minutes to soften the crusts, then rinse and brush the scalp with a soft brush. You could also massage the baby's scalp with nonperfumed baby oil or petroleum jelly and then comb it with a fine-toothed comb to remove the scales and oil. Cradle cap can get worse when the baby's scalp sweats, so try to keep your baby's scalp as dry and cool as possible. Avoid putting a hat on the baby indoors and in heated cars. If cradle cap lasts longer than 2 to 3 weeks or if it spreads to your child's neck, face, or buttocks, call the doctor. He or she may recommend using a medicated shampoo and/or ointment.

SUNBURN

Keep your baby out of the sun as much as possible between the hours of 10:00 AM and 4:00 PM when the sun's ultraviolet rays are strongest. Dress your baby in long-sleeved clothing, long pants, and a hat with a wide brim all the way around. Use a stroller with a shade on it. Don't use sunscreen on your baby until he or she is 6 months old. Before then, an infant's body is not able to handle the chemicals in the sunscreen.

Exercise

You don't have to sign up for baby exercise classes to promote physical development, but exercise is as good for babies as it is for everyone else. Help your baby exercise whenever you play together. In addition to stimulating development, play gives your baby physical exercise. In the first few months, before your baby gains control over his or her muscles, you can move your baby's muscles for him or her. For example, when your baby is lying on his or her back, rotate his or her legs in a bicycling pattern. Help him or her practice rolling over so he or she will be able to do it at about 4 to 6 months of age.

Placing your child on his or her stomach on a blanket on the floor will help him or her to lift up the head and use the arms (and eventually learn to crawl). To encourage your baby to lift up his or her head, attract his or her attention by making soft sounds with your voice, a rattle, or a bell, or by playing soft music. Exercise your baby's arms by playing patty-cake. Carefully manipulate your baby's arms to show how to reach and then provide toys to reach for.

Try not to confine your baby too much to an infant seat or carrier. Place him or her in different positions–for example, lying on his or her back or tummy or sitting propped up with pillows. When you put your baby to bed, don't swaddle or wrap him or her in a blanket, because it restricts movement. Try to spend as much time as possible outdoors, but remember to protect your baby from excessive heat or cold, the sun, and insects.

Your baby's physical growth

From birth to age 1, an infant triples in weight and grows 9 to 10 inches. The fastest rate of growth occurs during the first 3 months, after an initial loss of weight during the first few days after birth. On average, infants lose about 10 percent of their body weight after birth, so that, by the 10th through the 14th day of life, they weigh about the same as they did at birth. From then until about the end of the third month, most babies gain an average of an ounce a day whether they are taking breast milk or formula. Your child's growth during these early months will be influenced by his or her weight at birth, whether or not he or she was full-term or premature, and the intake of breast milk or formula. At each well-child visit, your doctor will evaluate your child's growth—checking his or her weight, length, and the head circumference—to make sure that your child is growing at a steady rate (see page 238).

Your baby's development

A baby's brain develops faster during the first year of life than at any other time. Parents have always known that newborns need nutrition, love, warmth, protection, and nurturing, but scientists have recently discovered an equally essential but less obvious need—mental stimulation. An infant's brain is a super-sponge that is most absorbent from birth to about age 12, especially during the first 3 years, when important connections between brain cells are made.

Just as all infants require food before their bodies can develop, their brains require "food" in the form of impressions—vision, hearing, smell, touch, and taste—before they can develop. A baby is eager to learn from the moment of birth. The more stimulation you give your infant from birth on—touching, talking, hugging, cuddling, responding to his or her needs, exposing him or her to visually interesting objects—the more connections will form in his or her brain. These connections translate into brain power, increasing your child's ability to think and acquire knowledge, and they influence his or her emotional well-being.

Experts used to advise parents to reserve childhood for "child's play" and put off "real learning" until their child entered school. But a child who has a chance to learn in infancy and early childhood begins school at a distinct advantage that will last for years. Young children have an inborn drive to learn; for them, learning and play go hand in hand. Benefits come from simple activities all parents can do with their children—such as talking, singing, reading, and getting down on the floor and playing. As your child interacts with you, he or she will gain confidence, will learn that people are responsive and helpful, and will find out that his or her actions have a predictable effect. Though simple, these measures are immensely enriching for your child's development.

Developmental milestones

Although every child develops at his or her own pace and interacts with the world in his or her own way, experts have established a range of skills, frequently referred to as developmental milestones, that most children achieve by specific ages. Children may develop these skills at varying ages, but they usually develop them in a predictable order.

A baby who was born premature, was of low birthweight, or had an illness or feeding problem, will probably need several months to catch up with other infants the same age. The milestones listed below are a very rough guide of what your baby may be able to do by the end of 3 months of age. If your baby has not reached any of these milestones, talk to your child's doctor:

- Raises his or her head up when lying tummy-down and supports the upper body with the forearms.
- Recognizes some sounds and turns toward familiar sounds and voices.
- Opens and shuts hands.
- Swipes at dangling objects.
- Grasps and shakes toys that are put in his or her hands.
- Starts using hands and eyes together; spends lots of time watching his or her hands move.
- Recognizes a breast or bottle.
- Watches faces intently.
- Watches objects move from one side to another in his or her field of vision (about 8 to 12 inches in front of his or her face).
- Smiles at the sound of your voice or in response to your smile when he or she is happy.
- Imitates some movements and facial expressions.
- Coos, laughs, or blows bubbles.
- Explores everything with his or her mouth.
- Holds head steady (when held) when sitting or while being carried.

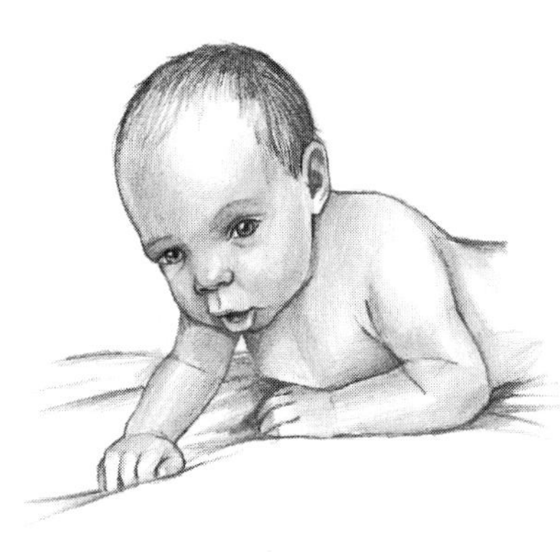

Supporting weight with forearms
Your baby may be able to hold his or her head up and support his or her own weight with the forearms by the third month of life.

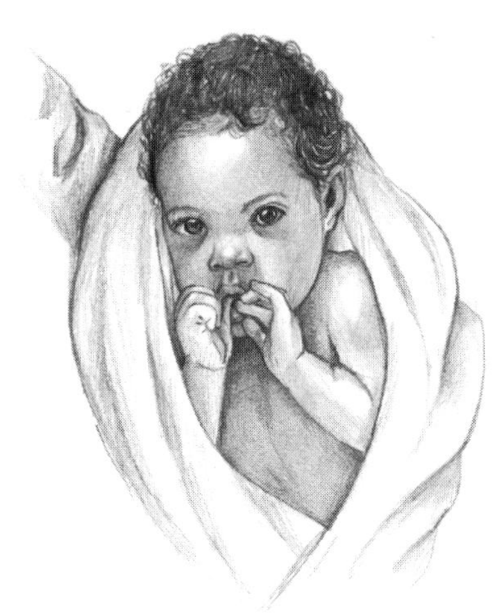

Everything into the mouth
Your baby will put his or her fingers and any objects he or she finds into his or her mouth at 3 months of age.

Talk to your baby

Studies show that spoken language is a powerful brain-builder. Hearing lots of words each day—from a parent or other caregiver who talks with love and meaning—can dramatically boost a child's intellectual and social development. In the early weeks, you will need to hold your face in your child's field of vision, about 8 to 10 inches in front of his or her face.

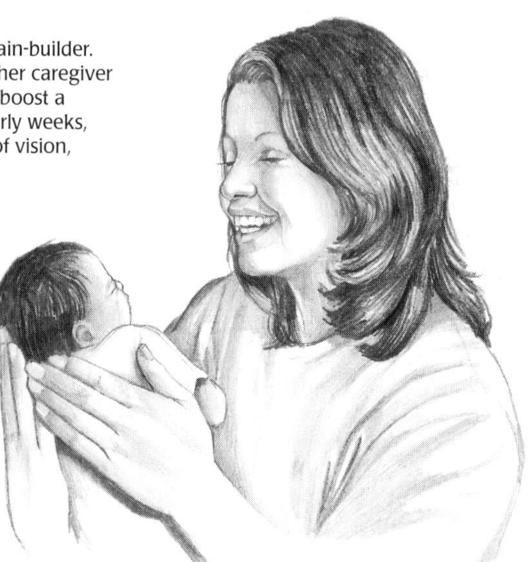

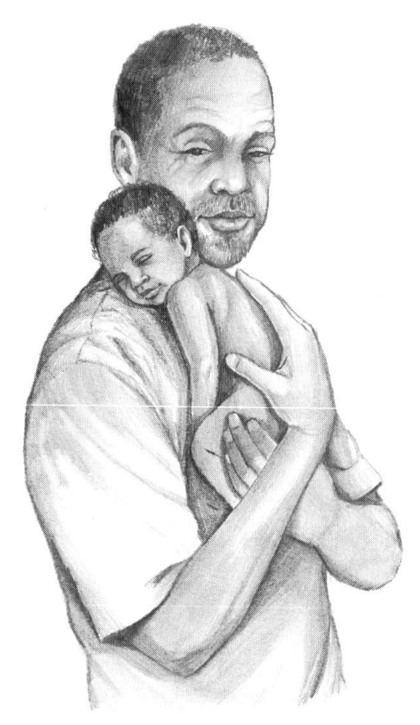

Massage your baby

Massage not only feels good to a young baby—it stimulates the development of his or her brain. Frequently massage your baby's back, abdomen, arms, legs, and feet.

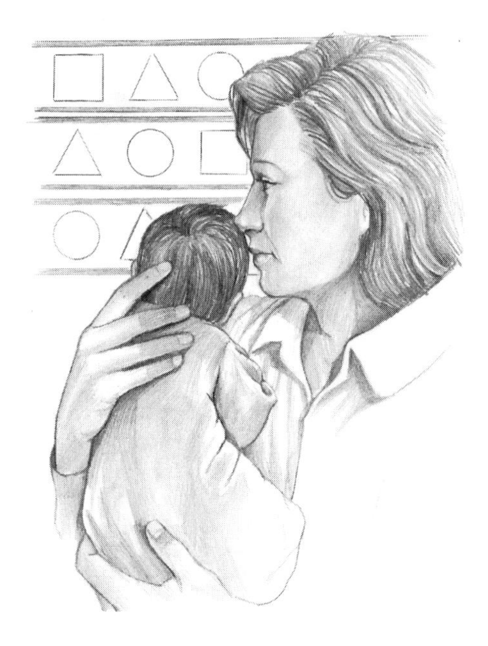

Show your baby different shapes

Show your baby light-dark contours, such as high-contrast pictures, objects, or shapes. Young babies are especially attracted to simple drawings of the human face and black-and-white patterns of stripes, checks, and bull's-eyes.

BOOSTING YOUR CHILD'S BRAIN DEVELOPMENT

Children love learning. A child's developing brain thrives on different kinds of stimulation at different ages. During the first few months of life, an infant can respond to things he or she can see, hear, and feel. Here are some things you can do to have fun with your infant while boosting the development of his or her brain:

- Respond to your baby's needs as quickly as possible.
- Smile at your baby often and call him or her by name.
- Look at your baby when you talk to him or her.
- Hold your baby close while you sing, dance, read, or talk; slowly and gently rock your baby in your arms several times each day. You can't hold your baby too much during these early months.
- Play a variety of music. Exposure to different types of music, such as classical, stimulates the same parts of the brain that are involved in learning and memory and can improve a child's ability to learn some subjects in school, especially math.
- Softly blow on your baby's hands, feet, and tummy during play.
- Provide interesting, textured, age-appropriate toys that make noise or are brightly colored–such as rattles and soft animals, dolls, or balls–to appeal to your baby's senses of sight, hearing, and touch.
- Place different soft and pleasant textures, such as wool, satin, flannel, or a fluffy toy, against your baby's skin.
- Keep the television off, especially when you are playing with your baby.

HOW BABIES LEARN LANGUAGE

Children first hear language in the uterus before they are born, giving them the ability to recognize their mother's voice at birth. Babies learn language by listening to people who talk to them. Their brain focuses on the sounds, acquiring a feel for how the language uses sounds to make syllables and sentences. By 6 months, long before a child can say or understand words, his or her brain has already built the foundation necessary for acquiring a language.

Could your child have a hearing problem?

Hearing problems are often difficult to detect until children are 12 to 18 months old, when they should start saying words. But the earlier in life any hearing problems are detected and treated, the better. Children with hearing deficits are at risk of having a delay in learning language. Although your child's doctor will evaluate your child's hearing at each checkup, watch for the following signs of hearing loss during the first 3 months:

- Your child does not startle in response to a sudden loud sound.
- Your child does not seem to recognize his or her mother's voice.
- When sleeping in a quiet room, your child does not move or wake up at the sound of voices or nearby noises.
- Your child does not respond to sounds, music, or voices.
- When crying or fussy, your child does not calm down when a parent speaks while out of sight.

You might feel self-conscious about talking to a newborn who doesn't understand what you are saying, but, as you talk, your child's brain is building a network of connections that will serve as the framework of your child's ability to learn to speak, read, and think. Turning on the television or radio won't help a child at this age learn language. In fact, excessive exposure to television can impair your child's language development. Babies learn best when you make eye contact and try to engage their attention. Your tone of voice is also important—be positive and animated. Speak slowly, carefully enunciating words, and emphasize or repeat certain words to make it easier for your baby to distinguish individual words.

CHAPTER • 2

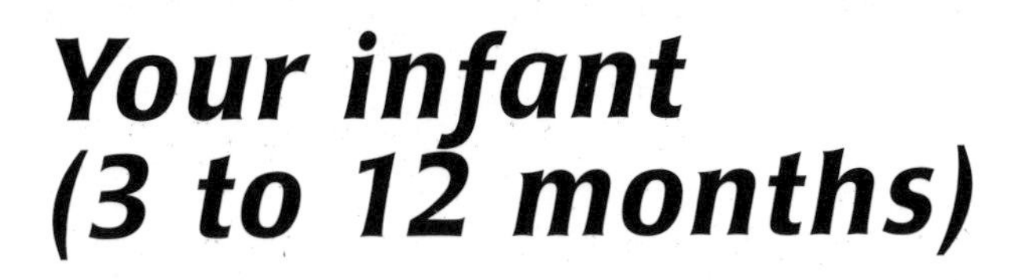

Your infant (3 to 12 months)

As your infant grows and develops, he or she will become more and more alert and interested in the world. You'll find it easier to engage your baby in communication and play and his or her unique personality will emerge before your eyes. By the end of the first year of life, your baby, so helpless as a newborn, will take his or her first steps toward toddlerhood and independence.

WHAT YOU CAN DO FOR YOUR CHILD NOW

Along with love and security, an infant needs a stimulating environment in which to explore and learn. The following list describes the most important things you can do for your infant from the fourth through the 12th month of life:

- **KEEP BREAST-FEEDING.** You can start introducing solid foods when your child is about 4 to 6 months old.
- **TALK TO YOUR CHILD.** Spoken language has an extraordinary effect on many aspects of intellectual development.
- **READ TO YOUR CHILD.** Reading accelerates the acquisition of language skills and presents a time for closeness.
- **HELP YOUR CHILD INVESTIGATE THE WORLD** by identifying objects and people.
- **STIMULATE YOUR CHILD'S DEVELOPMENT** during play with games such as peek-a-boo and pat-a-cake.
- **CHILDPROOF YOUR HOME** (see page 76).
- **ALWAYS PUT YOUR CHILD IN A SAFETY SEAT** whenever he or she is in a car or other motor vehicle (see page 294).
- **TAKE YOUR BABY TO THE DOCTOR** for the recommended checkups and vaccinations (see page 226).
- **DON'T PUT YOUR CHILD IN A WALKER, EXERCISE SAUCER, OR JUMPING HARNESS.**

Your child's physical growth

Children grow more in their first year than at any other time. All infants gain roughly the same amount of weight during their first year no matter what they weighed at birth—about 5 to 7 ounces a week in the first 3 months, 4 to 5 ounces a week between 3 and 6 months, and 2 to 3 ounces a week between 6 months and a year. But, because babies start at very different birthweights, their individual weekly weight gain will differ greatly. That means that a 7-pound baby will generally double his or her weight in 6 months and triple it in a year. But a 5-pound premature infant should double his or her weight in 3 months and triple it in 6 months (unless he or she has been undernourished). A large baby weighing 11 pounds at birth will come close to doubling his or her weight at 6 months, but, if the baby tripled his or her birthweight at 1 year, the baby would be considered obese. A child's weight gain will slow down at around the age of 1 year. The doctor will evaluate your infant's growth at each well-child visit to make sure your baby is progressing consistently from visit to visit (see page 238).

Your baby's first teeth

First teeth usually start coming in at about 6 months, although some children get them as early as 4 months or as late as 12 to 16 months. When your child is about 6 months old, if he or she is not drinking fluoridated water, your doctor or dentist may recommend giving your child a supplement of fluoride, a mineral essential for strong teeth. Never allow your baby to go to sleep in the crib with a bottle of formula or juice or carry a bottle around during the day because he or she could develop baby bottle tooth decay (see page 259). Tooth decay can also occur if your baby stays at your breast throughout the night. If you have any questions about your baby's first teeth, talk to your doctor or dentist. For information about teething and how to take care of your baby's teeth, see chapter 9.

Your child's development

Between 4 and 6 months, your baby will begin initiating contact with you and other people. He or she will smile more, laugh, and make "razzing" noises at you. Children this age often seem very demanding because they cry when left alone for too long and calm down immediately when you give them attention. They are not being manipulative; interacting with people is essential to their development, and they do not yet understand why you are not right there when they want you. By crying, your child is telling you to come and talk, socialize, and play—or that he or she is bored and needs a change of scenery or activity. He or she may need reassurance that you are still there to comfort him or her. Your child will also let you know when he or she is content to lie and stare at his or her hands or watch the world happily from an infant seat.

At about 8 months of age, your child may start being afraid of anyone other than you. He or she may not want to be left with the regular sitter and may cry when other people hold him or her. If your child has such "stranger anxiety," ask people to approach your child quietly while you're holding him or her, perhaps offering a toy. Tell them to avoid looking at or talking directly to the child until he or she gets comfortable with them and relaxes.

At 9 months, your child will learn that objects are permanent–that they exist even when he or she can't see them. Your child will now remember you when you are not present but won't yet realize that you will return; for this reason, he or she may not want to let you out of sight. This "separation anxiety" can be intense but will pass. A 9-month-old also has an intense curiosity and will begin to reach for objects or food (making even meals a time for discovery). He or she will also enjoy games of peek-a-boo.

During the second half of the first year, your child will likely spend much time and energy learning to walk, a skill that is achieved in three phases. The first phase is sitting alone without support. The second is creeping or crawling. Not all children crawl, nor does crawling predict your child's future ability to walk, move, or think. In the third phase, the child pulls up to a standing position by holding onto furniture, crib bars, or an adult's hands. The child then takes steps while holding onto furniture–a skill known as cruising. Eventually, the child can walk without help. It can take several months from the time a child first pulls up to a standing position to the time he or she begins to walk around freely. Most children walk by 16 months of age.

Learning to walk is a major leap in a child's development and the inner drive to master it shows the 1-year-old's desire for independence. At the same time that children learn to walk, they become increasingly skilled at using their hands. Before 6 months, your baby reached and grasped for an object in one motion. After 6 months, he or she will reach for an object without necessarily grasping it and can transfer it from hand to hand. By 9 or 10 months, he or she will likely be able to poke things with the index finger and pick up small objects between the thumb and index finger. This is the time when your child will want to learn how to eat with his or her fingers and use a spoon and a cup, so provide plenty of opportunity to practice (see page 91). By the end of the 10th month, your baby will begin releasing objects from the hands, initiating a new favorite activity of dropping things to the floor and watching you pick them up.

Because these activities consume so much of a child's interest and energy, they can interfere with his or her sleep routines and may even cause a temporary pause in learning other skills, such as language. Don't worry–once the excitement of learning one particular skill passes, your child will show renewed interest in other skills.

Certain toys stimulate an infant's development. From birth to 2 months of age, babies like crib mobiles, toys with black and white patterns, and musical toys. Give a 3- to 6-month-old infant stuffed animals and noisemakers that are easily grasped. Infants who are 6 to 12 months old are stimulated by large blocks, teething toys, nesting cups, soft balls, and push-and-pull toys.

Childproofing Your Home

A child's home should be a safe place to play and explore. But many children are exposed to unnecessary risks in their own homes. Before your child learns to crawl, get down on the floor and look around to see things from his or her point of view. You might be surprised at the number of potential hazards you find. Don't wait for something to happen—take action now. Make safety checks of your home every 6 months keeping in mind how your child has grown. Here are some room-by-room suggestions to help prevent accidents and injuries.

Stairs

- Use child safety gates (see inset). Avoid accordion gates, which can trap a child's head or fingers.
- Keep stairways well lit and free of clutter. Remove loose or worn carpeting. Don't allow children to play on stairs.
- Handrails should extend entire length of stairways.
- Install smoke detectors on each level of your home, especially near top of stairs on second floor. Check the batteries monthly. Replace them once a year.
- Install carbon monoxide detectors on each floor.

Garage

- Make sure electric garage door has a system that automatically stops and reverses door when electric eye beam is broken or door touches an object in its path.
- Store tools in locked toolboxes and lock away all chemicals.
- Lock freezers and refrigerators that are in use. Remove doors of those that are no longer used, and unplug them.

Kitchen

- Keep a fire extinguisher and first-aid kit in an easy-to-reach location, but out of the reach of children.
- Keep matches, lighters, sharp items, medicines, and household cleaners in a cabinet that an adult needs to reach with a step stool. Install safety locks (see inset) on cabinets that are at child level.
- Unplug small appliances when not in use and keep cords away from edges of counters.
- Never leave a hot liquid within your child's reach.
- Use the back burners of the stove and turn pot handles toward the back.
- Cook all meat, eggs, poultry, and shellfish thoroughly to prevent food poisoning. Wash knives, cutting boards, and your hands with hot, soapy water after preparing meat or poultry.
- Don't put tablecloths on tables; small children can pull items down.
- Keep stools and chairs away from counters and the stove.
- Keep alcohol out of the reach of children.

Living room

- Keep floors clear of tripping hazards, such as throw rugs or electrical cords. Route electrical cords along walls and tape them or secure them with plastic tubing. Check cords regularly to make sure they're not frayed.
- Put corner guards on sharp furniture edges.
- Cover all electrical outlets (see inset) when they're not in use.
- Keep potted plants out of reach of children and make sure that they are not poisonous.
- Avoid glass tops on tables. Remove heavy or breakable items from table tops.
- Make sure all furniture, shelves, and TVs on stands are stable and cannot be tipped or pulled over. Don't put furniture in front of windows; a child could climb on furniture and fall out.
- Put locks on doors you don't want opened.
- Install glass doors or screens on fireplaces.
- Keep floor clear of small items that a child could choke on.
- If you have a sliding glass door, put decals on it to prevent a child from walking into it.

Child's bedroom

- Use flame-resistant bedding and make sure your child has flame-resistant pajamas. Check labels when you purchase these items.
- Install safety locks on all windows throughout the house to keep them from opening more than 2 inches.
- Make sure all furniture is low; cover any sharp edges. Use shelves for toys or store them in a toy chest with a removable lid or a lid that stays open in any raised position. Watch out for hinges on a toy box that could pinch or squeeze small fingers.
- Place your baby's crib away from windows.
- Don't allow strings or cords longer than 7 inches to dangle near or into your child's crib. Lower level of mattress as your child grows and learns to stand. For more about crib safety, see page 300.
- Use only metal or wood window blinds; those made of vinyl can contain lead. Tie or hang up drapery or window-blind cords or install a special fixture to wrap the cord around (see inset).

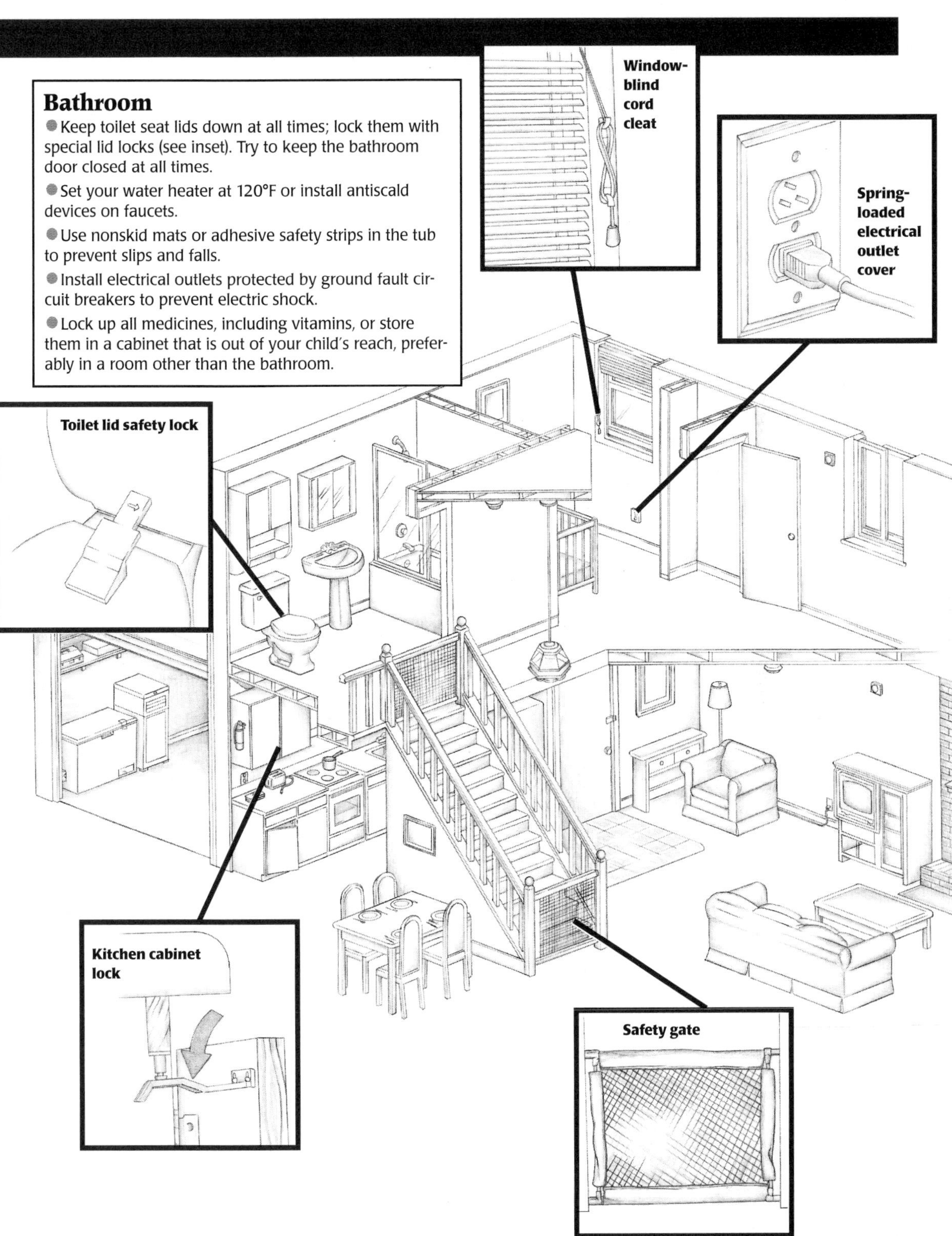
Bathroom
Keep toilet seat lids down at all times; lock them with special lid locks (see inset). Try to keep the bathroom door closed at all times.
Set your water heater at 120°F or install antiscald devices on faucets.
Use nonskid mats or adhesive safety strips in the tub to prevent slips and falls.
Install electrical outlets protected by ground fault circuit breakers to prevent electric shock.
Lock up all medicines, including vitamins, or store them in a cabinet that is out of your child's reach, preferably in a room other than the bathroom.
Window-blind cord cleat
Spring-loaded electrical outlet cover
Toilet lid safety lock
Kitchen cabinet lock
Safety gate

DEVELOPMENTAL MILESTONES

Each individual child develops some skills more easily than others. Your child may not reach all of the developmental milestones listed below at a particular age, but that does not necessarily mean that your child has a developmental delay. The doctor can evaluate your child and alert you to potential problems or recommend intervention if he or she thinks it is necessary.

Use these developmental milestones as a guide to help you understand the kinds of play and activities that your child might need and enjoy at a particular stage. Your interactions and the stimulation you give your child can greatly enhance his or her development (see page 81).

At 4 months:

- Makes swimming movements with the arms and legs.
- Supports head well.
- Opens hands more frequently.
- Grabs objects.
- Clenches a rattle, shakes it, and puts it in his or her mouth.
- Reaches with his or her arms.
- Makes different sounds for different needs.

Heads up

By about 4 months of age, your child will have good control of his or her neck muscles and will be able to hold up his or her head when sitting or being held. A child this age especially enjoys interacting with people and easily smiles, laughs, and babbles in response to playful attention.

At 5 months:

- Shows better control of the head, neck, and trunk.
- Sits with support.
- Grabs feet and brings them to his or her mouth when resting on back.
- Babbles and "razzes."
- Turns toward a sound.
- Laughs out loud.
- Investigates objects by putting them in mouth.

At 6 months:

- Rolls from back to stomach.
- Sits briefly without support but still leans for balance and may fall over.
- When sitting, reaches out for objects in a raking motion.
- Transfers objects from hand to hand.
- Holds bottle.

- Searches for lost objects.
- Smiles at the mirror.
- Imitates sounds.
- Makes consonant sounds such as "ba" and "da."
- Can tell the difference between a "friendly" tone of voice and an "angry" one.

At 7 months:
- Bounces when held in standing position.
- Sits without support.
- Pivots to reach objects when sitting.
- Clasps hands.
- Bangs objects together.
- Eats with hands (not using a fork or spoon).
- Rolls over well.
- Drinks from a cup.
- Imitates noises.
- Responds to his or her name.

At 8 months:
- Creeps (moves forward on stomach by pushing with the legs and feet and steering with the arms).
- Crawls backward.
- Rings a bell.
- Understands "no."
- Sits up independently.

At 9 months:
- Crawls (some babies crawl on their hands and feet or scoot around on their bottoms).
- Pulls up to standing position and sits back down after standing, without help.
- Opens fingers at will and can drop or throw objects.
- Picks up tiny objects with thumb and index finger (the pincer grasp).

Crawling
Your child will probably start crawling by about 9 months if you have given him or her the opportunity by providing lots of "tummy time" on the floor. Crawling exercises several muscle groups and lets a child explore independently. But always supervise your crawling child. Get down on the floor with him or her as often as you can.

- Puts fingers in holes in a pegboard.
- Enjoys toys with moving parts, such as wheels or levers.
- Plays peek-a-boo.
- Recognizes familiar words.
- Turns pages, many at a time.

At 10 months:
- Stands with support.
- Holds crayon and tries to scribble.
- Understands names of loved ones.
- Waves good-bye.
- Produces more and more consonant sounds.

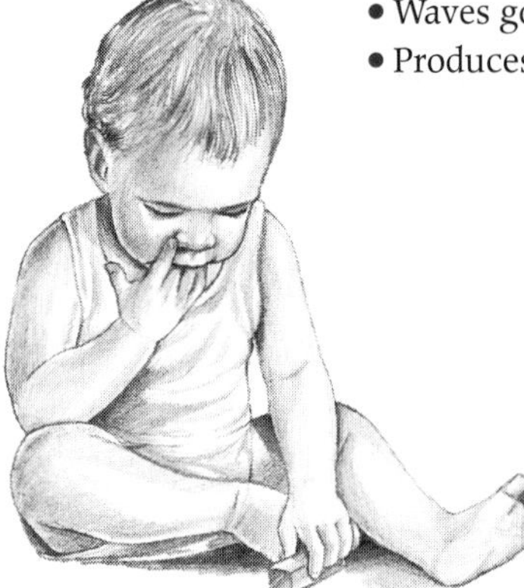

Cruising

When your child is about 11 months old, he or she will begin taking steps while holding onto furniture or your hands. This activity, called cruising, is good practice for learning to walk without help.

The pincer grasp

By about 11 months of age, your child will have refined the pincer grasp, the ability to pick up small objects between the thumb and index finger. Your child will want to practice this skill constantly and will look for tiny things to investigate—usually by putting them into his or her mouth. Baby-proofing your home is essential (see page 76).

At 11 months:
- Walks holding on to furniture (cruises) or when both hands are held.
- Shows fascination with hinges and swinging doors back and forth.
- Follows a command made with a gesture, such as pointing.

At 12 months:
- Takes first steps independently.
- Can put objects in container.
- Says two or three words.
- Points at things he or she wants.
- Understands and responds to simple questions.

BOOSTING YOUR CHILD'S DEVELOPMENT

As your child's first and most important teacher, you will lay the foundation for all of his or her future learning. The things you can do to improve your child's chances of being happy, smart, and successful are simple and enjoyable–and many parents have always done them instinctively. For example, just talking to your child can increase his or her intelligence and improve his or her ability to learn language, to think, and, eventually, to do well in school.

The most important things you can do to provide a loving and stimulating environment are to respond to your baby's needs with love and consistency, and to touch, play with, talk to, and sing to your child. Infants have a strong drive to practice new skills. Give your child as much freedom as possible to explore (with supervision).

Until children become mobile and skilled with their hands, they have to depend on others for stimulation and entertainment. Change your child's scenery throughout the day–for example, move the child from room to room, sit outside, or go for walks in the stroller. Vary your child's body positions frequently to give different perspectives and provide opportunities to exercise different muscles and learn different skills. Your child will have an easier time learning to roll over, sit up, crawl, and walk if you provide plenty of space on a safe floor than if you keep him or her in an infant seat. He or she will become skilled at picking up and handling objects if you provide a variety of interesting ones. Your child will talk more easily if you frequently speak directly to him or her.

Respond to your child's cues. He or she will let you know when boredom strikes. Watch for your child's readiness to perform a new skill and then provide the opportunity to do it. Helping your child learn new skills does not mean pressuring your child to do things he or she is not developmentally able to do or interested in. If your child does not respond to your encouragement to try something new, he or she is probably not ready for it yet. Try it again later.

This time of rapid development in your child's life will pass quickly. Take advantage of every opportunity to explore and discover new things together. Remember that play is learning for very young children. Not only are you and your child having fun together, but each new experience and interaction is forming the basis of your child's future intelligence, imagination, and creativity.

Toys for infants

Your child's toys need not be either expensive or educational. In fact, certain store-bought toys can be inappropriate for children this age and it can be very expensive to provide new playthings every time your child gets bored with old ones. Children this age are fascinated with ordinary household items such as pots and pans, measuring spoons, boxes with lids, plastic containers with lids, paper, and large pieces of fabric–and they love to play with blocks and look at pictures. They generally like new playthings that are only slightly different from their familiar ones. So, when your baby tires of playing with a furry ball, give him or her a rubber one, or a ball of a different size; replace a pot or pan with one of a different size or shape, or a foam block with a wooden one.

Brain-building activities for a 4- to 6-month-old

Work on some brain-building activities when your child is between 4 and 6 months old. You'll have fun getting to know each other and, at the same time, you'll be stimulating your baby's intellectual development. Let these suggestions inspire you to think up many more on your own:

- Cuddle, hug, massage, and say loving things to your baby; you can't do this too much.
- Talk to your baby often; when you do, make eye contact and exaggerate your facial expressions. Call your baby by name.
- Gently rock your baby back and forth as you make fun noises.
- Show your baby increasingly complex pictures of real objects. At this age your baby relies mostly on vision to acquire information about the world.
- Move interesting objects into your child's field of vision. Motion also attracts your baby's attention.
- Wiggle your baby's fingers and toes as you tell stories, count, or sing songs about each one.
- Give your baby safe objects he or she can use to learn about shapes and texture. Make sure the objects aren't a choking danger (see page 306).
- Encourage your infant to explore your face with his or her hands.
- Sing favorite songs to your baby using lots of facial expressions. Babies love repetition, so sing the same songs or nursery rhymes again and again.
- Take your child outdoors to experience various sights, sounds, and textures, pointing them out and naming them as you go.
- Hold your baby in front of a mirror. Let your child study the reflection of the two of you as you point to parts of the face.

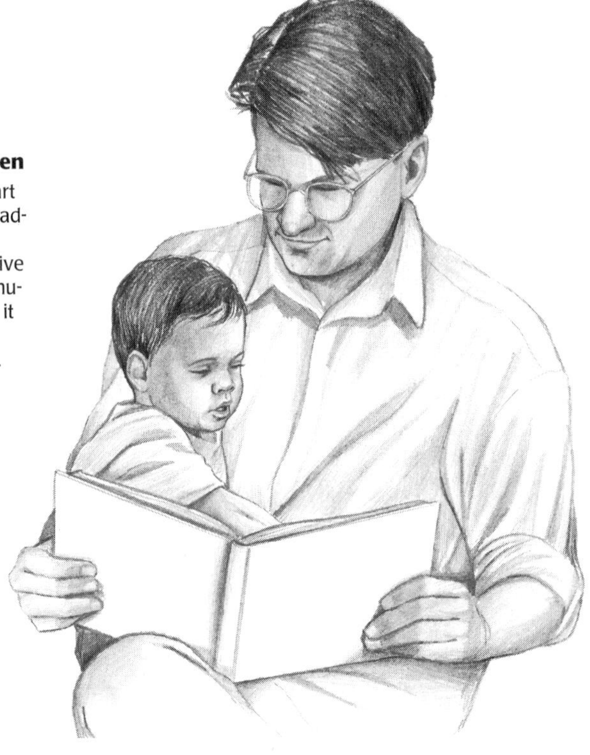

Read to your child often

It's never too early to start reading to your child. Reading aloud is one of the simplest and most effective things you can do to stimulate development. Make it a habit to read to your child at least once a day.

• Put colorful pictures or photos in places where your baby spends time (by the crib or changing table, for example) and vary them frequently. Look at photographs of family members and tell your baby what he or she is seeing.
• Let your baby touch toys and other objects as you raise them up and let them fall down. Then let him or her try. This will help your child learn about different sounds and the concepts of "down" and "drop" and will let him or her practice hand control.
• Use wooden spoons and other simple tools to count out rhythmic 1-2, 1-2-3, and 1-2-3-4 patterns. Encourage your baby to mimic the beat.
• Fill a container with cereal or other objects that will rattle when you close the lid and shake it. Ask your baby what's inside and let him or her peek and touch as you name the object. Change the objects as you help your baby discover different sounds and objects.

Brain-building activities for a 6- to 12-month-old As you and your child get to know each other better, you'll find many fun and stimulating things to do. These are just a few examples of the kinds of learning activities that are especially beneficial for children your baby's age:
• Cuddle, hug, massage, and say loving things to your baby often.
• Talk to your baby about the things you are doing–folding laundry, opening and closing doors, putting on socks and shoes.
• Sing lullabies and play music. Listening to music will teach your child about rhythm and melody and may make later learning easier. Music stimulates some of the same areas of the brain that are involved in math, language, and other skills.
• Stack spools, blocks, or plastic cups up and knock them down. Let your baby help. As you stack the objects, explain what you are doing to help your baby learn the meaning of "up" and "down."
• Hold your baby in front of the mirror and point out and name the parts of his or her face. Help him or her touch each part.
• Demonstrate and talk about cause and effect. For example, show your baby how turning the doorknob opens a door, flipping a switch turns on a light, and turning a faucet allows water to run. When your child is between 9 and 12 months, let him or her try these things under supervision.
• Expose your child to other children. If he or she is not in day care, join a play group, get together with other parents who have young children, and exchange baby-sitting with other parents.
• Roll a small ball around in a bowl or pan, and let your baby watch the circular movement and touch the ball.
• Crumple a piece of wax paper, foil, or gift wrap. Your baby will love the sounds.
• Use spoons, lids, and various size containers to help your baby experiment with sounds, fit lids onto containers, and stack small objects into larger ones.
• Use books, magazines, pictures, and newspapers to point out people and objects. This activity shows that pictures represent real things and that objects and pictures have names. Your child will also learn to love books.

- Kick or roll a ball back and forth to help build the baby's hand-eye coordination, motivation, and attention span.
- Play hide-and-seek by hiding an object under a towel or blanket; reinforce the name of the object and the concept of "under" as you play.
- Take your child with you to new places and expose him or her to new situations. Talk about the interesting things you see as you point them out.
- Place some of your baby's favorite toys within his or her view and ask where they are, watching to see if he or she will look for or move toward the object. Give your baby an object that you name, such as a book, and ask him or her to give it back to you. Then, hide the book while he or she watches, and ask him or her to find it.
- Tape a large piece of paper to a table and give your child a crayon. Demonstrate what the crayon can do.
- Encourage imitation. Clap your hands and say "clap," make kissing sounds

Learning "in" and "out"

Give your child lots of chances to learn the difference between something that is in and something that is out. Practice this skill by providing containers for him or her to drop things into.

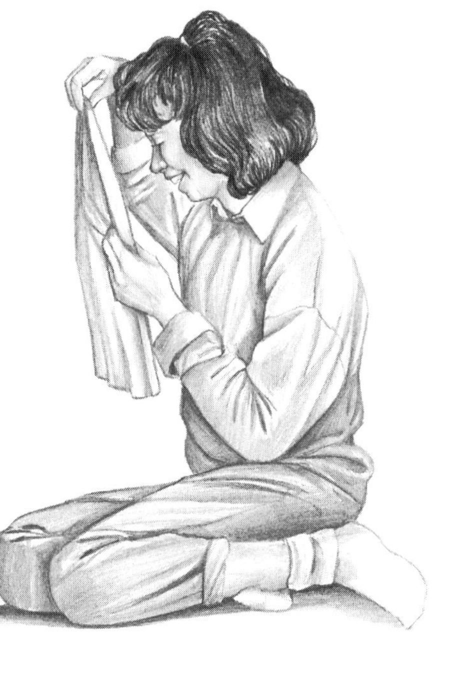

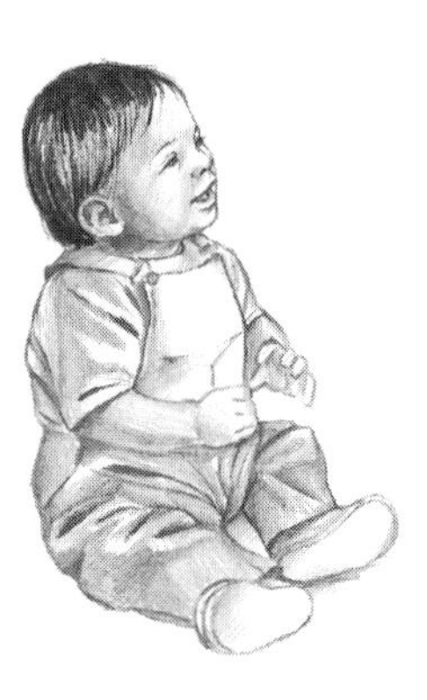

Peek-a-boo

Playing peek-a-boo with a 9-month-old is more than just fun. It tells your baby that you can be there even if he or she can't see you.

and say "kiss," and spread your arms wide and say "big." Wave and say "hi" when you greet your child and wave and say "bye" when you leave. Giving your child this practice will make it easier to acquire other skills that are also learned through imitation.

• In conversation, link sounds and an activity or object. For example, teach your baby that the sound of water running in the bathroom signals an impending bath or that the ring of the doorbell means a visitor has arrived.

• When your baby can eat finger foods, put different foods on the tray for touching and tasting. Talk about the "squishy" banana or the "crunchy" cereal. Letting your child make choices enhances curiosity and helps your child learn about differences using the senses of taste and touch together.

HELPING YOUR CHILD LEARN LANGUAGE

Listening to you and other people, your child learns language at an incredibly fast rate and with little effort. At 8 months of age, your baby will master the ability to pick out words from the rushing streams of speech he or she hears, detecting clear patterns in the sounds of the language. Scientists now believe that language is not learned in the usual way people learn—it's too enormously complex a task for children to accomplish in such a short time. Language seems to be an innate characteristic of humans, whose brains are genetically programmed to learn language in the same way their bodies are programmed to build a heart, lungs, and other organs.

Your child will understand the meaning of many words and phrases and will begin to try to verbalize by his or her first birthday. Here are some noticeable

Could your child have a hearing problem?

Although the doctor will evaluate your child's hearing at each checkup, you may want to watch for signs that your child cannot hear adequately. Hearing impairment can affect your child's ability to learn language. If you notice any of the following warning signs at the ages indicated, talk to your doctor immediately:

(Between 4 and 8 months)

• Your child does not turn his or her head or eyes toward a sound he or she can't see.
• In a quiet setting, your child's expression does not change at the sound of a voice or a loud noise.
• Your child does not seem to enjoy shaking a rattle, ringing bells, or squeezing noisemakers.
• At approximately 6 months, your child has not started to babble to himself or herself or doesn't seem to try to talk or babble back to people who are speaking directly to him or her.

(Between 9 and 12 months)

• Your child does not turn quickly or directly toward a soft noisemaker or to a "shush."
• Your child does not respond when his or her name is spoken.
• Your child's voice does not go up and down in pitch when babbling.
• Your child does not make several different consonant sounds (m, b, p, g) when babbling.
• Your child does not respond to music by listening, bouncing, or singing along.
• Your child does not understand what "no" means.

language breakthroughs your child will probably make this first year:
- Recognizing his or her name.
- Saying two or three specific words other than "dada" or "mama."
- Imitating familiar words.
- Clearly understanding and following simple instructions such as "bring" or "give."
- Recognizing words as symbols for objects; for example, pointing to familiar objects in a picture book when you say the word.

The more you talk to your child, the larger his or her vocabulary and the better his or her language skills will be. Here are some things you can do to enhance your baby's ability to learn language:
- When you have your child's attention, make noises and sounds or sing softly.
- Talk to your child as you care for him or her throughout the day. Speak slowly and in short sentences that describe the here and now, pointing to things you are talking about. Emphasize action words.
- Respond to your child's coos, gurgles, and babbling by imitating the sounds. His or her first words are likely to be "mama" or "dada." Each time you hear bits and pieces of longer words, say the whole word to help your child learn it.
- Read books to your child every day and let him or her see you reading for pleasure.
- Recite simple nursery rhymes.
- Play simple games with your child, such as "pat-a-cake."

Feeding your infant

In the next few months, your baby will begin eating with his or her fingers and might be able to use a spoon. He or she will also be ready to drink from a cup. Learning to eat and drink without help usually occurs toward the end of the first year. Until then, breast milk or formula will continue to be your baby's major source of nutrition. To avoid ending up with an underweight or overweight baby, let your child determine how much food he or she needs.

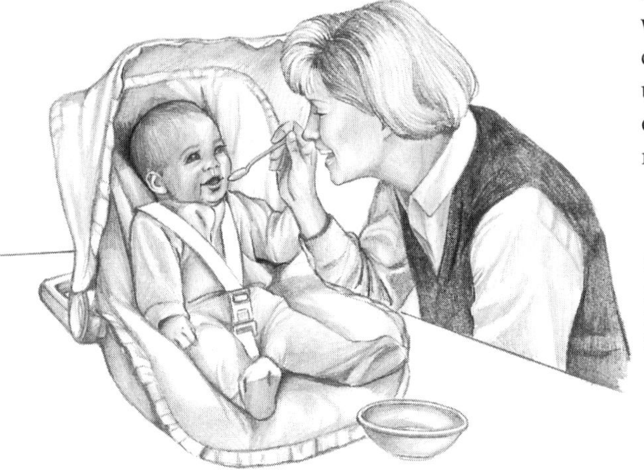

Starting on solid foods
Introduce solid foods one at a time so you can see whether your baby has a reaction to a certain food.

INTRODUCING SOLID FOODS

Your child's doctor will probably recommend waiting until your baby is between 4 and 6 months old before introducing solid foods–6 months if your baby is prone to allergies. (The earlier solids are introduced, the more likely they are to cause allergies.) A baby usually cannot swallow or digest solid foods well enough to benefit from them until after 4 months of age. Until then, breast milk and formula should be your baby's only source of nutrition because they are more balanced in nutrients than any other food.

Learning to eat with a spoon may take some time. Your baby won't lose the inborn reflex to push his or her tongue outward in response to a touch until the third or fourth month of life. The child should also be old enough to sit up and turn away from offered food. If your child still sticks out his or her tongue when you offer food with a spoon, wait a couple of weeks before trying again.

At each well-child visit in the first year, your doctor will advise you about introducing solid foods. Most doctors recommend giving a single-grain, iron-fortified cereal, such as rice cereal, as a baby's first solid food, because babies tolerate it well. Give your baby only baby cereal for about 2 weeks to 1 month before introducing another kind of food. Then add one food at a time, waiting a few days to a week before offering another food, so you can see whether the new food causes a digestion problem or allergy. Don't rush the introduction of solids; your baby is still getting the most important nutrients from breast milk or formula. Here are some tips for starting your infant on solid foods:

- Strap your baby into an infant seat or a high chair; it's easier to feed a baby if you have both hands free.
- Cover your baby's shoulders and chest with a large bib that has a pocket to catch any dribble. Put newspapers or a plastic mat under the high chair to make cleanup easier.
- Use a baby spoon; some come coated with rubber or plastic. Older babies may enjoy spoons specially designed for babies to grasp.
- For the first few times, give your baby a little breast milk or formula before offering solid foods. Extreme hunger may make your baby impatient and reluctant to try anything new or too frantic to settle down to eat.
- Place a small baby-spoonful of food on the middle of your child's tongue. Initially, your baby may want just a taste but will gradually accept a few small spoonfuls, eventually working up to about 2 to 3 tablespoons of each food per meal.
- End the meal when your child shows that he or she is no longer hungry by turning away from the spoon more than once. Don't worry that your child did not finish the portion of food you prepared.

After introducing cereal to your baby's diet, introduce puréed or strained foods–starting with fruits and vegetables at 5 or 6 months of age and strained meats at about 6 months of age. You can start meats later to minimize the risk of food allergies triggered by protein. Don't give up on vegetables if your child seems to prefer fruit–keep trying different vegetables. Increase the amount of food a bit at each meal. If your family is vegetarian, you can give your baby adequate protein with soy-based products. Discuss your vegetarianism with your child's doctor to ensure that your baby is getting adequate nutrition.

If your child spits up frequently after you introduce a new food or if he or she develops a facial rash, stop offering that food. The foods most likely to cause allergies in infants include dairy products, eggs, wheat and corn products, citrus fruits (such as oranges), tomatoes, peanut butter, and seafood. Your doctor will probably recommend waiting until your child is 9 to 12 months old before introducing or reintroducing these foods; the timing will depend on whether or not your baby has (or other members of the family have) a history of allergies. Wait until your child is 1 year old before giving regular cow's milk because it doesn't provide enough iron or other vitamins for an infant. A deficiency of iron can lead to anemia (see page 412). Milk may also cause allergies or irritate your child's intestines when given before age 1.

Some children take less breast milk or formula once they start eating solids; others don't. The important factor is balance: you want your child to get more and more nutrients from foods and less from milk. At about 9 months, a child needs at least 16 ounces of breast milk or formula, 2 to 4 ounces of iron-containing foods such as cereal or meat, and a multivitamin supplement. Limit your child's intake of fruit juice to less than 4 ounces of undiluted juice or 8 ounces of half-strength juice diluted with water per day. Drinking fruit juice at the expense of breast milk or formula can cause serious nutritional problems in infants, including diarrhea and failure to gain weight.

Feedings will not necessarily be smooth—and they'll certainly be messy—as your baby learns new motor skills and becomes increasingly interested in the world and less interested in sitting still in a high chair. Make mealtimes fun by talking to your child playfully or giving him or her a cup or spoon to hold.

FOOD SAFETY

Both homemade and commercial baby foods are healthful for babies, but any food's safety and nutritional value depend on safe handling and preparation. Many parents choose commercial baby foods as their baby's first solids because they are convenient. If you choose to give your baby commercial baby foods, you can feel confident that they are safe and nutritious because they must meet rigorous standards set by the federal government.

Food manufacturers use preparation techniques that preserve the food's nutritional content and they carefully test the level of pesticide residue in each food (which experts believe is probably lower than that in produce bought fresh and prepared at home). Manufacturers sometimes use small amounts of flour to thicken baby foods such as vegetables. These flours, which are the same flours that babies eat in cereals, are acceptable, safe, officially approved ingredients for baby foods.

Salt is no longer added to commercial baby foods and you shouldn't add any to the foods you give your baby. Unsalted foods contain enough naturally occurring sodium for your baby. Avoid getting into the habit of putting sugar or natural sweeteners such as applesauce into baby foods to persuade your child to eat them. If you sweeten everything your baby eats, he or she may resist accepting other flavors and have a more difficult time shifting to a balanced, adult-style diet later.

If you prefer to make your own baby food at home, ask your child's doctor for guidance. He or she may recommend a baby-food cookbook or child care manual. You should always follow safe handling procedures and be especially careful with foods–such as meat, poultry, seafood, and eggs–that carry the risk of contamination with disease-causing bacteria. Use nutrient-preserving cooking methods such as steaming, microwaving, baking, or broiling before puréeing or straining foods. Avoid boiling or frying–boiling causes the nutrients to leach into the water and frying adds too much fat and extra calories. Always cook food thoroughly and wash fruits and vegetables well to help prevent food poisoning.

Some vegetables–including beets, collard greens, spinach, and turnips–contain high levels of nitrate, a salt contained in soil and water, and may not be safe for infants when prepared at home. (The commercially prepared versions of these vegetables have safe levels of nitrates.) Excessive consumption of nitrates can cause a serious form of anemia in young infants. Ask your doctor about this risk if you prepare these vegetables at home.

The biggest risk by far is contamination with bacteria. Infants can get severely ill and develop life-threatening complications from some foodborne

Handling and preparing food safely

It's easy to recognize food that has spoiled because it looks and smells bad. But you might not be able to tell when food has become contaminated with dangerous bacteria. To make sure that the food you prepare for your baby and family is safe, follow these rules:

- Don't let uncooked meat, poultry, or eggs come into contact with cooked foods.
- Always wash your hands before preparing food.
- After using a cutting board for preparing raw meat or poultry, clean it thoroughly with detergent and water before using it to prepare other foods.
- After preparing poultry, which is a prime source of salmonella bacteria, thoroughly wash all cutting surfaces, knives, the sink, and your hands with hot, soapy water.
- Don't store raw meat in the refrigerator longer than 3 to 5 days; refrigerate raw poultry no longer than 2 days.
- Defrost foods in the refrigerator or microwave, not on the kitchen counter.
- Never refreeze frozen foods that you have thawed, except bread.
- Don't buy or use food in cans with bulging tops. Throw away foods in cans that hiss when you open them (unless they have been vacuum sealed). The food could be contaminated with a toxin that can cause a type of serious food poisoning called botulism.
- Cook beef, pork, and poultry until they are done in the middle. You should not be able to see any pink. That means all beef should be cooked until well-done. Cook all beef, pork, lamb, and veal to an internal temperature of 160°. Cook poultry, including stuffed poultry, to an internal temperature of 180°.
- Always cook eggs until the whites are firm and the yolks are thick.
- Refrigerate leftovers promptly.

diseases. Some foods are especially dangerous and should be carefully avoided. Never give your infant unpasteurized apple juice, juice blends that contain unpasteurized apple juice, or unpasteurized apple cider. (Check the label to make sure a product is pasteurized.) Don't give honey or corn syrup to an infant under 1 year of age because these sweeteners could be contaminated with bacteria that can cause a serious infection called infant botulism (see page 438).

Babies don't seem to mind food that is at room temperature or even cold. But if you want to heat baby food, test the temperature before giving it to your child by tasting it yourself to make sure it's not too hot. If you heat baby food in the microwave, stir it before testing the temperature because food warmed in a microwave heats unevenly.

To keep commercial baby foods safe:

- Store boxes of infant cereal in a clean, dry place. Put the boxes in containers with tight-fitting lids if insects regularly invade your dry foods.
- Serve infant cereal immediately after mixing it with liquid. Don't save leftover cereal for another meal.
- Don't buy or use baby food if the jar's vacuum seal has been broken.
- Refrigerate opened jars of baby food immediately after opening. You can store covered jars of fruit and small bottles of juice for 3 days after opening; large bottles of juice can be stored for 7 days. All other baby food should be stored in the refrigerator for no more than 2 days after opening.
- If you feed your baby from the jar, throw out any food left in the jar. To avoid waste, spoon a portion of food into a bowl and refrigerate the rest.
- Never put leftover baby food back in the jar, and don't save food from the infant's dish for another meal.
- Thaw frozen baby food in the refrigerator or microwave only—never on the kitchen counter.

To safely prepare baby foods at home:

- Before you start, thoroughly clean all utensils, work surfaces, and equipment—especially those used for raw meat, poultry, seafood, or eggs—with liquid dish soap and hot water and rinse them well. Wash your hands.
- Cook all foods of animal origin (meat, poultry, seafood, or eggs) thoroughly. To be absolutely safe, cook all foods thoroughly.
- Wash fruits and vegetables thoroughly.
- Don't refrigerate homemade baby foods for more than a day or two.
- On outings, take along jars of commercial baby foods instead of homemade ones—they're easier to keep safe from bacterial contamination.

WEANING

Weaning—the transition from breast or bottle to a predominantly solid-food diet—is a healthy, natural step in helping your child grow up. There is no right or wrong time to wean a child from the breast or bottle but doctors recommend weaning after the age of 1 year. Older children can become overly attached to the breast or bottle and resist giving it up. Between 6 months and a year, as children develop new skills and become more active in exploring their environment, they begin to lose interest in the breast or bottle and many will naturally and gradually wean themselves. For this reason, the easiest, most pleasant way to wean a child is to let the child control the process.

Watch for signs of your baby's decreasing interest–when he or she stops nursing frequently to look around or play, refuses the breast, tries to slide off your lap before the feeding is finished, throws the bottle down, or chews on the bottle nipple instead of sucking it. Respond by offering fewer feedings and encouraging the use of a cup. Be patient, because it can take a few months for a child to learn how to take all fluids from a cup or glass.

Eliminate one feeding every 4 days to a week (depending on your child's level of acceptance and cooperation), replacing the feeding with a cup of formula (or whole cow's milk if your child is older than 1 year). Eliminate the midday feeding first, then the afternoon feeding, and, lastly, the bedtime feeding, which is usually the hardest to give up. If your child sleeps through the night and does not wake up hungry, he or she doesn't need this last feeding. Gradually reduce the amount of formula or breast milk at bedtime or give a bottle of water instead or a drink of water from a cup. If you are breast-feeding and your breasts become engorged during the weaning process, express just enough milk to relieve the pain but no more. As you nurse less, your breasts will naturally reduce their production of milk. (For information about weaning a baby from breast to bottle, see page 52.)

Start offering a cup as early as the fifth month to get your child used to it, even though he or she probably won't be adept at using it until about the eighth or ninth month. Try different kinds of cups to see which your child prefers. Trainer cups with one or two handles, a lid with a spout, and a weighted bottom are good for beginners but your child may prefer a small plastic

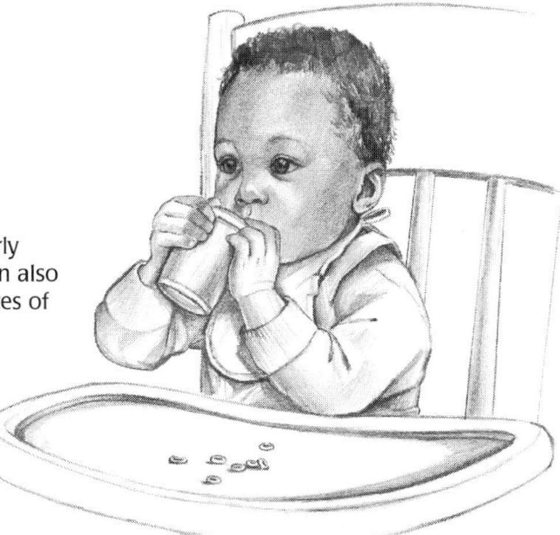

Learning to use a cup

Children can drink from a cup fairly well by 9 months of age. They can also pick up, bite, and chew small pieces of solid food.

glass with a lid and spout. The spout helps minimize spills, which is easier for you, too.

During the weaning process, spend even more time cuddling and playing with your baby. This closeness will make you both feel better as you adjust to this important change. Provide a stuffed toy or blanket for security if your child needs one.

FEEDING AN 8- TO 12-MONTH-OLD

Between 7 and 8 months of age, you can introduce your baby to mashed or coarsely puréed table foods. Commercial junior baby foods are unnecessary for most children, but they can be convenient for parents. Begin introducing bite-size pieces of soft foods such as bananas at 9 to 10 months, or whenever your child develops the pincer grasp (the ability to pick up objects between the finger and thumb). The best finger foods are those that will dissolve in the mouth or that a baby can chew (or gum) and easily swallow, such as small pieces of canned pears or peaches, O-shaped oat cereal, small pieces of crackers or toast, bits of cheese such as cheddar or American, and cooked vegetables. Cut foods into the size of a pea if they're firm or into the size of a marble if they're soft. Avoid foods that could cause choking (see page 305), junk foods (which lack nutrients), foods prepared with added sugar or salt, and cereals and breads made with white flour, which can get pasty in the mouth and cause gagging or choking.

Over the next few months, increase the amount of finger foods you give your child and decrease the amount of mashed foods that require spoon-feeding. Some children willingly accept and enjoy trying new foods; others are picky. Give small portions. Giving large portions to a child this age can cause feeding problems and make your child overweight. A baby will eat only as much as he or she needs, so let your child determine the amount.

Many children are more interested in playing than in eating at this age. Your child may throw food on the floor or squish it in his or her hand or hair while eating. Try not to worry too much about the mess and don't discourage your child's experimentation, which will probably only last for a few months.

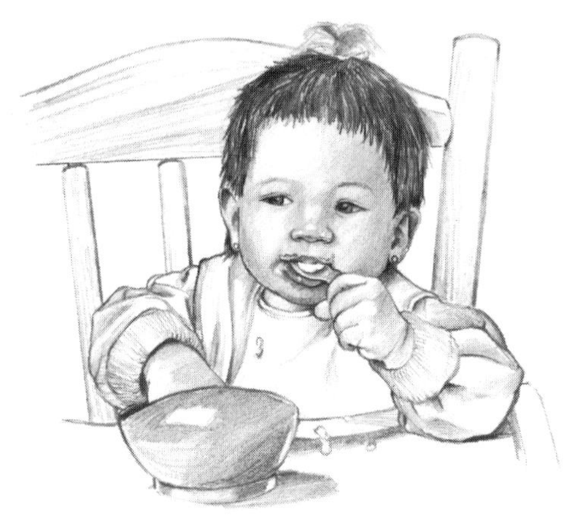

Eating without help
Children learn how to feed themselves between 6 and 12 months of age. Their attempts may be messy, but they accomplish the task all the same—often with great gusto.

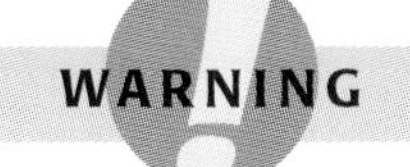

Some foods cause choking

To avoid the risk of choking, don't give your infant the following foods: raisins, popcorn, nuts, whole grapes (peeled grapes cut in small pieces are okay), whole peas, raw or firm vegetables or fruits (carrots, celery, bell pepper, apples, or unripe pears or peaches), large chunks of meat or poultry, pieces of bacon, sunflower seeds, or hard candies. Toast bread and cut it in small pieces before giving them to your baby. Hot dogs most often cause choking in infants, especially when they are cut into coin-shaped pieces. Give your child finger foods only under supervision when he or she is sitting in a high chair or other seat. Never leave him or her alone during meals. For more information about choking prevention, see page 304.

Self-feeding is an exciting new learning experience and an essential step in your child's development. If you don't allow your child to go through this phase now, self-feeding might be even harder to learn later. To minimize cleanup, put a large bib on your child, roll up his or her sleeves above the elbows, and provide a plastic cup or glass with a lid and spout. Place newspapers, a plastic mat, towels, or an old shower curtain on the floor under the high chair or table. Keep several rolls of paper towels on hand for cleanup. End the meal when your child spends more time playing with the food than eating it.

Instead of scolding your child for making a mess, reinforce good manners by praising your child each time he or she takes a polite, neat bite. Children this age like to eat with other people, which helps them learn table manners. Try feeding the baby first and then pull his or her high chair up to the table during the family meal and share some of your food. Always offer your baby a spoon and an unbreakable dish even though he or she probably won't be able to use them properly until about 15 to 18 months of age.

Once your baby begins eating three meals a day about 5 hours apart, offer a small snack in between meals. Make the snack a nutritious, nonmilk food, such as fruit or dry cereal. But if eating snacks ruins your child's appetite at mealtimes, stop offering them. Too many snacks in addition to meals promote excess weight gain. If your child is gaining too much weight, talk to the doctor. You may be overfeeding your child. The doctor will probably tell you to give only age-appropriate amounts of food at each meal (see page 113) and to stop when the child has had enough. Being overweight in childhood is linked to an increased risk of chronic illnesses such as heart disease, diabetes, and some types of cancer later in life. Obesity very commonly carries over into adulthood.

On the other hand, your child may be a picky eater and you may worry that he or she isn't getting enough nutrients. Although the nutritional requirements for a young child are surprisingly small, your child's doctor may recommend a daily multivitamin/mineral supplement to be safe.

HEALTHY EATING HABITS

You won't be able to influence your child's diet very much when he or she gets older and starts deciding what to eat independently. That's why you need to instill healthy eating habits now. Help your child acquire a preference for healthful foods using the following guidelines:

- Offer a variety of nutritious foods—even those vegetables, fruits, and grains that you personally don't like.

Fat: Essential for infants

Adults need to limit their intake of dietary fat to less than 30 percent of their total calories. But for children under age 2, fat and cholesterol are essential for proper growth and brain development. Too little fat in the diet could prevent your infant from growing properly. You won't see total fat, saturated fat, or cholesterol counts on baby-food labels because daily values for these nutrients have not been established for infants. When you introduce cow's milk into your 1-year-old's diet, provide whole milk. Low-fat and skim milk don't contain enough fat and calories to meet the nutritional needs of a 1-year-old. When your child is between 2 and 3 years of age, you can start limiting the amount of fat in his or her diet (see page 114).

- Hold off on giving your child overly sweet foods, such as baby-food desserts, candy, soda, and pastries during the first year. These foods have little nutritional value.
- Avoid foods that are high in sodium—and don't add salt to foods you give your baby.
- Serve only whole-grain bread, rolls, pancakes, and crackers. Your child will be less likely to accept them later, after getting used to white-flour products.
- Set a good example. Your child won't eat healthfully if no one else in the household does.

Exercise

In the next several months, your baby will learn to sit up, crawl, stand up, and walk and will become increasingly adept at fine motor skills. Your child will get plenty of exercise while learning these new skills as long as you provide the freedom and space to practice them. The least helpful thing you can do is to confine your baby to the crib, playpen, or an infant seat for long periods. You should also avoid putting your child in a walker. Walkers are dangerous (see page 299), and they inhibit learning to walk because they cause improper development of a child's legs and hips. The lower leg muscles develop but the hips and upper leg muscles do not. The same information applies to stationary exercise saucers, which can also adversely affect a child's posture. The best and safest place for a child this age is on the floor, as long as you have childproofed your home (see page 76) and supervise your child's floor time. If you must leave your baby alone briefly, put him or her in a playpen.

You can help your baby's muscles grow strong by including physical activity when you play with him or her. To help your baby learn to roll over (he or she will first learn to roll from stomach to back), place him or her on a blanket on the floor, alternating between the back-down, tummy-down, and side positions. Roll your infant over and back. Put the baby on his or her side and place a toy nearby to interest your child in rolling over to touch it. When the child is tummy-down, place toys or a mirror in front of your baby so he or she will look up; holding up the head strengthens the back and neck muscles. In the tummy-down position, he or she will also begin inching around to reach for toys.

When your child is learning to sit alone, hang some toys safely above your baby to look at and reach for. (Never tie toys across a crib or playpen, because the child could get tangled up in them and choke.) This effort helps the child learn to balance his or her body and manipulate objects with the hands. Once your child learns to crawl, he or she will pull up on furniture, strengthening the arm muscles, and then will start taking steps while holding on to furniture. Encourage this activity by putting toys or other interesting items on furniture that your child can hold on to while investigating the toys. A child this age learns how to support his or her weight and how to balance while playing with push toys, such as a toy lawn mower.

Sleep

After the first 3 months of life, your baby's sleep will become less and less linked to feeding. He or she will become increasingly active and want to stay awake longer and longer over the next several months. Some children sleep as little as 9 hours each day; others as much as 18. Your baby may sleep through the night, roughly 12 hours, and take two naps of a half hour to 3 hours each during the day. Keep a daily routine as much as you can.

Maintain your child's mid-morning and mid-afternoon naps for at least the first year, even if your baby doesn't actually sleep, because these breaks are good for you both. Put your baby in the crib or some other safe place with safe toys and let him or her play or go to sleep for about 1 to 3 hours. Your child won't protest these breaks if they're part of the daily routine. Be responsive to your child's needs for sleep and stimulation. Many babies are especially alert in the late afternoon. Recognize when your baby acts fussy, rubs his or her eyes, or sucks a finger or thumb–and put him or her to bed.

Young infants sleep as much as they need because they cannot yet keep themselves awake when they are tired. But at about 9 months of age, you may notice a change in your baby's sleep pattern. Your child may fight off sleep, sometimes becoming so exhausted that he or she cannot relax enough to fall asleep. A child this age wants to keep repeating newly learned skills and doesn't want the excitement to stop. To help your child get needed sleep, follow established bedtime routines, such as giving a bath, reading a story, singing a song, cuddling, rocking, or massaging. Be firm about bedtime; your baby is more likely to conform to routines if you are not ambivalent. It will get harder to establish a sleep pattern as your child gets older and more willful.

Your child may be afraid to separate from you at the end of the day and might wake up periodically during the night for reassurance. All babies alternate between periods of light sleep and deep sleep. Try to ignore your baby's whimpers or restlessness during periods of light sleep. If you rush in and pick up your baby to play, you're setting up expectations for the following nights. When the baby cries for you insistently at night for 5 or 10 minutes, go into the baby's room, make sure nothing is wrong, and rub his or her tummy to help the baby get back to sleep. Encourage your child to cuddle up to a favorite blanket or soft toy. Repeat the techniques you used earlier to get your child to sleep through the night (see page 57).

Discipline

Until your child becomes mobile and can get hurt or into trouble, little discipline is necessary. But once your baby starts crawling, you need to establish safety limits that you enforce consistently and firmly. For example, each time your child reaches out for the stove or an electric outlet, say "no," pick up the child, and firmly remove him or her. Discipline should be training, not punishment—the goal is to help a child learn how to control his or her behavior. Remember that it's always effective to reward your child for being good.

CHAPTER • 3

Your toddler (1 to 3 years)

The toddler stage, extending from ages 1 to 3, is a time of incredible learning, growth, and change. Commonly referred to as the "terrible twos," this stage can be exciting for both parents and children, but it requires lots of patience, watchfulness, and humor. Your compliant, agreeable infant may suddenly turn stubborn and resistant. Toddlers expend great energy learning to walk, run, talk, solve problems, and relate to people. They have a drive to be independent and carry strong ideas of how things should be done. Toddlers say "no" to almost every suggestion, insist on doing things for themselves, and refuse help, sometimes strongly. The more you know about how children develop during this stage, the better you'll be able to respond to your toddler's needs. Such knowledge can also make living with your toddler less stressful and much more fun.

WHAT YOU CAN DO FOR YOUR CHILD NOW

Toddlers tend to be rambunctious and rebellious—and altogether challenging. The learning your child does during these 2 years will contribute a great deal to his or her future success. Keep your child safe as he or she explores, give your child as much attention as you can, and, most of all, have fun together.

- **KEEP ALL MEDICINES, CLEANING PRODUCTS, AND OTHER HOUSEHOLD CHEMICALS LOCKED AND OUT OF REACH.**
- **KEEP BITES OF FOOD SMALL** to prevent choking and don't give your child small, hard pieces of any food (such as peanuts, popcorn, tortilla or potato chips, or candy).
- **TAKE YOUR CHILD TO THE DOCTOR FOR ALL HIS OR HER ROUTINE MEDICAL CHECKUPS AND VACCINATIONS.**
- **START THE PROCESS OF TOILET TRAINING ONLY WHEN YOUR CHILD SHOWS SIGNS OF READINESS,** such as telling you he or she has just wet the diaper.
- **ALWAYS PLACE YOUR CHILD IN A CAR SEAT,** put the car seat in the back seat, and make sure your car has childproof locks.
- **DON'T GIVE YOUR CHILD ANY TOYS WITH SMALL PARTS.**
- **PROVIDE NUTRITIOUS MEALS AND SNACKS.**
- **FEED YOUR CHILD A HIGH-FIBER DIET** rich in whole grains and fresh fruits and vegetables to prevent constipation while your child learns to use the toilet.
- **MINIMIZE YOUR CHILD'S EXPOSURE TO SMOKE;** second-hand smoke increases a child's risk for ear infections, colds, and asthma.

Your child's physical growth

Your child's growth will be slower during the second year than the first, but, by the age of 2, he or she will probably weigh four times more than at birth and will reach about half of his or her adult height. During the second year, children gain an average of about half a pound each month. Between ages 2 and 3, they gain about 3 to 5 pounds. Body proportions begin to change. The shoulders straighten out, the rib cage becomes progressively flatter, and the neck grows longer. The legs become longer and straighter and look more in proportion with the trunk; the feet develop arches.

Muscle mass, which up to now has been relatively low compared with bone and fat, increases at twice the rate of bone development during this period, making children look both thinner and more muscular. As their muscles develop, children gain more control over them. Toddlers learn to use their large muscles to walk, run, climb, throw, and dance. They use the small muscles of their hands to scribble and to pick up things.

Most children become pretty competent walkers by about 16 months. At first, they walk with a sway back–the stomach pushing out in front, the feet far apart and pointing out, and the arms held out for balance. As they develop better balance, the feet begin to turn in and become more parallel. It takes a few weeks or months of independent walking before toddlers can do other things at the same time, such as carry a toy, look up, reach up over the head, squat, or turn. They'll want to try new ways of moving and getting around, such as climbing stairs, stooping and getting back up, kneeling, and walking backward. By about 20 months, children can usually run and may even be able to jump up with both feet. Toddlers use their eyes, hands, feet, and body together in constant motion–climbing, pushing, pulling, kicking, throwing, dancing, chasing, falling down, and touching everything within reach. Such frenetic activity can make a watchful adult exhausted; even some professional athletes would have a hard time keeping up with a toddler!

Your child's development

The ability to walk gives toddlers an awareness of being a unique individual and instills a strong drive to become independent, which often looks like stubbornness or negativity. Toddlers insist on dressing and undressing themselves, holding their own cup, and using a spoon. They learn to snap, button, and zip clothing and get through a meal using a spoon, fork, and cup with fewer and fewer spills and messes. Some even use the toilet. The emotional changes that toddlers undergo as they struggle to take control of their actions, impulses, feelings, and body can cause sudden mood swings–from smiling and friendly 1 minute to sullen and tearful the next. These mood changes are normal.

Try to compliment and praise your child whenever you notice he or she is being good.

Toddlers are nonstop investigators—their explorations teach them about the world and help them develop their own way of approaching new problems and situations. They love to take out and put in, push and pull, open and close, fit together and take apart, stack up and knock down, and hide and find. Toddlers also love to grasp, squeeze, twist, and turn; roll, throw, catch, and bounce; and crawl over, under, and through. Each new object your child touches, tastes, smells, hears, or sees sparks fresh associations in your child's brain as he or she compares it with familiar objects.

The 12- to 18-month-old starts to do things more deliberately and learns the connection between cause and effect (if the stack of blocks gets too high, it falls over). He or she can have a goal in mind and make a plan for achieving it. For example, seeing a toy, he or she can decide to get it, pull up a stool or chair, and climb up to reach it. Getting up from a nap, an 18-month-old can think about the toy he or she was playing with right before the nap, remember where it was left, retrieve it, and start playing with it again. Your child's imagination starts to develop at this age too. He or she will use familiar toys, such as a pot, in new ways (for example, for a hat).

Your child's first concepts are broad, vague, generalized, and attached to concrete objects. For example, if the family pet is a dog, at this age your child may think all animals are dogs—whether they are real, toys, or in pictures. But by 2 years of age, he or she will recognize that dogs are different from cats, and will begin sorting them and all kinds of other things into their appropriate groups. Number concepts are simple at this age. Your 2-year-old may understand bigger and smaller and more and less but will probably comprehend any number more than one or two as "a lot." Concepts of time relate only to your child's own daily routine, such as going on an outing after lunch.

Toddlers are self-centered by nature, but they enjoy the company of children their own age. Even though they don't actually play cooperatively, but rather alongside one another, they may occasionally exchange a toy or word (especially "no" or "mine"). These interactions with other children are important because they teach social skills. When you invite another child over to play, it's a good idea to put away your toddler's favorite toys and books; he or she would be hurt and upset if you tried to force sharing, a social gesture he or she does not yet understand. Because toddlers see the world through their own needs and desires, they can't yet understand that other people may think and feel differently and you can't yet reason with them.

Toddlers are great imitators—that's how they learn to do things for themselves. You might notice your toddler feeding his or her dolls or putting them carefully to bed, even telling them to eat their vegetables or go to sleep using your exact words or tone of voice. Whenever you notice your child watching you, you can help him or her become a better imitator by doing your tasks with more deliberate movements. Let your toddler "help" you with chores around the house—putting groceries away, carrying items, and preparing meals.

If your child can't yet do a certain thing alone, suggest that you do it together—but first let him or her try.

Their self-centeredness also makes toddlers think that everything that happens—both good and bad—is the result of something they have done. Keep this in mind if something traumatic, such as a death or a divorce in the family, occurs. Help your child understand that he or she is not to blame. Although 2-year-olds have a strong desire to be independent, they still need the support and vigilance of their parents and other caring adults to keep them happy and safe. Help your child through major transitions, such as moving from a crib to a bed or using a potty-chair or a toilet instead of a diaper, with patience, reassurance, and kindness—and by planning ahead. Help your child learn to anticipate what comes next by preparing him or her for subsequent activities during the day—for example, give your child a warning about 10 minutes, then 5 minutes—perhaps even 1 minute—before meals, outings, and other activities to allow some transition time. Continue to supervise your child because he or she still lacks the common sense and foresight necessary to keep himself or herself out of danger.

DEVELOPMENTAL MILESTONES

All children develop in leaps and pauses and acquire skills at different rates in different areas. For this reason, it's best to observe how your child develops overall rather than to focus on particular skills, such as using a spoon or fork. Consider the following levels of development less as "milestones" than as suggestions of activities you can encourage your child to do.

At 13 to 15 months:
- Walks well alone.
- Climbs furniture and stairs.
- Stoops to pick up an object and gets back up.
- Imitates housework.
- Drinks from a cup.
- Points with his or her index finger.
- Cooperates with dressing.
- Removes socks and hats.
- Finds a hidden toy.
- Plays alone.

Undressing

Undressing is a step toward independence. Help your child learn to undress by loosening his or her clothes so they're easy to remove. For example, while your child is standing, help him or her push pants down from the waist to the knees and then have him or her sit down to pull the pant legs over the feet. Be patient and praise your child's efforts.

At 16 to 18 months:
- Walks backward.
- Walks up stairs holding someone's hand.
- Likes push-pull toys.
- Removes larger pieces of clothing.
- Takes toys apart and puts them back together.
- Sorts different shapes.
- Turns pages of books.

At 19 to 21 months:
- Kicks and throws balls.
- Builds a tower of three to four blocks.
- May start to show hand preference.
- Puts lids on containers.
- Shows independence.
- Puckers up to give a kiss.

At 22 to 24 months:
- Walks up and down stairs alone.
- Builds a tower of eight blocks.
- Helps undress.
- Uses spoon well.
- Unzips zippers.
- Does not share (everything is "mine").
- Plays with other children side by side—not together.
- May show readiness for toilet training.

Up and down stairs
Stair-climbing is great exercise for toddlers and one of their favorite activities—especially once they can do it without anyone's help. Let your child try to climb stairs whenever you get the chance. Resist the temptation to save time by carrying your child up and down.

At 2 to 3 years:
- Runs well.
- Balances on one foot.
- Bends over easily without falling.
- Alternates feet when walking up stairs.
- Pedals a tricycle.
- Dresses him- or herself.
- Feeds him- or herself.
- Opens door by turning knob.
- Turns book pages one at a time.
- Makes vertical, horizontal, and circular strokes with a pencil.
- Plays with others; can take turns.

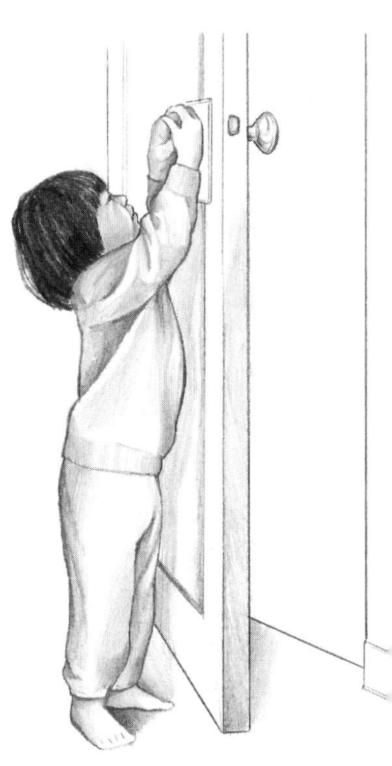

Opening doors
Curious 2-year-olds have a hard time ignoring closed doors and quickly figure out that all they have to do to open them is turn a knob. Once your child can open doors, make sure that any doors you don't want opened have childproof locks.

BOOSTING YOUR CHILD'S INTELLECTUAL DEVELOPMENT

Children are born with the potential to be curious, creative, and intelligent; it's up to parents and other caregivers to help them fulfill their potential. All children have a set routine or daily pattern. Recognize your child's pattern and try to fit in stimulating learning activities at the times he or she is most receptive and observant. Toddlers have short attention spans, but you can help increase your child's ability to concentrate by regularly sitting down with him or her for a few minutes and giving your complete attention to an activity he or she seems especially focused on. Playing side-by-side with your child will also instill trust, security, and a love of learning. During these early years, when your child's brain is developing rapidly, your participation in even simple daily activities with your child will make a lasting impression.

Brain-building activities for a 12- to 24-month-old Here are some suggestions for stimulating play:
- Talk to your child. Talking directly to your child is the simplest, most effective way to increase his or her intelligence.
- Read to your child every day.
- Respond to your child's natural curiosity by encouraging him or her to explore and interact with the world; let him or her bang, push, pull, dig, and draw.

• Count everything (fingers, toes, hands, and stairs) and name everything (bird, tree, shirt, airplane).
• Limit TV watching to less than an hour a day.
• Encourage your child to help undress him- or herself, to eat without help, to drink from a cup, and to wash his or her hands so that he or she learns confidence and independence.
• Memorize or make up rhymes and songs that capture your child's interest.
• Make all trips, such as going to the grocery store, learning experiences. Talk about what you're seeing and doing, shake containers to hear the sound they make, feel different items, and name colors.
• Give your child an open box or dish to put objects into and take things out of. Or provide a box with a lid and encourage your child to open and close it.
• Use household objects to show the concepts of "open," "closed," "inside," and "outside."
• Practice stepping with your child on stairs; stepping helps develop gross motor skills and the idea of "up" and "down."
• Provide opportunities for your child to be around other children. Because toddlers don't yet know how to share and play together, provide lots of toys for

Blocks stimulate learning

Building blocks are valuable learning tools. Blocks teach simple calculations. Give your child a set of various sizes and shapes and watch him or her make decisions about balance and learn about spatial relationships and shapes.

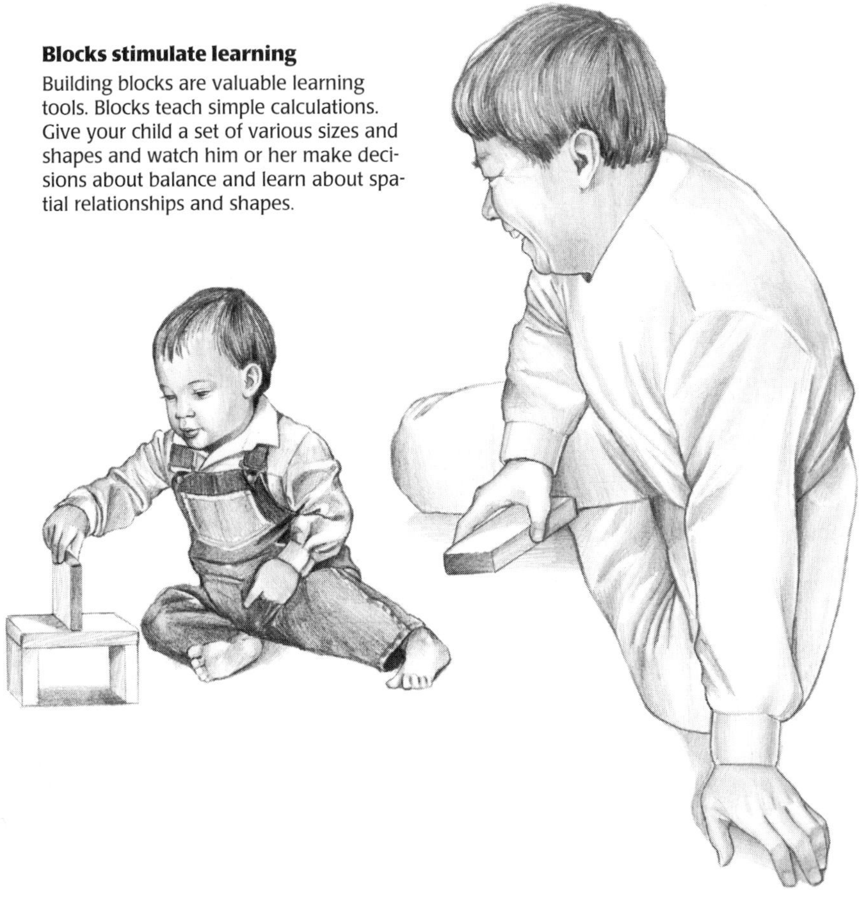

each child and put away your child's favorite playthings ahead of time to avoid squabbling.
• Give your child a large box to push around the room, to give a ride to a stuffed animal, or to climb into.
• Let your child practice throwing a soft ball into a large plastic laundry basket.
• Invent make-believe stories starring your child.
• Play games with your child that require the use of imagination and language skills.

Brain-building activities for 2-year-olds Two-year-olds love to learn new skills. The following are examples of the kinds of activities that can help your 2-year-old develop these skills:
• Read to your child every day. When you finish a story, ask your child simple questions about it such as "What did you like best?"; "What was the dog's name?"; or "Where did they go?" These discussions can help develop your child's listening and understanding skills.
• Let your child "read" a favorite book to you.
• Limit television viewing to less than 1 hour each day.
• Encourage your child to brush his or her own hair, dress and undress, feed him- or herself, and blow his or her nose (with only a little help from you). These activities will help develop your child's coordination, independence, and self-confidence.
• Constantly identify colors of household objects (when you're folding clothes, for example) and ask your child to point to something else of the same color; this helps your child learn to recognize, match, and name colors.
• Play creative, interactive games and plan activities with other children.
• Draw with your child using crayons, pencils, and chalk.
• Introduce the potty-chair and begin toilet training. Progress slowly—your child will master this skill at his or her own pace.
• Take walks and visit libraries, museums, casual restaurants, parks, beaches, and zoos.
• Have fun with finger-play songs and games (such as "Itsy Bitsy Spider"), which will reinforce your child's ability to imitate and make-believe.

Language development

The ability to talk opens up the world for children and adds a new dimension to their relationships as they learn to express their feelings and see people react to them. Language gives them the tools that will eventually enable them to control and understand their emotions, to think and remember, and to cooperate with playmates and other people.

Most children know only a few words between 12 and 17 months but, at about 18 months, an explosion of learning occurs—they start acquiring new words at an accelerated pace, and they start combining words into phrases. By their second birthday, most children have a 100-word vocabulary and by their third birthday many children have a vocabulary of between 1,000 and 2,000 words and have mastered most sounds and acquired the rules of grammar that enable them to speak the language fluently. Three-year-olds speak well in the present tense.

Your 15-month-old can understand just about everything you say. By the age of 2 years old, your child is putting two or three words together in phrases, usually the name of a familiar object and a word to describe it or what it does–such as "bad dog bite" or "read book." The way in which a child this age puts two words together, using only the most important words and getting their sequence correct, shows that he or she has already learned basic grammar. A toddler's grammatical mistakes are usually logical. For example, most children learning English will add "s" to the ends of all words to make them plural ("mouses" for "mice") and "-ed" to the ends of verbs to put them in the past tense ("goed" for "went"). Your role in helping your child learn language is to consistently provide examples of the rules of grammar. When your child says something incorrectly, such as: "There are lots of mouses," respond by repeating the sentence using the correct grammar: "Yes, there are a lot of mice." Many children have problems pronouncing r, l, s, th, and n, substituting one sound for another ("wabbit" for "rabbit"), omitting a sound ("han" for "hand"), or distorting a sound ("shlip" for "ship"). Repeat difficult sounds often so your child hears how they sound.

Encourage your child to use the words he or she knows by asking who, what, and where questions ("why" and "when" come later). Although you may be good at reading your child's gestures, provide words to help him or her verbalize his or her needs, desires, and thoughts. You can encourage your child's efforts to talk by listening carefully and showing respect for what he or she has to say. This attitude lets your child know that you like it when he or she uses words to tell you things. It also teaches the child proper listening skills: "while you talk I listen" and "while you listen, I talk." Not everything your child says requires a long conversation; sometimes a nod or smile is enough. Showing that you're listening teaches your child that talking is worthwhile and an effective way to communicate his or her needs and wants.

LANGUAGE MILESTONES

Just as some children learn to walk earlier than others, some children seem to pick up language more easily. But, in general, the more language your child hears, especially when it is directed at him or her and delivered in an animated way, the more examples he or she can use to develop the tools of language. You cannot talk too much to your toddler–this is the time when his or her brain is wiring itself for language. Think of the following milestones of language development as sparks to stimulate conversations and interactions with your child–and effective ways to nurture your child's verbal skills.

At 13 to 15 months:
- Says three or four words in addition to "mama" and "dada."
- Recognizes the names of familiar people, objects, and body parts.
- Responds to name.
- Follows one-step instructions, such as "Go get the ball."
- Names family members.

At 16 to 18 months:
- Says five to ten words.
- Can point to two or three body parts.
- Points to simple pictures.
- Gives kisses.
- Follows two-step instructions, such as "Go get the ball and bring it to me."

At 19 to 21 months:
- Says 10 to 15 words.
- Labels actions (such as says "Up" for "Pick me up").
- Asks "What's that?" frequently.
- Uses noun-verb combinations such as "Dog go."

At 22 to 24 months:
- Says about 100 words.
- Says two- to three-word phrases.
- Repeats what he or she hears.
- Uses "me" when referring to self.
- Listens to stories.
- Repeats nursery rhymes.
- Asks for food and drinks.
- Pretends to read.
- Associates names with familiar objects.

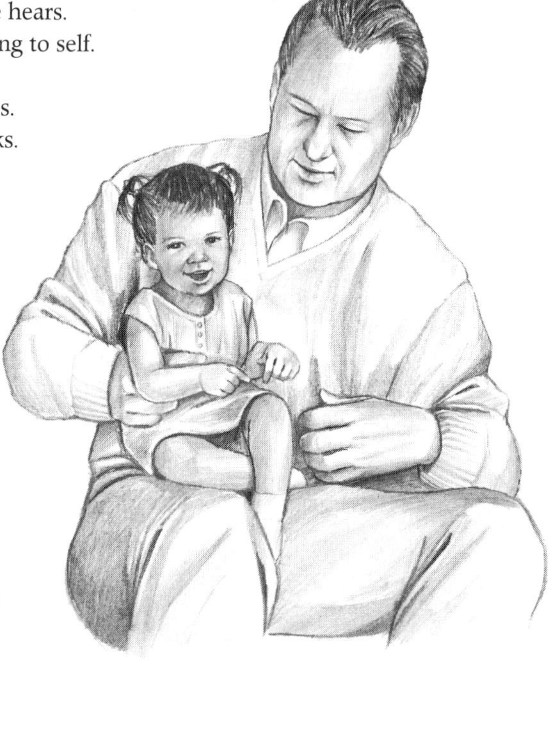

Where's your knee?

If you have been persistent at labeling everything, your 18-month-old will be able to point to a few body parts as you name them. Repeat the names of body parts whenever you have a chance, such as when you're bathing or dressing your child.

- Distinguishes "one" from "many."
- Communicates feelings using words and gestures.
- Lets you know when he or she has to go to the bathroom.
- Identifies body parts.

At 2 to 2½ years:
- Says two- to three-word sentences such as "Me want milk."
- Uses own name.
- Points to and names many common pictures and objects.
- Sings parts of songs.
- Uses two-word negative phrases such as "No want."
- May say "no" when he or she means "yes."

At 2½ to 3 years:
- Learns 50 new words every month.
- Can say three-word sentences.
- Can say full name, age, and sex.
- Understands concept of "two."
- Uses pronouns (I, you, me, we, they) and some plurals (cars, dogs, cats).
- Can be understood, most of the time, by other people.
- Carries on conversations with self and dolls.
- Understands some simple physical relationships (in, under, big, little).
- Follows simple instructions (such as "Put the book on the table").
- Understands simple time concepts such as last night and tomorrow.
- Likes to hear the same stories repeatedly.
- Knows own gender by age 3.
- Answers "where" questions.

Make-believe

Talking on the telephone is one of the grown-up activities that toddlers most like to copy. Listen to the animated "pretend" phone conversations of your toddler. Notice how your child handles the phone just like you, holds his or her head the same way, speaks with a similar inflection, or even repeats verbatim things you have said. The accuracy of your child's impersonation reflects his or her keen observation of you and underscores your importance as a role model.

STIMULATING YOUR CHILD'S LANGUAGE DEVELOPMENT

The best way to stimulate your child's language development is to talk to him or her–as much as you possibly can. Talk simply, clearly, slowly, and directly to your child. Describe what you're doing, feeling, and hearing when you're together. Talk about an event or outing before, during, and afterward. Reward and encourage your child's efforts to say new words and to communicate, looking directly at him or her when he or she talks to you, listening attentively and being responsive and enthusiastic. Show you understand what your child says by answering, smiling, or nodding your head. Here are some other things you can do to improve your child's language skills:

- Repeat new words and use them frequently.
- Read books to your child every day. Bring books with you wherever you go, turn yourself into an actor by reading with enthusiasm, and ask questions about the stories.
- Take your child on frequent, interesting trips (to the park, zoo, and museums or to visits with friends and relatives) and describe everything you're seeing and doing.
- Read a poem or story (such as "The Three Little Pigs") that repeats phrases, and have your child say a particular phrase each time you read a new part of the story. Act out the story with your child.
- Turn storytelling into a language partnership by letting your child fill in some of the words in a story or say the punch lines to familiar jokes. Help your child string stories together about what he or she has been doing by filling in the words he or she leaves out and by asking questions; this helps your child learn to tell complete stories and know that you are interested in what he or she has to say.
- Listen to, memorize, and repeat rhymes and songs; sing the same songs slowly, starting with simple melodies such as "Mary Had a Little Lamb" and say the same rhymes over and over. Look for poems or tongue twisters that repeat sounds and letters. Your child will learn to enjoy the sounds of words and will learn to make his or her voice go up and down.
- Help your child classify objects–such as toys, clothes, or dishes–into groups; this will help him or her understand that objects can look different but be in the same group.
- Use colors, numbers, and time in your conversations and during daily activities. For example, count toes as you dry your child after a bath or say "It's 8:00 at night, time for bed."
- Use descriptive language to explain what you are doing, planning, or thinking.

Could your child have a hearing problem?

Although children develop language at different rates, they should continually show progress. If your child has a speech or hearing problem, early treatment is essential. Talk to your child's doctor if you notice any of the following warning signs between ages 1 and 3:

- Your 1-year-old doesn't pronounce many different consonant sounds at the beginning of words.
- Your 1½-year-old doesn't say more than five words.
- You cannot understand your 2- to 3-year-old's speech most of the time.
- Your 2- to 3-year-old doesn't use two- or three-word sentences.
- Your 2- to 3-year-old cannot follow two instructions together (such as "Get the block and put it on the table").

- Have your child deliver simple messages from you to another person.
- Help your child listen and follow directions by playing games in which you give instructions such as "Throw the ball" or "Touch your nose."
- To get your child to think and talk, ask "what if" questions such as "What would happen if we didn't mow the lawn?"
- Sing, listen to music, and dance with your child.

Nutrition

Teaching your child healthy eating habits now will benefit him or her throughout life. In addition to preventing weight gain and obesity, a nutritious, balanced diet may help reduce the future risk for chronic diseases, including some cancers and heart disease. Toddlers benefit from structure and limits. Establish a regular schedule of three small meals a day and two or three healthy snacks–and avoid giving out any other food in between. Preventing children from snacking freely throughout the day will make them more likely to eat the nutritious foods provided at mealtime. Give nutritious snacks such as raw vegetables (except for carrots and celery, which can cause choking), fruit, and cheese and crackers; minimize cookies, candy, and soft drinks.

After your child's first birthday, you'll probably notice a drop in his or her appetite and a new pickiness about what he or she eats. Your child's appetite has decreased because his or her growth has slowed, reducing calorie requirements. Give your child a variety of healthful foods and let him or her choose which ones to eat. He or she should be able to handle most of the foods that you and the rest of the family eat. Toddlers tend to be naturally careful about trying new foods. If your toddler doesn't seem to like a new food, continue to offer it now and then at meals; he or she is likely to come to accept it as long as you don't pressure him or her to eat it.

Don't expect your toddler to eat some of everything on the table–and respect his or her food preferences. Children are usually more willing to eat starches (such as rice or pasta) and meat than fruits and vegetables, so it's a good idea to offer fruit and vegetables at the beginning of the meal and for snacks when your child is most hungry. Vegetables that children tend to like best include broccoli, thawed frozen peas, potatoes, corn, and sweet potatoes. A dip or a little grated cheese can make vegetables more attractive to some children.

Your child may resist certain foods, eat only one or two favorites for long periods and then tire of those, or eat large amounts of food at one meal and almost nothing at the next. View your child's nutrition in terms of his or her total diet–not necessarily one food, one meal, or one day at a time. If your child is eating a variety of foods over the course of several days, he or she is probably getting adequate nutrition.

Don't try to control the amount of food your toddler eats. Some toddlers react to this kind of pressure by overeating or refusing to eat. Your toddler can

Toothbrushing

Brush your child's teeth at least twice a day without toothpaste (see page 259). You can start using a pea-size amount of toothpaste when your child is about 2 or 3 years old).

regulate his or her food intake more accurately than you can, so don't worry if he or she isn't eating as much as you would like at a particular meal. If you think that your child isn't eating a variety of foods, write down what he or she eats for 3 days and ask the doctor about it. He or she may recommend a daily multivitamin-mineral supplement. Use the following general guidelines when giving your child food:

- Test the temperature of the food yourself because a toddler is unlikely to consider how hot a food may be before digging in.
- Avoid foods that are heavily spiced, salted, buttered, or sweetened.
- Mash or cut food into small pieces.
- Provide a variety of tastes, colors, and textures.
- Make sure your toddler eats only while seated and when supervised by an adult.
- Limit your child's access to sweets.
- Don't add sugar to food and don't make a rich dessert everyday.

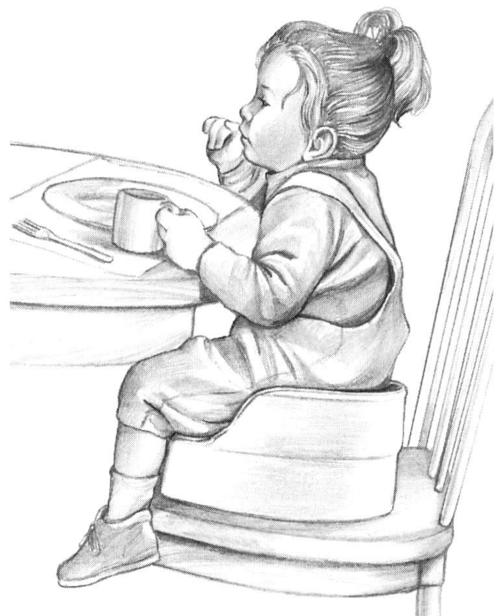

Table manners

Mealtimes are opportunities for toddlers to explore, test limits, and learn about independence, but meals should also be pleasant and relaxing for the whole family. Teach table manners by encouraging your child to drink all liquids from a cup or glass and use a spoon and fork. Although you will still be giving your child finger foods, provide appropriate utensils for him or her at meals and show how they're used.

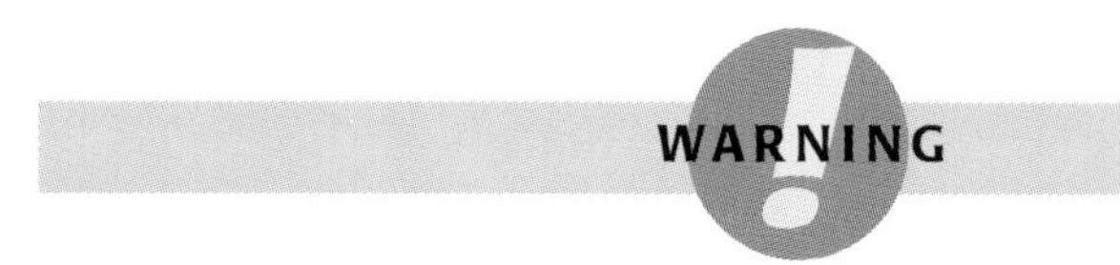

Certain foods can cause choking

Toddlers are still learning to chew and swallow efficiently and often gulp their food when they're in a hurry. Your child is still not old enough to have the foods that are most likely to cause choking (see page 305)—including hot dogs, nuts (especially peanuts), whole grapes, whole raw carrots, raw celery, round hard candies, spoonfuls of peanut butter, popcorn, and raw cherries with pits. For more about preventing choking, see page 304.

A BALANCED DIET

Given the freedom to choose from nutritious foods on their own, toddlers tend to eat a variety of foods and achieve a balanced diet—as long as it is provided to them. A balanced diet should include a combination of carbohydrates, protein, fats, vitamins and minerals, and fiber in appropriate proportions.

Carbohydrates Carbohydrates are starches and sugars found in fruits, vegetables, and starchy foods such as pasta, whole-grain bread, legumes (dried beans, peas, and lentils), brown rice, and potatoes. Carbohydrates are the body's best source of energy and they should make up about half of the calorie content of your child's diet.

Protein A child's body requires protein for growth and development and for maintenance and repair of muscles, skin, and other tissues. Protein should make up about 15 percent of your child's diet. Good sources of protein include milk, lean meat, cheese, eggs, nuts, legumes, and fish.

Fat Fat is an especially important part of the diet during the first 2 years of life. Because children grow at such a rapid rate during this time, they need the concentrated source of energy and nutrients that fat provides. Fat supplies substances that are essential to a child's growth and development and are especially important for the development of the brain and nervous system. Don't introduce a low-fat diet until your child is between 2 and 3 years old (see page 114). Until that age, give your child whole milk and don't worry about limiting his or her intake of other fats, except those in high-calorie junk foods. (Once you start giving your child junk foods, it will be hard to eliminate them later.)

If your child has a family history of heart disease before age 55 or if someone in your family has a high cholesterol level, your child's doctor may suggest testing your child's cholesterol level (see page 235) at age 2. If the level is found to be unusually high, your child's doctor may recommend a special low-fat, low-cholesterol diet for your child.

Fiber Fiber is the indigestible part of plant foods such as whole grains, legumes, vegetables, and fruits. These foods make up the largest portion of the Food Guide Pyramid (see page 113). Fiber provides important health benefits throughout life, including promoting normal bowel function and helping to reduce the risk for some diseases, such as cancer and heart disease. It's important to provide a variety of fiber-rich foods to your child each day because there are different types of fiber in foods and you want to be sure that your child gets a balance of them. Avoid foods such as white rice and white bread, which have been stripped of their fiber.

Vitamins and minerals The body needs vitamins and minerals to function well. A balanced diet provides all of the essential vitamins and minerals and

HEALTHY EATING

Serve your child a wide variety of nutritious foods to ensure that he or she gets all the nutrients needed for growth during childhood. The most widely accepted nutritional guidelines advise giving your child a balanced diet that is low in fat (begin to lower fat intake between ages 2 and 3); provides plenty of whole grains, vegetables, and fruits; minimizes sugar and salt; and provides enough calories for growth. A healthy diet can reduce a child's future risk of developing heart disease, some cancers, diabetes, obesity, and osteoporosis.

Healthy eating from the start

The eating habits your child develops now will last a lifetime. Use the following guidelines to instill healthy eating habits early:

- Buy only the foods you want your child to eat, including plenty of fruits, vegetables, and breads and cereals containing whole grains.
- Let your child make his or her own choices from the foods you provide.
- Involve your child in planning weekly menus and shopping lists.
- Establish set meal and snack times.
- Give your school-age child a good breakfast because it can improve school performance. Check breakfast cereal labels to avoid buying those with a high sugar content.
- Limit high-calorie, sugary, high-fat snacks and drinks. They usually have little nutritional value and leave no room for healthy foods.
- Don't add salt to food you're preparing and don't put the saltshaker on the table.
- Encourage your child to drink plenty of water.

Make mealtime a social time

Children learn about healthy eating from their families. Meals also provide a good opportunity to teach your children about your family's cultural and ethnic customs related to food.

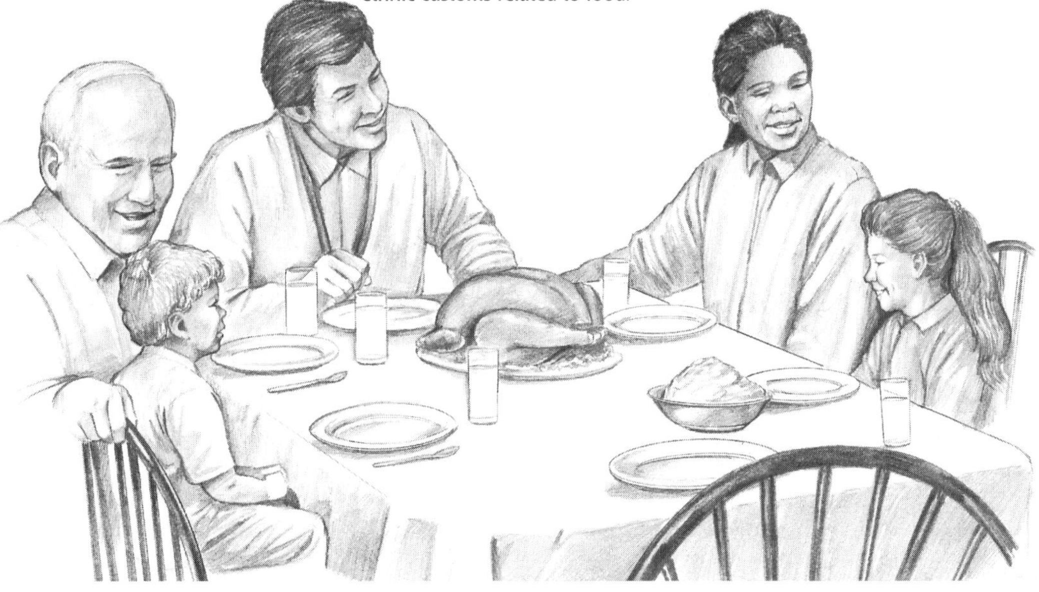

The Food Guide Pyramid

The US Department of Agriculture developed the Food Guide Pyramid to help you provide your family with healthful foods in the right proportions. The Food Guide Pyramid's food groups are organized to illustrate their proper proportion in your family's diet. For example, grains form the largest part of the Food Guide Pyramid because the greatest number of servings your family consumes should be from grain foods—such as whole-grain breads, pasta, rice, and cereals. The Food Guide Pyramid graphically shows that whole grains, vegetables, and fruits form the foundation of a healthy diet.

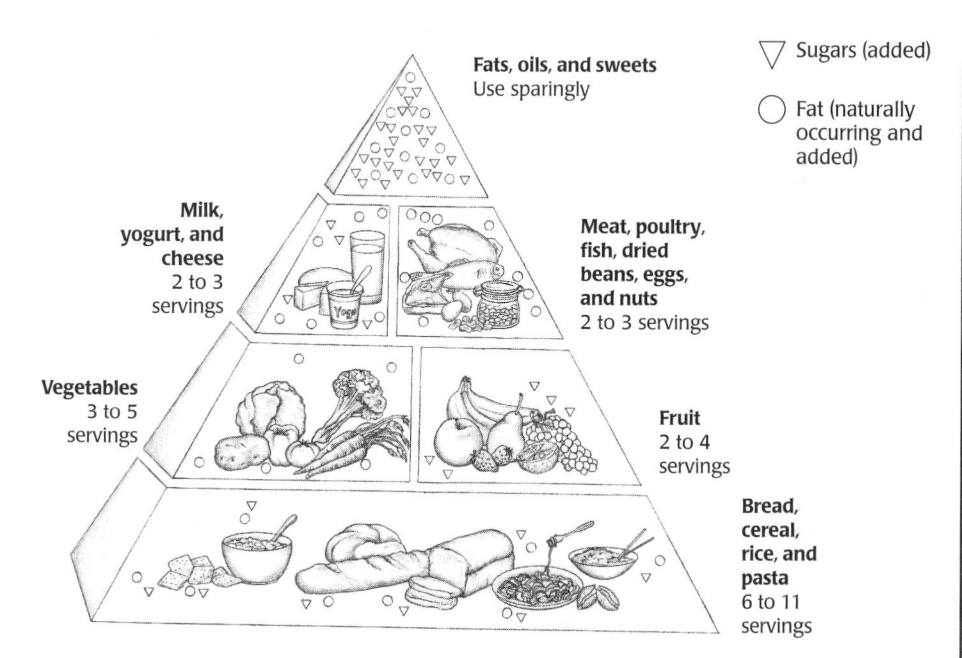

The Food Guide Pyramid illustrates that a diet should include plenty of grain foods, vegetables, and fruits, fewer dairy and other protein foods (meat, poultry, or fish), and very few fats and sweets. The range of servings recommended is for adults. The lower number of servings listed is generally suggested for children.

Food Guide Pyramid portions are smaller for young children than for adults—about half of an adult-sized portion for a school-aged child. That guideline translates into about ½ cup of lettuce, ½ cup of rice or vegetables, and ½ slice of bread. But, because your child needs to consume six servings of grains and three servings of vegetables each day, you can give your children two servings of grains—½ cup of rice or a whole slice of bread—at one meal. To make it easier to calculate, estimate the average young child's serving size of each food to be 1 tablespoon for each year of life. For a 5-year-old, that's 5 tablespoons or slightly more than ¼ cup. As your child grows, he or she will probably request larger servings. Offer one, small serving first—your child can always ask for more. One exception to the rule is protein. Growing children need 1½ times more protein per pound of weight than do adults. But adult protein requirements are low so, if your young child consumes 2 ounces of protein and drinks a couple of glasses of milk each day, he or she will easily meet or exceed the recommended protein requirement for toddlers.

Calcium: Essential for strong bones and teeth

Eating a diet rich in calcium, along with exercising regularly, helps build strong bones. The more bone density your child builds now, the lower his or her risk of osteoporosis (bone-thinning) later in life. Your child also needs calcium for strong teeth. Good food sources of calcium include low-fat or nonfat dairy products (such as milk, yogurt, or cheese), leafy green vegetables, and calcium-fortified fruit juices. Canned salmon and sardines are also calcium-rich. Your child needs adequate amounts of vitamin D, which is added to milk, to absorb calcium properly. The body also manufactures vitamin D when the skin is exposed to sunlight.

How much calcium does your child need each day?

Age	Amount in milligrams
Birth to 6 months	400
7 to 12 months	600
1 to 10 years	800
11 and older	1,200 to 1,500

Lower fat diet after age 2 or 3

Don't feed a child under the age of 2 years a diet low in fat because young children need dietary fat for growth and brain development. Recommendations vary about when to switch a child to a diet that is lower in fat. Most health experts agree that a child should begin to consume a low-fat diet (in which he or she gets 25 to 30 percent of calories from fat) starting at about 2 or 3 years of age. Children with a family history of either high cholesterol or an early onset of heart disease (before age 55) should be screened for cholesterol (see page 235) and should consume a generally low-fat diet beginning at age 2. Here are some ways to limit your child's intake of fat:

- Offer skim or 1 percent milk instead of whole or 2 percent.
- Serve more fish and poultry and less red meat (beef and pork). Use lean ground turkey in hamburgers and meat loaf. When serving red meat, choose the leanest cuts.
- Remove the skin from poultry and trim the fat from meats before serving.
- Serve lower-fat hot dogs, bacon, sausage, and sandwich meats and limit the amounts you serve.
- Use butter or margarine sparingly on toast or just use jelly or jam. Switch to soft, lower-fat margarine.
- Avoid frying foods. Use low-fat cooking methods such as baking, broiling, grilling, poaching, or steaming.
- Increase your child's intake of fiber. Most children consume way too little of this important nutrient. Fiber-rich foods include whole-grain breads and cereals, legumes (dried peas and beans), vegetables, and fruits.

Fruit juice: Too much of a good thing

Although fruit juice is a nutritious beverage, drinking an excessive amount (12 ounces or more a day) can lead to health problems in toddlers. Limit your child's intake of fruit juice to less than 12 ounces a day and dilute it with water. Fruit juice contains mostly sugar, so a child's natural preference for sweet-tasting foods can make him or her choose fruit juice over other nutritious but less sweet foods or can fill him or her up, leaving less of an appetite for other foods. Excessive consumption of fruit juice has been linked to obesity and short stature in some young children. Toddlers who drink large amounts of fruit juice that contains a substance called sorbitol (check the label) can develop chronic diarrhea, abdominal pain, or bloating. Giving fruit juice in a bottle, during naptime or bedtime, can lead to tooth decay (see page 259). In some cases, fruit juice may replace milk, a child's major source of calcium, in the child's diet.

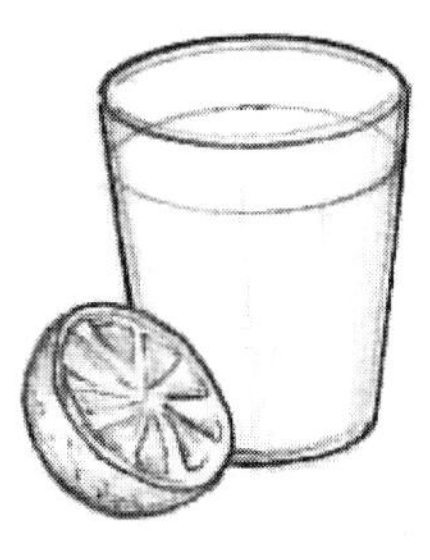

Healthy lunches

Whether you pack a school lunch for your child or serve lunch at home, follow these healthful tips:

- Use lean meats and poultry—such as white-meat turkey or chicken, lean roast beef, or tuna—in sandwiches and use low-fat condiments such as mustard or reduced-fat mayonnaise.
- Fill sandwiches with lettuce, tomato, sprouts, and other vegetables your child likes.
- Substitute sliced bananas, raisins, dates, or apple butter for jelly on peanut butter sandwiches.
- Use whole-wheat, rye, pumpernickel, or bran bread instead of white.
- Boost the calcium content of your child's lunch with low-fat mozzarella sticks, snack-size cups of yogurt, or a flavorful low-fat yogurt dip for cut-up vegetables.
- Add some fresh fruit and a small bag of carrot or celery sticks to your child's lunch.
- Substitute pretzels or graham crackers for potato chips and other high-fat snack foods.

Healthy snacks

If your child needs a snack between meals, make it a healthy one. Check this list of healthy snack foods before your next trip to the grocery store.

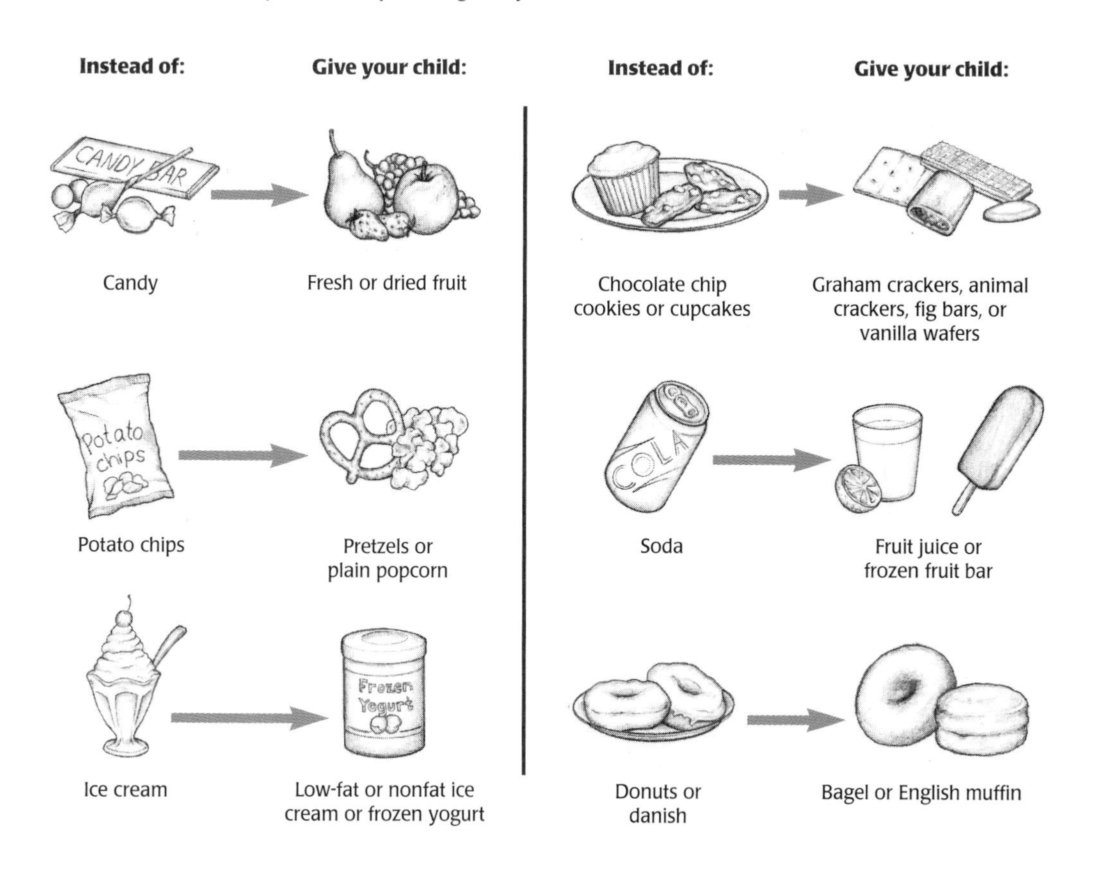

deficiencies are rare in this country. But certain disorders, such as malabsorption (see page 560), can cause a vitamin or mineral deficiency. Signs of a deficiency vary, depending on the lacking nutrient, but can include dry skin, night blindness or light sensitivity, cracked lips, bleeding gums, a fissured tongue, poor tooth development, soft bones, or fatigue. Following the recommendations of the Food Guide Pyramid (see page 113) is a good way to ensure that your child's nutritional needs are met. All fruits and vegetables are naturally rich in vitamins, minerals, and other health-promoting substances. Some fruits that are especially dense in nutrients include oranges, grapes, strawberries, kiwi, cantaloupe, peaches, and nectarines. Nutrient-rich vegetables include broccoli, tomatoes, spinach, peppers (especially red), sweet potatoes, and onions. Animal-food products (such as egg yolks and meats) are some of the best sources of vitamins and minerals, especially iron and calcium, so it's not a good idea to eliminate all of these foods from your child's diet.

CALCIUM Calcium is one of the most important nutrients for children because it builds strong bones and teeth at a time when they are developing rapidly. Your toddler should be getting about 800 milligrams of calcium each day (an 8-ounce glass of skim milk supplies about 300 milligrams and a cup of plain nonfat yogurt supplies 400 milligrams).

Encourage your child to drink plenty of milk with each meal and snack and serve other foods that are rich in calcium, including:

- Dairy products such as yogurt and cheese
- Dark-green leafy vegetables such as kale and mustard or turnip greens (spinach, although nutrient-rich, contains a substance that interferes with absorption of calcium)
- Tofu and soy milk processed with calcium sulfate (check the label) and other soybean products
- Broccoli
- Products made with legumes such as lentils, navy beans, and kidney beans

If your child dislikes many of the foods that are naturally rich in calcium and you are concerned that he or she is not getting sufficient amounts, make a point of shopping for calcium-enriched foods such as fortified orange juice, breads, and cereals. A calcium supplement is rarely needed because so many foods are calcium fortified. It also can be difficult for you to determine a safe level of supplementation; excessive amounts of calcium can actually be harmful.

IRON Lack of sufficient iron in a child's diet can cause iron-deficiency anemia (see page 412), a condition that can hinder physical and intellectual development. If your child is not getting enough iron from his or her diet, the doctor may recommend a supplement. But give your child iron supplements only if his or her doctor recommends them; excessive intake of iron is extremely dangerous and can be fatal.

What about vitamin supplements?

If your child is a picky eater, as many toddlers are, and you are concerned that he or she is not eating a variety of foods, you might want to give a daily multivitamin-mineral supplement prepared especially for children to help satisfy his or her nutritional needs. But continue to offer your child nutritious foods to choose from because supplements do not provide all the nutrients and other beneficial substances found in foods.

Good food sources of iron include:

- Meats, including beef, pork, lamb, and liver and other organ meats
- Poultry such as chicken, turkey, or duck, especially the dark meat
- Fish
- Leafy greens of the cabbage family, such as broccoli, kale, and turnip or collard greens
- Legumes, including lima beans, green peas, and dry beans and peas (such as pinto beans, black-eyed peas, and canned baked beans)
- Egg yolk
- Whole-wheat bread and rolls
- Iron-enriched white bread, pasta, rice, and cereals (check the label to determine iron content)

VEGETARIAN DIETS

Important nutrients are so widely dispersed among different foods that, even if a child doesn't eat particular foods, he or she is still likely to be getting adequate nutrition. But problems can arise when whole categories of foods are absent from the diet, such as can occur with various types of vegetarian diets. The traditional vegetarian diet, which excludes only meat, poultry, and fish and products made from them, is unlikely to cause any problems for children because they can still get sufficient protein from milk, cheese, eggs, vegetables, and cereals.

But the more restrictive vegan diet, which eliminates animal protein entirely—all dairy products and eggs as well as meat, poultry, and fish—often lacks a sufficient number of calories and essential vitamins and minerals and is, therefore, usually inadequate for growing children. A diet containing no animal food could be low in protein, calcium, and vitamins A, D, and B_{12}. Because a vegan diet's calorie count is low compared with its bulk, a child would need to eat a relatively large amount of food to meet his or her body's energy needs and have enough calories left over to promote growth and development. Discuss your child's calorie needs with a dietitian if you want your child to follow a strict vegetarian diet.

Toilet training

There is no specific age at which all children should be toilet trained. Some children show signs of being ready between 18 and 24 months; others may not be ready until they're 2½ years old or older. The right time depends on the child's readiness—both physically and emotionally—because the chances of success are best if the child has control. You can't force your child to use the toilet any more than you can force him or her to eat or sleep. You'll need lots of time, understanding, and patience. Be encouraging and quick with praise for even small progress and avoid pressure or punishment–and try to make the process as enjoyable as possible.

Avoid power struggles by not showing extremes of concern, anger, or irritation–it's easy to turn your toddler's temporary objection to using the toilet into a major problem. Your toddler is struggling to be independent and is likely to take issue with you on anything that comes up. Show your child the steps involved in using the toilet and then let him or her do them or refuse to do them. At the first sign of resistance or lack of cooperation, stop the training. Success depends on teaching at a pace suitable to your child and his or her level of interest.

When training begins after a child's second birthday, the process usually takes about 4 months. Many children become fairly reliable in the daytime by the age of 2½ years, no matter when they start training. Bowel training is often easier than training a child to urinate in the toilet because children usually have only one or two predictable bowel movements a day, while they may urinate eight to ten times a day. It's also usually easier to recognize the signs of an impending bowel movement, allowing the child enough time to get to the potty-chair. Urination is more irregular, urgent, and difficult for some children to recognize and control long enough to get to the potty-chair in time. But many children can and do control urination before their bowel movements. Either way, follow your child's lead. When a child feels in charge of the situation, he or she will be potty trained.

You can't even begin toilet training until your child realizes that he or she has wet or soiled a diaper. And then, to be able to use the toilet successfully, the child must be able to recognize the urge to eliminate. Your child may be ready for toilet training if he or she:

- Stays dry for at least 2 hours during the day or is dry after naps.
- Has bowel movements that are regular and predictable.
- Indicates through posture, facial expression, or words that he or she is about to have a bowel movement or urinate.
- Can follow simple instructions.
- Can walk to the bathroom, undress, and dress again with only a little help.
- Seems uncomfortable in soiled diapers and wants to be changed.
- Tells you when he or she has a wet or soiled diaper.
- Asks to use the potty-chair or toilet.
- Asks to wear "big-kid" underwear.

Treat bowel movements and urination in a simple, straightforward way. Before you begin toilet training, teach your child the words you want to use to describe body parts, urination, and bowel movements. Choose the words carefully because friends, neighbors, and your child's other caregivers and teachers will hear them; avoid words that could be offensive, confusing, or embarrassing to your child or others. Negative words such as "dirty," "naughty," or "stinky" can make your child feel ashamed and self-conscious.

Encourage your child to tell you when he or she is about to urinate or have a bowel movement. (Boys may initially learn to urinate sitting down.)

Before having a bowel movement your child may grunt or make other straining noises, squat, or stop playing for a moment. His or her face may turn red. Explain to your child that these are signs that he or she is about to have a bowel movement and it's time to try the potty-chair. Put the potty-chair in the child's room or wherever he or she spends the most time during the day. Having the chair in a convenient place will serve as a reminder and be less likely to interrupt play.

During the training period, your child's clothes should be loose-fitting and easy to pull on and off. Don't use diapers once your child has had repeated successes on the potty. Let him or her use cotton training pants or disposable "pull-up" trainers, or run around with a bare bottom. Disposable training pants may not be as effective as cotton ones because, for some children, they feel too much like diapers. Whenever your child is successful, give praise and encouragement but don't overdo it because too much praise can detract from the child's own excitement and pride in the accomplishment. Young children may want to watch the "action" in the toilet bowel as you flush the toilet or they may even want to flush the toilet themselves; some think the waste products are part of them and wonder where they go. Teach your daughter to always wipe from front to back in one downward motion (not in a back-and-forth scrubbing motion). This is a very important habit to develop because the female urinary opening is close to the anus, allowing bacteria to easily enter the urinary tract and cause infection.

Be prepared for "accidents" but don't punish or scold your child for them. Having a few accidents during the day means your child is trying, but consistent accidents or accidents right after getting up from the potty may indicate he or she is not

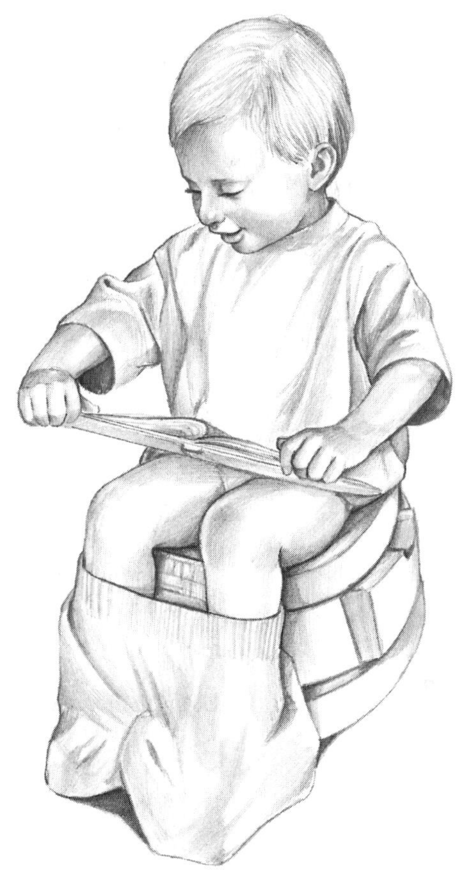

Toilet training

During toilet training, remind your child every hour to try to use the potty-chair. For small children, a potty-chair is easier to sit on than a regular toilet because their feet can rest on the floor, which makes them feel secure.

quite ready. Your child may need a little more time to learn how to relax the muscles that control the bladder and bowel. If your child seems worried or resistant to using the potty-chair or has too many accidents, postpone toilet training for a while.

To show resistance to pressure, children sometimes hold back bowel movements, which can lead to constipation (see page 284). The stool can become large and hard, causing pain during elimination. This may make your child even less receptive to using the potty. To avoid constipation, it's important to provide your child with a nutritious diet that contains adequate fiber (see page 111) to help produce soft, easy-to-pass stool. Talk to your child's doctor if your child seems uncomfortable during a bowel movement or if you notice a change in the stool. Never give your child laxatives, suppositories, or enemas unless his or her doctor recommends them. Children who are sick or hospitalized or under other kinds of stress (such as moving or the arrival of a new sibling) may regress in their toilet training. Wait until the illness or stressful situation is over before restarting training.

Many children do not stay dry through the night until age 4 or 5–and usually not before they are dry during naps and for at least 4 to 6 hours during the day. For unknown reasons, girls tend to achieve night dryness earlier than boys. Don't expect your child to stay dry during the night until your child is physically ready; the ability to control the bladder during sleep is regulated by a signal from the bladder to the brain. If this automatic signaling system has not yet developed in your child, he or she will not remain dry through the night. Keep your child in diapers at bedtime until he or she wakes up dry in the morning for several weeks in a row.

Your child will probably let you know when he or she is ready to move from the potty-chair to actually sitting on the toilet. Make sure your child is tall enough to sit on the toilet or provide a secure booster step and help him or her practice getting on and off before actually using it. Let him or her see you, older siblings, and other cooperative people use the toilet. Don't flush the toilet while the child is sitting on it because flushing can be scary to a youngster. Let your child first get used to the rushing water and the sight of things disappearing down the toilet by letting him or her practice flushing pieces of toilet paper.

Exercise

You don't have to do much to encourage a toddler to exercise. In fact, you'll have a much harder time getting him or her to slow down long enough to eat or get diapered or dressed. You're probably exhausted just watching your energetic toddler. Your job is to provide a safe environment for your child to explore and give him or her plenty of opportunity to move around. Encourage physical activity by going for walks and by spending as much time as you can outdoors. Keep the TV off. Allowing a toddler to sit for hours in front of a television can establish sedentary habits that can last a lifetime, leading to all kinds of health problems, including obesity.

Once your child has learned to stand and walk, he or she will want to be moving all day long. Let your child walk barefoot; shoes are necessary only for protection from the cold or from potentially dangerous surfaces. Walking barefoot is good exercise for the feet because the gripping action of the toes on the ground builds up the arches. There are some examples of things you can do to help your child develop strength and coordination and establish a lifelong habit of physical activity:

- Provide safe furniture and other objects for your child to practice climbing on. Pad sharp edges.
- Give your child push-pull toys; playing with these toys exercises most muscles (and also sparks a child's imagination). Let your child push the stroller.
- Make simple obstacle courses for your child to navigate; this helps improve coordination.
- Put pillows on the floor for your toddler to jump into.
- Walk, run, dance, step, jump, march, skip, and kick balls with your child to help develop his or her coordination and let him or her release energy.
- Let your child play outside on swings and slides, in sandboxes, and on riding toys or tricycles; help your child move along monkey bars.
- Practice catching, throwing, and retrieving balls of various sizes.
- Play music and encourage your child to move to it; show him or her how to twirl, spin, jump up and down, and sway.
- Give your child play objects–such as large cardboard boxes or plastic laundry baskets–that encourage crawling, climbing, and pushing.
- Gently roughhouse with your child on the floor.
- Play "Simon Says," giving simple instructions such as "Bend your knees."

Sleep

Between the ages of 1 and 3 years, most children sleep about 10 to 13 hours each day–but these hours aren't always consecutive. A toddler's energetic mobility and daily adventures are likely to disrupt his or her usual routine, including sleep. Children, like everyone else, vary in the amount of sleep they need; the best way to tell if your child may not be getting enough sleep is if he or she is tired or overly fussy during the day.

Most children give up their morning nap between 1½ to 2 years of age and take one long 2- to 3-hour nap in the middle of the day, usually after lunch. Some children continue to take two short naps; others give up naps altogether. There is often a transition period when two naps are too much but one is not quite enough. During this period, it's still a good idea to put your child down for at least one nap or for quiet time in bed with toys; he or she will usually sleep when tired and cranky enough, but don't worry if he or she doesn't. Once or twice a day, slow your child down with quiet times by engaging in calming activities such as sitting and reading a book together or going for a walk in the stroller.

Toddlers are notorious for waking during the night, often every night, and disrupting their parents' sleep. Your child may resist going to bed at night because he or she doesn't want to be away from you, doesn't want to stop the important learning he or she has been doing all day, or just needs to demonstrate the hallmark contrariness of being a toddler. A change in the normal routine—such as a new room or bed, loss of a favorite blanket or cuddly toy, or a trip away from home—can also cause your child to awaken during the night.

Keep up your usual bedtime rituals (see page 57), such as taking a bath. Read a book, sing a song, tell a story, talk over the day's events, play soft music, or massage your child when your child is already in bed and relaxed. Try to maintain the same bedtime every night, alerting your child half an hour and then again 10 minutes beforehand. Using an egg timer to indicate the actual time a child should be in bed can help reduce battles. Give your child some control by letting him or her pick out which pajamas to wear. Allow him or her to sleep with a favorite stuffed animal or other safe toy. Make it a habit to tuck your child snugly in bed and hug and kiss him or her good night.

If your child gets up after you have said good night, return him or her quickly to his or her bed without any conversation. Do this as many times as it takes. If your child gets up and walks around the house looking for things to do while everyone else is asleep, you'll need to put up a gate in the bedroom doorway. Allowing a toddler to explore unsupervised in the middle of the night can be dangerous. Once he or she stops wandering in the night, you can remove the gate.

During periods of light sleep or active dreaming, children may wake up or be restless. Some children will not awake fully and will be able to get themselves back into a deep sleep on their own. Other children become fully awake, often after a bad dream, and may cry out in fear. Nightmares are especially scary to toddlers because they cannot distinguish their imagination from reality. To help reduce nightmares, don't let your child watch any television before bedtime and don't let him or her watch potentially scary or violent shows (including cartoons) or movies at any time of the day. Restrict his or her viewing to age-appropriate educational or nature programs because many shows that you might consider safe can present images that are frightening to a child.

No one solution for night waking works for every child. What helps one child sleep through the night may have the opposite effect on another child. For example, eliminating the daytime nap may help some children sleep better at night but make other children overly tired and so tense they can't settle down enough to sleep soundly. Having a large dinner may help some children sleep better, but may give others indigestion that keeps them awake. For most parents of toddlers, it's a matter of trial and error as they respond to their child's personality and needs, their own needs, the needs of other family members, and their lifestyle. Many children have a favorite comfort object such as a blanket or a soft stuffed animal that is an adequate substitute for a parent's attention in the middle of the night, keeping them contented enough to put themselves back to sleep. A night-light in your child's room can be reassuring, especially when he or she awakens in the middle of the night.

Make it a point not to go into your child's room to check on him or her while he or she is settling down for the night unless he or she is actually awake and crying loudly—and then it's important to respond quickly. The longer the child cries, the more likely he or she is to work him- or herself up to a panic, and the harder it will be to calm the child back to sleep. Sometimes all that your child needs is a reassuring glimpse of a parent. Go in and pat your child for a while to help comfort him- or herself back to sleep. But keep any kind of stimulation to a minimum—avoid conversation, don't lie down with the child, and don't get him or her out of bed; he or she needs to know that this is the time for sleep, not play.

When your child wakes up in the middle of the night and seems to be afraid, hold, comfort, and reassure him or her. Encourage your child to talk about it. Never punish your child for being afraid or ignore his or her fears. Stay with the child until he or she has calmed down enough to go back to sleep. If he or she is persistently afraid to go to bed or has frequent nightmares, or you have other concerns about your child's sleep, talk to your child's doctor (see Sleep disturbances, page 627).

Early morning waking is common in toddlers. If your child wakes up at 5 or 6 o'clock—earlier than you want to start your day—let him or her play alone in the crib for an hour or so. Leave a safe toy or a favorite book in the crib at night so your child will have something to play with in the morning.

Most children are ready to switch from their crib to a bed at about the age of 2 years. It's best to wait until your child asks to sleep in a "big" bed like a grown-up. If your child learns how to climb out of the crib, you may want to move him or her to a bed earlier because you can't prevent a child from climbing out of a crib, and falls from a crib can cause serious injury. A good first bed is a mattress and box spring (no frame) placed on the floor, or a toddler bed, which is smaller and lower than a regular twin bed. Avoid bunk beds, because they are dangerous for young children. If you don't have a bed yet, put the crib mattress on the floor temporarily.

Most parents of toddlers complain that they feel exhausted most of the time—and can't remember their last relaxing evening or full night of sleep. But, as hard as it is to imagine now, your child will eventually become a better sleeper and will demand less middle-of-the-night attention. Talk to other parents and find out how they have coped. If you are feeling so tense and fatigued that you are afraid you might take your frustration out on your child, talk to your child's doctor.

Sexuality

Children develop their basic attitudes about sexuality during their early years, beginning at birth–from the way they are touched, caressed, cuddled, and cared for. As you hold and touch your baby, you are communicating and expressing love and acceptance and showing your baby how special he or she is. Toddlers are keen observers of how family members show affection for each other–and they quickly learn what is OK to do and what is not OK. Between ages 2 and 3, children become aware of being a boy or a girl and display this sexual identity by imitating the same-sex parent–for example, by copying the parent's walk, gestures, or smile.

Toddlers are intensely curious about their bodies. A child learns about his or her body by exploring it. When you change your child's diaper or give a bath, you'll notice him or her touching his or her genitals–because it feels good and it's comforting. Toilet training increases a child's natural interest in his or her genitals. Genital exploration and masturbation are normal and healthy for both girls and boys, who usually do it at this age when they're tired and trying to go to sleep. The pleasure young children get from touching their genitals is more general than sexual.

To keep your child from feeling bad about any part of his or her body and to promote healthy sexual attitudes, accept his or her genital play and ignore it. It's important for children to like all parts of their body and they can detect negative or positive attitudes by the way in which you, other family members, and caregivers refer to body parts. Teach your child the correct names of the genitals and other "hidden" body parts while you are diapering, dressing, and bathing him or her, and repeat the words often. Using the correct terms, such as penis or vagina, will make it easier to use these words in conversations about sex when your child is older.

Scolding or punishing your child for masturbating could instill lasting negative feelings or guilt about getting pleasure from genital play. If your child's attention to his or her genitals is disturbing to you personally, instead of scolding, try engaging his or her interest in another activity. If your child masturbates in public, tell him or her that it's fine to investigate and play with his or her genitals but that it's a private activity that people do only when they're alone in a bathroom or bedroom. Your child may not fully understand the concepts of modesty and privacy until he or she is 5 or 6 years old but you can begin teaching them now by being simple, direct, and honest.

Genital exploration or masturbation is not a cause for concern unless the child does it to the point that it interferes with daily activities or sleep or if he or she seems to be doing it to tease you. In some cases, excessive masturbation, just like excessive thumb sucking, can result from too much pressure on a child to master new skills such as table manners or using the toilet. Relax the pressure for a while and see if it helps. If the behavior continues, talk to your child's doctor about other things you can do that might be helpful.

Discipline

All children need discipline—it makes them feel secure and loved and helps them learn self-control and how to take initiative, solve problems, and get along with others. For toddlers, discipline involves setting firm limits and promoting good behavior by giving lots of positive attention and providing a loving, nurturing environment. Because toddlers talk, get around on their own, and generally participate in family life, people tend to assume they understand much more than they do about how they should behave. In reality, toddlers don't yet know that they are supposed to do what they are told; they may oblige only when they feel like it.

Unrealistic expectations can lead to constant scolding, which can make you both feel bad. Instead, respond to your toddler's needs. Spend lots of leisurely time with your child, play with him or her, and smile at, cuddle, kiss, touch, hold, rock, and hug your child often. Always keep in mind that your toddler is not deliberately being difficult or trying to make you angry. The more positive and available you are to your child, the more secure and responsive he or she will be to your requests and expectations, and the less likely he or she will feel the need to test your love and availability by acting out.

Communicate with your child in respectful tones and words—giving explanations rather than accusations. To get your child to do something he or she doesn't want to do, turn it into a game or challenge, such as "I bet you can't put your toys away before I finish folding these clothes." Instead of yelling at, threatening, ridiculing, or spanking your child for misbehaving, give positive feedback for good behavior—smiles, touches, hugs, and words of praise. Give positive reinforcement when your child shows caring behavior (such as politeness), responsibility (such as putting toys away), and following rules (such as not running with food in his or her mouth). Praise your child for learning new skills, and even for trying. The more you praise your child, the more he or she will want to try new things.

Negative approaches don't work to change behavior over the long term and can escalate to verbal and physical abuse, make your child afraid of you, and make you feel guilty and ashamed. Promises or bribes such as "If you do this, I'll do that" don't work with toddlers because they can't remember from 1 minute to the next what they agreed to. A misbehaving toddler will often respond to distraction. If the child is doing something you don't want him or her to do, offer an alternative toy or activity. You can often change a toddler's behavior by ignoring unwanted behavior and giving the child lots of attention at other times.

When setting limits for your child, choose them carefully—too many restrictions become meaningless. You can easily reduce the number of daily confrontations with your child by organizing your home and your routine as much as possible in ways that you, your toddler, and the rest of the family find acceptable—allowing your child to explore freely without being in physical danger or able to break anything valuable (see page 76). Put any objects you don't want your child to play with out of his or her reach, lock up forbidden cabinets, or block off the stairs or rooms you don't want your child to go into.

Many doctors recommend temporary time-out as an effective discipline technique, one that works for most children and parents. Time-out discourages unacceptable behavior by isolating the misbehaving child in an uninteresting (but not frightening) place, such as a chair or the corner of a room facing the wall. Decide ahead of time which behaviors will result in a time-out. Most people save time-outs for misbehavior that is potentially dangerous or that cannot be ignored, such as biting out of anger, teasing the family pet, or prolonged screaming or tantrums.

When the child misbehaves, calmly but firmly take him or her to the time-out area and set a timer (1 minute for each year of age) so the child will know when it's over. Stay within sight or hearing of the child but don't talk to him or her, and don't give him or her a toy, book, or security object. If he or she leaves the area, calmly return him or her and reset the timer. You may have to hold your child in the time-out area, but don't give him or her your attention–turn your head away and don't speak. When the time-out is over, treat the child normally, giving comfort if he or she comes to you. Don't insist that the child apologize for the misbehavior. However, you might want to restate the rule he or she broke and discuss appropriate behavior.

Here are some more ways to help reduce friction and make living with a toddler as fun and enjoyable as it should be:

- Give your toddler many opportunities to choose, but limit the number of choices. This increases his or her sense of freedom and control; for example, let him or her decide which book to read, which color cup to use, which toys to take into the tub, or which fruit to eat for a snack. But don't offer a choice when there is none, especially about safety issues such as whether or not to sit in the car seat.
- Don't have too many rules. Establish realistic expectations and avoid unnecessary arguments over issues that don't matter, such as which clothes to wear.
- Plan ahead and allow enough time for activities, such as dressing or getting into the car, so you're not rushed.
- Try to say "yes" to your child as often as you can. If you are unsure about granting a request, put off the decision for a while; otherwise, make a decision right away. When you do say "no," be firm and give a simple reason for your answer. Don't apologize to your toddler for setting limits.
- Praise your child often for good behavior. Be specific in your praise; for example, instead of saying "Good girl!" say "I'm happy you put all your toys away" or "I like it when you drink from your cup without spilling your milk."
- Be a good role model; even at 15 months, children copy aggression and other unacceptable behavior they see (including what they see on television).
- Show respect for your child and concern for his or her feelings when you have to correct him or her. Start sentences with "I" instead of "You," which is accusatory; for example, say "I feel bad when you. . ." instead of "You shouldn't. . ."

• Give simple, clear instructions to your child in a firm but friendly voice; this avoids confusion and will make your child more likely to comply.
• Instead of responding with anger when your toddler is asking for attention, give him or her a hug, a smile, or some other sign of recognition. Be aware of the times your child tends to be most demanding and difficult–such as at the end of the day when you're both tired, when you have a visitor, when you're on the phone, or when you go to the grocery store.
• Stick to your word so that your child sees the consequences of his or her behavior. If you say you are going to take something away or put your child in time-out, do so quickly if he or she continues to misbehave.

TEMPER TANTRUMS

Temper tantrums–which can take the form of crying and screaming, body-thrashing, head-banging, breath-holding, breaking objects, or jumping up and down–commonly begin between ages 1 and 2. These displays of frustration and anger reveal the toddler's inner struggle to become independent and are a normal part of development. Most toddlers throw tantrums only when they're with their parents or other caregivers, whose rules and limits they are testing. These challenges to rules and limits help toddlers learn to assert themselves. Toddlers want to be in control; they want to be independent and make their

QUESTIONS PARENTS ASK

Behavior problems

Q What do I do when my child bites or hits me?

A First and foremost, don't bite or hit back! Some parents wrongly think that biting or hitting the child back will teach a child not to do it. In fact, just the opposite is true–the child will get the message that hurting someone is acceptable behavior. Time-outs (see page 126) are effective with this kind of behavior. Also, since biting and hitting are attention-seeking devices, tell your child at a calmer time how he or she can get your attention in an acceptable way.

Q How do I get my toddler to share?

A Sharing is not a trait that most toddlers understand. It is a learned response that usually occurs when the child is a little older. When your toddler has other children over to play, put away any important toys that your child feels especially possessive of. Don't force your child to share at this age but periodically show your toddler how the process works and reinforce good behavior with praise.

own choices. They often get frustrated when their parents and other adults don't seem to understand their feelings or needs. They get angry when they don't get their way or are prevented from doing something. Simply being hungry, tired, or uncomfortable can lead to a tantrum.

You can head off many problems just by being alert to your child's moods or watching for other signs, such as sleepiness or hunger, that often precede tantrums. You can't always prevent temper tantrums but, by establishing priorities and setting reasonable limits for your child, you might be able to reduce their frequency. For example, avoid situations that could frustrate your child, such as long trips or visits during which your child has to keep still or can't play. Give your child a healthy snack if a meal is going to be late. Try to time busy or stressful activities or outings for when your child is rested. If your child is getting cranky or frustrated with a particular activity, draw his or her attention to a different one.

Children in the middle of a tantrum react differently to different approaches so you'll need to find what works best for you and your child. Generally, it's important to react calmly (reacting angrily is likely to reinforce the behavior) and avoid offering bribes to get your child to stop (or he or she will expect to be rewarded for every tantrum). Try to reduce the stress level, which will make both you and your child feel more in control. Some children respond to being picked up and held, rocked, or stroked. Others may do better being taken to a safe spot where they can work out their anger alone. Try distracting your child with something else, such as a new activity or toy, or by being funny (make a funny face or say something that usually makes your child laugh). If this doesn't work, don't persist; let your child have the tantrum. Try to ignore the behavior, unless the child is in danger of hurting him- or herself or others or if the tantrum is going on in a public place. In these situations, take the child gently but firmly to a quiet, secluded place to calm down. Some children, once they are out of control, don't know how to pull themselves together and need an adult to help them.

CHAPTER • 4

Your preschooler (3 to 5 years)

The preschool years are a period of intense and rapid intellectual and social development. Preschoolers are fiercely independent, very curious, adventurous, and often mischievous. They seem to be in constant motion but can focus on an activity longer and are more likely to cooperate when playing with other children. Preschoolers still need lots of love, attention, and firm but kind guidance from their parents. Give your child plenty of opportunities for stimulating play and allow him or her to be creative in developing new skills.

WHAT YOU CAN DO FOR YOUR CHILD NOW

Children need encouragement to grow and learn. You are your child's first and most important teacher so take advantage of every opportunity to teach your child and keep him or her safe.

- **ALWAYS PLACE YOUR CHILD IN A CAR SEAT OR BOOSTER SEAT.** Put the seat in the back seat of your car and use your car's childproof locks at all times.
- **LIMIT TV-WATCHING** to less than 2 hours of educational viewing a day. Encourage physical activities and share them with your child. Take walks, play simple outdoor games, or go to the park.
- **GIVE YOUR CHILD LOTS OF OPPORTUNITIES TO PLAY.** Children learn through play, which is a natural way for them to explore, be creative, learn to solve problems, cooperate with other children and with adults, and develop academic and social skills.
- **START LIMITING THE AMOUNT OF FAT IN YOUR CHILD'S DIET.**
- **TEACH YOUR CHILD HOW TO USE A TOOTHBRUSH** to promote good oral health.
- **ALLOW TIME FOR PLENTY OF REST**—10 to 12 hours of sleep a night and a "quiet time" or nap during the day.
- **SUPERVISE YOUR CHILD CAREFULLY** to avoid falls and other injuries.
- **INSIST THAT YOUR CHILD WEAR A SAFETY HELMET** whether he or she is tricycling or bicycling.
- **MAKE SURE YOUR CHILD HAS REGULAR MEDICAL CHECKUPS** and all the necessary vaccinations.
- **PRACTICE REGULAR HAND- AND FACE-WASHING** with your child to cut down on the spread of infectious diseases.
- **SET A GOOD EXAMPLE IN WHAT YOU DO AND SAY;** be kind, patient, and respectful to your child as well as to other people. The best way to learn consideration for other people is by example.

Your child's physical growth

Preschoolers grow at a steady but gradually slowing rate. Between 3 and 4 years of age, children gain about 5 pounds and grow 3½ inches; from the 4th to the 5th year of age, they gain about 4½ pounds and grow 2½ inches. Your child will continue to lose baby fat and gain muscle during this time, making him or her grow stronger and look more mature. The arms and legs will become thinner and the upper body narrower and more tapered. Some children who grow in height faster than in weight and muscle can look extremely thin and almost fragile at this age. This appearance is usually no cause for concern because they gradually fill out as their muscle development catches up to their height. You should be more concerned if your child gains weight faster than height because it can mean he or she may be getting too fat. If you are worried that your child's growth may not be on track, ask your doctor to measure and weigh your child every 6 months.

The length of your child's skull will increase slightly, and the lower jaw will become more prominent. The upper jaw will widen to allow room for the permanent teeth (see page 258), making your child's face look larger and the features more distinct.

Preschoolers' movements are graceful. They stand up straight, with their shoulders pulled back, and walk with an adultlike heel-to-toe gait. Stronger abdominal muscles make their abdomen look much flatter. Preschoolers enjoy activities that use their large muscles, such as running, skipping, swinging, riding a tricycle, and throwing or kicking a ball. They like to jump with both feet, dance to music, and balance on one foot. You will notice your child's increasing control over hand and arm muscles in the growing complexity of his or her drawings and in his or her skill at manipulating blocks and using scissors, modeling clay, and other materials.

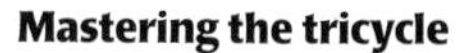

Mastering the tricycle

Preschoolers love to move around and are fascinated by their newfound ability to pedal a tricycle from one place to another. Riding a tricycle is not only fun, but it helps development of the large muscles of the arms and legs and hand-eye coordination.

Your child's development

A child's imagination begins to soar at about age 3 years when the child can originate thoughts that are not based only on the physical world. Preschoolers use their imagination in all kinds of ways–to give new functions and uses to objects and new identities to people they know. They use toys and dolls to act out events and interactions, they make up imaginary people, and they like to pretend to be someone else. These fantasies can take up much of a preschooler's time and energy and are a normal and healthy part of a child's development. Pretend play allows children to test their ideas about the world and learn about social interactions and relationships and helps them find creative ways to work out conflicts. Your 3-year-old's growing mental abilities can also bring on new fears and phobias. For example, the child's imagination can turn the shadows on the bedroom wall into a monster or convince him or her of the presence of a scary creature under the bed. By the time your child is 5, he or she will be better able to distinguish fantasy from reality.

Social interactions with peers become increasingly important. Preschoolers learn from each other how to behave. They tease, push one another to do daring things, and make each other angry or unhappy. They may treat each other as rivals one moment and babies to be mothered the next. These interactions help give a child a firmer sense of self and help him or her learn about fairness, taking turns, following the rules, negotiating, compromising, and cooperating–essential skills for success in school. Give your child lots of opportunities to be with other children.

Preschoolers are dealing with new feelings of anger. When your child lashes out, try not to react angrily. Instead, teach your child positive ways to deal with his or her feelings by talking about them. Some children find it easier to express their feelings in an indirect way. For these children it may work better to have them draw a picture and talk about it; feelings are often revealed in this way. Children who don't learn how to express their feelings in words often resort to aggression and other negative behavior.

Preschoolers still play side by side but are increasingly willing to take turns and cooperate with other children. For example, one child may cut out pictures while another glues them on a piece of paper to make a design. Reinforce cooperative behavior by telling the children how much you like the way they are working together on the project. Preschoolers are generally still too young to engage in more structured cooperative play such as that required by ball sports

The importance of friendships

A child's unique personality and temperament influence his or her social behavior. So do interactions and relationships with family members. If your child has a hard time forming attachments to other children or if you notice other children shying away from your child, your child may have a problem such as difficulty dealing with anxiety or anger. Children who are aggressive or disruptive, unable to sustain close relationships with other children, or unable to make a place for themselves in their peer group are at risk for serious problems, including difficulties in school. Talk to your child's doctor if your child is having trouble getting along with other children. If your child is naturally shy and has only one close friend, you probably don't need to be concerned, as long as your child's shyness doesn't keep him or her from enjoying fun activities such as birthday parties and family outings. Most shy children eventually outgrow their shyness.

Too much TV can be unhealthy

Good television programs can expose children to new worlds and promote learning and creativity. But sitting passively in front of a television for long periods can slow a child's social and intellectual development and contribute to being overweight. A preschool child is especially vulnerable to the influence of advertisements (especially those for junk foods and toys). Excessive exposure to violence on television can make a child extremely fearful, more tolerant of violent behavior, and more likely to imitate such behavior by becoming aggressive.

Limit your preschooler's television viewing to less than 2 hours a day and carefully monitor the content. Look for programs that will stimulate your child's interest and curiosity (such as shows on wildlife, natural history, and science) and encourage reading (such as dramatizations of children's literature). If a show could be scary to your child, sit and watch it together and talk about it afterward. These discussions can reassure your child and allow you a chance to share your values and viewpoint. Starting when your child is age 3, plan with your child which shows to watch; turn the television on when the show starts and off when it's over. Try to balance watching good television with other fun activities—and never use the television as a baby-sitter.

and board games. Sharing is one of the most difficult social graces for children to learn. Help your child learn to share by letting him or her choose some toys that don't have to be shared and help him or her understand that the other toys are to be shared. Praise your child each time he or she makes an effort to share.

Preschoolers learn differently than older children and adults—their intellectual development is tightly linked to their social, physical, and emotional development. They learn through play—their brain is eager to learn and it soaks up information about the world from hands-on experiences and interactions with other people. Even an activity as simple as stacking blocks, for example, helps a child learn about geometry, shapes, and balance. Don't dampen

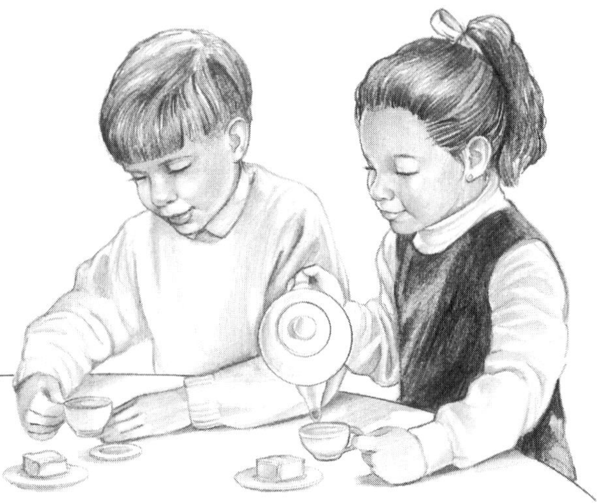

Child's play

Children learn social skills by playing with other children. Preschoolers begin to understand that it's more fun to cooperate and share than play alone and hoard their possessions. Give your child plenty of opportunities to be with other children.

your child's natural instinct to learn by forcing "academics" on your child before he or she is ready. (There is no evidence that formal instruction at an early age gives a child any lasting advantage in school.) The most effective ways to boost your child's intellectual development and guide his or her attempts to make sense of the world are to listen to your child, be in tune with his or her needs, read and talk to him or her, make him or her feel safe and loved, and encourage him or her to explore, experiment, and discover. Most importantly, have fun with your child.

DEVELOPMENTAL MILESTONES

The preschool years are a time of incredible social, emotional, physical, and intellectual growth. Each child develops skills in different areas at different rates. Use the following developmental guidelines to help you gauge whether or not you are giving your child enough opportunities to explore, experiment, and discover through play.

At 3 years:
- Knows shapes and colors.
- Can count to 10.
- Says the ABCs.
- Can ride a tricycle.
- Can copy a circle.
- Dresses him- or herself.

At 4 years:
- Moves forward and backward with ease.
- Walks up and down stairs without holding on.
- Hops on one foot.
- Throws a ball overhand.
- Catches a bounced ball most of the time.
- Dresses and undresses without help.
- Copies circles and squares.
- Uses scissors.
- Can copy some capital letters.
- Draws a person with two to four body parts in addition to the head.
- Engages in fantasy play.

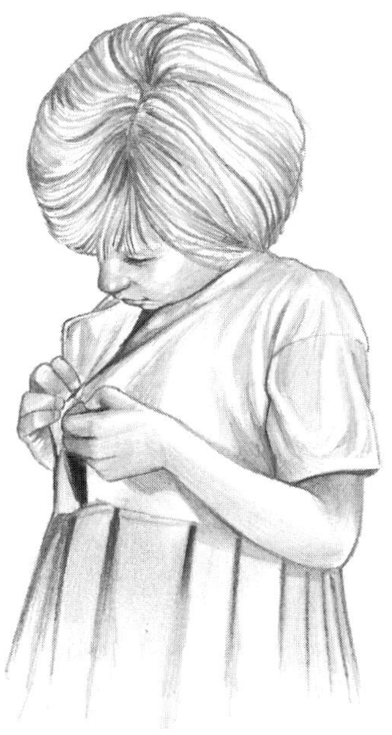

Dressing
By the time your child is 4 years old, he or she will be able to dress and undress without any help from you. This is an important step toward independence and you should encourage it by letting your child choose what to wear and by allowing sufficient time for getting dressed.

- Begins to play with other children and take turns and share.
- Enjoys silly humor, riddles, and practical jokes.

At 5 years:

- Skips.
- Hops and does somersaults.
- Swings and climbs on playground equipment.
- Uses a fork, spoon, and (sometimes) a table knife with ease.
- Draws a person with eight to ten body parts.
- Copies a triangle.
- Prints some letters.
- Uses the bathroom by him- or herself.
- Understands the meaning of numbers up to 10.
- Is very imaginative and likes to exaggerate.
- Likes to sing, dance, and act.
- Knows the difference between day and night, morning and afternoon.

BOOSTING YOUR CHILD'S INTELLECTUAL DEVELOPMENT

Throughout the preschool years, you can do many simple things to help your child grow, develop, and have fun learning. Your goal is to instill a love of learning that will last a lifetime–long after your child is out of school. Find activities that interest your child. An activity that is too difficult can frustrate and discourage a child; one that is too easy can cause boredom. If your child is not interested in a particular activity, try something else. Whenever possible, give your child a choice. Activities should be fun or they won't increase your child's excitement and love of learning. Following are some suggestions of the kinds of things you can do to promote your child's intellectual development. There are limitless ways to engage and stimulate a child in creative play; you'll be amazed at how many clever ideas you can think up on your own if you try. Remember, the brain develops most rapidly in the first 5 years of life and this is a critical time to "feed" your child's hungry brain.

- Read to your child and respond to his or her interest in learning the letters and words on the page.
- Talk to your child as you carry out everyday activities, describing what you're doing. Use numbers, shapes, and colors in your conversations.
- Shop wisely for toys; few toys hold a child's attention for long. Choose toys that have lots of uses and will spark your child's imagination and creativity. Look around your home for play items and let your child create new uses for them.
- Teach your child to do household tasks such as setting the table, washing and drying dishes, sorting

Teaching self-care

As your child grows, you can give him or her more responsibility for his or her health. When your child is in the preschool years, you still need to supervise these efforts. Preschoolers should learn to dress themselves, use the toilet on their own, and brush their teeth (see page 259) with a parent helping. Give gentle reminders to help your child develop the habit of washing his or her hands frequently, especially before and after meals and after using the toilet. Hand-washing is especially important for children who are in day care or preschool because germs spread easily among young children.

Developing skills through play

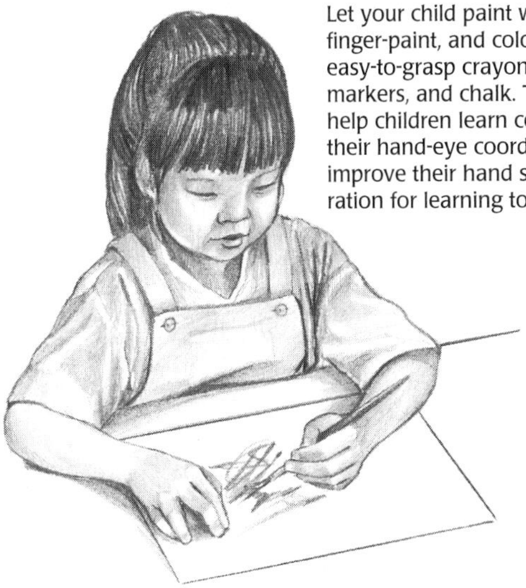

Building up to writing

Let your child paint with a brush, finger-paint, and color with fat, easy-to-grasp crayons, washable markers, and chalk. These activities help children learn colors, develop their hand-eye coordination, and improve their hand skills in preparation for learning to write.

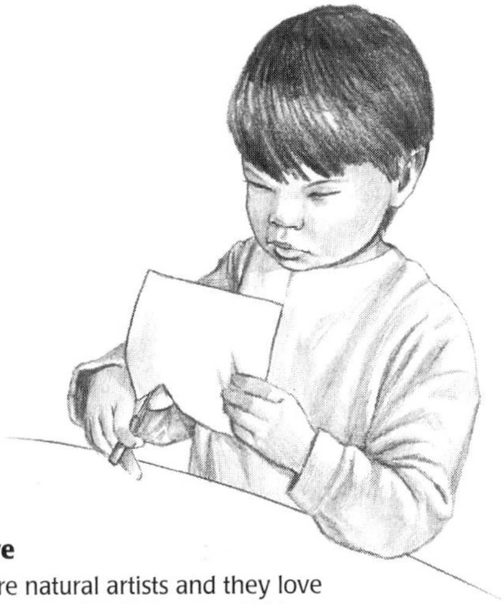

Being creative

Preschoolers are natural artists and they love to cut, scribble, and paint. Help your child develop his or her finger skills through creative play by providing paper, blunt scissors, pens, crayons, and other materials.

Sorting

Give your child opportunities to sort objects into groups according to how they look, how they are used, and other ways. The ability to categorize things into familiar groups sharpens a child's observation skills and enables him or her to learn about new objects more easily.

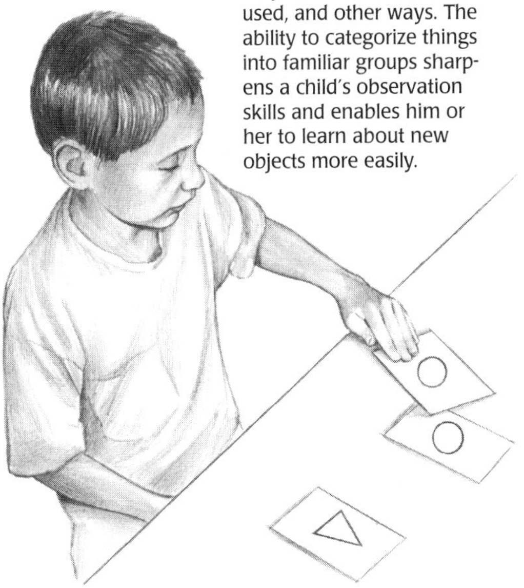

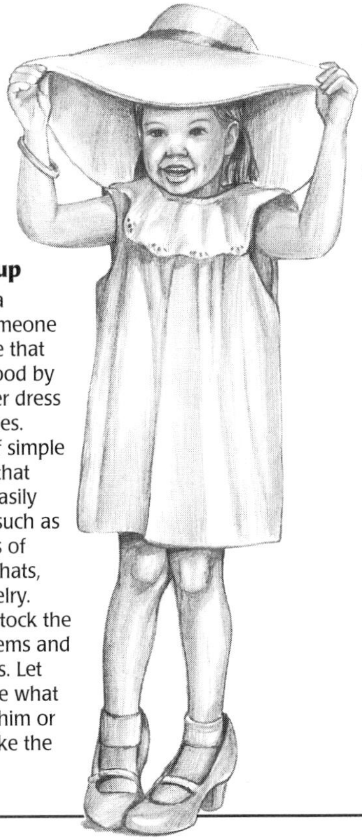

Playing dress up

Give your child a chance to be someone different and see that growing up is good by letting him or her dress up in adult clothes. Provide a box of simple dress-up things that your child can easily manage alone, such as interesting items of clothing, shoes, hats, purses, and jewelry. Occasionally restock the box with new items and remove old ones. Let your child decide what to wear and let him or her know you like the choice.

laundry, carrying out the garbage, and dusting. These types of activities help children learn new words, how to listen to and follow directions, how to count, and how to sort into groups. (Doing chores also helps children improve their physical coordination and learn responsibility.)

- Give your child building materials such as blocks and modeling materials such as clay, which teach concepts such as size, color, and shape.
- Go exploring with your child and talk about plants, trees, animals, and local geography.
- Listen to music with your child.
- Provide opportunities for your child to learn math. For example, playing with blocks can teach depth, width, height, and length, and games that have scoring, such as throwing balls into a basket, require counting. Help your child count his or her favorite toys.
- Use finger paints to show what happens when you mix colors.
- Provide opportunities for varied experiences. Go for walks in your neighborhood, take bus rides or train rides, and visit museums, libraries, and zoos in your community.
- Give your child dolls, doll clothes, play houses, dress-up clothes, and puppets to use for dramatic play. Participate in your child's imaginary scenes.
- Identify objects that go together, such as articles of clothing, animals, vegetables, fruit, and furniture. Cut out colorful pictures from magazines and catalogs and make a scrapbook, grouping them into categories. Mix and match pictures to create nonsense pictures such as placing a cat on a tricycle and talk about what's wrong with the picture and ways to fix it.
- Help your child sharpen his or her reasoning, thinking, and observation skills by asking him or her questions such as "What has four legs?"
- Engage your child in interactive play with simple games, puzzles, computer learning games, nursery rhymes, and songs.
- Discuss the weather. For example, as you look at different cloud formations, guess if it will rain that day.
- Talk about the numbers that matter most to your child–such as his or her age, home address, phone number, and height and weight–to help him or her learn important math concepts. In conversation, use expressions of time (hours, days, months, years; older, younger; yesterday, today, tomorrow), length (inches, feet; longer, taller, shorter), or weight (ounces, pounds; heavier, lighter). Answer questions about numbers simply and clearly.

Language development

Your child's language skills will blossom during the preschool years. His or her vocabulary will grow exponentially and he or she will speak in complete sentences that are several words long and follow grammatical rules. Your child will go from talking about the concrete to communicating ideas. He or she will learn abstract concepts by learning the words for them, such as round, square, tall, short, pretty, or ugly. He or she will recognize the characteristics that define a particular group and will then be able to tell or show you what they are. For example, children love learning the sounds different animals make by barking like a dog or quacking like a duck.

Preschoolers master the rules of grammar by picking out the important words from the language they hear. But, although your child's language skills sound advanced, he or she still understands things only on a literal level and is usually unaware that words can have many different meanings. Reward your child's efforts to speak by showing that you understand him or her. If his or her grammar isn't perfect, expand on what he or she has said using the correct grammar. For example, when your child says, "See dog," you might respond by saying "Yes, I see that big, brown and white dog with the long ears and I can hear him barking 'Woof-woof'. "

Preschoolers practice their new language skills by talking and asking questions endlessly, which feeds their rapid intellectual development and helps them learn about the world around them. Before, when your child asked you what something was, he or she would be satisfied with a name. Now he or she is looking for more information about the object, so try to be as descriptive as you can in your answers.

Preschoolers can pick up a foreign language readily and can learn to speak it fluently. If you have an opportunity to expose your child to a foreign language, including a preschool foreign language program, take advantage of it.

Constantly repeating the words they know helps preschoolers practice sounds and inflections and see the effects their words have on other people. They discover the words that evoke especially strong reactions and will use them again and again. If you scold your child, he or she will say the word all the more. The best response is to ignore your child's use of "naughty" words (which, at this age, are usually related to bodily functions) or say the words you would have preferred that he or she use to express feelings and thoughts. If your child realizes that the words have no special power over you, he or she will eventually get bored with them. Preschoolers learn what words are acceptable and what words are not acceptable by testing them out on people to see what reaction they get.

Preschoolers sometimes have a harder time expressing their ideas than coming up with them and, when they get excited or are in a hurry to say something, their speech may sound jerky and uneven as they search for the right words. They may even repeat words. Most preschoolers stutter occasionally–they usually outgrow this tendency as their language skills mature. Stuttering (see page 630) rarely turns into a real problem. It is best to ignore it, be calm and accepting, and try to get the child to speak more slowly. It also helps to talk to your child in a slow, relaxed way, listen to what he or she says rather than how he or she says it, give him or her plenty of time to talk without interruptions, and avoid filling in words while he or she is trying to tell you something. Don't allow anyone to tease or make fun of your child's speech. If your child continues to stutter for more than 6 months, talk to your child's doctor. He or she may recommend an evaluation by a speech and language specialist.

Unless your child shows a genuine interest in learning letters and numbers, don't bother trying to teach them formally. The eagerness to learn about letters should come from your child, not from you. You can, however, help your child understand some of the basic concepts of reading by, for example, following with your finger as you read to your child. This shows the child that words and pictures are different and that words are made up of letters, separated by a space, and go across the page from left to right. Letting your child help turn the pages will teach that pages turn from right to left.

LANGUAGE MILESTONES

The rate of children's speech development varies so widely that it's difficult to provide a timetable that applies to all children. At the same time, it's important to uncover any delays or speech problems as early as possible so that corrective measures can be taken. Talk to your child's doctor if your child does not seem to have acquired many of the following language skills.

At 3 years:

- Uses the present tense in sentences.
- Uses the concept of future tense correctly.
- Asks "what," "where," and "who" questions.

At 4 years:

- Knows own last name and several nursery rhymes.
- Says sentences of four or five words.
- Uses the concept of past tense correctly.
- Is understood by strangers.
- Names at least four colors.
- Shows an interest in schedules, such as Sunday, summer, in the morning.
- Begins to differentiate between fantasy and reality.
- Asks many questions, including "Why?"

At 5 years:

- Speaks sentences of more than five words.
- Knows street address.
- Understands spatial relationships such as on top, behind, far, and near.
- Follows three-step commands.
- Recalls part of a story.
- Likes making faces and being silly.
- Identifies coins.
- Asks questions for information.
- Uses all parts of speech.
- Tells stories.

STIMULATING YOUR CHILD'S LANGUAGE DEVELOPMENT

One of the most important ingredients for success in school is the ability to communicate. There are countless simple things you can do to help your child learn to communicate and develop a better understanding of the world. Here are just a few:

- Talk to your child. Expand your child's vocabulary and broaden his or her understanding of language and the world by explaining things in more depth and detail. For example, when talking about body parts, explain what they do. "These are my ears. I can hear music, your voice, the dog's bark, and the birds' chirping." When talking about objects, describe what they do in simple terms your child can relate to.
- Read to your child at least once a day. Talk about the stories when you're finished and encourage your child to make up his or her own scenarios.
- Visit your local library with your child and get a library card in your child's name. Spend time in the children's section browsing through books and let your child choose books to take home. Ask the librarian about story hours and other special programs for children.
- Listen to your child. Listening encourages your child to talk and helps you find out what your child knows and doesn't know, what he or she thinks or feels, and how he or she learns–and tells your child that his or her feelings and ideas are important.

Could your child have a speech problem?

Children develop language skills at different rates, so try not to constantly compare your child with other children the same age. A child who lags behind peers during the preschool years will usually catch up with them. Repeating whole words a few times is normal between the ages of 3 and 4 years. This speech pattern does not bother the child and usually stops within 6 months. True stuttering, which also first appears at this age, is characterized by repetitions of parts of words, and causes obvious distress to the child.

If your child has a speech or language disorder, a careful evaluation by a speech and language pathologist and early treatment are essential to help your child reach his or her full potential and achieve academic success. Talk to your child's doctor if you notice any of the following problems between ages 3 and 5 or if you have any concerns at all about your child's speech development. For more about speech problems, see page 630.

- Your 3-year-old says few sounds correctly.
- Strangers seldom understand your 3-year-old's speech.
- Your 3-year-old leaves out the initial consonant sounds from many words.
- Your 4-year-old leaves out final consonant sounds from many words.
- Your 5-year-old continues to substitute easy sounds for more difficult sounds.
- Your child's stuttering continues for longer than 6 months.
- While stuttering, your child grimaces, breathes faster, or shows other signs of distress.
- While stuttering, your child loses eye contact with the person to whom he or she is speaking.
- Your child stutters and a parent or sibling also stutters.

- Recite nursery rhymes and simple songs, incorporating finger plays, puppet shows, and props and music. Sing together in the car.
- Ask your child questions that require more than a "yes" or "no" response.
- Encourage your child to ask questions by always responding thoughtfully, even when he or she has already asked the same question 10 times. If you don't know the answer, say so and try to find the answer with your child.
- Keep supplies of paper, pencils, markers, and other writing materials within your child's reach. Experience with these tools will make learning to print letters easier.
- Let your child dictate a story to you and make a booklet of a few pages by punching holes in the pages and threading yarn through them. Suggest writing about members of the family, the child's favorite toys, friends, or pets.
- Print the letters of your child's name on paper, saying each letter as you write it. Whenever your child draws a picture, write his or her name on it. Spell your child's name on the refrigerator door with magnetic letters. Print your child's name on a card and put it on the door of his or her room or in a special place.
- Make an alphabet poster with your child and hang it on the bedroom wall. Label the things your child draws. Write out the names of various household objects on paper and tape them to the objects, emphasizing the sounds and the letters (start with one-syllable words). Let your child watch you writing out grocery lists, naming each word as you write it. If your child displays an interest, help him or her write his or her own list by showing how to form the letters and spell the words.
- When your child starts writing first words, respond to the content and don't be too concerned about misspellings. Make a book of your child's writings.

Feeding your preschooler

Your preschooler will continue with pretty much the same diet and daily pattern of eating he or she had as a toddler—three small meals and two or three snacks a day. Try to give your child four or more servings a day of fortified or whole grains (cereal, bread, or rice), at least five servings of fruits and vegetables, four servings of low-fat milk products, and two servings of protein (meat or legumes). That may sound like a lot, but children's serving sizes are small—an average of 1 tablespoon for each year of age. For a 4-year-old, that's 4 tablespoons or about ¼ cup (see page 113).

Food binges, food strikes, and other dietary idiosyncrasies are common during the preschool years and are a normal part of development. Preschoolers often go through food jags (periods during which they eat only a few foods for several days or weeks) and times when they eat greater or lesser amounts of food. The best way to handle food jags is to give your child the foods he or she is interested in eating but also provide other foods to encourage variety and more choices. Give your child very small amounts of new foods to taste; he or she will resist if you insist that he or she eat a large portion of an unfamiliar food. Avoid saying "Clean your plate" or "No dessert until you eat your vegetables." Using food as reward or punishment does little good and can lead to eating problems. If your child chooses not to eat at mealtimes or regular snacktimes, don't offer any foods in between. If you are concerned that your child isn't eating enough, take note of everything he or she eats over a 1- or 2-week period to get an idea of total intake, and ask your child's doctor about it.

Mealtimes are much more social now because preschoolers like the company of other people while they eat—and they are more enjoyable as meal companions than they were as toddlers. Preschoolers also like to help prepare meals and do tasks such as setting the table. (Take advantage of the times your child helps you to talk about issues such as kitchen safety, safe food handling, and cleanliness.) Your child will be more receptive to using table manners now, and the easiest way to teach them is to set a good example.

LIMITING FAT

If you haven't done so before, now is the time to start limiting your child's intake of foods that are high in fat, especially those from animal sources, such as red meat and whole-milk dairy products. Here are some tips for reducing the fat in your family's diet and helping your child develop healthy eating habits:

- Serve mostly fruits, vegetables, fortified whole grains, and legumes at meals and for snacks.
- Serve smaller portions of higher-fat foods.
- Choose low-fat or nonfat milk and other dairy products.
- When buying packaged foods, check the labels and buy those naturally low in fat—those that have less than 3 grams of fat for every 100 calories.
- For baking, cooking, and salad dressings, use monounsaturated oils such as olive, canola, and peanut oil. Avoid saturated fats (such as coconut, palm, and palm kernel oils) and hydrogenated fats, which are often used in packaged baked goods. Always check labels for the type of fat.
- Limit high-fat, high-calorie toppings such as butter, margarine, sour cream, and gravy.
- Choose lean cuts of meat and limit high-fat meats such as beef, pork, and lamb; trim the fat off the meat before cooking.
- Serve poultry, seafood, and legumes as a source of protein in place of meat; remove the skin from poultry.
- Use low-fat cooking methods such as baking, broiling, grilling, poaching, and steaming.
- Limit the number of eggs to three or four per week.
- Serve vegetable-based and broth-based soups. When making cream soups, use low-fat or nonfat milk.

ADDING FIBER

Few American children eat enough fiber (see page 111), a substance that is essential for good health throughout life. Generally, you can provide your child with an adequate amount of fiber by following the Food Guide Pyramid recommendations (see page 113) and giving your child a variety of fruits and vegetables, cereal (especially bran) and other whole-grain products, and legumes (dried peas, beans, and lentils). You still need to make sure your child is getting enough calories to provide sufficient amounts of essential nutrients to promote growth and development.

Don't give your child fiber supplements—fiber-rich foods are usually packed with lots of beneficial vitamins, minerals, and other nutrients that supplements don't provide. Fiber-rich fruits include apples, bananas, dried figs and dates, pears, oranges, prunes, and berries. Fiber-rich vegetables include broccoli, brussels sprouts, carrots, corn, peas, and potatoes with skins. Try serving legumes (good ones include pinto beans, lentils, chickpeas, and kidney beans) once a week. Milk and milk products and meat are low in fiber but fulfill other nutrient needs.

If your family is changing from a low-fiber to a high-fiber diet, increase the fiber gradually. To help reduce bloating, gas, or other problems that sometimes result from a high-fiber diet, add fiber-rich foods gradually and encourage your child to drink plenty of water and other liquids. (A good rule of thumb is to drink a glass of water for each additional serving of the drier sources of fiber such as whole grains.)

Exercise

Physical exercise is essential for good health—even in the preschool years. Preschoolers like to be in constant motion but they also love to watch television. For many, TV watching can become a deeply ingrained habit. The easiest step you can take to ensure that your child stays physically active is to keep the TV off or limit your child's viewing to less than 2 hours a day. Here are some other ways to keep your preschooler active and healthy:

- Spend lots of time together outdoors.
- Go for walks with your child.
- Go to the park or playground and let your child play on equipment appropriate to his or her age and abilities.
- Play active games with your child.
- Jump, hop, skip, dance, walk on tiptoe, and march to music with your child.
- Bounce, throw, kick, and roll balls with your child.
- Help form neighborhood sports teams and participate in them with your child.
- Be a good role model by being active yourself.

Sleep

Preschoolers generally need between 10 and 12 hours of sleep each night. Children who don't get enough sleep may be drowsy or irritable during the day and are more susceptible to illness. Like everyone else, children differ in their need for sleep. You can tell if your child isn't getting enough sleep if he or she is unusually fussy or crabby during the day, especially in the early evening. If your child attends day care or preschool, ask the teachers if your child appears tired; preschoolers who are fatigued during the day can miss out on some of the learning experiences these programs can provide.

Although many children stop taking naps at this age, it's still a good idea to put your child to bed with books or cuddly toys or have quiet times once or twice a day to calm the child down. Children this age can be overstimulated and have a hard time settling down enough to fall asleep at night even if they are tired. It is especially important at this age to establish a regular bedtime and be firm about enforcing it, even if your child doesn't always fall asleep right away. Maintain a regular bedtime routine, such as bathing and brushing teeth. Many children have an easier time falling asleep if their last 1 or 2 hours before bedtime are spent in low-key, comforting activities such as reading, telling stories, singing a favorite song, or sharing the best parts of the day. Avoid roughhousing or starting lengthy play activities right before bedtime. Turn the television off long before bedtime; some children have a hard time calming down after watching TV.

If you work full-time, it's especially important to put your child to bed at a regular time—even if it means spending less time with your child. Postponing bedtime can prevent your child from getting a sufficient amount of sleep and can turn him or her into a tired, cranky evening companion—and strain your relationship. However, focus all your attention on your preschooler at this time. You can prepare dinner and eat together, or just sit and read or talk about feelings, concerns, or each other's day. Give your child lots of lap time.

Most preschoolers sleep through the night, but they may wake up several times, check their surroundings, and fall back to sleep. If your child wakes up and calls for you, give him or her about 10 minutes to go back to sleep before you respond. If your child is still awake, go to his or her room, give reassurance that everything is all right, and leave; don't provide anything to eat or drink and don't bring the child to your bed.

Sometimes, preschoolers are awakened by frightening dreams that they think are real. If your child wakes up afraid and crying in the middle of the night, go to him or her and give comfort, support, and reassurance until he or she has calmed down. If your child seems to have frequent nightmares, talk about dreams and the fact that

Bed-wetting

Most preschoolers wet their bed at least occasionally while they are going through nighttime toilet training. Some children who have stayed dry for a number of days or weeks may suddenly start wetting the bed, often after a stressful event or change in their lives. In these cases, it's best not to make an issue of it; just go back to using training pants at night for a while. If the problem persists, talk to your child's doctor; he or she may recommend an enuresis (bed-wetting) treatment program (see page 429).

Bedtime rituals

Children thrive on daily routine, and one of their favorites is being read to at bedtime. Try to read to your child every night; it's a chance to be close, share an experience, and relax—and it stimulates the development of your child's brain.

everybody has them. You can even read stories together about dreaming and sleeping. If the nightmares become so frequent that your child is afraid to go to sleep, talk to your child's doctor; he or she may be able to determine the underlying cause and recommend things you can do to help your child overcome his or her fears (see Sleep disturbances, page 627).

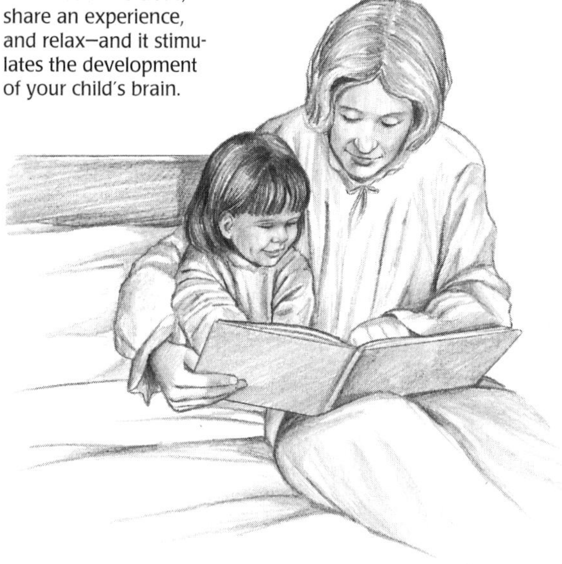

Some preschoolers experience sleep disturbances called night terrors (see page 627)—the child wakes up an hour or so after he or she has fallen asleep and appears to be awake and very upset, even screaming, kicking, or thrashing. This disturbance can go on for 10 to 30 minutes until the child calms down and goes back to sleep (and remembers nothing of the incident in the morning). A child having a night terror will not respond to anything; all you can do is hold the child to prevent him or her from getting injured. Some children have just one episode of night terrors while others have several. It's rare for night terrors to occur frequently or over a long period. In most cases, they are no cause for concern and stop as the child grows older. But, if your child has frequent night terrors, talk to the doctor.

Sexuality

Preschoolers are intensely curious about sex. Sexual exploration with peers is common among 3- and 4-year-olds, usually taking the form of playing "doctor," getting undressed together, and looking at each other's genitals. This is how they learn about sexual differences. If you come upon your child and a friend playing in this way, don't overreact by scolding. Instead, suggest that both children ask you questions about their bodies. You might explain that they are getting older now and older children and adults are expected to keep their bodies covered in public.

You can foster healthy feelings about sex by answering your child's questions as they come up. Being open and responsive now will make your child more likely to continue to communicate with you about sex and other personal issues as he or she gets older. You want your preschooler to learn about sexuality from you rather than from friends, television, or movies. Answer your child's questions honestly, in straightforward, simple terms, using the correct names for body parts and providing only as much information as you think he or she can understand. Don't explain sexual intercourse at this point. Gradually add new details as your child gets older and understands more. It's more important to set aside a child's misconceptions by asking "What do you think happens?" than to spell out more details than a child can absorb.

If you are uncomfortable discussing sexuality with your child, read a picture book about the subject together. When choosing a book, go through it first to make sure you are comfortable with it. The book should be written in a tone acceptable to you, in language your child can understand, and should not stereotype men's and women's roles. Help your child see that sexuality is a valuable part of a loving, trusting relationship between two people; set a good example by exchanging warm hugs and kisses with your partner in front of your child.

When your child is about 3 years old, depending on your family's feelings about nudity and privacy, stop bathing and showering with your child, especially a child of the opposite sex. Four-year-olds start showing some modesty about their bodies and an understanding of the difference between private and public behavior. Close the bathroom door when you use the toilet and close the bedroom door when you get dressed. Suggest that your child do the same. Teach your child that masturbation is fine to do when he or she is alone in the bedroom or bathroom, but not in front of other people.

Three years of age is also a good time to teach your child the difference between good touching (friendly hugs and pats on the back) and bad touching (the touching of private parts of the body that are usually covered by a bathing suit). You may also discuss unwanted touching (such as kissing or rubbing anywhere on the body that might make your child uncomfortable). Make sure your child understands that his or her body is private and no one should be allowed to touch it without his or her permission. For more about preventing sexual abuse, see page 327.

By about age 4, girls may become intensely attached to their father and boys to their mother. This behavior is a normal part of personality development and will pass with time, especially if you overlook it. If you are the parent who is being temporarily ignored, be patient and try not to take it personally or feel rejected–it will pass. Make an extra effort during this time to plan special outings alone with your child.

Discipline

If you have been firm, reasonable, and consistent in setting limits and disciplining your child up to now, he or she is probably beginning to show more self-control. Continue the discipline techniques (see page 126), such as time-outs, that have worked for you and your child. For preschoolers, time-outs are still usually more effective in changing problem behaviors than verbal explanations, warnings, and instructions. But, as your child's language skills develop,

QUESTIONS PARENTS ASK

Behavior problems

Q How do I get my child to listen?

A First, make sure your demands are reasonable. Keep instructions simple and direct by telling your child exactly what you want him or her to do (don't complicate matters by describing what you don't want). If your child persistently disregards you, use time-outs for a younger child and loss of a privilege for an older child. Use rewards as simple as praise when your child complies.

Q How do I get my 4-year-old to play with other children?

A Children vary in the ages and manner they can cooperate with other children. Encourage your child to play with other children whenever possible to develop his or her social skills. Have periodic play dates with one or two children in your home so that you can observe your child on familiar ground. Intervene if a touchy situation occurs by explaining the proper behavior in that instance, but don't interfere too much in minor squabbles. Understand that children this age often have a hard time sharing toys. They are often better behaved at other children's homes. Reassure your child that he or she will make more friends as time goes on.

reasoning should play an increasingly large role in improving your child's behavior. Give positive reinforcements for your child's good behavior; preschoolers often respond to visual rewards such as stars or check marks on graphs or calendars.

Take advantage of your preschooler's growing understanding that actions have consequences and help him or her take increasing responsibility for his or her behavior. When disciplining your child, offer alternatives that are logically related to the child's behavior and give the child a choice. Present the consequences of inappropriate behavior in a firm, but gentle voice. If you speak angrily, your words become a threat. Always be prepared and willing to follow through. Choose your battles carefully–decide ahead of time what issues are important to you and which ones you're willing to be flexible about. Remember that you are the most important role model your child has, so always be fair and controlled in your own behavior and treat your child with respect.

Temper tantrums

Temper tantrums usually occur less often and are less severe by about age 4 years. Tantrums that continue frequently well into the fourth year may be a sign of emotional problems. Talk to your child's doctor if:

- Your child's tantrums continue or get worse.
- Your child destroys or damages things during tantrums.
- Your child injures himself or herself or others during tantrums.

CHAPTER • 5

Your school-age child (5 to 11 years)

School-age children have a growing need for privacy and independence from their parents. At times, this changing relationship can be confusing, causing tension and conflict between you and your child. The best way to prevent or reduce problems is to keep the lines of communication open, be available, and stay emotionally connected. Your child will go through a number of transitions, such as starting school, changing classrooms and teachers, making new friends, and trying new activities. As your child faces these challenges, give him or her your love, support, and attention. Keep in mind that your major goal as a parent is to prepare your child to eventually succeed in the world outside the family.

WHAT YOU CAN DO FOR YOUR CHILD NOW

School-age children spend more and more time away from home, but they still need the care and love of their parents to feel safe, secure, and happy.

- **SPEND TIME WITH YOUR CHILD.** Find enjoyable activities to do together, and attend your child's athletic games, music recitals, or other special events. The time and energy you give to your child represents your love and acceptance.
- **PROVIDE YOUR CHILD WITH THE RIGHT KIND OF SAFETY GEAR AND EQUIPMENT** such as a helmet for biking, and knee pads, elbow pads, wrist braces, and a helmet for in-line skating or skateboarding.
- **BE SURE YOUR CHILD IS ALWAYS BUCKLED UP** in the back seat of the car.
- **ENCOURAGE PHYSICAL ACTIVITY;** set a good example by walking, running, biking, skating, swimming, dancing, or participating in a sport with your child.
- **SET CLEAR EXPECTATIONS FOR SUCCESS IN SCHOOL.**
- **ACCEPT YOUR CHILD'S INDIVIDUALITY, TALENTS, AND PERSONALITY.**
- **TEACH YOUR CHILD THE TRAFFIC SAFETY RULES** and show him or her how to cross the street (when he or she is over 7 years old).
- **KEEP HEALTHY FOODS AROUND THE HOUSE FOR NUTRITIOUS SNACKS.**
- **WHENEVER POSSIBLE, LET YOUR CHILD MAKE DECISIONS** and assume more and more responsibilities to show your trust.
- **EDUCATE YOUR CHILD ABOUT SUBSTANCE ABUSE.**
- **WARN YOUR CHILD ABOUT TALKING TO STRANGERS;** play act handling an uncomfortable or threatening situation.
- **KEEP THE LINES OF COMMUNICATION OPEN ABOUT SEX.**
- **BY AGE 8, PREPARE YOUR CHILD FOR THE CHANGES THAT PUBERTY WILL BRING.**

Physical growth

Children continue to grow gradually but steadily between ages 5 and 10, gaining an average of about 3 to 6 pounds a year and growing in height by about 2 inches a year. Most children alternate between growth spurts and periods of little growth. Boys and girls remain similar in size and body proportions. School-age children tend to look thinner than they did as preschoolers because their entire body size increases while the amount of body fat stays about the same. The long bones in the legs continue to grow, making the legs longer in proportion to the rest of the body. Muscle mass increases during this time, making children stronger and more coordinated. You will notice gradual improvements in your child's motor skills such as tying shoes, riding a bicycle, or catching a ball.

Your child's ultimate height depends primarily on heredity. If both you and your partner are short, your child is likely to be short too. Nutrition and exercise also play a role. Children this age need a nutritious, well-balanced diet (see page 112) and lots of physical activity. Physical activity makes the bones denser and stronger and promotes normal growth. If your child seems unusually short or tall compared with other children the same age, talk to your child's doctor. He or she may recommend testing to determine if your child has a growth disorder (see page 513).

The first signs of puberty (see page 165) can appear as early as age 8 in girls and 9 in boys (or as late as 13 in girls and 13½ in boys). Keep track of the changes in your child's body (while respecting his or her need for privacy). Keep in mind that there are wide variations in the normal pattern of development during this time. If your child is growing more slowly or faster than other children the same age, explain that these variations are normal and all children eventually catch up with each other. However, if you notice pubertal changes in a daughter before age 8 or in a son before 9, talk to your child's doctor. He or she will need to examine your child to rule out a problem, such as a hormone imbalance.

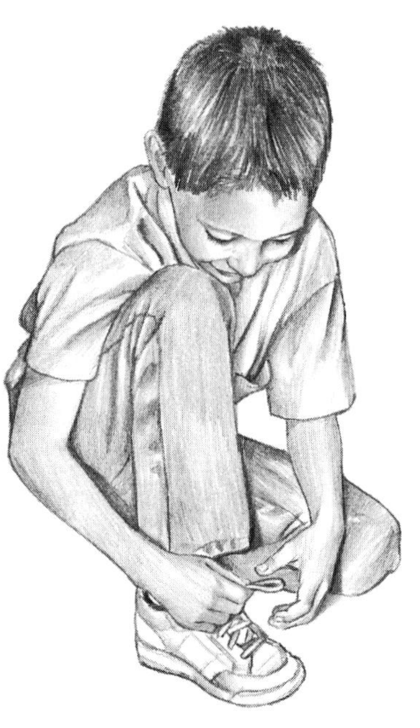

Tying shoes
A 5-year-old's finger skills and hand-eye coordination are developed enough that he or she can learn the complicated task of tying shoes.

Emotional, social, and intellectual development

Recent research on the brain shows a dramatic spurt in learning between ages 4 and 10—when the brain is most biologically equipped to learn. Although the brain can learn new skills throughout life, it will never again be quite as active and receptive as it is during these years. During this time the brain eagerly seeks information from the senses as it decides which brain cell connections to keep and which ones to eliminate. Connections that are not reinforced by stimulation from the outside world are trimmed away until, by about age 12, the brain's basic architecture has been formed.

Learning a foreign language and other skills such as playing a musical instrument become more difficult after age 12 because the brain has to work harder and more indirectly to commit these skills to memory by building new connections and breaking apart old ones. For instance, a child under 10 years old who moves to the United States from a foreign country can pick up English with ease, while his or her parents struggle to learn the language and, if they do, never completely lose their native accent. Music lessons affect the physical wiring of the brain by increasing spatial reasoning (the ability to recognize variations in the shapes and positions of physical objects), a skill that is used in physics, mathematics, and engineering.

While you should expose your child to learning opportunities—such as music lessons, athletics, dance, and foreign languages—don't overload him or her with too many activities or force him or her to do them. Let your child choose the activities he or she enjoys. One or two extracurricular activities is plenty for a school-age child because most activities require a degree of emotional and physical investment. Praise your child's achievements—successful experiences create a positive self-image. Children this age tend to take criticism personally and don't know how to accept

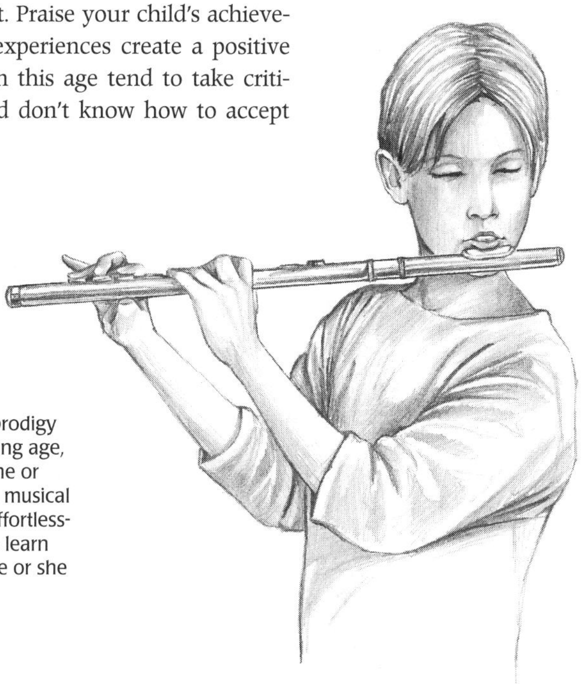

Music lessons stimulate the brain

Although you can't guarantee your child will be a prodigy by signing him or her up for music lessons at a young age, learning music will be a lot easier now than when he or she gets older. Although people can learn to play a musical instrument at any age, they can do it much more effortlessly before age 12. Give your child the opportunity to learn to play an instrument—but don't force the issue if he or she isn't having fun.

Encouraging good hygiene

School-age children become increasingly independent and take on more and more responsibility for their self-care. They learn to bathe themselves and wash, comb, and brush their own hair. Continue to reinforce your child's good habits, such as hand-washing, tooth-brushing, and flossing. Remind your daughter to always wipe from front to back after using the toilet to avoid urinary tract infections (see page 657). To avoid soreness around the anus in either a son or daughter, make sure your child does a good job wiping after using the toilet (check underwear for stains). By about age 10, children become much more focused on their appearance, paying increasing attention to the style of their hair and clothes.

failure, so try to concentrate on your child's successes and teach him or her how to learn from criticism.

School-age children need time to play with their friends, so they can learn to socialize. They begin to spend more and more time with their peers and less with their family. At 6 or 7, most children have one or two close friends of the same sex. As they get older, they generally have a few close friends, but these preferences tend to change frequently. Children usually befriend other children who are like them, with a similar temperament or similar interests or hobbies. Know the children your child makes friends with. A healthy friendship is one in which both children are on equal ground—neither one dominates the other or makes all the decisions. If your child has only one very close friend, don't worry about it as long as the relationship is positive for them both and doesn't limit their range of experiences.

Peer influence becomes stronger at around age 8, when children may form groups, or cliques. Membership in a group makes children feel secure and gives them a sense of identity, sometimes pressuring them to take on similar characteristics, such as dressing or talking in a particular way. If your child is spending time with children whose values you question, try to encourage friendships with other children whose behavior you approve of. You might suggest inviting another child over to play or to go on an outing. Instead of forbidding your child to play with a child, talk about the aspects of the child's behavior you don't like, without criticizing the child's person or character. Discuss the consequences of such behavior.

HELPING YOUR CHILD SUCCEED IN SCHOOL

Helping your child embrace a positive attitude toward learning and school is one of your most important jobs as a parent. You can do this by conveying a positive attitude yourself and making your home a place that accommodates and encourages studying and learning. Provide a quiet place for your child to study and help him or her plan and schedule daily activities such as studying, playing, and doing chores. Review your child's homework but resist the temptation to do it for him or her because this deprives the child of the opportunity to learn and progress academically. Instead, encourage him or her to solve problems independently. Teach the importance of striving to learn something new and interesting, or something that seems difficult at first. If your child has trouble with homework, talk to his or her teacher.

Keep in contact with your child's teachers. Monitor your child's progress through reports from teachers and by attending school open houses and parent-teacher conferences. If you are worried that your child is not doing well,

Is your child ready for school?

Starting school is one of the major transitions in a child's life and, for many children, it can be daunting. You can make your child's first days easier by visiting the school ahead of time to let your child see his or her classroom and meet the teacher. Take the walk to school several times in the weeks before school starts, pointing out landmarks along the way.

The skills listed here are common indications that a child is ready for school. If your child cannot perform some of them, it doesn't necessarily mean that he or she is not ready for school. It may simply mean that he or she hasn't had the opportunity to try them. Work with your child on the skills he or she doesn't have yet. If your child cannot perform most of the skills, talk to your child's doctor. Or ask the school principal and kindergarten teacher for their feedback.

A school-age child usually:

- Knows his or her first and last names.
- Knows his or her home address and phone number.
- Pays attention when read to.
- Follows instructions.
- Dresses without help.
- Can hold a pencil.
- Likes to write and draw and may write his or her own name.
- Can count (and may be able to count by twos, fives, or tens).
- Can copy shapes such as circles, squares, and triangles.
- Can sort objects by color, shape, and kind.

talk to the teacher or principal about special resources such as a reading specialist, guidance counselor, or tutor who can give your child the extra help he or she may need.

Your child's success in and enjoyment of school depend in large part on his or her language skills, particularly the ability to understand speech and to read. The kind of support and encouragement you give in helping your child become a reader will change as he or she gets older. Children who become skilled readers and who enjoy reading in their free time are likely to succeed in school, especially if their parents show they expect them to be successful.

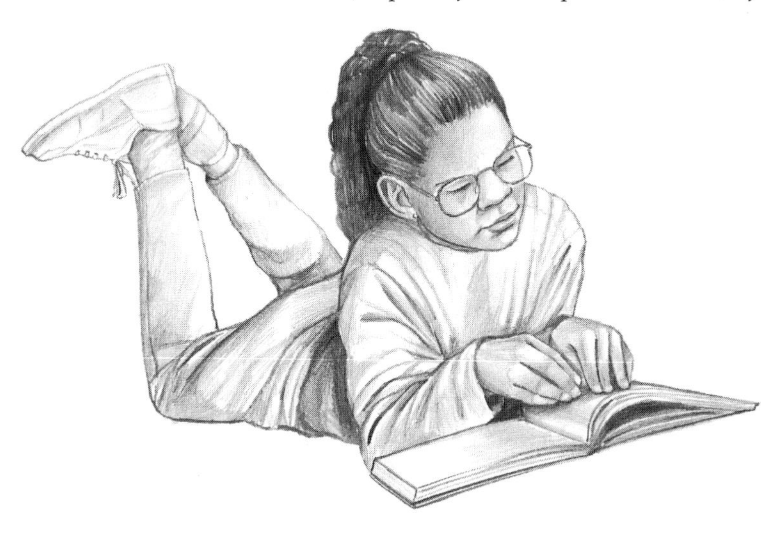

The joy of reading
Instill a love of reading by giving your child a wide range of reading materials, including books, comics, newspapers, and magazines (children love having a subscription to a magazine geared to their interests). Make them available throughout the house and let your child choose what to read. Let your child see you reading for pleasure.

Here are some things you can do to instill a love of reading in your child:

- Read with your child whenever you get a chance.
- Set up a bookcase in your child's room. Put a reading lamp next to your child's bed and let him or her read in bed.
- Take your child to get a library card and visit the library frequently.
- Suggest reading whenever your child is bored and looking for something to do.
- Encourage your child to write; for example, suggest corresponding with pen pals (even by e-mail), keeping a journal, and writing stories (on paper or on the family computer).
- Let your child see you reading for enjoyment. Take the time to read a book your child enthusiastically recommends.
- Look up words in the dictionary with your child.
- Help your child learn to use an encyclopedia or the Internet to gather information.

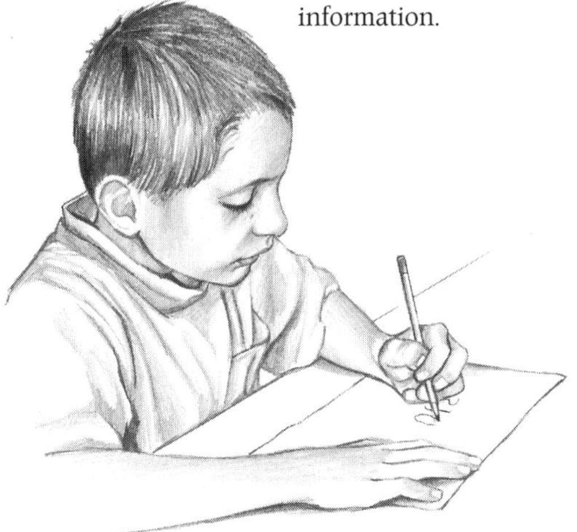

Learning to write
By the time your child is ready for school, he or she will probably be able to print his or her name. Once able to do this, your child will probably want you to show him or her how to write other words as well. Provide plenty of chances to practice this essential skill by placing labels on objects throughout the house.

Feeding your child

Once children start going to school and getting involved in after-school activities, it becomes increasingly difficult to schedule family meals together. Try to have at least one meal a day with your child and continue to provide a nutritious, well-balanced diet following the Food Guide Pyramid recommendations (see page 113). Whenever possible, involve your child in meal planning and preparation and take advantage of trips to the grocery store to teach the basics of nutrition by reading labels.

Many school-age children are tempted to eat high-fat, high-calorie, high-sodium foods that have little nutritional value and often take the place of more healthful foods. You can't always control what your child eats outside the home, but you can limit his or her consumption of junk foods by not making them available in your home. Many children this age are picky eaters and have unpredictable preferences for certain foods and dislikes of others. Don't worry about picky eating and don't give in to your child's desire for junk food because you think he or she is not eating enough. Serve a variety of foods and encourage your child to taste them. Most children outgrow this pickiness with no harm to their growth or development. If your child is losing weight or gaining too much weight, talk to your child's doctor. On average, school-age children should eat the following foods for optimum nutrition and health; older school-age children will eat more than younger ones:

- Six or more servings a day of whole grains such as breads, cereals, or pasta. One serving is equal to one slice of bread, 1 ounce of ready-to-eat cereal, or ½ cup of cooked cereal or pasta.
- Three or more servings of vegetables, especially leafy dark-green ones or deep yellow ones. One serving is equal to 1 cup of leafy greens or ¼ to ½ cup of chopped raw or cooked vegetables.
- Two or more servings of fruit, especially citrus fruits, melons, or berries. One serving is equal to one small fruit, ½ cup of chopped or cut fruit, or 1 cup of berries.
- Two or more servings a day of dairy products such as milk, cheese, or yogurt. A serving is equal to 1 cup of milk or yogurt or 1½ ounces of cheese.
- Two servings of lean meat, poultry, or fish, or alternatives such as eggs, legumes (dried peas and beans), nuts, or seeds. A serving is equal to 2 to 4 ounces of cooked meat. One egg, ½ cup of cooked dried beans, or 2 tablespoons of peanut butter equal 1 ounce of meat.

A good breakfast is essential—it provides energy, improves concentration, and sharpens performance in school. Serve foods for breakfast from as many different groups as your child will accept—especially milk, whole grains, fruit, and protein. Try combinations such as peanut butter or cheese slices on toasted whole-wheat bread, a shake made with milk or yogurt and fresh fruit, or sliced fruit on cereal. (Choose cereals that contain 6 grams or less of sugar per serving; check the label.) For ideas about healthy snacks and lunches to pack for school, see page 115.

SCHOOL LUNCHES

If your child's school provides breakfast or lunch, make sure that the meals are nutritious and well-balanced by asking for a weekly menu of school meals. The biggest problem with school lunches is likely to be an excess of fat and sodium, not the lack of sufficient nutrients. If you don't feel that the school meals are up to your standards, express your concerns to the principal, other parents, members of the parent-teacher group, and the school board and encourage them to take steps to provide healthy school meals. Efforts such as these have sparked many school food service departments to take healthful measures such as revising recipes, using lower-fat cooking methods, reducing sodium, replacing whole milk with low-fat or skim milk, and reducing the serving sizes of meats. If the school is unwilling to change its lunchtime offerings, pack a healthy lunch for your child yourself. Continue to teach your child to make healthy food choices and make sure he or she understands the importance of a healthy breakfast and lunch.

DISCOURAGING OVEREATING

American children are becoming fatter and fatter. If you think your child is overweight (see page 580), don't put him or her on a diet. Talk to your child's doctor, who can determine if your child is truly overweight and who can recommend a sensible, healthful weight-loss plan. Discourage your child from eating while watching TV, reading, studying, or riding in the car (children who are distracted by other activities while eating tend to eat more). Allow eating only when your child is sitting down at the kitchen or dining-room table. Try to persuade your child not to eat on-the-run and to eat only when he or she is hungry. The goal is to help your child develop good habits that can be followed throughout his or her lifetime.

First concerns about body image

Although body image and self-image do not seem to be as closely linked in boys as in girls, changes in the size and shape of their bodies strongly affect how both boys and girls feel about themselves. Many girls who are diagnosed with eating disorders (see page 478) actually developed their distorted body image as early as age 7. Even at this young age, some girls become preoccupied with their weight and try to limit their intake of food in unhealthy ways.

Nurture in your child a healthy body image and attitude toward food. Consider your own body image and feelings about food and eating. Children are very good at tuning in to their parents' unspoken values. Praise your child for accomplishments, not appearance, and avoid using food as a reward or punishment.

Exercise

Exercise is as essential to good health as eating and sleeping. Exercise boosts the heart's endurance by making it pump more efficiently, improves the strength and endurance of the large muscles in the legs and arms, increases flexibility, helps maintain a healthy weight, and reduces stress. Children who develop a habit of physical activity at a young age are more likely than sedentary children to be physically fit adults.

Encourage your child to be physically active. Good activities for school-age children include cycling, brisk walking, jogging, soccer, swimming, basketball,

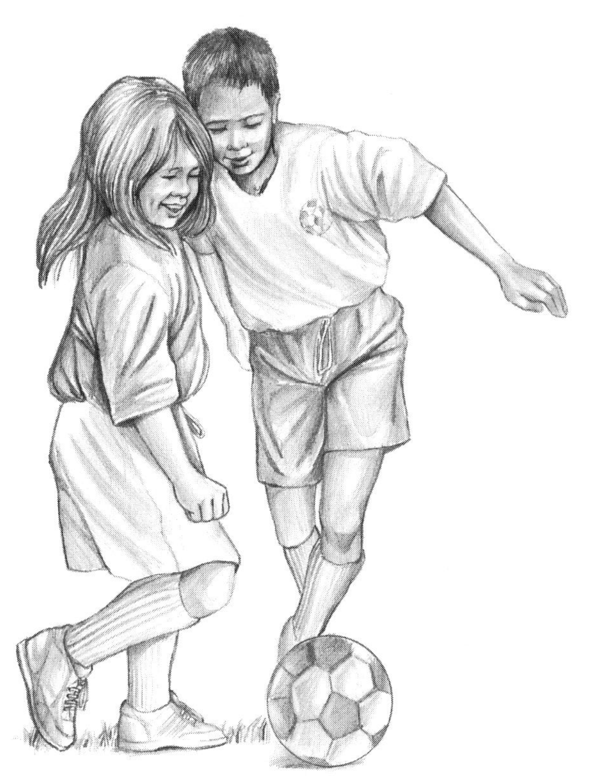

The benefits of exercise

Your child needs to exercise often and vigorously. For some children, participating in an organized sport is a fun way to exercise and can help them learn about teamwork and sportsmanship. The important thing is to encourage your child to participate in a physical activity he or she truly likes.

dancing, and skating. Suggest walking or biking instead of riding in a car. Make walking the dog one of your child's chores. Give your child opportunities to participate in recreational sports activities that develop his or her athletic skills.

Don't force your child to participate in an activity he or she doesn't enjoy, or one that doesn't suit his or her abilities. Let your child choose. Many team sports involve some physical impact (contact) with another person. If your child chooses to participate in a high-contact sport, make sure he or she wears the appropriate protective equipment, and that it fits properly. When choosing an athletic program for your child, look for programs that give all team members equal playing time, regardless of their skill level, and that emphasize learning good sportsmanship, mastering the skills of the sport, participating, and having fun–not just winning. Safety rules should be followed during practices and games and use of appropriate protective equipment should be required. Coaches should have a strong knowledge of the sport (which tends to reduce the risk of injury).

LIMITING SEDENTARY TIME

Although television offers many high-quality educational programs and can open up the world for children, it can also become a habit that does more harm than good to a child's social, emotional, and intellectual growth. Time spent watching television can stunt creativity and language development by taking the place of activities that nurture these skills, such as playing, reading, doing homework, and interacting with other children and adults. The amount of time a child spends watching TV is strongly related to his or her performance in school. Excessive television viewing can interfere with homework assignments, reduce the amount of sleep a child gets, and discourage the habit of reading. Viewing violent programs can make children afraid, worried, or suspicious and can increase aggressive behavior. Television tends to depict sexual behavior and the use of alcohol, cigarettes, and illegal drugs in seductive ways. Watching television can also affect a child's physical well-being and development because it prevents him or her from participating in more active types of recreation.

Other types of inactive pursuits can also be harmful. Video games and computer programs (even educational ones) may engage a child's mind more actively than watching television but have the same drawbacks.

Try to limit your child's television viewing (and video-game playing) to less than 1 or 2 hours a day, or 1 hour or less on school days and 2 hours a day on weekends. Set a good example and limit your own television viewing. Keep the TV off during meals and don't allow your child to watch it until he or she has completed homework or household tasks. Encourage other activities such as reading, sports, conversation, games, or hobbies. Help your child plan which shows to watch and encourage a variety of programs appropriate to his or her age and level of understanding.

Sleep

Although children vary widely in their need for sleep, school-age children generally need about 10 hours each night. A lack of sleep can interfere with a child's ability to learn and succeed in school. Consistently enforcing a regular, not-too-late bedtime, especially on school nights, helps children develop a healthy sleep pattern and improves their ability to cope with the day's challenges. Most children stay in their room and sleep well through the night by age 6 or 7. By 7 or 8 years old, they have developed a sense of feeling tired and are more likely to go to bed voluntarily. Although sleep problems are uncommon at this age, many children may have occasional nightmares or other sleep disturbances (see page 627). Try to calm your child down before bedtime or

Bed-wetting

Most children who have an ongoing bed-wetting problem have never been consistently dry at night, usually because of a delay in physical development. Persistent bed-wetting is more common in boys than girls and tends to run in families. Most girls outgrow it by age 5 and boys outgrow it by age 6. If your child continues to wet the bed after those ages, talk to your child's doctor; he or she may recommend a treatment program (see page 429). Try not to make your child feel ashamed or embarrassed by criticizing or punishing him or her. Keep in mind that your child is not wetting the bed on purpose or out of laziness—to your child the situation is already distressing enough and your criticism may make the problem worse. Praise your child whenever he or she stays dry all night and try positive reinforcement strategies such as a calendar or chart that records and (psychologically) rewards dry nights.

when your child is overly tired by encouraging quiet activities such as reading, playing board games, drawing, or working puzzles. Even after your child learns to read, continue the habit of reading to him or her at bedtime. Let your child read in bed for a certain amount of time before lights go off.

Sexuality

School-age children are naturally curious about sex–but most parents have a difficult time discussing the subject with their children. It's much better for your child to learn about sex from you than from other children (who are likely to give lots of misinformation) or the media (who are likely to portray sex in a sensational manner or in a way that may go against your values). A sound basic knowledge of sexuality will influence your child's attitudes, beliefs, and values and his or her self-image, relationships, and intimacy throughout life. Make the effort to be your child's primary source of sexual information, keeping in mind that curiosity about sex is not the same as sexual activity. In fact, children who have accurate information about sex are less likely to engage in sex at an early age than those who lack such knowledge–and less likely to acquire sexually transmitted diseases and become pregnant as teenagers.

If your child has not asked questions about sex by age 5, bring up the subject. Take advantage of teaching opportunities such as talking about the pregnancy of a friend or relative or discussing a television show or movie that has some sexual content. As a general rule, you should answer questions about sexuality with truthful, straightforward explanations, providing only as much detail as you think your child can understand and always using the correct language for body parts and processes. As your child gets more mature, he or she will be able to accept more detailed answers. Be sure to convey that sexual feelings are normal and natural.

Find out what your child is learning in the sex education program at school and expand on it. If you are uncomfortable discussing sex, you might ask a close relative or friend to help you convey the information that your school-age child needs. Before 8 or 9 years old, a child may know some sexual facts such as how babies are born or how they are conceived but may not have come to a cohesive understanding of basic sexuality. By age 10, both girls and boys should know all of the following about sexuality:

- The correct names of genitals and other body parts
- How the reproductive system works
- How babies are conceived and born
- The physical and emotional changes both sexes undergo in puberty
- The process of menstruation
- What masturbation is
- The function of birth control
- Sexually transmitted diseases (see page 183) and how they are contracted

Masturbation is a normal and healthy way for children to explore sexual sensations. By age 6, children are aware that masturbating in public is not socially acceptable, although most will continue to masturbate in privacy in their bedroom or in the bathroom. Don't make your child feel that masturbation is bad or dirty; feelings of guilt and secrecy can impair a child's sexual development. Talk to your child's doctor if you are concerned that your child masturbates excessively or if he or she does so in front of other people.

Discipline

Your school-age child still needs your guidance to help him or her learn the self-control that is necessary to become a responsible person capable of making wise decisions and showing consideration for others. Continue to give your child lots of praise for good behavior. Positive reinforcement builds a child's confidence and promotes communication, while unkind words make children feel bad about themselves. Keep in mind that it's a lot easier to prevent unwanted behavior than to stop it.

As your child gets older, it becomes increasingly important to set clear expectations. Accept your child's input when making rules and determining consequences for unacceptable behavior. School-age children tend to be self-righteous and concerned about fairness, and like to debate and negotiate to get their way. When you and your child disagree about the rules, have an

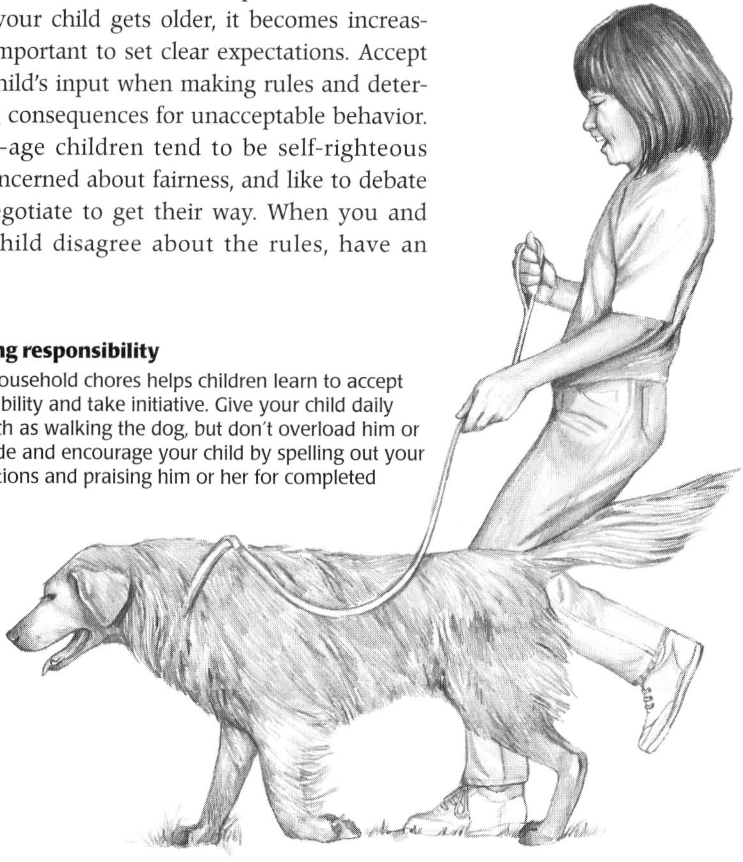

Learning responsibility

Doing household chores helps children learn to accept responsibility and take initiative. Give your child daily jobs, such as walking the dog, but don't overload him or her. Guide and encourage your child by spelling out your expectations and praising him or her for completed tasks.

Discipline at school

The discipline and self-control a child learns at home form the basis of his or her behavior at school. Children benefit when their parents get closely involved with their school, especially with teachers. Listen carefully to your child's teacher, because teachers often spot problems or warning signs of problems before parents do. If your child's teacher reports a discipline problem with your child, make an appointment to meet with the teacher and your child to work out a solution together.

open exchange of ideas and learn each other's point of view, always keeping in mind that it's your responsibility as the parent to set the family rules and values and enforce them. Never negotiate rules at the time of an infraction—stay firm on what you've said and follow through with the agreed-upon consequences.

Time-outs (see page 126) can continue to be effective with your school-age child, but you may want to add other methods such as time away from a favorite activity. You might try requiring your child to accomplish a certain number of tasks before he or she can resume a privilege.

If your attempts to guide your child's behavior don't seem to be working, ask for help. Sometimes people outside the family can see things more objectively and can offer helpful tips about discipline and other child-rearing practices. Professionals who are trained in child development and behavior can give you helpful information and recommend different approaches to try to change your child's undesirable behavior.

QUESTIONS PARENTS ASK

Behavior problems

Q How can I stop arguing with my child about every little thing?

A Pick your battles. Save your disagreements for important matters, such as safety. Don't have too many rules. Encourage your child to express his or her opinions but make it clear that the rules you do decide on must be obeyed. In spite of your child's argumentative attitude, your child cares what you think. He or she is just testing the waters and you should encourage this independence because it is necessary for your child's growth. However, insist that your child go to school and show you (and others) respect. Be firm about other issues you feel strongly about.

Q How do I get my child to help around the house?

A Tell him or her what you expect. If he or she should be taking out the garbage, walking the dog, or cleaning up the dinner dishes, say so. Don't overburden your child and don't expect perfection. But spell out the consequences of inaction or "forgetting." Loss of a privilege is a helpful way to get a child to accept more responsibility.

Helping your child resist cigarettes and alcohol and other drugs

Drug use occurs among children of all racial, ethnic, and socioeconomic groups. American children are bombarded by messages that subtly and often not-so-subtly encourage the use of cigarettes, alcohol, and other drugs. The most effective way to reduce your child's risk of using drugs is to be a good role model. Children get confused when they are presented with antidrug education and prevention programs in school but witness use of these substances at home. Children whose parents use alcohol and other drugs are much more likely to use them than are children whose parents don't use them—and children who use alcohol and tobacco at a young age are more likely than other children to go on to use other drugs.

It's never too early to educate your child about ways to resist peer pressure to smoke cigarettes or use other drugs. Start talking about these issues when your child is 5 years old–and keep talking. Don't wait until your child has a drug problem. Teach your child the health, safety, and legal consequences of using drugs and explain that, just like other drugs, alcohol and marijuana can be dangerous. School-age children are very curious and concerned about their bodies, so emphasize staying healthy and avoiding substances that might harm them. Explain how both prescribed and nonprescription medicines that may be of help during illness in the proper dosages can be harmful if misused–by being taken for wrong or misguided reasons, at inappropriate times, or in excessive doses.

If you smoke, try to quit. Never smoke in the house. Try to get family members who smoke to quit. Stress smoking's harmful effects on a person's appearance and athletic performance, and the powerful addictive hold tobacco can have on the body. Discuss adults your child knows who are trying hard to quit, often without success. Children tend to think that people can quit smoking whenever they want. Point out that chewing tobacco and snuff are just as addictive and harmful as tobacco that is smoked.

Children who start drinking alcohol at a young age are more likely to use alcohol heavily, to have alcohol-related problems, to abuse other drugs, and to get into trouble with the law. Because a child's body is smaller than an adult's, alcohol can build up more easily in a child's blood, making a fatal overdose more likely. If you have an occasional cocktail or a glass of wine with dinner, make sure your child understands the differ-

Resisting peer pressure

Help your child deal with peer pressure to use drugs. Practice role-playing with your child so he or she can learn ways to refuse drugs. When offered cigarettes, alcohol, or other drugs, suggest that he or she:

- Say "no" and show that he or she means it. This is the easiest and most direct method to use. Tell him or her not to argue about it or discuss it further with the person offering the drug.
- Give reasons. Tell him or her to say that drugs are dangerous; they can be physically addictive; and they interfere with school, family, and relationships.
- Suggest other things to do. Tell him or her that it's sometimes easier to recommend other activities–such as going to a movie or working together on a project–than say "no" to a friend who wants to experiment with drugs.
- Leave. If none of the above has worked, tell him or her to get out of the situation immediately. Go home, go to class, join a group of friends, or talk to someone else.

ence between what adults can do legally and what is appropriate and legal for children to do. Maintain this distinction by not getting your child involved in your drinking; don't ask him or her to mix a drink for you or bring you a beer, and never offer sips of your drink. Although you may think this type of behavior is harmless, a small child will not be able to distinguish the boundaries between adult behavior and his or her own.

Explain that smoking marijuana is illegal for anyone, even adults. Marijuana smoke contains more cancer-causing agents than tobacco smoke and damages the lungs and respiratory system. Smoking marijuana can reduce a person's concentration and coordination and impair motivation and learning. Over time, a person can become psychologically dependent on marijuana and the drug can become the center of his or her life.

School-age children need rules to guide their behavior, and parents need information to help their children make good choices and decisions. Use the following guidelines to help you talk honestly and forthrightly with your child and spot any potential trouble, and to help your child develop the proper attitude toward the use of drugs:

- Set and enforce rules against the use of alcohol and other drugs. Be specific in explaining the rules and the expected behavior and clearly define the consequences for breaking the rules. Be consistent in enforcing the rules; turning your head occasionally sends mixed messages to your son or daughter.
- Learn about the effects on the mind and body of alcohol and other commonly used drugs and educate your child about them, in terms of the short-term impairment and long-term health problems they can cause. Learn the symptoms of drug use so you'll be able to recognize them if your child is using drugs. Get to know the street names of drugs and what they look like and be able to recognize the drug paraphernalia associated with each one.
- Make your child feel comfortable about bringing problems or questions to you. Then he or she won't hesitate to come to you if he or she has concerns about or problems with drugs or alcohol. Listen carefully and don't allow your anger over something your child says to end the conversation. When responding to your child, avoid being judgmental or accusatory.
- Get your child involved in a variety of activities and work with other people in your community—through clubs, schools, churches, and neighborhood groups—to sponsor and promote safe, healthy programs for preteens and teenagers.
- Talk with your child about the glamorous images of drug use in the movies, on TV, and in rock music lyrics. Ask your child's opinion about these messages. Help your child recognize that these messages do not present the other side—the harmful effects of drugs.
- Know where your child is at all times and get to know your child's friends.
- Ask for help if you need it. Many hospitals, community colleges, and other organizations offer classes to help parents communicate with and understand their children. You can get information from your local library, school, or community service organization.

If you suspect that your child is using alcohol or other drugs and you feel that you can't talk to him or her about it, ask the doctor to speak to your child in private. Should your child's drug use escalate into abuse or addiction, the doctor can refer your child to the appropriate treatment program. Treatment encourages a drug-free lifestyle and seeks to nurture family relationships and teach strong coping skills.

CHAPTER • 6

Your preteen and adolescent (11 to 21 years)

Adolescence is a time of rapid physical, intellectual, social, and emotional growth. It can also be a time of increased stress because teenagers have to cope not only with the changes in their bodies, but also with the pressure to conform to social trends and higher expectations from adults. Parents and family are the most important influences for most teenagers, despite the increasing importance of their peers. Educate yourself about adolescent development so you know what to expect and can watch for signs of problems early, when they are easiest to address.

WHAT YOU CAN DO FOR YOUR CHILD NOW

Although your child is becoming more independent and mature, he or she still needs your love, guidance, and patience. Help your teenager learn to be a responsible, self-disciplined adult who will use good judgment about his or her life.

- **TALK WITH YOUR CHILD ABOUT WAYS TO HANDLE THE PRESSURE TO ENGAGE IN RISKY BEHAVIORS,** such as using alcohol or other drugs, smoking, or having sex (see page 195).
- **PROVIDE NUTRITIOUS, WELL-BALANCED MEALS** and snacks (see page 112).
- **ENCOURAGE YOUR CHILD TO BE PHYSICALLY ACTIVE.** Plan family activities—such as swimming or taking walks—that involve exercise.
- **MAKE SURE YOUR CHILD GETS ENOUGH SLEEP,** especially on school nights (see page 193).
- **TEACH YOUR DAUGHTER HOW TO DO A BREAST SELF-EXAMINATION** (see page 173) **AND YOUR SON HOW TO DO A SELF-EXAMINATION OF HIS TESTICLES** (see page 175).
- **TALK ABOUT TAKING RESPONSIBILITY FOR CONTRACEPTION AND PROTECTION AGAINST SEXUALLY TRANSMITTED DISEASES** (see page 180) before your child becomes sexually active.
- **IF YOUR DAUGHTER BECOMES SEXUALLY ACTIVE,** tell her that she needs to practice birth control and have regular pelvic examinations (see page 254), Pap smears, and tests for STDs.
- **MAKE SURE YOUR ADOLESCENT SEES A DOCTOR IMMEDIATELY IF HE OR SHE HAS SYMPTOMS OF STDs** (see page 183).
- **SHOW AFFECTION.** Use words that show you care about and are proud of him or her.
- **LEARN THE SIGNS OF DRUG USE** (see page 197), **DEPRESSION** (see page 467), **AND EATING DISORDERS** (see page 478) so you can get help right away.

Your child's development

Preteens and teens face numerous choices and decisions as they learn to become independent and express their individuality—often by exploring different clothes, hairstyles, friends, music, hobbies, religions, political issues, and social causes. They have an innate need to find things out for themselves—to test their feelings and ideas about life. They may reject their parents' values and challenge their rules, often pushing the limits placed on them by adults and society.

Teenagers change constantly. They may be helpful and kind 1 minute and cross and rude the next. Adolescents sometimes want to be alone and keep their thoughts to themselves; at other times they want to be with their parents and share their feelings. Let your child know that his or her ideas and feelings are important to you by spending more time listening to your child than talking. Listen actively by nodding and reflecting your child's words periodically to show that you're really hearing what's being said.

Teenagers get conflicting messages from their parents, their peers, and the media. As they struggle with the increasing need to "belong" socially, they may also feel pressure to perform academically. For some adolescents, these challenges are complicated by difficult family situations, dangerous neighborhoods, or exposure to alcohol or other drugs. Without support or guidance, many teens fall victim to behaviors that place them, and others, at risk. Dropping out of school, running away from home, joining a gang, or using alcohol or drugs can jeopardize a child's ability to mature—physically, emotionally, and intellectually. These risky behaviors can sometimes lead to depression, social isolation, and suicide.

Show confidence in your child and expect the best. Praise your child often for jobs well done. Teenagers are less likely to engage in high-risk behavior if their parents set clear expectations for success and are emotionally available. Stay in contact with your child's teachers and school and encourage your child to be involved in positive activities such as sports, music, theater, or academic clubs. Teenagers who are busy with activities that require a commitment tend to do better in school and are more likely to have the self-confidence to resist negative peer pressure.

One of the hardest parts of being a parent is that, in spite of all your knowledge and experience, you can't always prevent your child from making mistakes. Children have to learn many things for themselves—often the hard way. As your child gets older, your ability to manage or control his or her behavior steadily diminishes. Your child begins to learn more from his or her own experiences, observations, and peer group. This does not mean that you should be passive in your relationship with your child. What teens need most is reliable information but they accept it best when you give it in the form of advice rather than orders.

Your teenager needs your guidance so he or she can learn to make good decisions and acquire sound judgment. This guidance requires open communication, which shows your child that he or she can trust and confide in you. Praise your child when he or she does the right thing and let him or her know when you think he or she has done something wrong. But refrain from lecturing, preaching, shaming, or embarrassing your child, especially in front of others. Be a good role model; behave in the way you want your child to behave and, when you do something wrong, admit it and talk about it.

Spend as much time as you can with your teenager. It isn't always easy, especially if you work outside the home–and teenagers like to spend time with their friends or on their own. Insist that your child take part in family activities. Include his or her friends sometimes. You will be able to enjoy something together while letting your child know you want to be with him or her.

Puberty

Puberty is the body's natural transition to physical and sexual maturity, marked by dramatic growth and the development of adult physical sexual characteristics. Puberty can begin as early as 8 years of age in girls and 9 years of age in boys. It can start as late as 13 to 13½ years of age in either sex. Both early onset of puberty, otherwise known as precocious puberty, and late onset need to be evaluated by a doctor.

Puberty is marked by a dramatic increase in physical growth in both boys and girls. During puberty, your child will gain weight and grow in height much more rapidly than during childhood. This period of rapid growth is known as a growth spurt.

The growth spurt usually begins in girls between 10 and 11 years of age and ends at about age 13 or 14, on average. Girls grow 3 inches per year for the first 2 years of the growth spurt and then grow only 1 to 2 inches after they begin menstruating, reaching their maximum adult height by about age 15. Boys enter their growth spurt at about 12 to 13 years of age. It lasts until about 15½ years of age. Boys grow around 4 inches per year for 2 years and most reach their adult height by the time they are age 19.

Girls can gain 15 to 20 pounds during the initial part of the growth spurt and boys gain about 30 pounds. Final adult weight depends on a child's genetic makeup and his or her eating and exercise habits.

PUBERTY IN GIRLS

As girls go through puberty, they need to know how their reproductive system works. Prepare your daughter for her first period by explaining what happens during the menstrual cycle and why. Be straightforward so your daughter will feel comfortable about asking questions. Use the correct terms for parts of the body to give your daughter the vocabulary she needs to understand and talk about reproduction.

External female genitals Much of the female reproductive system lies inside the body, but certain structures are external. The entire outer genital area is called the vulva and is covered by pubic hair. The two flaps of skin that join at the top like an inverted "V" are the labia majora, the outer, larger set of lips that cover and protect the opening to the vagina, the muscular passage that leads from the uterus to the outside of the body. Just inside the labia majora are smaller, hairless lips called the labia minora, which protect the opening to the vagina. At the top of the labia minora, where the inner lips join, lies the clitoris, a pea-sized mound of tissue that is extremely sensitive and plays the most important role in female sexual arousal. During sexual arousal, the clitoris, the labia minora, the vagina, and the surrounding network of connecting blood vessels and muscles swell with blood.

Just under the clitoris lies the opening of the urethra, a short tube through which urine travels from the bladder and passes out of the body. The vagina opens just below the opening of the urethra. The vagina is surrounded by a delicate, elastic, mucous membrane called the hymen, which is open enough to allow menstrual blood to flow out each month. An area of skin and underlying muscle called the perineum lies between the top of the labia and the anus.

Learning about external anatomy

It's important for girls to familiarize themselves with their genital area so they can recognize any changes that might signal infection. The easiest way to see the external genitals is to sit cross-legged holding a small mirror in front of the genital area. The external genital area, including the anus, is called the perineum (inset).

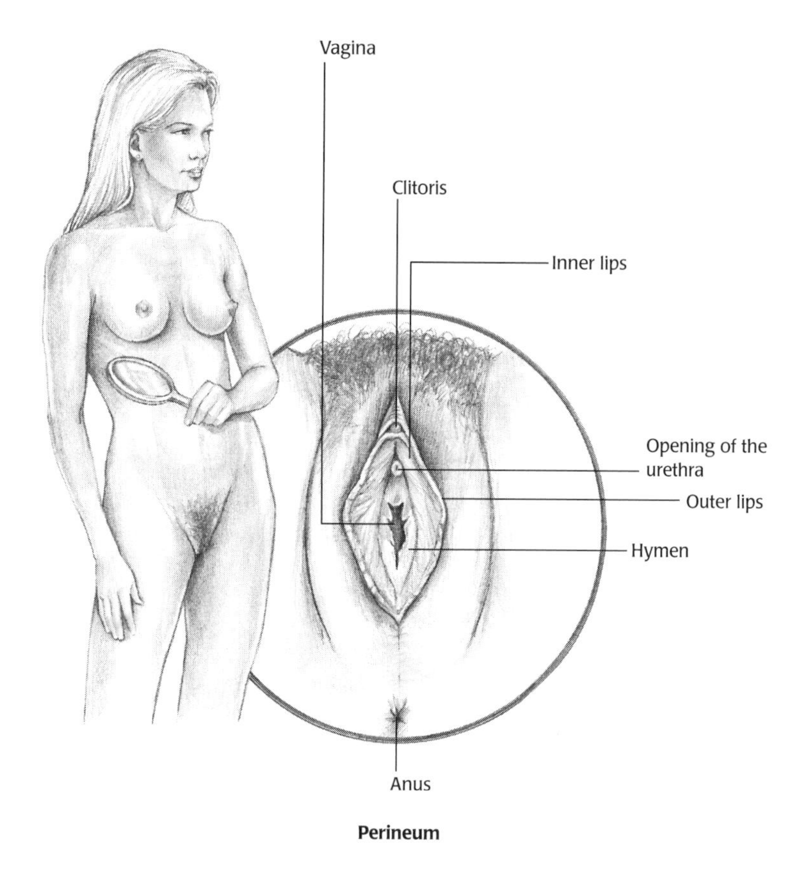

Perineum

Internal female reproductive organs The female reproductive organs lie in the lower abdomen. To help you visualize their exact location, see the color illustration on page 22. Here are brief descriptions of their functions:

VAGINA The vagina is a muscular tube, about 3 to 5 inches long, that leads from the external genitals into the internal female reproductive organs. The inside of the vaginal opening is partially covered by a membrane called the hymen, which may stretch and tear the first time a woman has sexual intercourse. The vagina constantly produces secretions that maintain a naturally moist environment and a balance of helpful bacteria. (Some vaginal discharge is normal but, if it causes irritation, has a strong or unpleasant odor, or increases significantly, a doctor should examine it to rule out an infection.)

CERVIX The cervix is the bottom of the uterus and opens into the vagina. Glands inside the cervix produce mucus, which increases in the middle of the menstrual cycle around the time of ovulation (when an ovary releases an egg). During menstruation, blood and tissue from the uterus pass through the narrow cervix into the vagina.

UTERUS The uterus is a small, hollow organ, about the size of a closed fist, that lies in the center of the pelvis. Its thick, muscular walls are lined with tissue called the endometrium, which builds up and sheds during each menstrual cycle. During pregnancy, a fertilized egg implants into the endometrium. In most girls, the uterus tips slightly forward; in some it tips backward. The position of the uterus does not affect fertility.

FALLOPIAN TUBES The fallopian tubes extend about 4 to 5 inches from either side of the uterus to the ovaries. The ends of the tubes closest to the ovaries

Sex hormones

Sex hormones work together to direct the dramatic changes that occur in boys and girls during puberty and to orchestrate the workings of the reproductive system throughout life. Learning about these hormones and how they work together can help young people understand how their reproductive system works. The sex hormones include:

- **Estrogen** Produced mainly in the ovaries, estrogen is the principal female sex hormone. It is responsible for normal female sexual development and ensures the healthy functioning of the female reproductive system.

- **Progesterone** This hormone is produced in the ovaries during the second half of the menstrual cycle, after an ovary has released an egg. Progesterone stimulates the lining of the uterus (the endometrium) to become thick and spongy in preparation for a fertilized egg. The hormone is also essential for sustaining a healthy pregnancy.

- **Testosterone** Testosterone is the principal male sex hormone. Testosterone carries instructions for normal male sexual development and plays a key role in bone and muscle growth. The hormone is produced in small amounts in the ovaries and adrenal glands in females and influences the sex drive in both males and females.

- **Follicle-stimulating hormone (FSH) and luteinizing hormone (LH)** These two hormones are produced by the pituitary gland in the brain in both males and females. In females, the hormones regulate the menstrual cycle by stimulating the ovaries to produce the hormones estrogen and progesterone. In males, FSH and LH regulate the production of testosterone in the testicles.

flare out to receive an egg from one of the adjoining ovaries once every menstrual cycle. An egg travels through a fallopian tube into the uterus. If the egg is fertilized by a sperm, it implants and a pregnancy ensues. An unfertilized egg is eliminated in menstrual blood.

OVARIES On each side of the uterus are the ovaries, which are about the size of walnuts. Girls are born with hundreds of thousands of eggs inside each ovary, but only about 500 develop into mature eggs that are released at ovulation. The eggs lie in tiny cavities called follicles. The follicles and supporting tissues produce estrogen and other hormones that play important roles in the reproductive cycle.

Early or late development in girls The timing of your daughter's puberty is likely to be the same as yours or that of other women in the family, but she should show signs of sexual development by age 13 and begin to menstruate by 15. Development of sexual characteristics before age 8 or the beginning of menstruation before age 10 is known as precocious puberty, which can be caused by a brain tumor, a tumor of the ovary or adrenal gland, other disorders, or hormone use. If your daughter shows early or late signs of puberty, she should see a doctor, who can determine the cause and recommend treatment if necessary. Girls who mature early or late often feel different from their peers. Give your daughter lots of loving reassurance until she catches up to her peers or they catch up to her.

Menstruation Menstruation is the cyclical shedding of blood and cells from the lining of the uterus. The brain and its intricate hormone signaling system regulate the menstrual cycle. A girl usually gets her first period between ages 11 and 14 (2 to 2½ years after the onset of puberty) but may get it as early as age 10 or as late as age 15. Thin or very athletic girls often start menstruating later than other girls because their bodies may not produce as much estrogen. Many girls have irregular periods when they first start menstruating and the amount of blood may be extremely small or unusually heavy. (Periods usually become regular 2 to 3 years after the onset of menstruation.) The length of periods can vary from girl to girl, lasting from 1 to 7 days. The average menstrual cycle is about 28 days (counting the first day of a period as the first day of a cycle) but it can range from 24 to 35 days. A girl's own menstrual cycle may vary by 3 to 7 days each month.

Girls who are adequately informed and prepared for their first period are more likely to view it in a positive light. Long before your daughter begins to menstruate, talk to her about menstruation in the context of other health and sex education topics, including reproduction, intercourse, contraception, and sexually transmitted diseases. Emphasize that menstruation is a normal body process that all girls and women experience and that no two people experience in exactly the same way.

The major menstrual concern of young girls is hygiene and the embarrassment of soiling their clothing. Reassure your daughter that her first period is

Stages of puberty in girls

After age 10, girls begin a rapid period of weight gain, usually doubling their weight by age 18. Girls develop a greater proportion of fat to muscle and bone than do boys because estrogen adds body fat while testosterone builds muscle. Girls usually start their growth spurt earlier than boys, so they are temporarily heavier and taller than boys the same age. Puberty usually proceeds in the following stages:

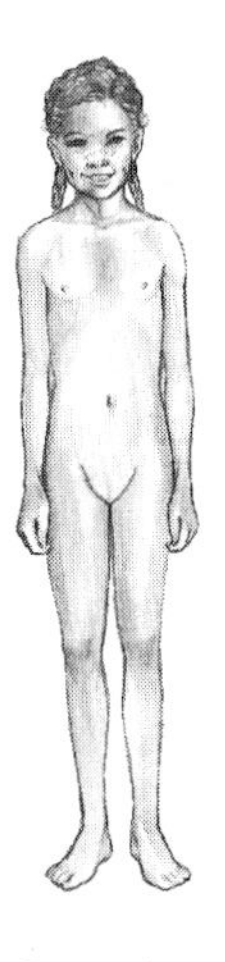

Stage 1

The first stage of puberty, referred to as prepuberty, is the period preceding the onset of puberty. No sexual development has yet occurred.

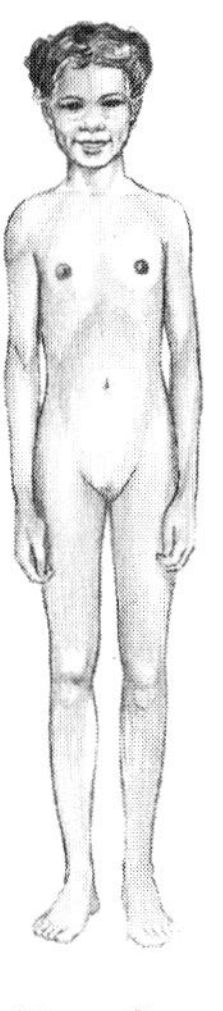

Stage 2

Puberty begins when the pituitary gland and hypothalamus in the brain signal the ovaries to start producing hormones. The first outward sign of puberty will be enlargement of your daughter's nipples and the appearance of breast buds. Sparse amounts of pubic hair also appear. Your daughter will also experience a rapid increase in height and weight.

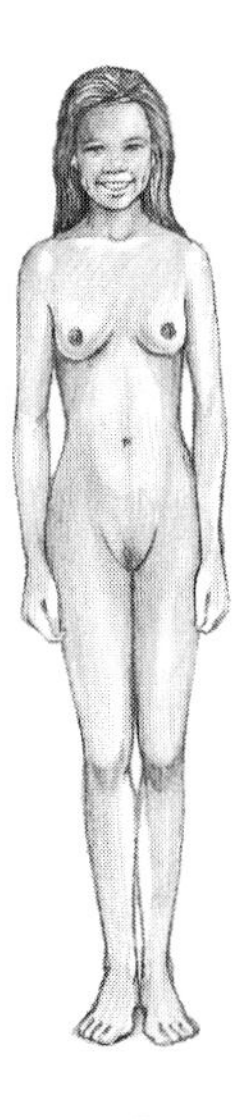

Stage 3

Your daughter's breasts gradually begin to grow fuller. More pubic hair appears and starts to curl. Underarm hair begins to grow about a year later and sweat glands under your daughter's arms cause an increase in perspiration. The higher production of hormones causes her skin to produce more oil, especially on her face (see page 401).

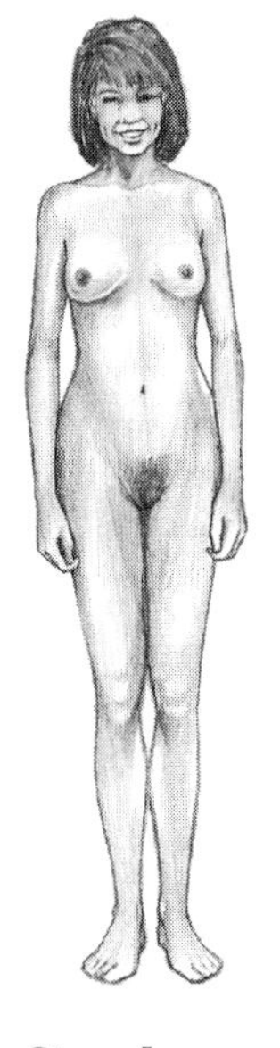

Stage 4

Your daughter's height and weight increase steadily. Her breasts continue developing and the nipples may protrude. Pubic hair grows in almost fully. A white, creamy discharge often appears 6 to 12 months before menstruation begins. Your daughter's ovaries start releasing an egg each month and, once this process begins, she can become pregnant.

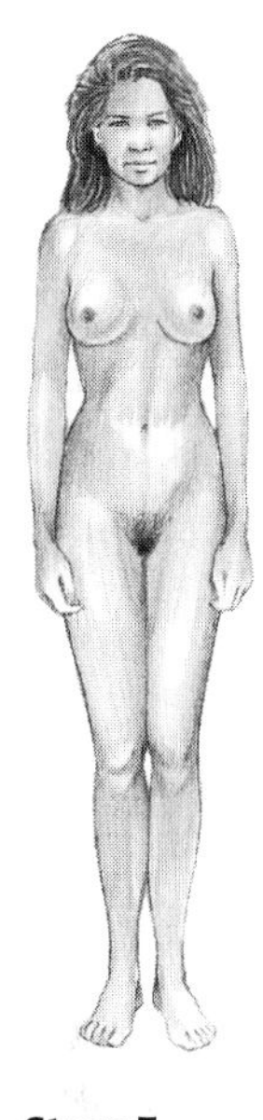

Stage 5

In the last stage of puberty, your daughter reaches physical and sexual maturity. Her periods become regular and her breasts and internal organs reach full size.

likely to be very light and will probably start with a wet feeling or a few drops of blood on her underpants, giving her plenty of time to get to a washroom. Once your daughter has shown signs of starting puberty, suggest that she prepare for her first period by keeping a couple of pads in her school locker or book bag, or buy them from a washroom vending machine. Shop with her for the basic supplies and make sure she knows how to use them. Today, some products are specifically designed for young girls.

Most girls feel more comfortable using pads when they first start menstruating but there's no reason they can't use tampons. Pads should be changed every 2 or 3 hours because menstrual blood develops an odor when exposed to air. Tampons eliminate the odor problem because they absorb blood inside the vagina but they need to be changed at least every 4 to 8 hours to avoid a potentially serious bacterial infection. If your daughter wants to try tampons, recommend the thinner ones at first because they're easier to insert. To insert a tampon most easily, tell her to relax and to gently push the tampon in following the natural tilt of the vagina, toward the back.

Explain to your daughter that tampons and pads come in varying degrees of absorbency. It's important to use the tampon with the least amount of absorbency, but also one that doesn't need to be changed more frequently than every 4 hours. Tell her always to check to make sure she hasn't left a tampon in her vagina after her period ends.

Show your daughter how to keep track of her periods on a calendar so she can figure out how long her usual cycle is and notice anything unusual, such as a change in the length of her cycle or a missed period. Once a regular cycle has been established, your daughter should notify the doctor immediately if she has missed a period. Missed periods can be a sign of pregnancy or serious medical problems. Some girls who are excessively thin, who have an eating disorder such as anorexia nervosa (see page 414), or who exercise excessively (see page 192) may stop menstruating, a possible indication that the ovaries have stopped producing enough of the hormone estrogen. A lack of estrogen, which is essential for building strong bones, can prevent the bones from growing and lead to the bone-thinning disorder osteoporosis at a young age. If your daughter usually has heavy periods, as many teenagers do, the doctor may give her a blood test to check for iron-deficiency anemia (see page 412), which can result from heavy blood loss. Once menstruation starts, all teenage girls should take a multivitamin with iron daily to avoid iron-deficiency anemia.

Many girls experience menstrual pain during their periods. If your daughter has severe pain during her periods, she should see a doctor to rule out an underlying medical problem. Your daughter can take ibuprofen for menstrual pain or try the following suggestions:

- Exercise, through brisk walking, jogging, biking, swimming, or aerobics.
- Take a warm bath or place a heating pad on her abdomen.
- Limit intake of caffeine in foods such as coffee, tea, cola, and chocolate.
- Limit consumption of salt.
- Get enough sleep before and during her periods.

The menstrual cycle

The average menstrual cycle is about 28 days long but can vary because of the lengthening or shortening of the time before ovulation. Ovulation always occurs 14 days before the start of the next cycle, but the time before ovulation can vary. For example, in a 35-day cycle, ovulation does not occur until day 21, but in a 23-day cycle, it can occur on day 9. Many factors can affect the length of the time before ovulation, including stress, so it can be difficult to predict exactly when ovulation will occur. An average menstrual cycle begins on day 1, the first day of a girl's period. It can take 2 to 3 years before a girl's menstrual cycle becomes regular. A girl can become pregnant even if her menstrual cycle is irregular.

Fallopian tube
Endometrium shedding
Ovaries
Uterus

Day 1

On the first day of blood flow, the lining of the uterus (endometrium) starts shedding. This is considered day 1 of the menstrual cycle. Bleeding can last up to about 5 days.

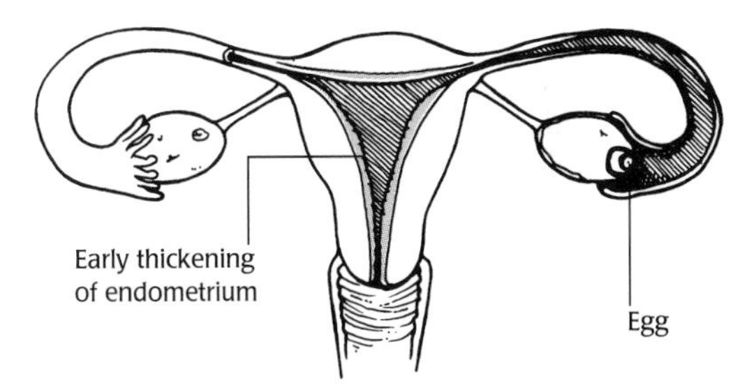

About day 9

The endometrium starts thickening in response to hormone signals from the ovaries and continues to thicken until about day 14 (in a 28-day cycle).

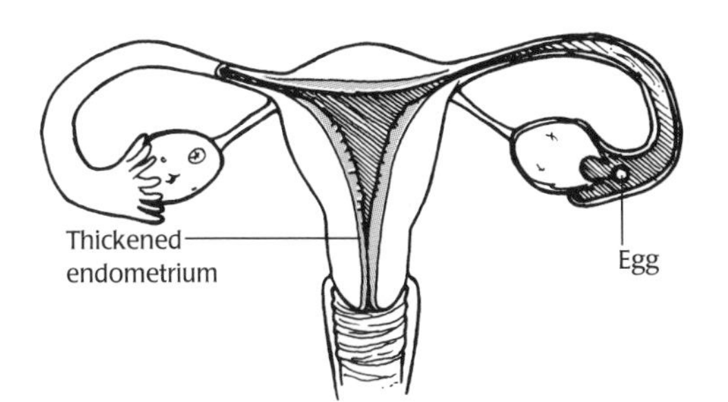

Day 14 (in a 28-day cycle)

An ovary releases a mature egg into a fallopian tube. This process is known as ovulation. The egg starts to travel down the fallopian tube toward the uterus. Pregnancy is most likely to occur around this time. Ovulation always occurs 14 days before the start of the next menstrual cycle.

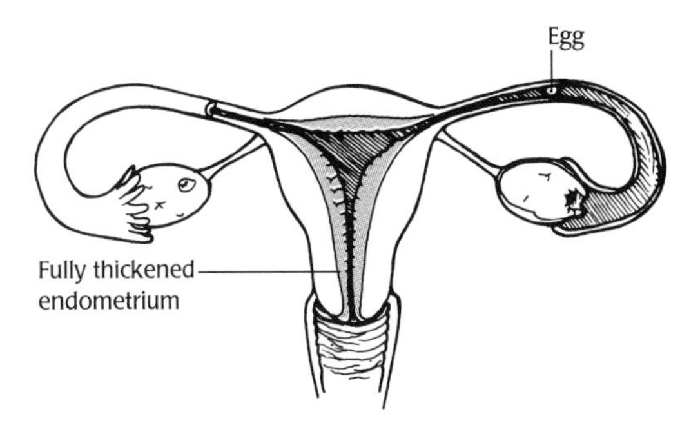

About day 19 (in a 28-day cycle)

The egg approaches the uterus. The endometrium has thickened so it can accept an egg that may have been fertilized. If the egg is not fertilized or cannot sustain a pregnancy, the menstrual cycle begins again on day 1.

Questions your daughter might ask about menstruation

When first learning about menstruation, your daughter will have lots of questions. It's much better for your daughter to get accurate information from you than wrong information from other sources. The more straightforward and open you are with your daughter, the more comfortable she will feel about asking you questions.

Q How much will I bleed during my period?

A Although the amount of blood flow varies from girl to girl, the average amount of menstrual blood each month is about 4 to 6 tablespoons. If you're soaking several pads or tampons and have to change tampons more frequently than every 4 hours, you should see your doctor. Excessive bleeding can lead to iron-deficiency anemia (see page 412) or indicate another medical problem.

Q Which feminine hygiene products are best to use during my period?

A Different products are better at different times during your period. Maxi pads are best for the heaviest days of blood flow, usually at the beginning of the period. Overnight pads are longer than usual to give protection while you sleep. You can use pantiliners for the light days of your period or for absorbing normal vaginal discharge between periods. If you're physically active, or just don't like wearing pads, you might prefer tampons. Sometimes you might have to use both to absorb a heavy flow of blood. Just use whatever products make you feel most comfortable. Avoid douches, which can wash away the helpful bacteria in the vagina. Shower or bathe daily to stay fresh. Powders and sprays can irritate your genitals.

Q Is there anything I shouldn't do during my period?

A No. You can do everything you normally do, including bathing and playing sports. Even swimming isn't a problem if you use tampons. For many girls, physical activity helps relieve mild cramps.

Q Could I lose my virginity using tampons?

A The hymen, a thin, flexible membrane, only partially covers the vaginal opening, allowing enough room for menstrual blood to flow out and for a tampon to be inserted. Even if tampon use does tear the hymen, it does not reflect on your sexual experience. The only way you can lose your virginity is to have sexual intercourse for the first time.

Q Why do I feel so fat when I have my period?

A Your body retains water just before and during your periods, which can make you feel fat. Your breasts may also feel tender. It's normal to gain a couple of pounds of water weight during this time and lose them right after the period ends. If you feel bloated, you may be more comfortable wearing loose clothing. Try limiting the amount of salt you eat for a few days before and during your period because salt increases water retention.

Routine checkups for girls Your daughter should start having regular pelvic examinations when she's 18—earlier if she is sexually active. Doctors routinely do a pelvic examination as part of the female reproductive system examination (see page 254). Many serious health problems, such as cancer of the cervix, can be detected at an early, more easily treatable stage by having routine screening tests such as a Pap smear. Tell your daughter what to expect during the examination and suggest that she ask the doctor to explain each step to make it less intimidating.

Pelvic examination The pelvic examination usually follows the breast examination in a gynecologic checkup. Tell your daughter about your own experience with pelvic examinations so she knows what to expect. Explain to her that it's not as scary as it seems and that it shouldn't hurt, although she may feel some discomfort. During the examination, a female attendant will be present. The doctor will ask your daughter to lie with her knees apart and relaxed or with her feet in metal stirrups at the end of the examining table. To do an internal pelvic examination, the doctor will insert a thin metal or plastic instrument called a speculum into her vagina to open it and examine it inside.

The doctor performs a Pap smear by inserting a tiny brush or swab through the speculum to take a sample of cells from the cervix. This procedure does not hurt. The cells will be sent to a laboratory to be examined under a microscope for changes that could lead to cancer. The cells will also be tested for some sexually transmitted diseases, especially genital warts (see page 500), which increase a woman's risk of developing cancer of the cervix.

The final step in the checkup is a manual internal pelvic examination. While your daughter is on the examination table, the doctor will insert one or two fingers of one hand into her vagina and place the other hand on her abdomen. Although it may seem difficult, relaxing as much as possible can make this procedure less uncomfortable. With the fingers, the doctor lifts up the cervix to feel the size, shape, and position of the uterus and ovaries. This action also enables the doctor to note any tenderness the patient may have in her pelvic area. The doctor may then place a finger in her rectum and compress her abdomen to further examine the uterus, ovaries, and lower pelvis.

Breast self-examination The doctor will teach your daughter how to examine her breasts for lumps and other changes that could indicate breast cancer. Encourage your daughter to develop the habit of doing the self-examination once a month as she gets older and her risk of breast cancer increases. The best time to do the examination is right after her period. Teach your daughter the following basic steps in a breast self-examination:

1. Standing in front of a mirror, look for any irregularities in your breasts—such as puckering, dimples, changes in size or shape, or pushed-in or misshapen nipples—while resting your hands on your hips and while holding your hands behind your head.

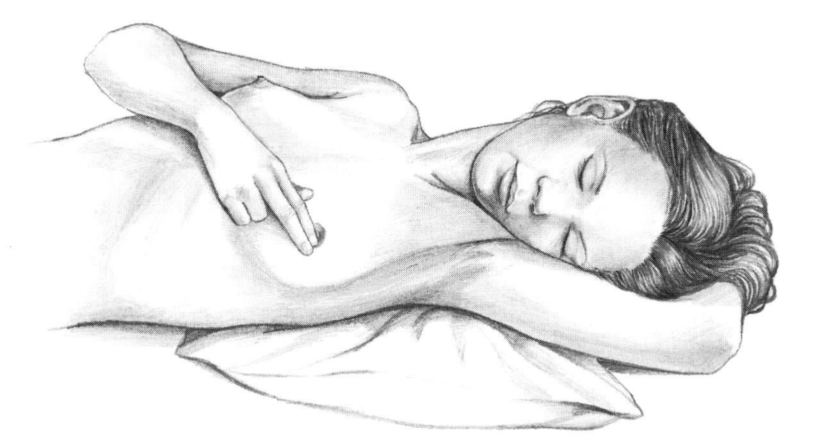

Make a habit of breast self-examination

During a breast self-examination, feel your breasts with the index and middle fingers of your hand, moving in smaller and smaller circles from the outside of your breast in.

2. Lie on your back, put a pillow under your right shoulder, and place your right hand under your head. Feel your right breast with the index and middle fingers of your left hand, moving in increasingly smaller circles from the outside of the breast in. Pushing the breast in gently, feel for any lumps or other abnormalities and for discharge near the nipple. (This can be easier to do while standing in the shower, when your skin is lubricated by soap.) Feel the area next to the breast and below the armpit for any lumps or abnormalities.
3. Repeat the above steps on the other breast.

Puberty in Boys

As boys go through puberty, it's helpful for them to know how their reproductive system works. Be straightforward and open so your son will feel comfortable asking you questions as they come up. Use the correct terms for parts of the body to give your son the vocabulary he needs to understand and discuss this important time of his life.

The male reproductive system Unlike the vagina and ovaries in girls, a boy's penis and testicles lie outside his body. Inside his body are glands and ducts that produce the fluid semen, the medium for transporting sperm, the male reproductive cells. From the time of puberty, sperm is continuously produced in the testicles. Each sperm cell consists of a head that contains hereditary information, and a long, whiplike tail that propels it. Sperm are so tiny that 500 million of them could fit in a teaspoon.

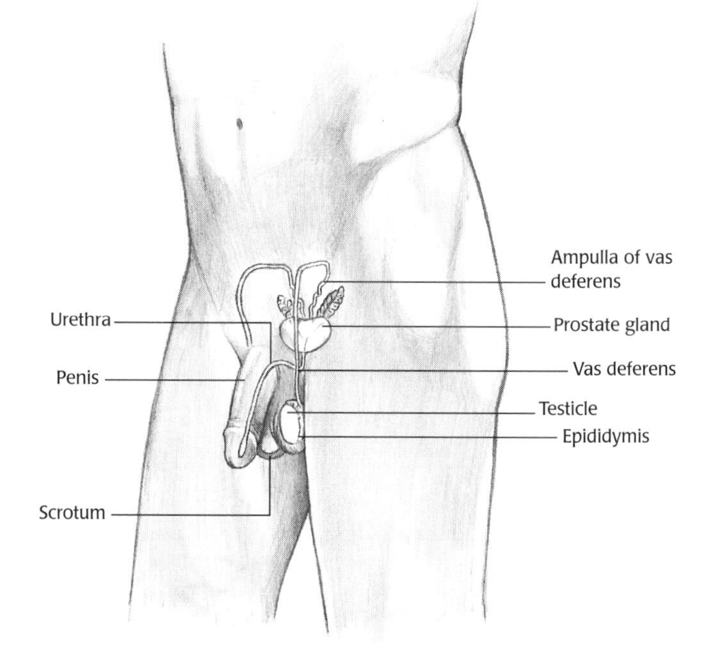

Understanding the male reproductive system

Sperm are produced in the testicles and stored in the epididymis, where they mature for about 2 weeks. Mature sperm travel from the epididymis to the vas deferens, a tube that transports them through the seminal vesicles and the prostate gland. The seminal vesicles and prostate gland secrete fluids that mix with the sperm to nourish them and increase their mobility. The resulting fluid, called semen, travels through the urethra and penis and out of the body during ejaculation.

Your son's reproductive system is located both outside of his body and inside his lower pelvis. Here are brief descriptions of the functions of each part of his reproductive system:

PENIS The penis is the male sex organ. It functions for both urination and sexual intercourse. During sexual arousal, the penis becomes engorged with blood, making it hard. This hardening is called an erection. An erection usually precedes ejaculation, the forceful release through the urethra just before orgasm of a thick, milky fluid called semen (which contains sperm).

URETHRA The urethra is a tube that runs from the bladder through the penis. The urethra carries urine from the bladder out of the body and also transports semen during an orgasm. A valve at the base of the bladder prevents urine and semen from going through the urethra at the same time.

SCROTUM The scrotum is an external pouch of skin that holds the testicles.

TESTICLES The testicles are two oval glands suspended in the scrotum. They produce sperm and testosterone and other male sex hormones. The testicles lie outside the body because sperm need a cooler-than-normal body temperature to survive. The left testicle normally hangs lower than the right one.

EPIDIDYMIS Located on top of each testicle, the epididymis stores sperm.

VAS DEFERENS The vas deferens is a thin tube that carries sperm from the epididymis on each testicle to a seminal vesicle and the prostate gland.

AMPULLA OF VAS DEFERENS This structure is used for long-term sperm storage.

SPERMATIC CORD This cord contains nerves, blood vessels, and the vas deferens.

SEMINAL VESICLES The seminal vesicles are two sacs, located behind the bladder, that produce a fluid that combines with sperm to form semen.

PROSTATE GLAND The prostate is a solid, chestnut-shaped organ located beneath the bladder and around the upper urethra. The prostate produces a fluid that mixes with semen, increasing its volume.

Testicle self-examination Cancer of the testicle is the most common cancer in young men between ages 15 and 35, so doctors recommend that boys start examining their testicles every month starting at puberty, around age 13 or 14 to familiarize themselves with the usual feel and appearance of the anatomy. Most cancers are found during these self-examinations. When detected and treated early, the cancer is highly curable.

Signs of testicle cancer include a painless, hard lump on the surface of a testicle, painless increase in the size of a testicle, unusual tenderness or pain, or a feeling of heaviness. The best time to do the examination is during or right after a shower or bath when the skin of the scrotum is relaxed and changes are easy to feel. To do the examination, a boy should gently roll each testicle between his thumbs and fingers, feeling for any lump or abnormality in texture or shape.

Early and late development in boys

If your son goes through puberty late—that is, if the size of his testicles measures less than 1 inch at age 14—take him to the doctor for an evaluation. About 2 percent of all boys go through puberty late with no known cause. They generally go on to develop normally. Early onset, otherwise known as precocious puberty, occurs if a boy starts going through puberty before age 9. Precocious puberty also needs to be evaluated by a doctor to rule out abnormalities of the testicles, adrenal glands, or brain.

Stages of puberty in boys

In boys, puberty can begin any time between ages 12 and 16. Because boys start their growth spurt later than girls, they are temporarily smaller and shorter than girls the same age. The male hormone testosterone increases their proportion of muscle and bone to fat. Puberty starts at different ages in different boys and progresses at varying rates but it develops in the following predictable stages:

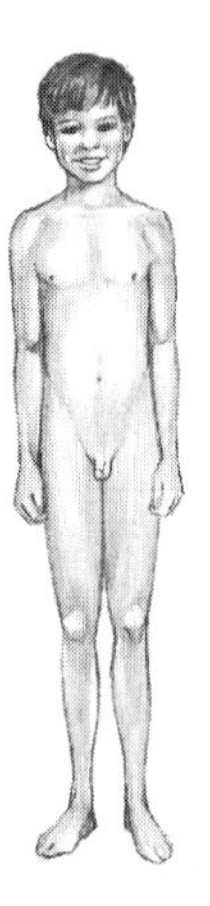

Stage 1
The first stage of puberty, referred to as prepuberty, is the period immediately preceding the onset of puberty. No sexual development has yet occurred.

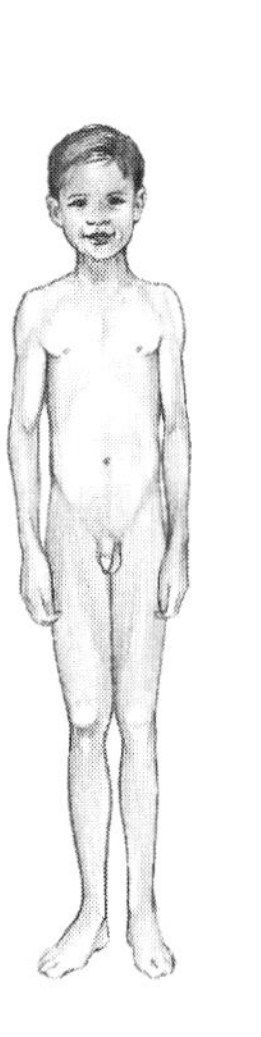

Stage 2
Puberty begins when the pituitary gland and hypothalamus in the brain start producing hormones that trigger the testicles to begin producing testosterone and other male hormones. The first noticeable sign of puberty is enlargement of the testicles and scrotum (the pouch holding the testicles). Sweat glands in the body increase their activity, producing a body odor.

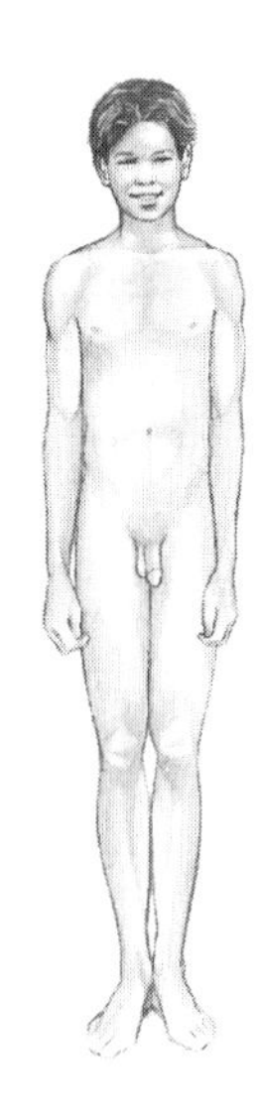

Stage 3
Pubic hair begins to grow sparsely on the skin around the base of your son's penis, which starts to grow longer. Boys usually begin to ejaculate around this time, either during masturbation or sleep. Your son's voice deepens as the vocal cords grow; for a few months this growth can cause the voice to change pitch suddenly, or crack.

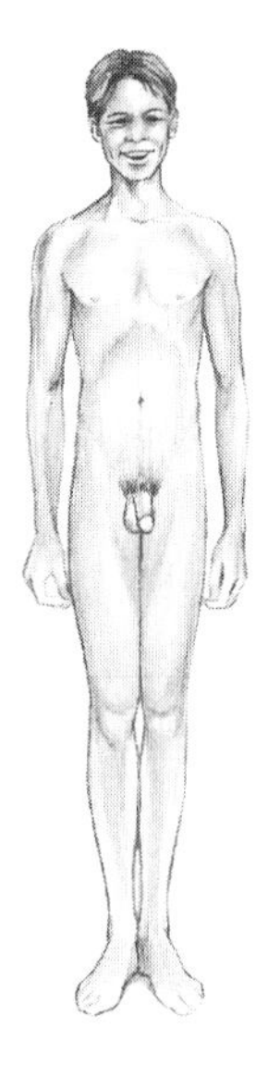

Stage 4
Your son's testicles continue to grow and his penis becomes longer and thicker. His penis and scrotum get darker and his pubic hair gets curlier and coarser and starts filling in. Hair starts growing under his arms and may appear on his chin and upper lip. A great spurt in height frequently occurs at this time.

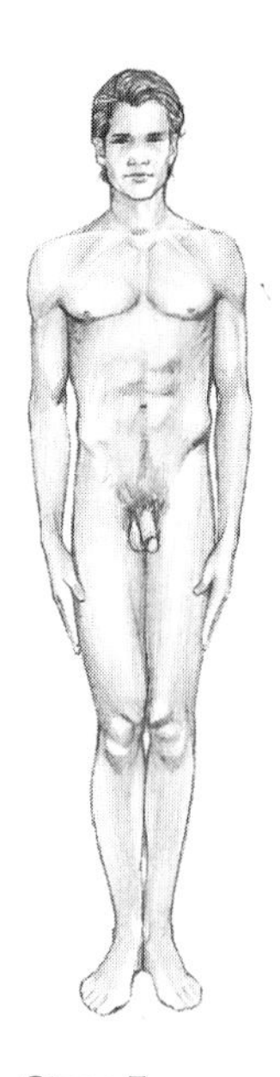

Stage 5
In the last stage of development, your son reaches physical and sexual maturity. Pubic hair extends to his inner thighs and hair may begin to grow on his chest. His growth in height starts slowing down until adult height is reached, usually between ages 16 and 18, but sometimes as late as age 21.

Questions your son might ask about puberty

Q My penis is smaller than the other boys' my age. Will I have a problem having sexual intercourse when I get older?

A No. The size of a penis has nothing to do with a man's ability to experience or give sexual pleasure. Just as other body parts can differ greatly from one person to another, the size and look of penises and testicles can vary too. Also, the size of a nonerect penis differs greatly from the size of an erect penis.

Q Sometimes I'll be sitting in class and, all of a sudden, I have an erection. I'm always worried that other people can tell.

A You're not alone—all boys have spontaneous erections at some time or other during puberty. Erections usually occur when you think about something sexy or exciting, but they can also occur for no apparent reason. Stay calm, try not to worry about it, and make yourself think of something not so sexy. Your erection is likely to go away.

Q Sometimes when I wake up in the morning I find a wet spot on my sheets or pajamas. Why does this happen?

A Doctors refer to this occurrence as nocturnal emission; most people call it a "wet dream." Wet dreams are common and normal during adolescence and usually result from sexually stimulating dreams. As you get older, you will have them less frequently.

Sexuality

The hormonal changes of puberty trigger intense sexual urges and desires and many teenagers respond to them by becoming sexually active. Two out of three teens are sexually active by their senior year in high school. Many experts believe that teenage sexual behavior may be encouraged by powerful influences such as television and other media, which associate sex with excitement, humor, and sometimes violence. The media unrealistically glamorize casual sex without love, consequences, or commitments.

Some teens become sexually active because they are curious about the physical changes they're experiencing and want to try out their "new" body. Others lack self-esteem and self-confidence and give in to pressure from a boyfriend or girlfriend because they're afraid of losing the relationship. For some teenagers, becoming sexually active is a way to rebel against their parents' values or to act out against their parents. Teenagers who feel distanced from their family often become sexually active to feel close, intimate, and affectionate with another person or to belong to a peer group that encourages sexual activity. Early sexual activity is sometimes a cry for help.

But even though teenagers are physically able to act on their strong sexual desires, few have the emotional and intellectual maturity necessary to deal successfully with sexual relationships—nor do they understand the potentially harmful consequences of such relationships. While having sex can be pleasurable, exciting, and healthy in a loving, trusting, mature relationship, its emotional and physical risks can outweigh the benefits, especially for teenagers, who are in the process of forming their identity and learning how to manage relationships and intimacy. Having sex is not proof of maturity. Mature relationships are based on caring, closeness, intimacy, and mutual respect. Introducing sex into a relationship can change it, often complicating it and adding stress—especially if one of the partners is not yet ready to have sex. Many teens who start having sex feel guilty about it and find their relationship unsatisfying.

Although there is little you can do to prevent your child from becoming sexually active, communicating your values and feelings about sex in ongoing conversations will help prepare your child to act responsibly. Explain to your child that intercourse isn't the only physical way to share love. Holding hands, kissing, and hugging can be satisfying ways to show affection. Express your hope that your child will wait until he or she is older before having sex. Bring up the subject whenever you can—for example, while commenting on a television show or an article you have read. Provide age-appropriate articles or books about teenage sexuality for your child to read. Be open and available to discuss these issues and answer your child's questions. Teens need information about their changing bodies and emerging sexual urges in early adolescence. If you haven't already educated your child about his or her sexuality, do so now so he or she can get sound, accurate information from you, instead of questionable ideas from peers.

Masturbation

Masturbation is a normal way for your child to explore his or her sexual feelings, express the natural sexual response, and relieve sexual tension. Masturbation is not harmful, either emotionally or physically. Many people of both sexes masturbate at least occasionally; others never do. Either is normal. Girls often masturbate by rubbing the clitoris until they reach orgasm. Boys masturbate by stroking or rubbing their penis until ejaculation. For teenagers, masturbation is a safe way to relieve sexual tension without having to worry about pregnancy, having a sexual relationship with another person, or sexually transmitted diseases.

Teens who have high self-esteem, a close relationship with their parents, important goals for the future, and who are informed about reproduction, sexuality, safer sex, and contraception are more likely to resist peer pressure to have sex or postpone having sex—or to be responsible when they do become sexually active. Sexual responsibility means making decisions that respect each partner's values and goals and promote self-esteem, not guilt. This responsibility also requires both partners to cooperate in practicing safer sex (see page 182) and using reliable contraception to avoid pregnancy (see page 184).

Most first sexual encounters are unplanned. Teach your teenager to think about how he or she will deal with a situation in which the opportunity or pressure to have sex arises. Encourage avoiding situations that might put him or her at risk of having forced sex, such as being alone with the person in a home or isolated setting. Make sure your child knows that drinking alcohol or using other drugs can affect his or her judgment. Although boys are usually the aggressors, adolescent girls are generally more physically mature than boys of the same age and can be just as sexually aggressive. Regularly remind your adolescent that he or she has much more than sex to offer as a person.

How conception takes place

Conception is most likely to occur around the time of ovulation. Few women know exactly when they are ovulating and the timing can fluctuate from month to month, influenced by factors such as stress, illness, sexual activity, or changes in routine. A woman can get pregnant at any time in her cycle, even during her period, so the only safe way to prevent pregnancy is to always use effective contraception (see page 185), although no method of contraception is 100-percent effective.

Reproduction is a complex process in which cells from a male and female combine after sexual intercourse to form an offspring. A comprehensive, basic understanding of how reproduction takes place can help your child make responsible decisions about his or her sexuality.

Conception

1. One of the woman's ovaries releases a mature egg into the adjacent fallopian tube.
2. During sexual intercourse, a man's erect penis enters his female partner's vagina and, when he has an orgasm, his penis releases semen, a thick fluid that contains sperm. Sperm in the semen travel up into and through the uterus into the fallopian tubes. Fertilization takes place when one of the sperm penetrates the egg in the fallopian tube.
3. The fertilized egg divides from one cell into many as it makes its way through the fallopian tube toward the uterus.
4. About 5 days after fertilization, the egg implants in the wall of the uterus, where it will develop into a fetus and continue to grow for the next 9 months.

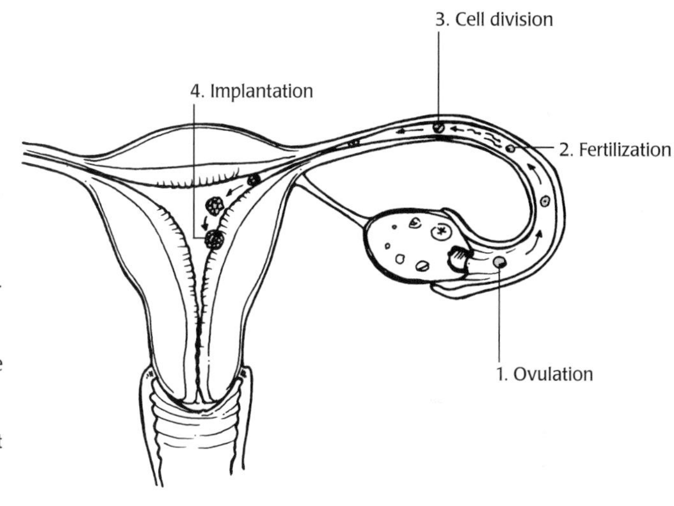

MALE SEXUAL RESPONSE

During the early stage of sexual excitement, when a male is stimulated physically or emotionally, his blood pressure, heartbeat, and breathing increase. More blood flows into the blood vessels of the penis, causing it to become larger and harder. The scrotum (the sac that contains the testicles) contracts and raises the testicles closer to the body. As the erection continues, the head of the penis may become larger and darker and a drop of clear fluid may appear at the tip. This fluid, called pre-ejaculate, contains some sperm (and therefore can cause pregnancy). It may also contain sexually transmissible organisms.

In males, ejaculation, the forceful release of semen from the penis, occurs in two stages: first sperm mix with fluid from the seminal vesicles to form semen and then muscle contractions occur in the penis and urethra to propel the semen out of the body. After ejaculation, blood gradually flows away from the penis and the penis softens. The man's heart rate and breathing slow down and his blood pressure returns to normal.

Female sexual response

During sexual excitement, the vagina secretes a lubricating fluid, the nipples may become erect, and the skin may become flushed. As blood pressure and pulse rate increase, the breathing becomes more rapid and the muscles may get tense. The clitoris (a small, very sensitive mound of tissue above the vaginal opening) may enlarge slightly; the inner, upper part of the vagina grows longer and wider and the lower part narrows.

This state of excitement may or may not culminate in orgasm, a reflexive response that is accompanied by pleasurable sensations and a series of muscle contractions in the vagina and uterus. Contractions last only a few seconds and come less than a second apart, sometimes accompanied by contractions of muscles in the hands, arms, legs, feet, spine, face, or neck. The woman's pulse, blood pressure, and breathing rate all increase. Some women experience multiple orgasms, one after another. Afterward, blood flows out of the genital area, and the pulse, blood pressure, and breathing return to normal.

Preventing sexually transmitted diseases

Sexually transmitted diseases (STDs) are infections that are spread during sexual activity–vaginal or anal intercourse or oral sex. Some STDs are caused by bacteria and can be cured with medication; others are caused by viruses and are incurable. Many cause long-term problems such as infertility. Each year, 3 million new cases of STDs are diagnosed among teenagers. Two of the most common STDs–chlamydia and gonorrhea–are more prevalent among sexually active teens than among any other group of people. One in five Americans over age 12 has genital herpes, an incurable STD that can cause recurring outbreaks throughout life and can be life threatening to a baby at birth if the mother has an outbreak at the time of delivery. Infection with the human immunodeficiency virus (HIV) continues to increase among teenagers–most young people who develop full-blown cases of acquired immunodeficiency syndrome (AIDS) in their 20s were infected with HIV when they were teenagers. AIDS is nearly always fatal. Many STDs cause no symptoms, so people don't know they have been infected.

These facts underscore the importance of talking to your teenager about how STDs spread and how they can be prevented. Young people need this information long before they become sexually active. The only way to completely avoid the risk of acquiring an STD is not to have sex, but educational programs that emphasize abstinence and don't mention protection against STDs and pregnancy have not reduced sexual activity among teenagers. Experts are concerned that giving the abstinence message without discussing the need to use latex condoms and safer sex will prevent teenagers from knowing how to protect themselves when they start having sex–at whatever age. Finally, many teenagers view abstinence as unrealistic, and reject it.

Next to abstinence, the most reliable way to protect against STDs is for boys to use latex condoms correctly during every sexual encounter (see page 184). Only condoms made of latex protect against STDs. The effectiveness of the female condom in protecting against STDs is not yet known, but if the girl's partner refuses to use a condom and she still intends to have sex with him, she needs to take responsibility for protecting herself. (Make sure your teenager knows that many contraceptive methods, such as birth-control pills, do not provide any protection against STDs.)

Adolescents who use condoms may have a false sense of protection—even condoms do not completely prevent STDs (or pregnancy). Although latex condoms provide some protection against the spread of HIV, they don't work as well against viruses such as herpes or genital warts that grow on areas not protected by a condom.

Educate yourself about STDs, how they are spread, and how they can be prevented. Get information from your doctor's office, health clinic, local library, or public health department. Have several conversations with your child, conveying your values as well as the facts. You might feel more comfortable bringing up the conversation casually, such as while riding in the car or doing a chore together. In general, try to keep your tone simple and direct, using specific, clear terms—and don't preach. Provide information based on your child's age and level of development. Listen carefully to any questions your child might ask. You may pick up clues about specific concerns or misinformation that you can clear up. If you don't know something, admit it and find out together with your child.

Don't assume that you will know when your child becomes sexually active—and don't take it for granted that your child isn't already having sex. Make sure that whenever your child chooses to become sexually active, he or she already knows the following facts about STDs:

- Most STDs are easy to acquire during intimate sexual contact.
- Having oral sex is not necessarily safer than having sexual intercourse. Some STDs can be spread through oral sex.
- The more people a person has sex with, the greater the risk of acquiring an STD. But don't let your child play a "numbers game." It only takes a single partner to get infected.
- A person can be infected with an STD and not know it. These infections often don't cause symptoms and, even without symptoms, a person can spread the infection to a sex partner.
- Having some STDs—including syphilis, genital herpes, gonorrhea, chlamydia, and trichomoniasis—increases the risk of becoming infected with HIV.
- The anatomy of the female reproductive tract puts girls at risk of developing fertility problems as a result of untreated STDs.
- In girls, one STD—genital warts—can lead to cervical cancer. Having many sexual partners increases the risk of developing cancer of the cervix.
- Without treatment, some infections can lead to serious health problems—including infertility (from chlamydia) or personality changes (from syphilis)—or even death (from AIDS). It is extremely important to see a doctor immediately

when symptoms first appear. Most infections can be cleared up with medication.

Teenagers may be afraid to see a doctor about symptoms that might have been caused by sexual activity, or they may not know how to see a doctor on their own, so they often don't get needed treatment for an infection. Make sure your child understands that all doctor visits are confidential. You might even consider offering to provide transportation to the doctor's office and payment for the visit. When diagnosed with an STD, teenagers are often reluctant to tell their sexual partner, putting the partner at risk for infection, preventing him or her from getting treatment, and risking reinfection for themselves. If your teenager cannot talk to you, he or she should talk to another trusted adult such as the doctor or a school counselor or nurse and ask for help to get the medical care he or she needs. The local office of Planned Parenthood (a national organization that provides education about reproductive issues and medical care for sexually active teenagers and adults) is a good source of useful information, counseling, and other services.

Safer sex It only takes one sexual encounter to contract an STD. Although not foolproof, the most effective protection against STDs is a latex male condom used correctly every time a person has vaginal or anal intercourse or oral-genital contact. The female condom may prove to be a reliable second choice. Tell your teenager the following facts about STDs and safer sex guidelines before he or she becomes sexually active:

- Don't have sex if you or your partner has symptoms of an STD (see page 183).
- Always use a latex male condom for every sexual encounter–vaginal intercourse, anal intercourse, or oral sex. For oral sex with a female, the condom should be split lengthwise and placed over her genitals. Make sure the condom does not contain a spermicide.
- In addition to a condom, use a spermicide containing nonoxynol 9, which provides additional protection against STDs. Spermicides are available over the counter and come in foams, gels, creams, or suppositories. Teenagers usually prefer foam because it doesn't leave a residue after intercourse.
- Use only water-based lubricants with latex condoms because oil-based ones–such as petroleum jelly, lotions, or oils–can damage the latex, making it permeable to an infection-causing organism.
- Avoid letting another person's body fluids–including semen, blood (including menstrual blood), and vaginal secretions–enter your body through the vagina, penis, urethral opening, anus, mouth, or a cut or open sore.
- Avoid situations in which you are under the influence of alcohol or other drugs, which can impair your judgment and make it more difficult to practice safer sex.
- Girls should not douche after having sex because douching can transfer germs into the reproductive tract, causing a more serious infection that could lead to infertility.

Symptoms of Sexually Transmitted Diseases

Many sexually transmitted diseases (STDs) don't cause noticeable symptoms. When left untreated, they can lead to more serious health problems, including infertility in females and painful swelling of the tubes that carry sperm from the testicles in males. If your child complains about any of the following symptoms, he or she could have an STD and should see a doctor immediately.

STD	Symptoms in Females	Symptoms in Males
Chlamydia	Often no symptoms at first. Later symptoms include vaginal itching; yellow, odorless vaginal discharge; pain during intercourse; frequent urination; and pain during urination. Possible bleeding between periods.	Pain or burning during urination; a watery, milky-colored discharge from the penis.
Trichomoniasis	Often no symptoms. Within 4 to 20 days after exposure, can produce a yellow-green, unpleasant-smelling vaginal discharge; itching and irritation in the genital area; pain during urination; discomfort during intercourse; and, sometimes, more frequent urination.	Often no symptoms. Can produce a clear discharge from the penis and pain during urination.
Genital warts	Growth of soft, flesh-colored, painless warts around the genital area. Warts can also appear on the cervix (the opening from the vagina into the uterus), which can be detected visually or by a Pap smear (see page 255).	Growth of soft, flesh-colored, painless warts around the genital area.
Gonorrhea	Seldom causes symptoms. Can produce a white, green, or yellow discharge from the vagina; pain during urination; spotting between periods; heavy bleeding during periods; and, occasionally, fever and abdominal pain.	Thick, yellow discharge from the penis; pain during urination; soreness at the opening of the penis.
Herpes	Genital tingling or itching; small blisters that pop open, causing burning, especially during urination. Sores turn to scabs. During the first outbreak, can produce swollen glands, fever, and body aches. Outbreaks can occur throughout life.	Symptoms same as for females.
HIV/AIDS	Often starts with a flulike illness. Symptoms may take years to develop and can include unusual or recurring infections and weight loss. Usually fatal.	Symptoms same as for females.
Syphilis	A painless, red sore in the area of sexual contact; swollen glands near the sore. In a few months, a fever, sore throat, headache, loss of appetite, or joint pain occurs and a flat, red rash appears over the body. Symptoms can disappear for years but return and can affect the brain, spinal cord, skin, and bone.	Symptoms same as for females.
Hepatitis B	Muscle aches, fever, fatigue, appetite loss, headache, and dizziness. Later, dark urine; loose, light-colored bowel movements; yellowing of the eyes and skin; and tenderness just below the ribs on the right side.	Symptoms same as for females.

Using condoms correctly

Condoms are inexpensive and available in most drugstores, supermarkets, and convenience stores. Buying condoms does not require a parent's permission or a doctor's prescription. Condoms come in various types, price ranges, and materials, and are lubricated or unlubricated. The most reliable condoms are made of latex or polyurethane. Natural materials such as sheepskin are more porous and can allow microscopic germs, including the human immunodeficiency virus (HIV), which causes acquired immune deficiency syndrome (AIDS), to pass through. Condoms also provide some protection against pregnancy and reduce a girl's risk of cancer of the cervix, which has been linked to sexual activity at a young age. Once a teenager becomes sexually active, he or she should carry a condom at all times, even when not expecting to have sex.

Male condoms protect against sexually transmitted diseases better than female condoms, but using a female condom is a good choice for girls who want to feel more in control. The female condom has other advantages. Unlike the male condom, the female condom protects the external genitals from infections such as herpes and genital warts. Its use does not depend on cooperation from a male partner. It can be used by a person who is allergic to latex, can be inserted up to 8 hours before having sex, does not have to be removed immediately after sex, and can be used with oil-based lubricants. Disadvantages include a higher price, a visible outer ring that may not appeal to a sex partner, and an increased risk of slipping or breaking during intercourse. The female condom also requires practice to learn how to insert it properly.

Before teenagers begin a sexual relationship, they need to talk to each other about using a condom. Refusal to use a condom shows a lack of maturity—a good indication of not being ready to take on a sexual relationship. To use a male condom correctly:

- Put it on an erect penis—before any contact with a partner's genital area or mouth.
- Place the condom over the tip of the penis, lubricated side out, and roll it downward toward the base of the penis, leaving about half an inch of space in the tip of the condom to hold ejaculated semen. A condom that is tight-fitting at the tip is more likely to tear.
- Withdraw the penis immediately after intercourse to prevent the condom from slipping off as the penis loses the erection. Dispose of the used condom and wash your hands.
- Never reuse a condom.

PREVENTING PREGNANCY

Nearly 1 million teenage girls get pregnant every year in the United States—a rate far greater than that of any other industrialized country despite equal rates of sexual activity. This high rate may stem from difficulty in accessing reliable birth control (which usually requires doctor visits and prescriptions), a lack of information about the availability of birth control, and unwarranted fears about its use. Inappropriate depiction of sex in the media and inadequate sex education of children can also be blamed.

Young people who engage in unprotected sex generally feel invulnerable to both pregnancy and STDs. Many teenage girls who are sexually active fail to see a doctor to obtain reliable contraception because they worry that the examination will be painful, that their parents will find out, or that the contraceptive method will cause health problems. They often don't see a doctor until they suspect they are pregnant. Younger teens usually don't use contraception because they think that their first sexual experience is a one-time event that won't lead to pregnancy. But half of all unintended pregnancies among adolescents occur within approximately 6 months of their first sexual encounter.

Most boys don't consider contraception their responsibility. Many don't understand that the risk of getting a girl pregnant without any protection is 90 percent; they don't ask a girl if she's using birth control before they have sex; and they don't have sufficient knowledge about reproduction, the female reproductive system, or the menstrual cycle. Make sure your son understands how conception occurs (see page 179) and that there is no safe time to have sex during a woman's menstrual cycle without the risk of pregnancy. Teach your son that withdrawal is not a reliable form of birth control because sperm can be released from the penis before ejaculation. Even if his partner uses the birth-control pill, he should always use a latex condom and spermicide for each sexual encounter to protect against STDs. Instill the idea that your son bears an equal responsibility for an unwanted pregnancy, which could affect his entire life.

In general, unmarried teenage girls who have babies are less likely to complete their education. Teenagers are also less likely than older women to have the emotional maturity to properly nurture and care for an infant, so their children often do not reach their full potential.

Girls younger than age 16 are at high risk for serious health problems during pregnancy, including STDs, anemia, high blood pressure, or prolonged or difficult labor. Compared with babies born to adult women, babies born to teenagers are more likely to be premature and of low birthweight, and to require intensive care after birth. These babies are also at increased risk of dying at birth. Most of these problems result from inadequate prenatal medical care; poor nutrition; and unhealthy habits such as smoking, drinking, or using drugs.

If your daughter becomes pregnant, talk to her about her options, including raising the baby, adoption, or abortion. Explain your feelings about each of these options and what you see as the advantages and disadvantages. Share books on the subject with your child. Suggest that your daughter talk to a friend who has had a baby as a teenager and ask her what it's like. Many pregnant teens decide to keep their babies rather than give them up for adoption. In this case, it's essential for a girl to finish her education and learn suitable parenting skills. Many high schools now offer on-site day care for the children of teenagers to allow the teens to finish high school. Parenting and child development classes can help them learn how to raise their children well.

Nearly half of pregnant teens choose to have an abortion. If your daughter is considering having an abortion, suggest that she talk to a gynecologist, an abortion counselor at a family planning clinic, or a member of the clergy.

Effective contraception Birth-control pills and condoms are the contraceptives used most often by teenagers. For girls who engage in sex regularly, the birth-control pill is probably the best choice. (But birth-control pills offer no protection against STDs—a latex condom must be used in addition to birth-control

Emergency contraception

If your daughter has had unprotected sexual intercourse, call her doctor right away. She can get emergency contraception from the doctor within 72 hours of the sexual encounter. Emergency contraception usually consists of taking two birth-control pills within 72 hours of the unprotected encounter and two more pills 12 hours later.

pills.) Along with being about 97-percent effective, birth-control pills provide some health benefits, including a reduced risk of iron-deficiency anemia (by making periods lighter), ovarian cancer, endometrial cancer, and osteoporosis. Birth-control pills also regulate the menstrual cycle, reduce cramps during periods, and improve acne.

The biggest problem with birth-control pills is that teenage girls often forget to take them. Adolescents also tend to have short sexual relationships, stop taking the pills as soon as a relationship ends, and often don't resume taking them when they start a new relationship. For this reason, many doctors recommend the longer-lasting hormonal methods of contraception–hormone shots or hormone implants. Hormone shots are given by a doctor every 3 months. Hormone implants consist of six matchstick-sized hormone-containing capsules placed just beneath the surface of the skin on the inside of the upper arm. They provide protection for 5 years. Birth-control methods such as the diaphragm require planning so they are not used frequently by teenagers. Natural family planning, or the "rhythm method," which restricts sexual intercourse during a woman's most fertile days of the menstrual cycle, has a high failure rate among young people who practice it because the exact time of ovulation is so hard to predict (see page 171).

Using a male condom with contraceptive jelly is almost as effective as using the birth-control pill, as long as both the condom and jelly are used each and every time the person has intercourse. But this method of birth control requires cooperation and a sense of responsibility in both partners.

HOMOSEXUALITY

Young people form their sexual identity during adolescence. By their early teens, most know whether they are sexually attracted to people of the opposite sex or their own. They may feel confused if they are sometimes attracted to members of both sexes. During adolescence, having sexual feelings for members of the same sex does not necessarily mean a person will be gay or bisexual (attracted to members of both sexes) later in life.

The biggest problems facing homosexual teenagers are social and emotional ones–including dealing with the negative attitudes of parents and other family members and friends. Adolescents who are questioning their sexual identity often feel lonely and rejected by family and friends, which puts them at increased risk for depression and suicide. Developing a network of friends within the homosexual community can give gay teenagers the emotional and social support they need. A child who has difficulty accepting his or her sexual orientation should get help from a school guidance counselor or social worker or a mental health professional at a local youth or counseling agency who can help him or her learn to deal with his or her sexuality in a positive way.

If your child tells you that he or she is homosexual, give him or her your love and support, no matter how you feel personally. Being supportive means accepting your child the way he or she is. At the same time that your child is risking your rejection, he or she may feel relieved of the heavy burden of guilt and shame that made him or her keep this major part of his or her identity from you. You now know more about the complete person your child is than you did before.

Many parents initially feel hurt or angry. They may think that they did something that caused their child to be homosexual. In fact, scientific evidence shows that parents have very little influence on their children's sexual orientation. Although the factors that influence sexual orientation are still unclear, most experts agree that it is determined very early in life and that biology plays a major role. No one makes a conscious choice to be gay—or heterosexual for that matter. Most parents, especially those who are surprised, upset, or angry that their child is gay, benefit by educating themselves about homosexuality and by participating in a support group for parents whose children are gay.

The same diseases that can be transmitted during heterosexual encounters can also be spread during homosexual encounters. Make sure your child is aware of how sexually transmitted diseases are spread and how to protect against them (see page 180). Give your child the same message about the importance of love, commitment, trust, and respect in relationships that you would if he or she were heterosexual.

Nutrition

The tremendous physical growth during puberty requires extra calories and good nutrition. Calorie needs can vary widely, depending on a child's growth rate and level of physical activity. For example, during the rapid growth spurt between ages 15 and 19, boys can eat enormous amounts of all kinds of foods—up to 4,000 calories a day. Even if they eat some junk food, many boys still get enough of the nutrients they need. Because girls usually stop growing at about age 15, they can easily become overweight if they consume more than 2,000 calories a day. Girls can't afford to eat as much junk food as boys because of their lower calorie needs.

To meet their energy needs throughout the day, preteens and teenagers need to eat at least three meals a day, starting with breakfast. Eating breakfast improves both physical and intellectual performance, making children more alert in school and better able to learn and perform in physical activities. Your child's increasing independence, active social life, busy schedule, and easy access to fast foods probably keep him or her from eating the way you would like. Because you now have little control over your child's overall diet, it's especially important to provide a wide variety of healthful foods at home, including nutritious snacks such as fresh fruits, cut up raw vegetables, cheese, and yogurt. Resist the temptation to buy high-fat, high-calorie foods that provide little nutrition because a teenager looking for a snack is likely to reach for them first.

Continue to follow the recommendations of the Food Guide Pyramid (see page 113). Carbohydrate-rich whole grains, fruits, and vegetables are the foundation of a healthy diet. Eating lots of fruits and vegetables is beneficial at any age, although fewer than 10 percent of adolescents eat the recommended five or more servings of fruits and vegetables each day. Fruits and vegetables contain antioxidants and other substances that help reduce the risk of heart disease, stroke, cancer, and other illnesses. Dairy products, fish, legumes, nuts, poultry, eggs, and lean meats are also important because they provide nutrients that promote proper growth and development.

One of the most serious adolescent health problems, obesity, results from consuming too many calories and getting too little exercise. Being overweight during adolescence is a major risk factor for health problems–including heart disease, stroke, high blood pressure, or type 2 diabetes–later in life. If you think your child has a weight problem, talk to his or her doctor before you try to put your child on a diet. Consider your own attitudes toward body image and diet. If you are preoccupied with thinness and communicate it to your child, you may be setting him or her up for a lifetime of disordered eating. For more about how to help an overweight child, see page 580.

BODY IMAGE

Many children develop a poor body image during adolescence. At a time when girls' bodies are naturally adding fat, they often feel the need to be unrealistically thin. Boys may feel pressured to look muscular and strong and engage in strenuous weight-lifting programs or use dangerous hormonal drugs, such as steroids (see page 201) or human growth hormone, to build up their muscles.

Teens who are overweight often become obsessed with dieting, which gives them an unnatural attitude toward food that can last a lifetime. Help your child diet in a sensible way by promoting the basics of a healthy lifestyle–eating a nutritious, balanced, low-fat diet rich in fruits, vegetables, whole grains, and legumes (dried beans, peas, and lentils) and exercising regularly. Gradually incorporate nutritional techniques into your cooking (see page 141) that can benefit everyone in the family. Regular exercise can help your child lose weight and maintain a healthy weight throughout life.

Although increasing numbers of adolescent boys of normal weight want to lose weight, girls are much more likely than boys to think they are overweight even when they aren't. Some girls starve themselves or force themselves to vomit or use laxatives or diuretics (drugs that cause the body to lose water through increased urination) to eliminate excess calories after eating enormous amounts of food. Although eating disorders (see page 478) are increasing among teenage boys, they are still much more common among preteen and teenage girls. Eating disorders can be life threatening. If you notice any changes in your child's eating behavior, an excessive concern about losing weight, overexercising, use of diuretics or laxatives, unusual sluggishness, or withdrawal from friends and family, talk to the doctor immediately.

CALCIUM: ESSENTIAL FOR TEENS

An increasing number of women are developing osteoporosis at younger and younger ages—primarily because they haven't built up their bones to their peak strength during childhood and adolescence. To try to reverse this trend, the federal government has increased the daily calcium requirement from 1,200 milligrams to 1,300 milligrams each day for children over 10. Most teenagers consume less than 800 milligrams a day.

During the teen years, girls tend to drink less milk and avoid other dairy products because they think these foods are too high in fat. In fact, dairy products are the highest quality source of calcium because the body most easily absorbs the calcium in these foods. Provide low-fat and nonfat versions of milk products—and stress, especially to a daughter, the importance of building up bone density during the teen years.

It's not hard to meet the daily calcium requirement (see chart on page 190). But if your child is not getting sufficient calcium from his or her diet, the doctor may suggest using calcium supplements to reach the recommended daily level.

Adolescence: An Important Time for Bone Growth

Nearly half of a person's total bone mass is formed during the teenage years. Bones reach their peak strength and density by about age 18. Along with exercise that puts weight on bones, getting enough of the bone-strengthening mineral calcium is essential. Teenagers, especially girls, who don't reach their full potential bone strength are at high risk of developing osteoporosis and disabling fractures later in life.

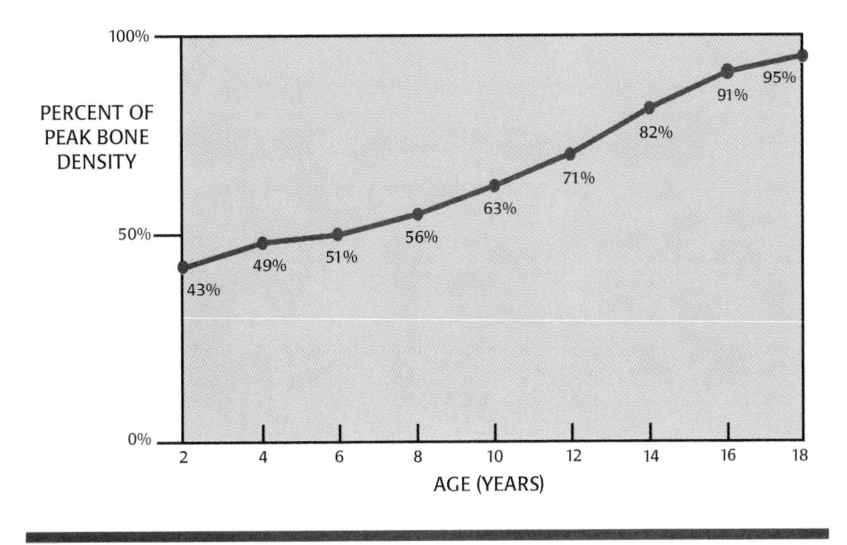

Good Sources of Calcium

The best way to get calcium is to eat foods that are rich in the mineral. Encourage your children to get the equivalent of a little more than four servings of calcium a day (with a serving providing about 300 milligrams of calcium) to reach the recommended 1,300 milligrams every day. Not all foods provide equal amounts, as you can see from the examples shown here. For example, you would have to eat 4 cups of broccoli or 2 cups of cottage cheese to obtain the same amount of calcium you would get from an 8-ounce glass of skim milk or fortified orange juice or a cup of fruit yogurt.

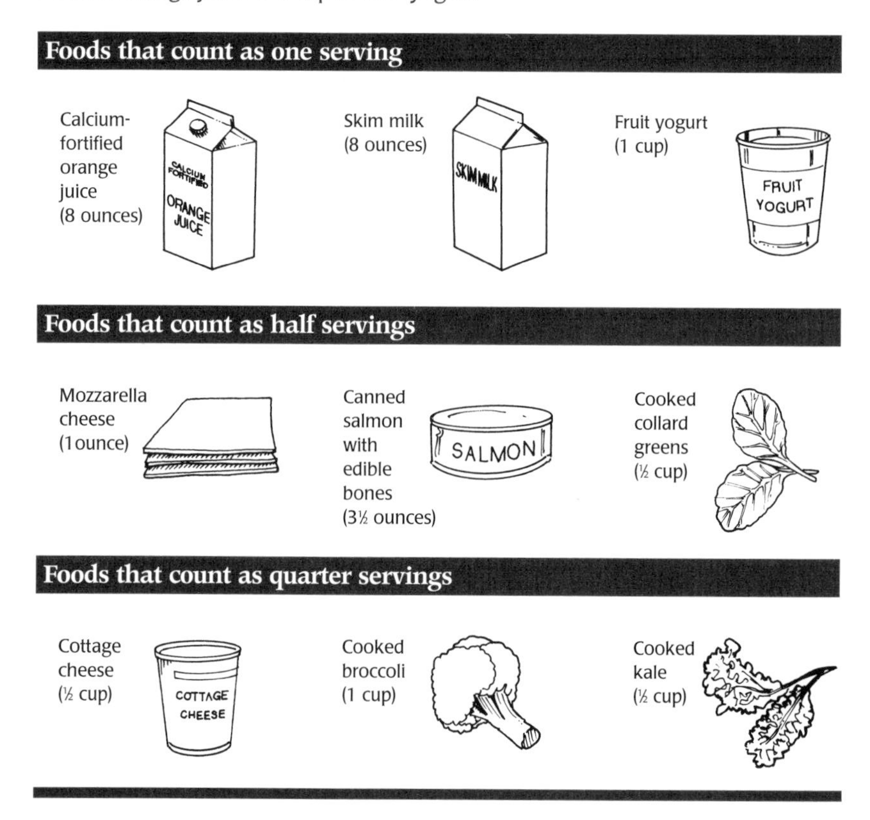

Why iron is important for teens

The daily requirement for iron jumps 50 percent after age 10—from 10 milligrams a day to 15. Teenage boys need more iron to meet the extra demands of their rapid growth. Girls need more iron after they start menstruating to replace the iron naturally lost in menstrual blood. If your daughter has unusually heavy periods, she may be at risk of developing iron-deficiency anemia (see page 412) from excessive iron loss during menstruation. Teenage girls who exercise intensely can also develop iron-deficiency anemia. The symptoms of iron-deficiency anemia include fatigue, irritability, headaches, lack of energy, and tingling in the hands and feet. If your daughter has any of these symptoms, talk to her doctor. He or she may recommend supplements to restore her iron to a normal level. Iron found in animal foods such as beef, chicken, tuna, and shrimp is more easily absorbed by the body than that found in plant foods such as dried beans, nuts, and dried fruits. For other sources of iron, see page 117.

Exercise

Exercise is beneficial throughout life–it improves strength, builds muscle, strengthens bones, lowers blood pressure, reduces body fat, and increases the "good" blood cholesterol levels while decreasing the "bad" blood cholesterol levels. Exercise also improves mood and lowers stress and anxiety. Weight-bearing physical activity makes bones strong and helps them take in the bone-strengthening mineral calcium. The bone-building effects of exercise are especially important during adolescence because this is the time when bones reach their peak strength and density. Being fit also helps children develop a positive self-image. Everyone should work toward a goal of exercising for at least 30 minutes almost every day. Exercising longer and harder provides additional health benefits.

The lack of exercise among American children is beginning to take its toll. Two out of three adolescents can't pass a basic fitness test. Fewer and fewer American schools require daily participation in physical education classes and many children spend more time watching television than doing anything else, including attending school. Teenagers who are not physically active are also more likely than active teens to engage in behaviors that are potentially harmful to their health–including smoking cigarettes, using marijuana, eating a poor diet, or failing to wear seat belts.

A person who establishes the habit of physical activity during childhood and adolescence is more likely to stay active and healthy as an adult. If your child has been sedentary, help him or her gradually become more active. Suggest ways to fit exercise into your child's daily routine. Have your child walk or ride a bike to school instead of riding in a car. Or suggest taking the stairs instead of an elevator whenever possible. Limit the time your child watches television, uses a computer, or plays video games. Be a good role model and engage in regular exercise yourself. Plan fun activities such as games, bike rides, or walks with family and friends.

Being physically fit means having good endurance, strength, and flexibility. Your child can develop each of these abilities through different types of activities.

Endurance Endurance, or aerobic fitness, is achieved through exercise that increases the heart rate, training the heart and lungs to work more efficiently. Aerobic exercise involves sustained, repetitive motion of the large muscles, such as those in the legs, and includes brisk walking, jogging, cycling, swimming, aerobics, skating, and stair climbing.

Female athlete triad

Adolescent girls who exercise too much and eat too little can develop a condition known as female athlete triad, characterized by three medical problems: an eating disorder (see page 478), the cessation of menstruation, and premature osteoporosis (bone thinning), similar to that which occurs after menopause. This condition is especially prevalent among girls who engage in gymnastics, endurance running, and figure skating. The disordered eating can cause near starvation and dehydration, while the osteoporosis can predispose an affected girl to recurrent stress fractures. Athletic performance is also adversely affected. If your daughter exercises so much that she stops menstruating, don't hesitate to take her to her doctor for a physical examination and evaluation. The bone loss produced by overexercising and disordered eating can be irreversible.

Strength Strength training, also called weight training or resistance training, is the use of free weights, weight machines, or resistance exercises such as push-ups to increase muscle strength and endurance. Young people should not begin a weight-training regimen until their body has reached full maturity (usually between ages 15 and 18) because weight training can interfere with the development of the bones and muscles or cause serious injury. Before your child begins strength training, make sure that he or she is trained properly by an expert, such as a physical education teacher or a trainer at a local health club, and that he or she learns the appropriate techniques and safety measures under close supervision.

Flexibility Flexibility is the ability to move the joints through their full range of motion, making it easier to do everyday activities and protecting the joint-supporting muscles from injury during exercise. It's a good idea to do stretching exercises for a few minutes before and after doing other kinds of exercises to maintain flexibility.

Getting exercise through sports
Your preteens or teenagers might enjoy exercise more by participating in team or individual sports. Involvement in activities in which they can feel a sense of accomplishment increases their self-esteem and their enjoyment of exercise. The most successful sports programs are those that present challenges to help children develop skills while having fun.

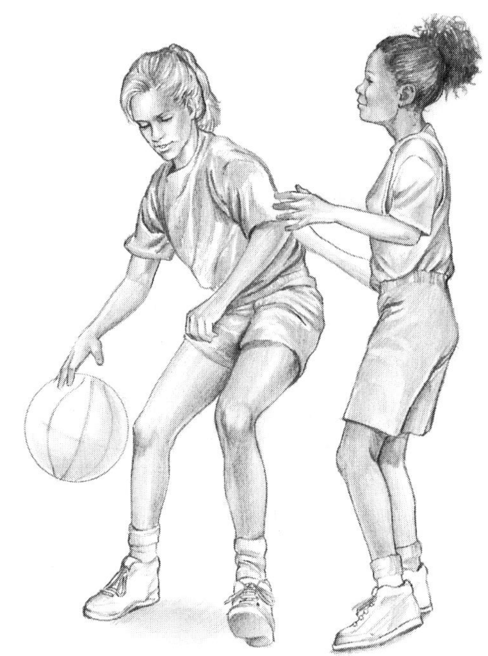

Sleep

The need for sleep increases during adolescence as puberty resets the biological clock. Teenagers begin to go to bed later and need to sleep later in the morning. To be as alert as possible, most teenagers require more than 9 hours of sleep each night–but many average 6 to 7 hours or less, especially on school nights. The lack of sleep can make a teenager moody, depressed, and tired during the day. Many teenagers fall asleep in class, which interferes with their ability to learn. They are also more likely to fall asleep driving a car, increasing their risk of causing a motor vehicle collision.

Children who consistently go to bed early and wake up early on both weeknights and weekends tend to do better in school than those who go to bed late. But it's not easy to get teenagers to go to bed early when their biological clock is telling them to stay up later. For as long as you can influence your child's daily schedule, help your child to maintain a regular bedtime on school nights. Establish a routine for everyone in the household–such as no television watching or talking on the telephone after 10:00 PM. Be a good role model and get a sufficient amount of sleep yourself.

Self-care

By age 11, children can manage most of their own personal hygiene, including showering or bathing daily and washing their hair. They should also wash their hands frequently to prevent the spread of infection. Increased hormone levels during puberty cause the sweat glands to produce more perspiration, which may now have an odor. Talk to your child about using deodorant or antiperspirant regularly.

Greater oil gland activity increases the risk of acne (see page 401). Pimples, whiteheads, or blackheads can form when oil gets blocked inside hair follicles (the cavities in which hairs grow). The tendency to develop acne is inherited and usually peaks between ages 16 and 19 in boys and 14 and 17 in girls. (There is no evidence that specific foods, such as chocolate or fried foods, cause acne.) If your adolescent is

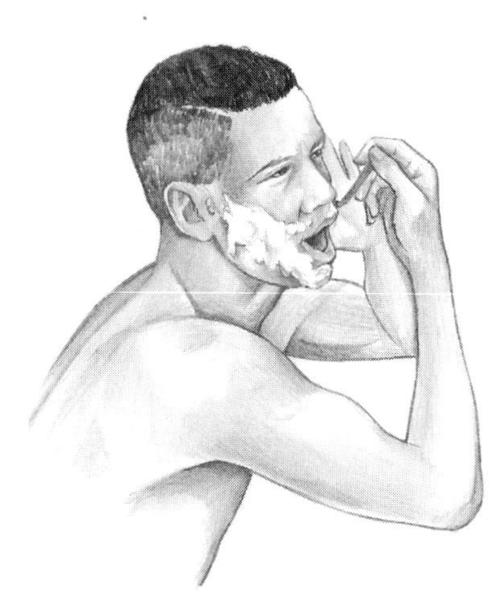

Starting to shave

Many boys need to shave by the time they leave high school. Teach your son the basics of shaving as soon as you notice hair appearing on his face. Tell your son never to share razors because of the serious infections that can be transmitted in blood, including hepatitis B and the virus that causes AIDS.

prone to acne, remind him or her to wash his or her face two or three times a day. Keeping the skin clean does not prevent acne, but it can keep it from getting worse. Your child should avoid using oil-based moisturizers or makeup on blemished areas. If blemishes are severe or don't go away on their own, take your child to the doctor, who can prescribe appropriate treatment (see page 401).

Continue to stress the importance of toothbrushing at least twice a day and flossing once a day to keep your child's teeth and gums healthy (see page 259). Encourage your child to wear ultraviolet light-screening sunglasses and to always wear sunscreen (with a sun protection factor of at least 15) to protect against the damaging effects of the sun (see page 287). Discourage sunbathing and the use of tanning beds, which are just as harmful as the sun.

School

When children reach high school, their parents sometimes become less involved with their schooling. Children whose parents stay involved tend to have better grades and a more positive attitude toward school than those whose parents are less active. Show an interest in your child's classes and encourage him or her to share information about school. Your enthusiasm lets your child know how important you consider his or her education.

Convey high expectations for your child's learning and behavior both at home and at school. Emphasize effort and achievement and praise your child for showing progress. Establish rules and routines for doing homework and provide a quiet place for study, away from the television, telephone, or loud music. Promote reading by reading yourself and by having interesting and appropriate reading materials available at home. Teach your child how to use the library and help him or her apply for a library card.

If your child is not doing well in school, contact his or her teachers or school counselor right away. Ask all of your child's teachers to call you immediately if they see a problem developing. It's important to clear up problems as early as possible. Ask about specific things you can do at home to help your child. Give teachers any information that might help them work with your child to improve performance.

Balancing School and a Job

Many teenagers successfully balance part-time jobs and school. At the same time, many parents wonder if it's a good idea for their children to work. Work provides many long-term benefits for adolescents but it also can have some drawbacks. Consider your child's individual situation to determine if work is beneficial for him or her.

The advantages of work include helping teenagers develop responsibility, learn to manage their time and money, and achieve some financial independence. Some jobs teach skills that can be used in future jobs and most jobs improve a child's social skills because they require interaction with other people. Being employed during high school also enables teens to acquire employer references that can be helpful in getting jobs later.

On the other hand, work takes time away from homework, which can hinder a child's success in school. Work also leaves less time for extracurricular and social activities that are important to an adolescent's development. Working late can also prevent teenagers from getting enough sleep. Employers may also take advantage of an adolescent's youth and inexperience.

If your teenager wants to work, establish guidelines that you both agree on. For example, make sure your child understands that schoolwork is the main priority and that keeping the job depends on maintaining good grades. Establish clear expectations about what you consider acceptable employment—such as the type of work, the safety of the work setting, and the maximum number of hours per week. You might suggest that your child work only on vacations or weekends. If your teenager doesn't need to work mainly to earn money, he or she might benefit from an unpaid internship that teaches skills that can transfer to a career.

Risky behavior

Every day, your child makes choices that may be good or bad for his or her health. Many of these choices involve potentially dangerous behaviors, such as using alcohol or other drugs, driving after drinking, or failing to wear a seat belt or a bike helmet. Help your child understand the impact that these behaviors could have on his or her future.

ALCOHOL AND OTHER DRUGS

Many teenagers experiment with alcohol and cigarettes. Alcohol is the most commonly abused drug and nearly half of all teens have tried marijuana by the time they leave high school, but only a few go on to stronger drugs such as cocaine. Adolescents start using drugs for a number of reasons. Some are curious about what it feels like to get "high," or they think that drugs will relax them, boost their self-confidence, or make them more social. They may use alcohol and other drugs to assert their independence or to fit in with a particular group of friends.

Children whose parents smoke or use alcohol or other drugs are more likely to see drug use as a normal step toward adulthood. If you drink, drink in moderation (one drink a day or less for women and two or less for men)—and never include your child in your drinking (for example by asking him or her to mix a drink for you). If you smoke cigarettes, quit now for your own health and to set a good example for your children. If you can't quit, talk to your child about how addictive nicotine is and how, when you were younger, you

Resisting peer pressure

Teenagers always want to do what their friends want to do. They can put pressure on each other to do things they know are wrong or risky, such as drinking alcohol or using other drugs, cutting school, cheating on a test, or having sex. Teach your child that he or she has a right to:

- Decide what he or she thinks is right and express his or her opinions.
- Be responsible for his or her own feelings.
- Say "no" and mean it.
- Leave an undesirable situation or suggest doing something else.
- Change his or her mind.

thought you could quit any time you wanted. Avoid smoking in the house and car.

To help your child resist drugs, take an interest in his or her activities. Have discussions about drug use, get to know his or her friends, and try to understand his or her problems and concerns. Emphasize that drugs do not help problems disappear and always show strong disapproval of drugs. Help your child understand that young people are especially vulnerable to the physical, psychological, and social effects of drug use because their brains and bodies are still developing.

A teenager's exposure to drugs usually follows three stages. The first stage is experimentation, when the child uses drugs as a form of recreation. This stage is the least dangerous. During this stage, a parent probably wouldn't notice any obvious changes in his or her child's behavior. Many teenagers remain at the experimental stage or stop using drugs altogether.

Teenagers who progress to the second stage become psychologically addicted to drugs, and actively seek them out. The drugs become more and more

Drug Use Among Children

This chart shows the percentage of American students who have tried these common drugs at least once. Alcohol and cigarettes are the drugs most often used by American teenagers, but marijuana is becoming increasingly popular. Children are experimenting with drugs at younger and younger ages, usually starting at about age 10. More and more younger children are using inhalants.

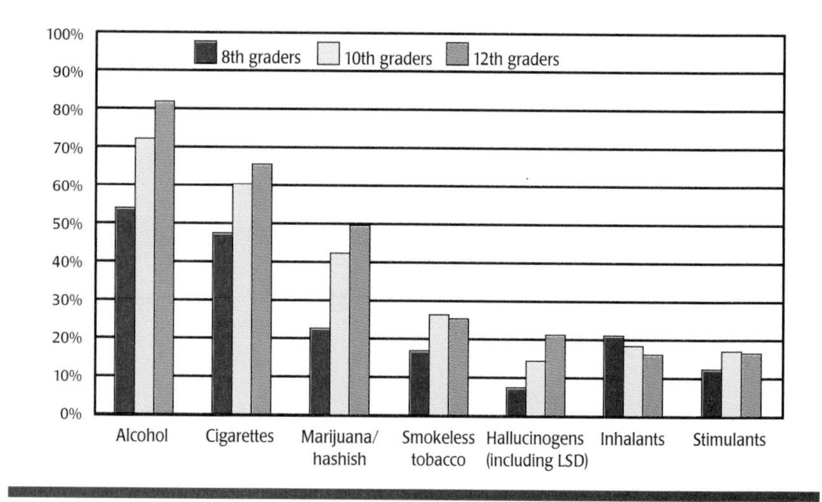

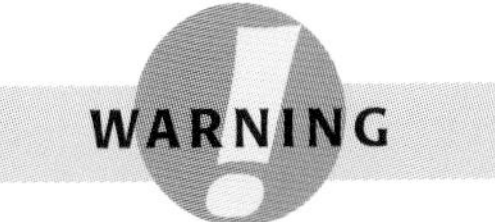

Your child could be using drugs

If your child is using alcohol or other drugs, get help right away to avoid serious problems. Call the doctor if you notice any of the following signs of possible drug use:

- Spending large amounts of time alone, or becoming isolated, withdrawn, or secretive.
- Drop in grades or other change in school performance.
- Drastic mood swings or changes in behavior or personality, such as violent temper outbursts, depression, lack of motivation, belligerence, irritability, apathy, hostility, or paranoia.
- Changes in your child's peer group, such as giving up longtime friends.
- Lack of interest in hobbies or social and recreational activities.
- Poor personal hygiene.
- Unusual odors on his or her clothing.

important, and the child may start avoiding old friends who don't use drugs or may give up activities, hobbies, and other interests. You might notice changes in your child's behavior at this point. If you do, get help immediately, because the next, more serious phase of drug use–abuse–is more difficult to reverse. A child who is abusing drugs becomes preoccupied with them and may lose interest in any other type of activity. His or her grades fall and he or she may get into trouble with the law.

When investigating your child's possible use of drugs, take an indirect approach. Ask about a friend's drug use or about drug use at school in general. Be nonjudgmental; you want to maintain a trusting relationship so your child will continue to be open with you. If you suspect your child is using drugs, talk to his or her doctor, who may refer you to a professional who specializes in counseling and treating adolescents who have a substance abuse problem. For more about drug abuse and treatments, see page 475.

Alcohol Alcohol is the drug that children most often use and abuse. Advertisements suggest that alcohol will give them more friends, greater prestige, more fun, and more sex appeal. Children often get mixed messages about alcohol that say it's OK to drink as long as they aren't using illegal drugs or driving after drinking. Talk to your child about the dangers of alcohol, treating it as seriously as you do other drugs.

Alcohol affects girls more strongly than boys because girls are usually smaller and because they lack certain digestive enzymes that help break down alcohol before it enters the bloodstream. For these reasons, girls can become dependent upon alcohol sooner than boys and are more susceptible to liver damage and other alcohol-related health problems that stem from long-term alcohol use.

Alcohol affects every organ of the body, but one of its most profound effects is on the central nervous system. Drinking just one or two alcoholic beverages can affect coordination, slow reaction time, distort vision and hearing, block memory, and impair judgment. Teenage alcohol use has been linked to poor academic performance, motor vehicle collisions, injury, blackouts, acquaintance rape, unplanned pregnancy, suicide, and homicide. Regular use can retard an adolescent's social, emotional, and intellectual development. Long-term use can cause serious health problems, including alcoholism, appetite loss, vitamin deficiencies, stomach ailments, skin problems, liver damage, sexual impotence, permanent damage to the heart and central nervous system, and memory loss.

Unsupervised parties

Teenagers often have parties at their homes when their parents are away. These parties almost always involve alcohol and, sometimes, other drugs. When your child tells you he or she is going to a party, find out exactly when and where the party is taking place. Get the name, address, and telephone number of the host, call and talk to the parent, and drop off and pick up your teen, if necessary. If your child refuses to cooperate, don't allow him or her to go to the party. To check on your child's activities, show up unexpectedly occasionally or arrive about 20 minutes early when picking him or her up.

Binge drinking—having five or more drinks in a row—is one of the most disturbing and dangerous aspects of adolescent drinking. Teenagers who binge drink are much more likely than nondrinkers to engage in risky behaviors. Drinking an excessive amount of alcohol all at once can cause alcohol poisoning, which can be fatal. Alcohol poisoning is more common among preteens and teenagers than any other group and drinking more than one drink in an hour increases the risk. Teach your child never to let anyone force him or her to drink alcohol and never to take part in drinking games or contests.

Cigarettes Nearly all adults who currently smoke became addicted to nicotine by age 17. After several years of decline, the numbers of children who smoke are increasing. Teenagers are easy targets for advertising that links smoking with toughness in males, glamour and thinness in females, and sophistication in both sexes. The average smoker starts at age 12 and becomes a daily smoker by age 14.

When you talk to your child about the harmful effects of smoking, stress its effects on appearance because teenagers are more likely to respond to messages about the unattractiveness of smoking than to those about health. Smoking causes dry skin and wrinkles, bad breath, stained teeth, and smelly clothes. Many people avoid being around smokers and both girls and boys say they would rather date a nonsmoker. Talk about how difficult it is to quit smoking because few children understand the strong addictive hold of nicotine. Most think they'll be able to stop whenever they want.

Smoking increases heart rate and blood pressure, reduces the senses of smell and taste, and increases the risk of respiratory infections, asthma, chronic bronchitis, emphysema, and stomach ulcers. The typical smoker's cough is actually a sign of a serious condition called chronic bronchitis, which eventually leads to irreversible lung disease unless the person stops smoking. Of the more than 1 million children who start smoking each year, one third will eventually die of it. A teenager who smokes is five times more likely than a nonsmoker to have a heart attack in his or her 30s or 40s. Smoking is a major cause of lung cancer, which kills more women than any other type of cancer (including breast cancer) and is the second leading cancer killer of men (after prostate cancer). Smoking also contributes to other cancers, including cancer of the mouth, throat, esophagus, bladder, and uterus. Smoking may also reduce fertility in both men and women and causes a low birthweight in newborns. If your child smokes, encourage and help him or her to quit. Talk to the doctor about techniques for quitting. Don't allow smoking at home or in the car; secondhand smoke can increase the risk of respiratory problems, heart disease, and cancer in nonsmoking members of the household.

Smokeless tobacco Smokeless tobacco refers to both chewing tobacco, a form of leaf tobacco, and snuff, finely ground tobacco that is inhaled. The number of young people, nearly all male, who use smokeless tobacco products is on the rise. The use of smokeless tobacco can cause nicotine addiction because the nicotine is absorbed into the bloodstream and affects the brain. Nicotine can increase the heart rate and blood pressure, cause an irregular heartbeat, and constrict blood vessels, which can slow reaction time and cause dizziness. Smokeless tobacco products can make the gums and lips sting, crack, bleed, and wrinkle; stain the teeth; cause bad breath; and reduce the senses of taste and smell. Sores and white patches may appear in the mouth. Constant irritation can damage the lining of the mouth and throat, increasing the risk of gum disease (which can lead to tooth loss) and cancer of the mouth and throat.

If your child uses smokeless tobacco, try to convince him or her to quit. Talk to the doctor about methods your child can use to quit. At the very least, make sure your child has dental checkups every 6 months to watch for early signs of potentially cancerous changes in the mouth.

Marijuana Marijuana comes from the leaves of the hemp plant (*Cannabis sativa*) and is usually smoked. All forms of marijuana, or cannabis, produce physical and mental effects, including bloodshot eyes, a dry mouth and throat, sleepiness, increased heart rate, difficulty keeping track of time, impaired or reduced short-term memory, and reduced ability to perform tasks that require concentration and coordination, such as driving a car. In some people, the drug can cause paranoia (excessive fear), mild hallucinations, and panic attacks. Frequent use can reduce the sex drive and increase the risk of male and female infertility. Long-term use damages the lungs and respiratory system and progresses to chronic bronchitis and emphysema. Marijuana smoke contains more

Could your child be using marijuana?

If you notice any paraphernalia designed for marijuana use—rolling papers (for making marijuana cigarettes), clips (for holding a marijuana cigarette), pipes, or bent paper clips (for cleaning pipes)—in your child's room, book bag, or pockets, your child may be using marijuana. Other evidence of marijuana use includes a distinctive odor on your child's clothes or in his or her room, use of incense or other room deodorizers, use of eyedrops, and wearing clothing or jewelry that promotes drug use.

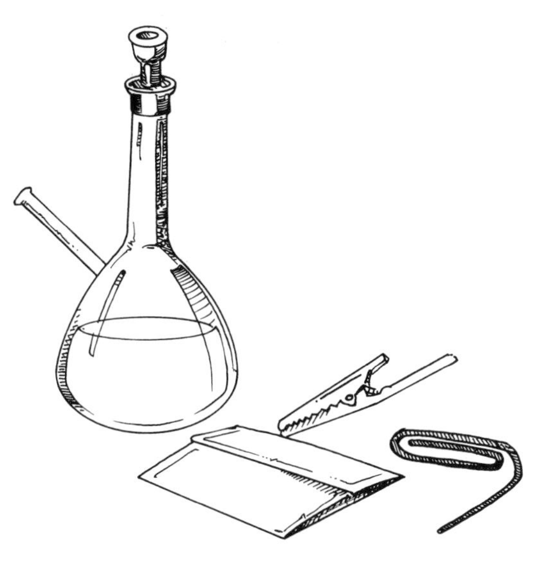

cancer-causing agents than tobacco smoke, increasing the risk of lung cancer. Heavy, chronic use can cause psychological dependence that can lead to loss of energy, ambition, and drive.

Inhalants An increasing number of children inhale chemicals found in common household products to get high. Inhaling such chemicals is attractive to children because they produce a feeling of euphoria immediately, cost little, are easily obtained, and their possession is not illegal. Inhalants can be found in glues and adhesives, nail polish remover, marking pens, paint thinner, spray paint, butane lighter fluid, gasoline, propane gas, correction fluid, household cleaners, cooking sprays, deodorants, fabric protectors, whipping cream aerosols, and air-conditioning coolants.

Using inhalants even once is extremely dangerous because they can cause sudden death in a number of ways–asphyxia (from inhaling solvent gases that limit available oxygen in the air), suffocation (from inhaling a chemical through a bag), choking on vomit, or reckless behavior in life-threatening situations. While using an inhalant, or just after, a child can fall victim to a syndrome called sudden sniffing death, in which the heart begins to overwork, beating rapidly but unevenly and causing cardiac arrest. Short-term effects of inhalant use include hallucinations, severe mood swings, numbness and tingling of the hands and feet, heart palpitations, breathing difficulty, dizziness, and headaches. Prolonged use can cause short-term memory loss, muscle spasms, an irregular heartbeat, liver and kidney failure, and permanent brain and nerve damage.

If your child uses inhalants, you might notice an unusual breath odor or a chemical odor on his or her clothing; slurred or disoriented speech; a drunk, dazed, or dizzy appearance; red or runny eyes or nose; spots or sores around the mouth; or loss of appetite. Long-term users may display anxiety, excitability, irritability, or restlessness. Other clues to inhalant use include frequently holding a pen or marker near the nose; smelling clothing sleeves; having paint or stain marks on the face, fingers, or clothing; or hiding rags, clothes, or empty containers of chemical-containing products. Talk to the doctor immediately if you notice any of these signs; your child needs immediate intervention.

Hallucinogens Hallucinogenic drugs are substances that distort a person's perception. The most well-known hallucinogens include lysergic acid diethylamide (LSD or acid), phencyclidine (known as PCP or angel dust), mescaline and peyote, and psilocybin ("magic mushrooms"). The effects of hallucinogens can last for as long as 12 hours. Physical effects can include increased heart rate and blood pressure; sleeplessness and tremors; lack of coordination; sparse, incoherent speech; decreased awareness of touch and pain (which can result in self-inflicted injuries); convulsions; coma; and heart and lung failure. The user may experience panic, confusion, suspicion, depression, anxiety, paranoia, violent behavior, disorientation, and loss of control. Delayed effects, or flashbacks (recurring memories of the experience) can occur more than a year after taking the drug. Everyone reacts differently to hallucinogens and there is no way to predict who will or won't have a "bad trip," which can produce terrifying thoughts and feelings or lead to injury and fatal accidents.

Anabolic steroids Some teenagers use anabolic steroids to increase their strength, obtain a hard-bodied appearance, and improve their athletic performance. The practice is most prevalent among boys who are varsity athletes in sports such as football, rugby, and wrestling. The use of anabolic steroids has also been rising in girls in recent years. These drugs can be taken in pill form or by injection (which increases the risk of HIV infection if needles are shared). Anabolic steroids can cause numerous harmful side effects, both physical and psychological. The liver, cardiovascular system, and reproductive system are affected most severely. In males, steroids can cause the testicles to shrink, breasts to develop, and increase the risk of baldness, infertility, and impotence. In females, the drugs can stimulate the development of irreversible masculine traits including growth of facial hair, breast reduction, and deepening of the voice. Steroids can also cause irregular menstrual periods and infertility. In both sexes, steroids can cause or worsen acne. In both sexes, the drugs induce extremely aggressive behavior and depression. Some side effects occur quickly; others, such as heart attacks and strokes, may not occur until years later.

Signs of anabolic steroid use include a rapid increase in weight and muscle bulk, aggressiveness, hostility, excessive moodiness, severe acne, baldness, and yellowing of the skin and whites of the eyes (jaundice). If you suspect your child may be using steroids, talk to the doctor and to your child's athletic coach (if your child is an athlete). Ask them to recommend ways to build muscle and strength without using steroids.

Driving

Motor vehicle collisions are the leading cause of death among all 15- to 20-year-olds, primarily because of the child's lack of experience and tendency to take risks. Once your child has his or her driver's license, gradually give him or her more driving privileges as he or she gains the experience necessary to drive safely. Set a good example by not speeding, following all traffic laws, always wearing your seat belt and requiring everyone else in the car to wear theirs, and never drinking alcohol or using other drugs when you drive. Tell your child to always call you or someone else you trust for a ride any time he or she or any other driver has been drinking or using drugs–no matter what time it is, no questions asked.

Establish house rules for safe driving and stick to them. Take away driving privileges if your child breaks any of the rules and don't give in–your major concern is your child's safety. Regularly remind your child of the importance of staying focused on driving and not getting distracted by playing the radio excessively loud or talking on a cellular phone. Here are some general rules that can help your child become a safe, responsible driver:

- The driver and all passengers must wear seat belts.
- No one in the vehicle may use tobacco, alcohol, or other drugs.
- Driving privileges will be taken away if the child gets a ticket, has a collision, or drives after drinking alcohol or using other drugs.
- Good grades must be maintained in order to drive. (Many auto insurance companies give "good student" discounts to full-time students; check with your agent.)

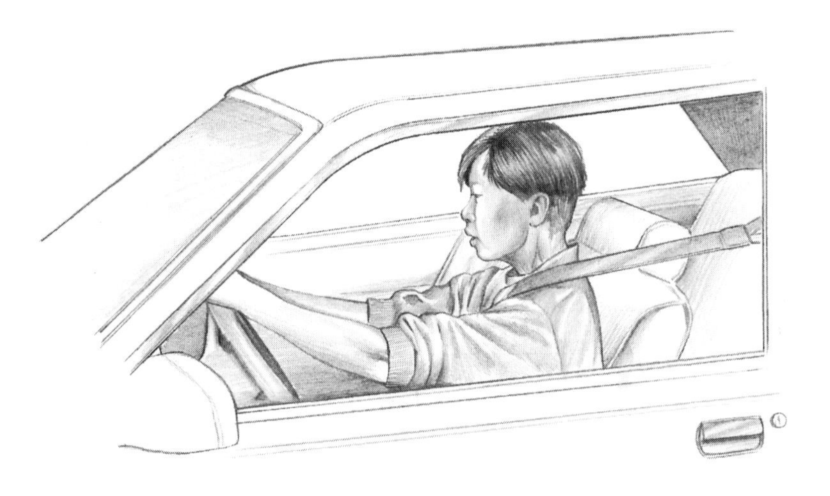

Buckle up every time
By the time your teenager gets his or her driver's license, he or she should already have established the habit of buckling up every time he or she rides in a car.

TATTOOS AND BODY PIERCINGS

Tattooing and body piercing are becoming increasingly popular among preteens and teens of all socioeconomic, racial, and ethnic groups. Both tattoos and body piercings carry certain long-term health risks.

Infection with hepatitis B (see page 517) is the most common serious health problem caused by tattoos and body piercings, but the risk of infection with HIV (the virus that causes AIDS) or tetanus also exists if the instruments used have been contaminated. Pigments used in tattoos can cause allergic reactions in some people and the Food and Drug Administration has approved no pigments for injection under the skin.

Younger adolescents between the ages of 10 and 14 who don't have easy access to money or transportation frequently tattoo or pierce themselves or have a friend do it. Older adolescents between 14 and 18 years of age often obtain tattoos or body piercings from artists in studio storefronts or temporary booths set up at rock concerts. No public health regulations exist to monitor tattooing or body piercing safety practices. Artists are generally not licensed or certified and are usually uninformed about sterilization and infection-control procedures. Many use unsterilized instruments.

Complications from piercings are most likely to occur in the mouth and in the upper part of the ear, sometimes causing permanent damage and cosmetic deformities. Serious infections are more common in piercings high on the ear because the tissue doesn't heal very easily. Tongue piercing may cause permanent numbness, speech difficulty, loss of taste, or swelling that can interfere with breathing and eating. Piercings adjacent to the teeth, gums, or cheek can cause tooth fractures, or inflammation and infection inside the mouth.

Piercings in areas such as the navel, nipples, and genitals take longer than usual to heal (up to 5 months) because they are shielded from light and air and are exposed to body moisture and irritation from clothing. Because of their location, body piercings are prone to recurring infections. In some body piercings, the hole never heals and scarring results.

Talk to your child about tattoos and body piercings in a straightforward, factual way by the time he or she is 10 years of age. If you know ahead of time that your child is planning to get a tattoo or body piercing, make sure he or she knows the risks and is vaccinated against hepatitis B. Discuss the permanence of tattoos and the cost of having them removed in the future. Although newer techniques for removing tattoos cause less scarring, these procedures are not easy to obtain, are very expensive, and are not covered by health insurance.

If your child has already gotten a tattoo or body piercing, try to be as nonjudgmental as you can, no matter how angry and upset you are. Make sure he or she takes the proper precautions to promote healing and prevent infection. Have the doctor examine the tattoo or piercing and instruct your child in proper care.

BELONGING TO A GANG

Gangs are no longer just an inner-city problem—they are attracting boys and girls from all socioeconomic and racial groups in smaller cities and towns and suburbs across the country. Gangs are characterized by their involvement in illegal behaviors such as violence, stealing, vandalizing, and using drugs. Most of the violence is carried out against other gangs. Gangs fill a void for some children who are searching for something, or someone, to connect with—to fulfill their need for recognition, to be part of a group, or to have a relationship with someone who "cares" for them. The gang relationship often serves as a substitute for the family, especially if the child's family isn't providing security, love, discipline, or monetary rewards.

If you suspect that your child might be involved with a gang, talk to his or her doctor, school counselor, principal, teachers, or other people who might be able to suggest ways to intervene. Community antigang interventions are most successful when parents, teachers, and other school personnel work together to reach a child individually. The following signs indicate that your child might be involved with a gang:

- A sudden drop in grades, discipline problems at school, or lack of involvement with school

- Tattoos or burns on the body
- A new nickname
- Gang graffiti on book covers or folders
- Wearing clothing of one color (especially blue or red)
- Using hand signals
- Making new friends and avoiding old ones
- Being unusually secretive
- Using tobacco, alcohol, or other drugs
- Signs of unexplained affluence, such as money and new clothes
- Negative contact with police or teachers
- Unexplained use of pagers
- Possession of guns or knives

If your child is depressed

During the transition from childhood to adulthood, the risk for depression rises. Teenage girls are twice as likely as boys to experience serious depression, but the numbers are increasing in both sexes. Suicide is the third leading cause of death among adolescents after motor vehicle collisions and homicide. Girls are more than three times as likely as boys to attempt suicide, but boys are four times more likely to be successful because they use more deadly weapons, such as guns. For every teen suicide, there are up to 200 suicide attempts.

Symptoms of depression in preteens and teenagers include talk about being sad, bored, or empty; extreme mood swings; engaging in dangerous activities; failing in school; running away from home; abusing drugs; stealing; or lying. If you recognize any of these symptoms in your child, get help right away. The treatment of depression is successful in most cases, especially when started in the early stages.

Left untreated, depression can worsen and lead to suicide. If your child ever talks about wanting to die, even in a joking way, take him or her seriously and get help immediately. Contrary to popular belief, talking about suicide is not an empty cry for help. You must take immediate action. Call your child's doctor or a local hospital emergency department, where a suicide crisis worker should be available 24 hours a day to evaluate the situation and intervene. If you think your child is in imminent danger, call 911 or your local emergency number. Remove from your home or lock away all guns, pills, kitchen knives, household chemicals, and ropes. To learn more about depression and its treatment, see page 467.

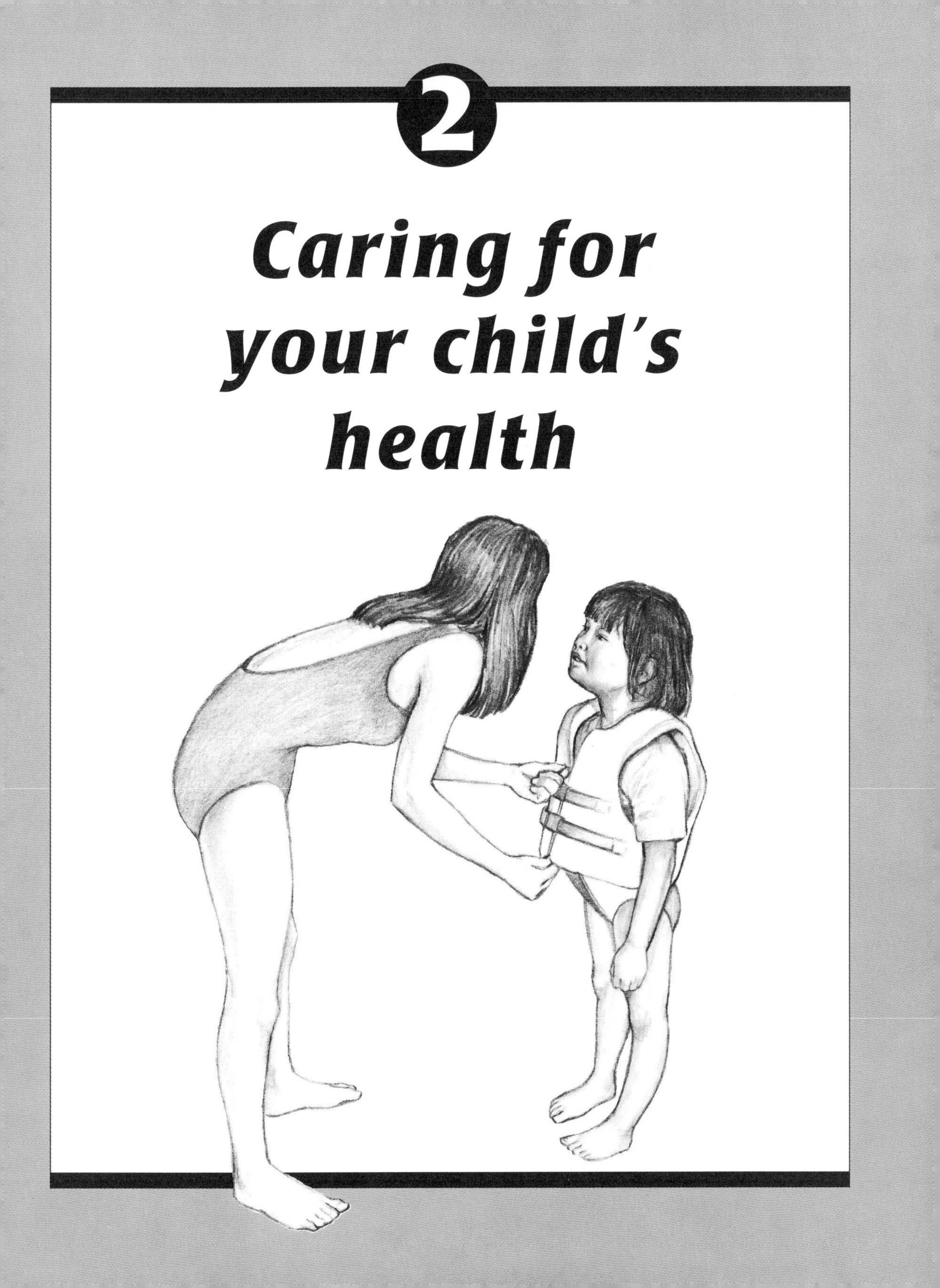
2
Caring for your child's health

CHAPTER • 7

Finding quality child care

Finding quality day care for your child is important not only for your peace of mind but also for your child's healthy development, especially during the first 3 years of life when warm, responsive care is especially crucial. You want to find a caregiver who understands that talking, cuddling, playing, and reading can stimulate the development of a child's brain and ensure his or her emotional health and well-being. During the first year, a baby thrives on concentrated attention from a loving caregiver who responds promptly to the baby's needs. Toddlers need a knowledgeable caregiver who encourages them to explore their environment safely and nurtures their growing independence. Preschoolers learn by doing and need both quiet and active play, so a preschool child-care setting should provide lots of toys, games, crafts, and other enjoyable and stimulating materials.

Each type of child care—a baby-sitter or nanny in your home, a day-care home, a day-care center, or a preschool—has its advantages and disadvantages and every family must weigh them carefully to determine the type of care that best suits their child's needs. Many families hire a single caregiver or arrange for their child to be cared for in a day-care home until their child is about 3 years old and then place him or her in a preschool program. (The fewer caregivers a child under age 3 has, the better.) After age 3, children benefit from a preschool program that allows them to socialize and provides a broad range of stimulating activities.

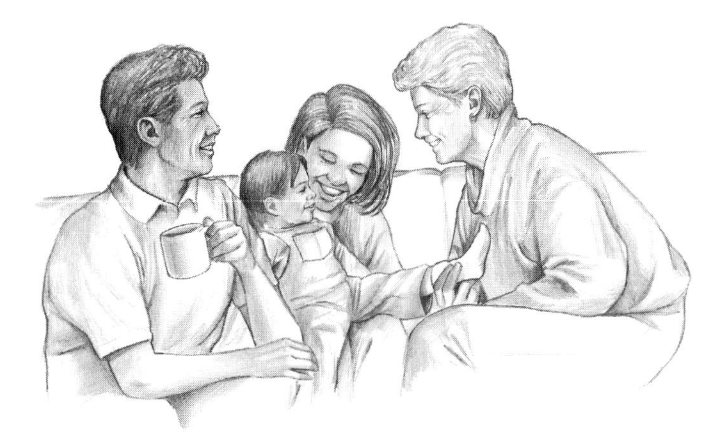

Look for a loving caregiver

Your child needs to form an emotional bond with the caregiver you hire—similar to the strong bond he or she has with you. Look for a person who will cuddle, hold, talk to, read to, and play with your child while you are away. Before hiring a caregiver, watch how he or she interacts with your child and how your child responds.

Baby-sitters and nannies

Many parents prefer to choose a baby-sitter or nanny to care for their child if he or she is under age 3. This option can be the most convenient, because the caregiver comes to your home. Your child will also be in a familiar environment and will avoid exposure to colds and other infections from other children. Hiring a nanny is one of the most expensive child-care arrangements, but the biggest difficulty is finding a reliable, well-qualified person. Because in-home care is not regulated in any way, you are the sole judge of a caregiver's character, knowledge, and skill.

Start your search at least 2 to 3 months before you go back to work so you have enough time to make a thoughtful decision. Ask friends and neighbors for recommendations. Before hiring or accepting an offer to baby-sit from relatives or friends, be sure they are qualified to care for your child and that you would feel comfortable giving them instructions or disagreeing with them on child-care issues that are important to you. Avoid hiring someone who is looking for something to do until a better offer comes along. To find candidates, check with a local agency that provides training and placement for in-home providers. Ask your doctor for names. Check child-care ads and place your own help-wanted ad in your local newspaper, local college career services office, and community bulletin board or newsletter. Specify the hours and days you need child care, your child's age, the general area in which you live (but don't give your address), and whether or not you want the sitter to live in or have a driver's license. If you require a nonsmoker, say so.

Your child's caregiver should have training in child development or have experience taking care of children. The caregiver should also appreciate the importance of stimulating your child's intellectual, social, and emotional development. He or she should be able to communicate well so your child can build his or her language skills. Your caregiver should respect your philosophy of child rearing and understand that you are the ultimate authority for making decisions about the care of your child. He or she also needs to guide your child's behavior with positive reinforcement rather than physical punishment.

Even if you work with a child-care agency that prescreens candidates, you should participate in the screening process. First, screen candidates over the phone to eliminate those who don't seem right. Listen to your gut feeling, even if you are under the gun because you need help immediately. Ask whether or not they're available the hours you need them, their salary needs, how long they can commit to the job, what interests them about child care, what kind of work they have done in the past, and when they can start. Invite the best candidates to your home for an interview. Some parents develop a job application form to make the hiring process more formal and professional.

Once you have a candidate in mind, contact at least three former employers and three personal references. Ask former employers about the candidate's responsibilities, his or her strengths and weaknesses, the ages of the children he or she cared for, absenteeism, how long the person worked for them, why he or she left, the kinds of activities he or she engaged the children in, problem areas, and whether they would hire the person again. Some parents hire corporate investigators to perform background checks on the candidate's criminal history and to verify his or her social security number. Such background checks do not require an applicant's consent, but if you want to obtain a copy of the person's driving record or credit history, you must first get a signed release.

Make sure your child is home during the interview with the prospective baby-sitter so you can see how the two interact. Prepare a list of questions in advance to help you stay focused on getting information; don't turn the interview into a conversation or social event. Include the following questions in your interview:

- What is your educational background in child development and your experience in child care?
- Why did you leave your last job? (Look for a candidate with a long history with one family, if possible.)
- What do you like most about your work?
- What do you know about nutrition and feeding children, especially infants and toddlers? Are you willing to cook and what can you cook?
- Have you cared for children the same ages as our children? (This is especially important if you need care for a newborn.)
- What activities would you engage my children in? (He or she should show enthusiasm.)
- How much television do you allow a child to watch daily? What shows do you think are appropriate for children?
- How would you handle a misbehaving child? (Listen for references to physical punishment or use of the word "punish.")
- Do you watch daytime television? Do you have other time commitments?
- Do you have any health problems?
- Have you ever been convicted of a crime?
- Do you know other baby-sitters in the area? (Look for someone who has connections to your neighborhood so you can call the employers of the other baby-sitters to get their impression.)

After hiring your baby-sitter, train and manage him or her like you would any employee. To avoid future misunderstandings, many experts recommend writing up a contract that describes the position and its responsibilities and is signed by both parties. Include the days and hours of work, salary and payment schedule, overtime rate, form of payment, holidays and vacation, job responsibilities, house rules, and rules for giving notice of termination by either party. The terms of the agreement can change as your needs change.

Describe your expectations in detail. State your rules about such things as meal and snack preparation (and any special dietary restrictions), watching television and listening to music (for both the caregiver and your child), playmates, housework, personal use of the telephone and message-taking procedures, per-

PREPARING YOUR BABY-SITTER

When you need to go out for a few hours or for an evening, you'll want to hire a baby-sitter you can trust. The best way to find a good sitter is to ask people you know for names of sitters they have used. You can also call the baby-sitter training program at your local school district or hospital for a recommendation. Ask if the instructors are trained by the Red Cross.

Your house rules

Your sitter needs to know your house rules. Go through them in the presence of your children so everyone hears the same message. Include information about:

- What meals and snacks are allowed and where they can be eaten.
- The TV programs your child can watch and for how long.
- How you want the sitter to handle discipline.
- Where they can go (the park, for example) and for how long, or whether they should stay at home.
- The usual cleanup and bedtime routines.

Your sitter needs to keep his or her attention focused primarily on your children. That's why you should also tell your sitter that:

- Phone calls should be kept short.
- You don't allow visitors, drinking, smoking, or drugs.
- He or she should not let strangers into the house.

Before you leave, be sure to show your sitter how your stove, microwave, thermostat, TV, and alarm system work.

Interviewing a prospective sitter

Check your sitter's references before you meet him or her. If possible, have the sitter spend some time with your children before you leave so he or she can get to know them and their routines. It helps your children to get to know the sitter too. A sitter should be 13-years-old or older and ideally should be trained in first aid and cardiopulmonary resuscitation (CPR). When you meet the sitter, ask him or her the following questions:

- Does he or she have experience or any younger brothers or sisters?
- Has he or she had any formal training?
- Does he or she do housework?
- How does the sitter handle discipline?
- How does he or she keep the children occupied?
- What are his or her rates?

Your sitter needs to know a number of things about your children and your household. Don't forget to give the sitter the following important information:

- Your children's ages and their favorite things to do.
- How long you will be away and how you can be reached.
- Any special needs your children have (such as diet) or any medical conditions (such as allergies).
- Whether or not you expect the sitter to do any housework.
- If you have any pets, whether or not the sitter needs to feed or walk them. Find out if the sitter is allergic to any of your pets.
- Your children's play, bath, and bedtime routines.
- Make sure your sitter knows the location of the phone and any safety hazards the children should avoid, such as steps.

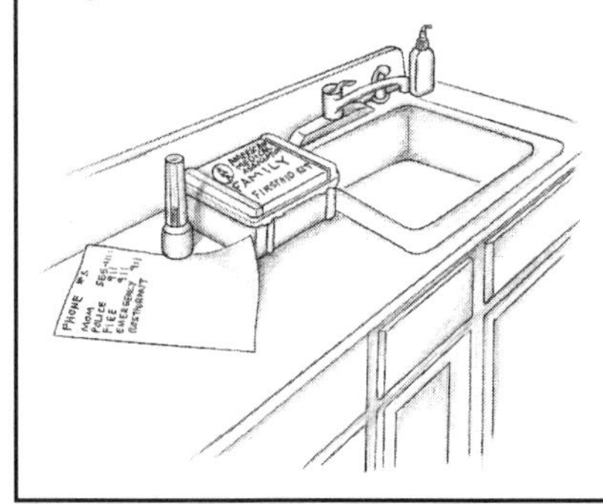

Before you leave

It's a good idea to leave a first-aid kit and a flashlight on the kitchen counter before you leave the house. Let the sitter know where you store extra batteries.

Your baby-sitter's checklist

Where you will be ______________________________

____

Address ______________________________

Phone number ______________________________

Time you will return ______________________________

Your home address ______________________________

Phone number ______________________________

Your cellular phone number ______________________________

Your pager number ______________________________

Emergency contact person (neighbor, grandparent)

____

Phone number ______________________________

Local emergency medical system phone number

____

Police phone number ______________________________

Fire department phone number ______________________________

Poison center phone number ______________________________

Doctor's phone number ______________________________

While you are away

The baby-sitter needs to be active while watching your children—not passively sitting in front of the TV. Depending on your children's ages, the sitter can engage in a variety of activities that will be fun for both the sitter and your children.

- **Infants** Infants sleep a lot but they need plenty of care and attention when they are awake. Your sitter will be busy changing diapers, feeding and burping the baby, and figuring out what to do when the baby cries. Infants like to be held, walked, and talked to. And remind your sitter that it's never too early to start reading to your baby. But it's probably safest not to ask your sitter to bathe your infant because of the risk of drowning and burns from hot water.

- **Toddlers** Keeping a toddler occupied is a never-ending job. Toddlers have short attention spans and a tendency to get into mischief. They enjoy games of pretend, nursery rhymes, and singing, and they love it when someone reads to them. Toddlers lose their tempers easily, so tell your sitter how you want him or her to handle your toddler's temper tantrums. Time-out (see page 126) is a good way of responding to a toddler who misbehaves.

- **Older children** Instead of just watching TV, your sitter should interact with your older child. The sitter can play board games or cards, read, draw, or go outdoors with your child, with your permission. Discipline may become more complicated with an older child. Be sure to tell your sitter exactly how you want him or her to enforce your rules.

Having fun together

The sitter you hire should be active with your child, not just passively sitting in front of the TV. Young children enjoy reading, games, rhymes, and singing.

What to do in an emergency

In an emergency, your sitter will have to try to stay calm even though he or she feels afraid. The first thing the sitter should do is assess the seriousness of the situation. Is your child breathing? Conscious? If there is a fire, can everyone get out safely? The sitter needs to get help fast by calling the local emergency medical services or fire or police department. Only then should the sitter call you.

If the sitter has had baby-sitter's training from a local hospital or school district, he or she will be better equipped to handle an emergency. Leave this book out for the sitter, with the first-aid section marked.

sonal visitors, smoking, and off-limit areas of your home. Make clear your position on discipline and physical punishment. Generally, it's not a good idea to insist that the baby-sitter do housekeeping—his or her full-time job is to care for your child. Have a backup plan in case the sitter is sick or goes on vacation.

Carefully go over the steps the caregiver should take in an emergency. Keep important telephone numbers posted by the telephone: your own and your partner's work, pager, and cell phone numbers; the child's doctor's number; the local emergency number; and the numbers of neighbors or nearby relatives who might be available to help out in an emergency. Prepare a medical release that authorizes the baby-sitter to sign forms in case of a medical emergency.

Find out your tax responsibilities by contacting the Internal Revenue Service. You might want to discuss tax issues with an accountant or lawyer because tax laws on child care vary from state to state and from year to year. In general, you are required to pay the prevailing minimum wage to a baby-sitter who works in your home on a regular basis and whose primary job is baby-sitting. You are also required to pay Social Security taxes for your caregiver. You may be eligible for a tax credit on your federal and state income taxes; check with an accountant or tax lawyer before filing your income tax forms.

Once you have hired a sitter or nanny, spend a few days at home with him or her and your child so you can observe their interaction and see the way the caregiver handles common situations. This extra time will ease the transition for your child and should reassure you that you made the right choice.

Communication is an important part of your relationship with a caregiver. Try to deal with conflicts and misunderstandings as soon as they arise; don't allow them to fester and turn into anger and resentment. One of the best measures of a baby-sitter's performance is your child's response. Is your child happy and content? Is he or she growing and developing at a healthy rate? Are his or her language skills developing as they should? Is he or she happy and responsive when the baby-sitter arrives?

Day-care homes

Many parents choose day-care homes for children under age 3. This type of day care takes place in the home of the caregiver, who looks after a number of children, sometimes including his or her own. The children may be of different ages. Many parents prefer day-care homes to day-care centers because the atmosphere is more like home and their child has one consistent caregiver who is more likely to give individual attention. This situation generally offers more flexible hours than a center; a more relaxed, natural environment; and a less formal relationship with the caregiver. The major disadvantage of day-care homes is that caregivers are unsupervised, making it hard to judge the quality of their work. You might also need to make other arrangements if the provider becomes ill or goes on vacation.

Day-care homes should be licensed by the state. Call the agency responsible for licensing child care in your state and ask for a copy of the state licensing regulations. Licensing shows that a child-care home has passed minimum standards, including adequately insuring the health and safety of children and not exceeding the child-to-adult ratio. State regulations vary, but a day-care home should not have more than six children per adult caregiver, including the caregiver's own children. If the children are infants or toddlers, the ratio should be no more than two children younger than 2 years old for each caregiver. (This ratio is smaller than that for day-care centers.)

When looking for a quality day-care home, visit several and compare them. Look for a setting you are comfortable with and a provider who shares your values and child-raising philosophy, and with whom you would feel at ease sharing your concerns about your child. When interviewing caregiver candidates, ask if they are accredited by the National Association for the Education of Young Children or the National Association for Family Day Care, organizations that impose standards of quality. Some providers may have a child development associate credential, indicating that they have training in child care, have passed a written examination and an oral interview, and have been observed and evaluated by a professional.

Make sure the home is warm, cheerful, clean, and safe. Check to see that the home has been childproofed (see page 76). Smoke alarms and carbon monoxide detectors should be present and in working order. Diapering and toilet areas should be clean and you shouldn't see any children with soiled diapers or training pants. Adults and children should always wash their hands after using the toilet and before handling food. Ask if there is a quiet area that can be used for naps, with clean bedding for each child.

The children should be able to get play materials for themselves, and the caregiver should encourage them to take care of the materials they use and put them away when finished. There should be enough toys and other materials to allow each child to play without having to wait more than a few minutes. The toys should be clean and in good condition and appropriate for the children's ages, interests, and abilities. Look for stimulating and creative materials such as books, blocks, puzzles, crayons, paper, paste, modeling clay, children's scissors, and pencils. There should also be lots of toys for active play, such as riding toys and push-pull toys. The television shouldn't be on for more than an hour during the day and the caregiver should plan daily activities that include free play, rest or naps, and outdoor time. He or she should encourage listening and talking through activities such as storytelling, word games, and imaginary play.

Observe the caregiver's interaction with the children to see whether he or she is patient, consistent, and fair. Does he or she have a sense of humor, show affection, and seem to genuinely enjoy being with the children? Do the children seem happy, comfortable, and relaxed? Does the caregiver hold infants while feeding them rather than propping up their bottles? Does he or she talk to infants and cuddle and play with them?

Find out if the caregiver uses discipline and guidance methods similar to yours. Does he or she use simple, positive directions and speak to the children in a friendly manner at their eye level? (Watch out for a provider who frequently says "no," "don't," or "bad.") Does the caregiver provide individual attention when necessary and praise children for their successes and good behavior? Look to see whether he or she encourages them to do certain things for themselves, such as getting a drink, washing their hands, or putting away a toy. Observe snack and meal times to see if they seem relaxed and enjoyable. Ask the caregiver for a typical weekly menu of meals and snacks. Check to see if the meals are nutritious and contain foods your child likes.

Once you have made your choice, maintain a good relationship with the provider by respecting the business aspect of the arrangement. Your responsibilities include picking up your child on time (many caregivers charge late fees), paying on time, and giving enough notice before your child goes on vacation or leaves the person's care. You should also notify the provider when your child is sick and will be staying home. Make sure you know the provider's policy about caring for a sick child.

It can take weeks for your child to adjust to the new sitter and environment. If your child is happy and looks forward to going to the caregiver's home, you know you've made a good choice. Frequently ask your child how he or she feels, what he or she has been doing, and what he or she likes or dislikes. If your child is too young to talk, monitor his or her emotional state, behavior, and cleanliness after being with the caregiver.

Day-care centers and preschools

Day-care centers–which are often called child-care centers, nursery schools, or early learning centers–can be operated by churches, schools, universities, social service agencies, the federal government (Early Head Start and Head Start), independent chains, and employers. Day-care centers care for children of all ages, although most are between ages 3 and 6. A major advantage of day-care centers is that parents don't have to worry about a particular caregiver's illness or vacation because several caregivers share responsibilities.

Preschools provide a more formal structure than day-care centers and emphasize educating children, usually those between the ages of 3 and 5 years. Preschools are usually staffed by teachers with training in early child development. They group the children according to their age and social skills and teach them fundamentals such as letters, numbers, shapes, and colors.

Start your search for a day-care center or preschool by asking other parents, friends, and coworkers about the ones they use. Look through community parent publications and newspaper ads and check the yellow pages under "child care" or "day care" or look up "preschools" under "schools." Ask your county child-care resources and referral agency for a day-care directory. Once you have narrowed down your search, check with a social services or child-care agency to see if the center has a current license and if there are any complaints, accidents, or closures on file. The National Academy of Early Childhood Programs can give you a free list of accredited centers grouped by state. Contact the National Association for the Education of Young Children for a list of accredited day-care centers in your state. Ask if staff members have Child Development Associate credentials or other early childhood certification. Caregivers and center directors should have basic training and experience in early childhood development. The lead teacher in a preschool program should be trained in early childhood education or child development.

State regulations vary about the number of caregivers needed to adequately care for children in day care, but most experts consider the best ratios to be one caregiver for every three infants, one caregiver for every three to six toddlers, and one caregiver for every seven preschool children. Many programs take only children of a certain age or accept only children who are toilet trained.

In your search for a quality center, visit several and ask if you can check all the areas your child would use. The center should be bright, cheerful, and well ventilated. It should have lots of books, toys, and play equipment, including games, blocks, sand, water, art supplies, and props for make-believe play. All materials should be accessible, clean, safe, well maintained, and appropriate for children of various ages. The center should have a written plan for play and learning activities that includes active play, quiet play, nap or rest time, and snacks and meals; ask to see it. Find out whether the children can explore in clean, safe areas—both indoors and outdoors. Make sure the children are supervised at all times.

Discipline at the center should aim to develop self-control through positive encouragement, giving praise and rewards for success. Caregivers need to correct unwanted behavior privately and kindly. They should never compare one child to another, criticize, ridicule, threaten, or physically punish a child. Caregivers need to explain the center's rules in easy-to-understand terms and the rules should be easy to follow for children of various ages.

Look for the following features in a quality child-care center:

- A current license or registration from the local government and evidence that the facility has been recently inspected.
- Staff members who have had training in child development, first aid, and injury and infection prevention.
- Clear posting of the telephone numbers of the local poison control center and ambulance service.
- Smoke alarms and carbon monoxide detectors that are in working order throughout the building.
- Rules about careful and frequent hand-washing after diapering a baby or wiping a nose, and before fixing a meal or snack.
- Clean, easy-to-reach toilets and sinks, towels, liquid soap, and toilet paper. A clean diaper-changing area for infants, with a sink within the caregiver's reach.
- Nutritious, well-prepared, and well-served food.

Finding a good day-care center

When looking for a quality day-care center for your child, visit several. Bring your child with you and watch to see what he or she likes and how he or she responds to the adults, other children, and activities. Try to visit at different times of the day, such as during lunch, naps, and outdoor play times.

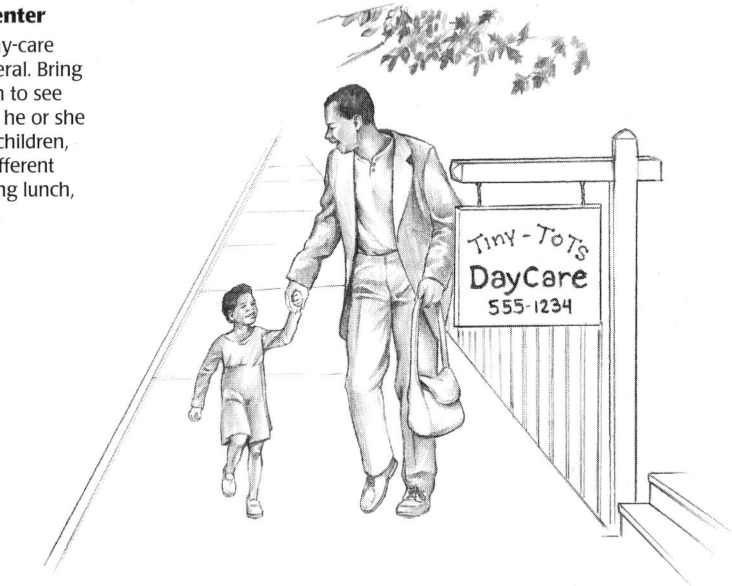

• An outside play area with no sharp edges, sharp rocks, hard surfaces, high climbers, tall slides, or unsafe swings (see page 315). Closely supervised outdoor activities.
• Children who seem happy and caregivers who spend lots of time telling stories and reading to the children.
• Assignment of each child to one caregiver who is primarily responsible for his or her care.
• A sleeping or quiet area that is large enough for all the children to rest during nap time. One bed, cot, or mat for each child with at least 3 feet between them.
• No television on site.
• Open visitation and regular meetings with parents.

Problems with your caregiver can arise because of miscommunication, a "bad fit," or your child's unreadiness for preschool or outside care. It's not always easy to tell, but follow your instincts and investigate further. Try talking things over with the caregiver or speaking with his or her supervisor. If you suspect a serious problem with your child's caregiver, call the agency that regulates child care in your state and express your concerns. The following warning signs may indicate problems with your child-care provider:
• He or she does not answer your questions or address your concerns.
• Your child persistently tells you about problems, is not happy, cries about or fights being left, or is afraid to go to the caregiver.
• Your young child is not eating well, is irritable, or develops nightmares, appetite loss, or personality changes.

Easing the transition

Some children show changes in behavior when they enter child care or have a new caregiver. Older infants may get upset when they're left with strangers. Toddlers may cry, pout, refuse to go, or act out in other ways. Preschoolers may regress or have trouble sleeping. These changes usually go away after a few days or weeks. Prepare your child before the new day-care situation starts. Visit the day-care center or child-care home with your child. Show your child that you like and trust the caregiver.

Let your child bring along a reminder of home, such as a family photo or a favorite stuffed animal or blanket. Talk about the new situation and the caregiver frequently. Don't make any other major changes, such as toilet training or moving to a new home, during the adjustment period. Set aside time each day to give your child your undivided attention—give him or her lots of hugs and kisses, read stories together, or just talk about each other's day.

You may need to spend some time with your child at the day-care center or preschool during the first few weeks to help ease your child's transition to the new environment. For example, you could stay for a few minutes at drop-off time to read a book or do a puzzle together.

Listen carefully to your child's descriptions of the caregivers and the other children. If his or her comments are always negative, talk to the caregiver about any problems your child may be having or ask your child's doctor for advice.

- Your child has unexplained injuries more than once.
- The staff at the center changes often.
- The center cannot give you a written copy of its policies.
- Other parents tell you about problems or concerns.

After-school programs

Regardless of their age, children and adolescents need to be in a safe, structured, and stimulating environment after school is out and while their parents are still at work. Lack of structured time can make a child bored or promote inactivity. Some children may try to find stimulation in unsafe behaviors such as drug and alcohol use, sex, or gang involvement. Public awareness of the importance of safe, enriching environments during children's out-of-school time has produced a growing number of before- and after-school child-care programs.

School-age child-care programs are designed for children between the ages of 5 and 14 years and can be housed in school buildings, recreation facilities, religious institutions, social or community service facilities, or existing day-care centers. They generally provide supervision during nonschool hours when parents' work schedules prevent them from being with their children—including before school, after school, and during school holidays and vacations, sometimes including summer vacation. The most common after-school care programs are located in schools but are usually sponsored by outside

When school is out

Most children benefit from organized after-school programs, where adults supervise them and encourage them to participate in constructive activities, such as art projects, music, or games. Good quality programs help children gain social skills, develop new interests, and improve their performance in school.

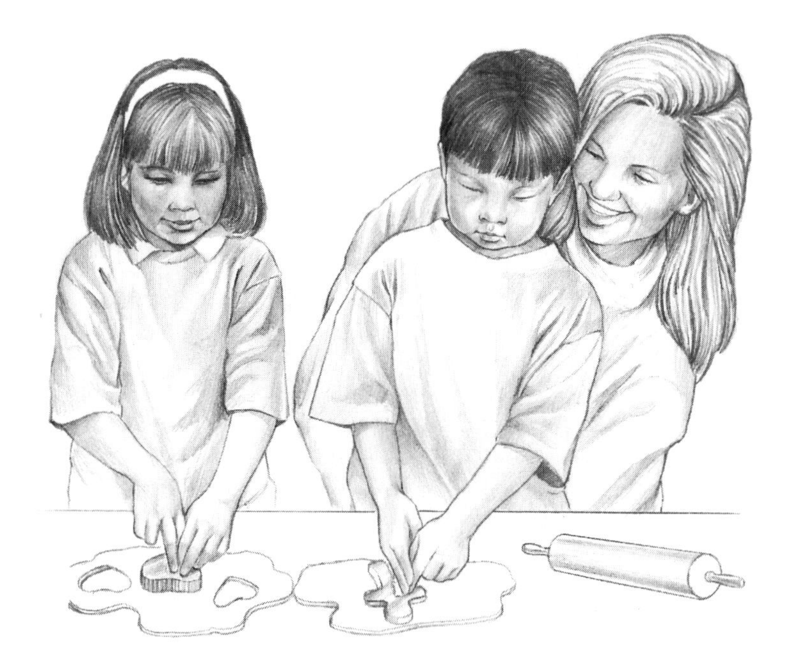

not-for-profit community organizations such as parks and recreation agencies. Many day-care centers provide services such as picking children up after school or transporting them from the center to school in the morning. Churches, civic groups, and agencies such as the YMCA also have programs for children after school. The costs of the programs vary widely.

Start looking for a good out-of-school program several months to a year before your child begins elementary school. Your preschooler may already be enrolled in a day-care center that has an after-school program for older children. Investigate both school and community programs. Ask about the hours, the training of staff members, types of activities, snacks, and whether or not holiday care is provided. Discuss the programs with your child to find one that fits his or her interests as well as your needs.

Well-planned activities are essential to the success of any after-school program. A good program is organized to be distinctly different from the regular school day, while still promoting a child's development. A stimulating after-school environment should enable children to pursue their own interests, learn new skills, and develop socially. High-quality programs give children access to a variety of enriching activities, help with homework and reading, and offer the opportunity to build meaningful relationships with peers and caring adults. Look for a program that provides a variety of activities, both physical and educational–ranging from sports, karate lessons, or dance to art, crafts, computer games, theater, and music lessons. Meet the staff people who supervise these activities so you will know who to contact if problems arise in the future.

Staying home alone

An estimated 5 to 7 million American school-age children go home to an empty house after school and fend for themselves. Some people say that being alone promotes responsibility and independence; others argue that the lack of supervision fosters delinquent behavior and hampers emotional and social growth. It's impossible to make a general statement about when a child can be left home alone safely. Usually children are not mature enough to be considered for self-care until they are 11 or 12. Some states have made laws that specify an age below which it is illegal to leave children alone, while other states don't set a specific age but consider the maturity level of the child. Ask your child welfare agency about the regulations in your state. Before letting your child come home to an empty house, explore other options such as supervised after-school programs.

The decision to allow your child to stay alone is complicated and depends on his or her maturity level and the conditions under which he or she will be alone. Children do best if they are mentally and emotionally ready to stay alone, have learned the skills and knowledge necessary to deal with the responsibility, and can talk easily with their parents about their fears or concerns. Even if your child is ready, other factors, such as an unsafe neighborhood, may prevent you from letting him or her stay alone. Consider how your child handles responsibility, follows directions, and uses good judgment. Does he or she want to stay home alone? Is the amount of time your child will be alone reasonable? Is your child resourceful enough to find something constructive, safe, and helpful to do if he or she is bored? Is he or she self-disciplined enough to do chores or homework without supervision?

Before leaving your child alone, carefully consider the potential problems and develop a plan with your child to address them. Make your home as safe as possible from obvious dangers. Check doors, windows, locks, and lighting; trim the bushes near doors and windows; and make a thorough home inspection to detect fire hazards. Make sure the batteries in your smoke alarms and carbon monoxide detectors are in working order.

Rehearse the family emergency plan (see page 312). Your child should be able to identify two escape routes from the house in case of fire and name two adults to contact in case of an emergency. He or she needs to be able to give his or her phone number, address, and directions to the house. Post your work number and the numbers of neighbors or nearby relatives or friends, 911 or your local emergency number, local police and fire department numbers, and the number of a poison control center near the telephone. Your child should know how to handle simple first aid for cuts and scrapes, burns, nosebleeds, poisoning, bites, choking, and eye injuries (see First Aid and Emergencies on page 666)—and should know where the first-aid supplies are kept.

Plan a trial period of self-care to see how he or she adjusts to the situation. Initially, you may want to present it as a temporary arrangement so that the child knows he or she can choose not to continue if it's uncomfortable and so you can end the arrangement easily if you feel the child is not handling it well. Establish a set of rules but limit the rules to important things and make sure they are clear and enforceable; write them down and post them in your home. Important standing rules are to phone you when he or she arrives home, to avoid entering the house if anything looks suspicious (he or she should go to a neighbor's instead and call you from there), and to always clear all after-school visitors with you in advance. Make sure your child knows not to open the door to strangers. Develop a plan for what he or she should do if someone comes to the door when you're not at home. Avoid arranging for service calls or deliveries while you are away. Tell your child never to let a caller know that you are not at home; he or she should simply say that you're busy and take a message.

While you are away, discourage excessive TV watching and computer game playing. Call your child as often as possible and make sure your child can easily reach you or another responsible adult by phone. Many communities have set up hotlines for school-age children who care for themselves after school. Volunteers provide comfort and support to children over the phone, which is especially helpful for parents whose work environment makes it difficult to receive calls.

Allowing your child to take care of him- or herself bestows a lot of responsibility. You have just as much responsibility for making this arrangement beneficial for your child. Most of all, be dependable. Be home when you say you will; if you're going to be late, call and tell your child. Make sure your child knows how to reach you at all times and give a backup person to call if you can't be reached. Keep nutritious snacks at home and teach your child how to prepare foods and safely use equipment such as cheese graters, peelers, and the microwave or toaster oven.

CHAPTER • 8

Routine health care

The doctor will want to see your child regularly for checkups to make sure that your child's growth and development are on track. The doctor will also give your child all the recommended vaccinations and treat any disorders or physical problems. During these checkups, talk to the doctor about your concerns and ask any questions you might have. Because you know your child better than anyone else, your doctor will rely on your insight and observations to help evaluate your child's health.

Your child's pediatrician

Take some time a few months before your child is born to seek out the doctor who will be the best "fit" for you and your child. Doctors can differ from one another considerably, including the way they interact with children and parents, their attitude toward preventive health or discipline, and their ability to communicate. Before choosing a doctor, consider your own personality and needs and clarify your attitudes toward parenting and important issues such as breast-feeding. You want your child's doctor to have a philosophy about child care that is much like yours. The doctor should also be someone you trust, have confidence in, and feel comfortable with–someone who can work with you to make sure that your child reaches his or her full potential.

PEDIATRICIAN OR FAMILY DOCTOR?

Your child's doctor should be either a pediatrician–a physician trained in the development and care of infants, children, and adolescents (usually to age 18)–or a family physician–one trained in the care of the entire family. Both types of doctors have had advanced training (known as a residency) in their specialty for 3 or more years after medical school. Your child's doctor should also be board certified–that is, certified by the American Board of Pediatrics or the American Board of Family Physicians. This certification means that the doctor has passed a detailed test covering all aspects of medical care for his or her specialty.

Some pediatricians have additional training in a subspecialty such as pediatric cardiology (the diagnosis and treatment of heart problems in children) or neonatology (the care of sick and premature newborns). If your child has a problem that requires more specialized treatment, your pediatrician may refer you to a subspecialist.

You may have a health insurance plan that requires you to choose a doctor from those participating in its network. If so, learn as much as you can about the available doctors so you can make an informed choice. If you have recently moved into a new area, call a nearby university teaching hospital, community hospital, or the local medical society and ask for a list of pediatricians or family doctors. One of the best ways to find a doctor for your child is to ask friends who have children if they would recommend their own child's doctor.

INTERVIEWING THE DOCTOR

Once you have the names of a few doctors, call their offices to set up an interview appointment. It's a good idea for both prospective parents to participate in this initial get-acquainted visit. Some doctors charge for the visit so ask ahead of time about fees.

At your initial meeting, get a feel for the office and how it is run. Check out the waiting room. Is there a separate area for very sick or contagious children? Is it clean? Are the nurses and receptionists friendly and helpful? Ask them about office hours, how they handle billing, insurance claims, phoning in prescriptions, and which managed-care plans they participate in. Find out about the fees, including those for immunizations. Ask about appointment scheduling and double booking. What is the average waiting time? How are emergencies handled? When talking to the doctor, find out these important points:

- The doctor's medical training and whether he or she is board certified.
- The hospital the doctor admits patients to.
- How soon after birth the doctor will see your baby.
- How you can reach the doctor after office hours or during an emergency.
- If the doctor has set aside a time each day to take phone calls from parents.
- Who you can talk to if the doctor is not available to answer your questions.
- If other doctors in the practice might sometimes see your child; you should meet them too.

After your interview, think about how comfortable you felt with the doctor. Was he or she easy to talk to? Did the doctor listen to your concerns? Can you play an active part in your child's health care? Do you have confidence in the doctor's medical expertise? Trust your instincts when making your decision–your comfort level and rapport with the doctor are crucial indicators of your future relationship.

Ultimately, the most important measures of a good doctor are the way the doctor relates to your child, communicates with you, and responds to your con-

Getting a second opinion

If you have an ongoing relationship with a doctor, you won't often need to seek a second opinion from another doctor, especially for minor health problems. However, you may want to consult another doctor under the following circumstances:

- Your doctor has recommended that you get a second opinion from a specialist.
- Your doctor has not been able to diagnose a health problem in a reasonable amount of time.
- Your child has been diagnosed with a serious, chronic, or rare illness.
- Your doctor recommends surgery. Find out if surgery is the only option.
- The diagnosis of an illness is uncertain.
- You are having trouble getting information from your doctor.
- Your child is not feeling better after the recommended treatment and the doctor does not have another approach.

cerns. If you have problems with any aspect of the medical care your child is receiving, speak frankly with the doctor. Don't hesitate to change doctors if the problems are not resolved. The relationship with your child's doctor is too important for you to feel uneasy.

Newborn screening tests

Every state requires testing of newborns for a variety of disorders 24 hours after birth and before the child is released from the hospital. Some disorders have no immediate visible effects on a baby but can cause physical problems, mental retardation, or even death unless they are detected and treated early.

To be most reliable, newborn testing must be done after the first 24 hours of life. If your child is being discharged from the hospital, make sure he or she has been tested before you leave. If your child was born at home, needed to be placed in a neonatal intensive care unit of the hospital just after birth, or was transferred between hospitals, he or she may not have had newborn screening. Ask your doctor to check your child's records to make sure all the proper testing was done. Try not to be too alarmed if the results of a first screening test are abnormal. The tests are preliminary and must be followed by more precise evaluation. For many children, the results of subsequent testing prove to be normal. Required screenings vary by state, but common tests screen for PKU, hypothyroidism, galactosemia, congenital adrenal hyperplasia, and sickle cell anemia.

• **PKU** Babies with PKU (phenylketonuria) (see page 595) cannot process a substance in food called phenylalanine. Without treatment, phenylalanine builds up in the bloodstream, causing brain damage and mental retardation. A PKU test that is done earlier than 24 hours after birth may not give accurate results. If your baby was tested within the first 24 hours of birth, your doctor will recommend having another test.

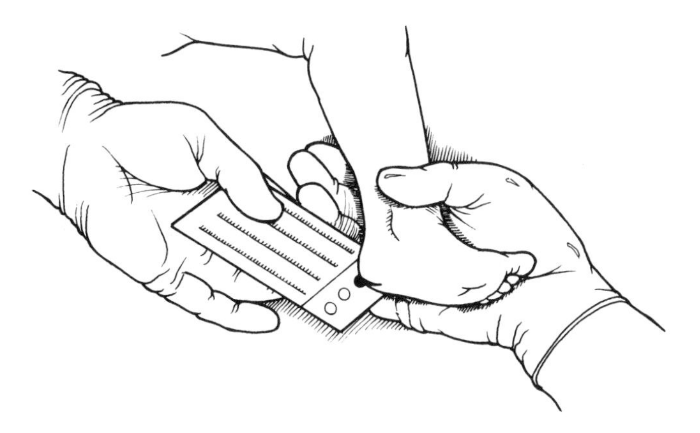

How newborn testing is done

To test a newborn for a number of life-threatening but treatable disorders, a doctor needs only one sample of blood, taken from the baby's heel. The blood sample is sent to a laboratory for testing and the laboratory then sends the results back to the doctor.

YOUR CHILD'S FAMILY HEALTH HISTORY

Your child's family health history holds important information for you, your child, and your child's doctor. It can help the doctor detect an abnormality or diagnose an illness early, when it is more easily treated. It can also guide you in helping your child prevent or delay a future health problem. For example, adjusting your child's diet or level of activity may help prevent the early onset of heart disease in adulthood. Use the form below to research your family health history before your child is born, and then make a family tree like the one on the next page. Include the health histories of both yourself and your partner, both sets of grandparents, aunts and uncles, and sisters and brothers.

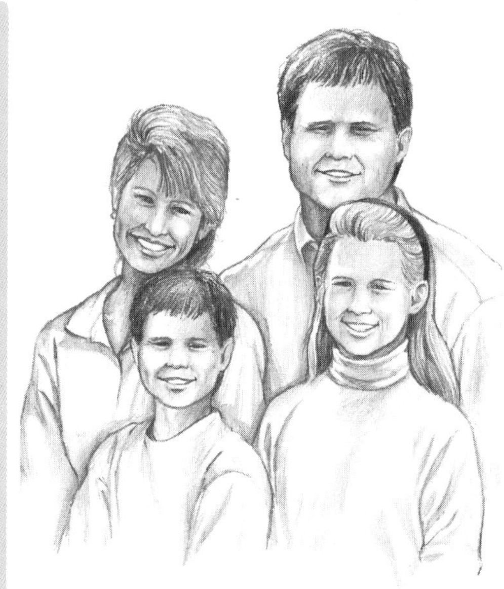

Family health history form

Name of relative ______________________ Relation to child ______________________

❑ Male ❑ Female Year of birth __________ Year of death __________ Cause of death __________

Ethnic background ______________________

If the person was ever diagnosed with any of the following health problems, note his or her age at the time of the diagnosis:

❑ Allergies
❑ Asthma
❑ Heart attack
❑ High blood pressure
❑ Heart disease
❑ Stroke
❑ Cancer (what type?)
❑ Diabetes
❑ Mental disorder (what kind?)
❑ Vision disorder (what kind?)
❑ Hearing problem
❑ Blood disorder
❑ Addiction to alcohol or another drug
❑ Seizures
❑ Early death (infant or child)
❑ Immune deficiency
❑ Rheumatoid arthritis
❑ Emphysema
❑ Mental retardation or illness
❑ Genetic disorder
❑ Chronic illness (what kind?)
❑ Rare or unusual illness

Lifestyle factors—smoking, eating a poor diet, being inactive, or alcohol or drug abuse—can also influence a person's risk of dying prematurely. Try to find out the following information about the lifestyle of each of your child's relatives.

Weight __________ **Height** __________

Smoking How long? __________ How many packs per day? ____ Never smoked __________

Drinking Heavy __________ Moderate __________ Never drank __________

Drug use Heavy __________ Moderate __________ Never used __________

Learning from your child's family health history

Once you have researched your child's family health history, use the information to construct a family tree like the one below. Give a copy to your child's doctor, who will discuss your child's risk factors with you and recommend steps to reduce those risks. Most illnesses are caused by genetic damage triggered over a lifetime by environmental factors such as a high-fat diet, smoking, or excessive exposure to sunlight. Understanding your child's susceptibilities to certain diseases can help you to reduce his or her risk of developing them in the future.

Let's say you have compiled the family tree below for your children. It shows that they are at increased risk of developing heart disease as adults because you have a high cholesterol level, your husband has high blood pressure, and his father had a heart attack before age 55. Your children also carry a risk of developing colon cancer as adults because your mother had colon cancer, which tends to run in families. The fact that you have polyps (abnormal growths that can become cancerous) in your colon increases the risk more.

You can take steps now to lower the risk of both heart disease and colon cancer in your children. Provide a nutritious diet that is low in fat and high in fruits, vegetables, and other high-fiber foods, such as whole grains and dried peas and beans. Encourage your children to exercise regularly so they can avoid becoming overweight. Preventive measures are most effective if begun early in life.

The family tree also shows that your brother has a son who was born with the genetic disorder sickle cell anemia. This disease occurs when a child receives one defective copy of the sickle cell gene from each parent. Both your brother and his wife carry one copy of the gene. Because your brother is a carrier, you might be too. Consider being tested for the gene. If a test shows that you carry the sickle cell gene, ask your partner to be tested before you have more children (see page 498). Otherwise, you risk passing on the disease.

YOUR PARTNER'S MOTHER
Type II diabetes; overweight
YOUR FATHER
Heart disease (diagnosed at age 70); high blood pressure; smokes cigarettes
YOUR PARTNER'S FATHER
Died at age 48 of a heart attack; overweight
YOUR MOTHER
Died at age 67 of colon cancer; overweight
YOUR BROTHER'S WIFE
Carries sickle cell gene
YOUR PARTNER
High blood pressure; smokes cigarettes
YOUR BROTHER
Carries sickle cell gene
YOU
High cholesterol level; polyps in colon; may carry sickle cell gene
YOUR NEPHEW
Sickle cell anemia (diagnosed at birth)
YOUR SON
YOUR DAUGHTER

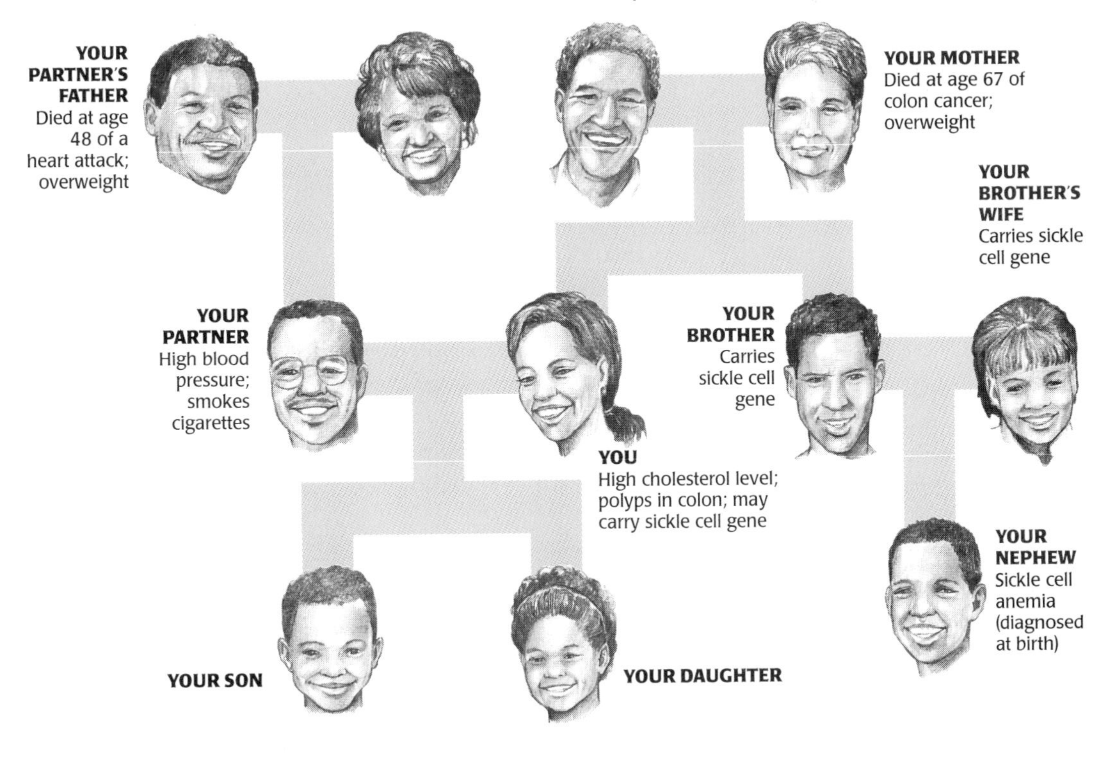

- **Hypothyroidism** Hypothyroidism (see page 530) is a disorder in which the thyroid gland does not produce enough thyroid hormone, which is essential for growth and development. Without prompt treatment, a child with hypothyroidism that is present at birth can have irreversible mental retardation, growth failure, breathing problems, and brain and nervous system abnormalities.
- **Galactosemia** Babies who have galactosemia (see page 493) cannot convert the sugar galactose into glucose, the sugar that the body uses for energy. Galactose builds up in the body, leading to liver disease, severe mental retardation, failure to thrive, cataracts, life-threatening infection, and death.
- **Congenital adrenal hyperplasia** Characterized by the abnormal production of certain hormones secreted by the adrenal glands, congenital (present at birth) adrenal hyperplasia (see page 459) causes the body to lose salt and water. If the disorder is not detected at birth and treated, an infant can suddenly go into shock and die or experience abnormal sexual development.
- **Sickle cell anemia** Sickle cell anemia (see page 624) is an inherited form of anemia (see page 412) in which red blood cells have an abnormal shape (like a crescent or sickle). A child has to inherit two copies of the defective gene (one from each parent) to be affected by the disease.

Vaccinations

Vaccinations, also called immunizations, can protect your child against a number of dangerous and extremely contagious infections, including polio, pertussis (whooping cough), and diphtheria. These diseases once killed thousands of children each year and left many more with life-threatening or disabling complications. Routine immunization of children has made these infections rare in the United States today. Taking your child in for vaccinations on schedule is one of the most important ways you can safeguard your child's health.

Vaccines give your child immunity to diseases by stimulating the immune system to produce substances called antibodies that fight disease-causing organisms. To protect against some infections, your child may need more than one vaccination. The initial vaccination triggers the body's production of antibodies, and later vaccinations, called boosters, reinforce the protection.

Your child needs to have a specified series of vaccinations (see page 227) during the first 2 years of life, usually starting at birth. Your doctor will tell you when your child needs the next vaccination and will keep a record of each shot, but you should also maintain a current record of all your child's vaccinations. You will need to provide this documentation before your child can be admitted to a day-care center, school, or camp. Ask your doctor or your health department for a vaccination record card or booklet and bring it with you to each of your child's doctor visits, even if a vaccination is not scheduled for that checkup.

Most vaccinations are given by injection, usually into the outer, upper part of the child's thigh or arm. The only exception is the oral polio vaccination, which is a liquid vaccine given by mouth with a dropper. Some vaccinations, such as those for diphtheria, tetanus, and pertussis (DTP) or measles, mumps, and rubella (MMR), are combined and given in a single injection.

Some vaccinations can cause reactions, but they are usually mild. The risk to your child of a severe reaction from a vaccination is much lower than the risk of getting one of the dangerous infections if he or she is not immunized. Before your child receives a vaccination, your doctor will describe possible reactions and tell you how to treat them. Applying cold compresses may help relieve swelling or irritation at the site of the shot.

Following are brief descriptions of the vaccinations your child needs and their possible side effects. If you notice any serious side effects after a vaccination, call your doctor immediately. If your child has already had a reaction to a vaccination, tell the doctor or nurse before the next shot in that series is given.

Recommended Schedule of Childhood Immunizations

This chart shows the recommended schedule of immunizations for all children. Your child's doctor can suggest the exact timing that is best for each vaccination. The schedule will vary if the child is underimmunized or has a serious illness, such as cancer.

Child's age	Vaccine
Birth-2 months	Hepatitis B (1)
1-4 months	Hepatitis B (2)
2 months	DTaP or DTP, Hib, polio
4 months	DTaP or DTP, Hib, polio
6 months	DTaP or DTP, Hib
6-18 months	Hepatitis B (3)*, polio
12-15 months	Hib, MMR (1)
12-18 months	Chickenpox
15-18 months	DTaP or DTP
4-6 years	DTaP or DTP, polio, MMR (2)
11-12 years	MMR (if not given previously), chickenpox (if not given previously, two injections needed if child is over age 13)
11-16 years	Diphtheria, tetanus

Key		
	DtaP	Diphtheria, tetanus, acellular pertussis
	DTP	Diphtheria, tetanus, pertussis
	Hib	*Haemophilus influenzae* type b
	MMR	Measles, mumps, rubella

* If not given during infancy, the hepatitis series must be completed by age 10 in some states. In others, the series is given at ages 11 or 12 years.

HEPATITIS B

Hepatitis B (see page 517), an inflammation of the liver, can cause liver disease, liver cancer, and death. The hepatitis B vaccination is given in a series of three shots: the first at birth or by 2 months, the second between 1 and 4 months, and the third between 6 and 18 months. Babies born to mothers infected with hepatitis B need to receive hepatitis B immunoglobulin (antibodies to fight the disease) at birth in addition to the hepatitis B vaccine. An older child who has not yet had the vaccination should receive the shots beginning at age 9 or 10. Some states require a hepatitis B vaccination by the fifth grade. The hepatitis B vaccination rarely causes any side effects.

DIPHTHERIA, TETANUS, PERTUSSIS

Diphtheria (see page 473) causes a thick membrane to develop in the nose, throat, or airway. The disease can lead to breathing problems, heart failure, paralysis, and death. Tetanus (see page 645) causes severe, painful muscle spasms that can prevent the jaw from opening and make swallowing and breathing difficult. Pertussis (see page 591), known more commonly as whooping cough, causes severe coughing that can interfere with eating, drinking, or breathing and can lead to pneumonia, brain damage, and death, especially in young infants.

The vaccination for diphtheria, tetanus, and pertussis is given in a combined injection (referred to as DTP) in a series of five shots: at 2 months, 4 months, 6 months, between 15 and 18 months, and between 4 and 6 years. For diphtheria and tetanus, the vaccination provides protection for only 10 years so your child will need subsequent booster shots. Booster shots for diphtheria and tetanus are given between ages 11 and 16 and then every 10 years throughout life. If your child gets a deep, dirty wound, he or she may need to have a tetanus shot again if it has been more than 5 years since the last one.

Most side effects from a DTP vaccination are mild: soreness, redness, or swelling at the site; fever; fussiness; or sleepiness. These symptoms usually begin soon after the vaccination and can last from 1 to 2 days. Ask your doctor about giving your child acetaminophen or ibuprofen to minimize side effects.

In rare cases, the DTP vaccination can cause extreme irritability, excessive sleepiness, a poor appetite, a high fever (103°F or higher), or seizures. A new form of the vaccine called DTaP is available that greatly reduces the risk of side effects. If your child has any of these symptoms after the DTP vaccination, call your doctor immediately or take your child to the doctor's office or emergency department.

POLIO

Polio (see page 597) is a serious disease that can cause muscle pain and paralysis. Polio was once very common in the United States but widespread immunization has made it rare today. If you hear about a case of polio in your area, ask your doctor if your child should have an extra dose of polio vaccine. Most children are given a series of four doses of oral polio vaccine: at 2 months, 4 months, between 6 and 18 months, and between 4 and 6 years.

In extremely rare cases, the oral vaccine can cause polio in the child receiving it or in a person who has had close contact with the child. For this reason, children who have a weakened immune system and are less able to fight infection are given an injection of inactivated polio vaccine, which does not ever cause polio. (The oral form is given more frequently than the inactivated form because it is easier to give and it provides better protection.) Tell your doctor if your child or anyone in close contact with your child has a weakened immune system from a disease they were born with, is undergoing long-term treatment with corticosteroids (synthetic hormones that reduce inflammation), has cancer, is undergoing radiation therapy or chemotherapy for cancer, has HIV (human immunodeficiency virus–the virus that causes AIDS), or has had organ transplantation.

HAEMOPHILUS INFLUENZAE TYPE B

Haemophilus influenzae type b (Hib) can cause meningitis (see page 564), pneumonia (see page 595), and epiglottitis.

The Hib vaccination is given in a series of three or four shots, depending on the type of vaccine used. The Hib vaccination causes no serious side effects. Possible mild side effects include soreness at the site, a slight fever, and fussiness within 24 hours of the injection. Symptoms usually subside within 48 to 72 hours.

MEASLES, MUMPS, RUBELLA

Measles (see page 562) causes fever; a rash; a cough; a runny nose; and red, watery eyes, all of which can last for 1 to 2 weeks. Measles can sometimes lead to ear infections, pneumonia, and, in rare cases, brain swelling and death.

Mumps (see page 572) causes fever, headache, and painful swelling of one or both saliva-producing glands in the cheeks and under the jaw. Mumps can progress to meningitis (see page 564) and, in rare cases, swelling of the brain. In males after puberty, the infection occasionally affects the testicles and can cause infertility.

German measles (see page 501), also called rubella, is usually not serious except to women who become infected during pregnancy. Their babies are at risk of being stillborn or of having birth defects such as visual impairment, deafness, mental retardation, and heart disease.

The combined vaccination against measles, mumps, and rubella (MMR) is given twice, the first shot at 12 to 15 months and the second shot either between ages 4 and 6 or ages 11 and 12. The most common side effect is a rash or fever that starts 1 or 2 weeks after the vaccination and can last a few days. The child is not able to spread measles while having these side effects.

If your child has a serious allergy to eggs, he or she should not receive the MMR vaccination without prior skin testing because the vaccine contains egg products. If the skin testing is negative, the child can receive the MMR vaccine. A child with a weakened immune system from cancer or organ transplantation should not receive the vaccine because it could cause disease in the child. However, most children with HIV (human immunodeficiency virus) should get the MMR vaccination. The vaccination is not given to pregnant women because of the risk of injury to the fetus.

Chickenpox

Chickenpox is a common infection that once affected most children in the United States by age 10. A vaccine became available in the United States in 1995. Chickenpox causes fever, a blisterlike rash, and itching that usually lasts about a week. Scratching the rash can cause scarring.

The chickenpox vaccination, called the varicella zoster virus vaccine, is given in a single dose to children 12 months or older. If an older child has not

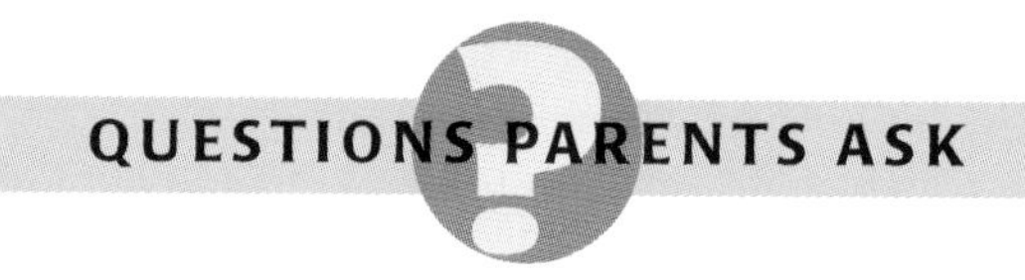

Vaccinations

Q What should I do if my child isn't feeling well on the day he or she is scheduled for a vaccination?

A For vaccinations to be effective, they need to be given on the recommended schedule, so take your child in for her scheduled shot. Children can usually get a vaccination if they have a minor illness or slight fever. Your doctor will determine whether your child can still have the vaccination.

Q My child is terrified of shots. Why can't all vaccinations be given to children by mouth?

A The digestive tract would destroy most vaccines. Most vaccines are injected into a muscle or into fat underneath the skin so they can be absorbed into the bloodstream.

Q I can't afford to pay for my child's vaccinations. What should I do?

A Check your health insurance policy; many health plans pay for vaccinations. If your health insurance does not cover vaccinations or if you do not have health insurance, talk to your doctor or call your local health department. Community health centers, medical school clinics, children's health clinics, public health clinics, and some pediatricians' offices provide vaccinations free or at a very low cost.

had chickenpox or been vaccinated against it, the doctor may recommend vaccination. In children older than 13 years, the vaccination is given in two shots 1 to 2 months apart.

Most children have no side effects from the chickenpox vaccination. Mild and temporary side effects include soreness, swelling, redness, or stiffness at the site within 2 days of the vaccination; or fatigue, fever, fussiness, nausea, or a mild rash within 3 weeks of the shot. If your child develops a rash, he or she may be able to give the infection to other people until the rash goes away.

INFLUENZA

Influenza, commonly known as the flu, is a respiratory infection caused by a virus. An influenza vaccination is available but, because new strains of the virus develop every year, the vaccination must be given every year—in the fall—to protect against the new strains.

Preparing your child for a shot

All shots hurt a little. Babies will cry for a few minutes, but they quickly forget the experience if you console them right away with a feeding or a hug. Try to divert attention away from the needle by holding or comforting the child. A reward can help make the experience less upsetting. Explain to an older child what to expect from a shot and why he or she is getting it.

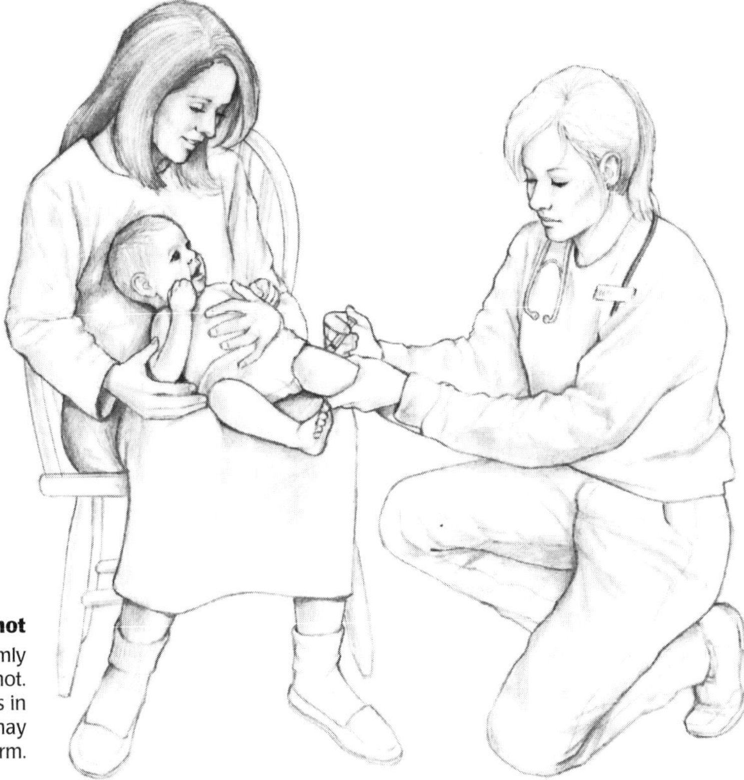

Getting a shot
Hold your child gently but firmly while he or she is getting a shot. Babies usually receive injections in the thigh; older children may receive them in the upper arm.

Because the flu is not serious for most healthy children, flu shots are not required childhood vaccinations. They are recommended for children over 6 months of age who have a chronic health problem and are at high risk of complications from the flu. But because the flu can keep a child out of school for up to a week, many parents are choosing to have their children (and themselves) immunized each fall when the new flu vaccine becomes available.

Flu shots seldom cause any side effects. Because the vaccine is made with egg products, a person who has a severe allergy to eggs should not have the shots.

Routine childhood tests and screenings

Doctors monitor a child's health through routine screening tests. Many serious illnesses, such as lead poisoning (see page 550) and high blood pressure (see page 520), cause no early symptoms. Routine tests can detect them before symptoms appear so they can be treated early.

BLOOD PRESSURE READING

Blood pressure is the force created in the bloodstream when the heart pumps blood into the vessels. A blood pressure reading shows how hard the circulating blood pushes against the vessel walls. Using an inflatable cuff and stethoscope, the doctor or nurse takes your child's blood pressure the same way as an adult's blood pressure is taken.

Normal Blood Pressure in Children and Adolescents

Your child's blood pressure (BP) can vary greatly within a normal range.

Age	Average BP for Girls	Upper End for Girls	Average BP for Boys	Upper End for Boys
2	90/56	110/74	92/56	110/72
4	92/56	114/74	94/56	112/72
6	96/58	116/74	96/58	116/74
8	100/60	118/76	100/60	118/76
10	102/62	122/80	102/62	122/78
12	108/66	126/82	108/64	126/82
14	112/68	130/86	112/64	130/82
16	112/68	132/86	118/68	136/86
18	114/66	132/86	122/70	140/88

Blood pressure is recorded in two measurements. The first, higher number is called the systolic pressure; it reflects the pressure in the blood vessels when the heart pumps blood. The second number, the diastolic pressure, records the pressure in the vessels when the heart rests between beats. The harder it is for the blood to flow, the higher both numbers will be.

The doctor will check the measurement of your child's blood pressure against a chart of normal blood pressure for children of similar age and same sex. Blood pressure in children can vary greatly within a normal range.

Your child will have a blood pressure measurement at each annual checkup beginning at age 3. The doctor routinely takes your child's blood pressure because high blood pressure can signal a serious illness that requires treatment, such as kidney disease, heart disease, and thyroid disorders (see page 648). If your child has high blood pressure, the doctor will evaluate it to rule out any disorders and recommend treatment. In most cases, once the condition that caused the high blood pressure is treated, the blood pressure returns to normal.

Being overweight puts a child at risk of developing high blood pressure at some time in life. If your child is overweight and has high blood pressure, the doctor will recommend a program of weight loss and exercise.

Scoliosis screening

Scoliosis is a condition in which the spine is curved either to the right or left side of the body. Scoliosis may be present at birth or it may develop as a child grows. Prompt treatment can prevent severe curves or complications such as lung and heart disease. Screening is recommended for the two most common forms of scoliosis–juvenile scoliosis and adolescent scoliosis–at each well-child checkup beginning at age 3.

To test for scoliosis, the doctor looks at the child's back and spine and evaluates posture while the child stands and then leans forward at the waist. The doctor examines the child's upper and lower back to make sure that the

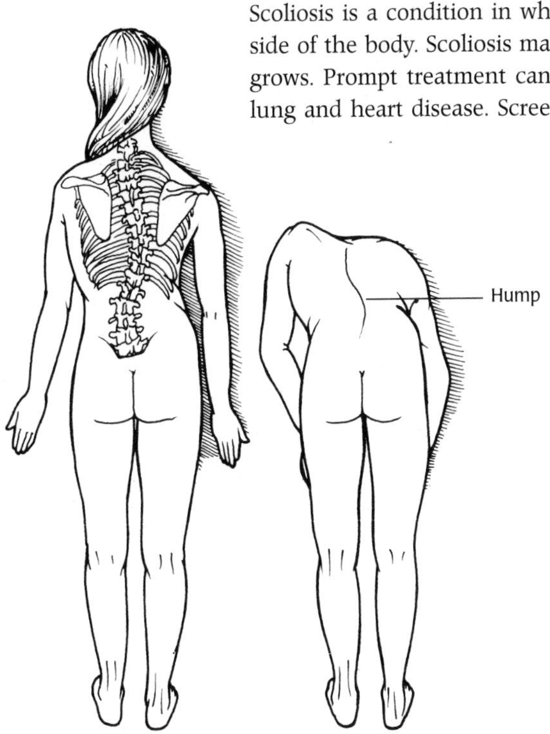

Testing for scoliosis

While a child stands (left), the doctor looks at the child's back to make sure that the spine forms a straight line from the center of the head to the center of the buttocks. He or she also checks to see that the shoulders, the shoulder blades, the hips, the creases at the waistline, the creases under the buttocks, and the backs of the knees are even on both sides. Then the doctor asks the child to bend forward at the waist (right). The doctor looks for a characteristic hump in the ribs or uneven shoulders and hips, which indicate scoliosis.

shoulders, shoulder blades, hipbones, creases at the waistline, creases under the buttocks, and the backs of the knees are aligned on either side of the child's body. He or she also checks the child's arms to see if they are hanging at equal distances from the trunk.

TUBERCULIN SKIN TEST

Tuberculosis (TB) (see page 652) is a highly contagious bacterial infection of the respiratory system. Without antibiotic treatment, the infection can become long term and life threatening.

The vast majority of American children are at low risk of becoming infected with TB, but some states or schools require frequent testing. If your child has contact with people who are recent immigrants from countries with a high incidence of TB, are infected with HIV (human immunodeficiency virus), are homeless, or are residents of nursing homes, you should talk to your doctor about how often the child should be tested.

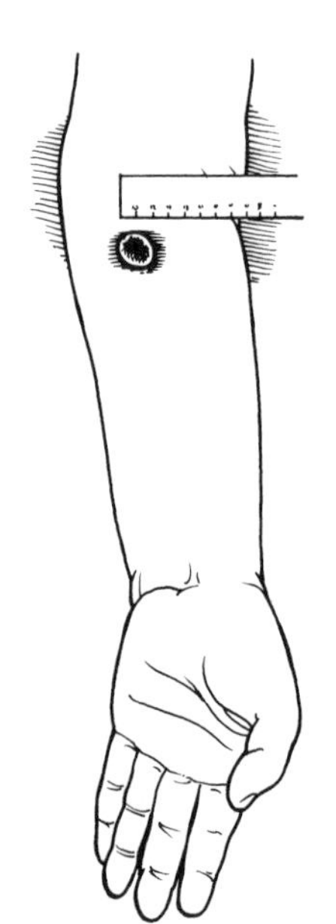

To administer a tuberculin skin test, the doctor or nurse injects a tiny amount of the TB bacterium protein under the skin of the inner part of the child's arm. A reaction in the form of swelling and redness at the site indicates that your child has been exposed to or infected with the bacterium. A positive reaction will require a physical examination and chest X-ray to determine appropriate treatment.

mm
10 20 30 40 50
5 15 25 35 45

Actual size

Results of the tuberculin skin test
If your child has been exposed to the tuberculosis bacterium, the area around the site of the skin test will become red, raised, or hard. In a low-risk, otherwise healthy child under the age of 4, the area will measure 10 millimeters or more; in an older child, the area will measure at least 15 millimeters.

BLOOD TESTS

Changes in the blood can be a sign of disease anywhere in the body. To detect any changes, the doctor will draw blood from the child's arm or finger for testing.

Complete blood cell count A complete blood cell count measures the main components of blood, including red cells, white cells, and platelets. A complete blood cell count can detect such disorders as anemia or infection.

Hemoglobin or hematocrit test A hemoglobin test measures the level in your child's blood of iron-rich hemoglobin, which carries oxygen to all the tissues of the body. A hematocrit test is a blood test that shows the percentage in the blood of red blood cells, the cells that contain hemoglobin. A child will be given one of these two tests to screen for anemia (see page 412). Children are likely to have a hematocrit or hemoglobin test between birth and 12 months of age and then periodically throughout childhood and adolescence.

Cholesterol screening A cholesterol test measures the level of fats in the blood. A person's total cholesterol level is used as an indicator of his or her risk of developing heart disease. Some doctors recommend that all children have a cholesterol test at age 6 and a follow-up test at age 8; others recommend the test only for those children considered to be at risk. Doctors may recommend

What Does a Cholesterol Profile Show?

A cholesterol profile measures the various types of fats in the blood—both harmful ones and helpful ones. Low-density lipoprotein (LDL) cholesterol is the "bad" cholesterol that causes fatty deposits to build up along blood vessel walls, increasing the risk of heart disease. High-density lipoprotein (HDL) cholesterol is the "good" cholesterol that cleanses the blood vessels of fats, reducing the risk of heart disease. This chart shows how doctors interpret cholesterol levels in children between ages 2 and 18. The relationship of these numbers to each other can also indicate risk of heart disease. Your doctor will carefully discuss any significant findings with you.

Level (milligrams per deciliter)	Future Risk of Heart Disease
Total Cholesterol	
Less than 170	Low
170-199	Borderline high
200 or higher	High
Low-density Lipoprotein	
Less than 110	Low
110-129	Borderline high
130 or higher	High
High-density Lipoprotein	
Less than 35	Low
35-45	Borderline high
46 or higher	High

testing for children over age 2 who have either of these inherited risk factors for heart disease:

- A parent with a total cholesterol level over 240 milligrams per deciliter (mg/dL)
- A family history of heart disease at an early age (a parent, grandparent, aunt, or uncle who had a heart attack or symptoms of heart disease before age 55)

Discuss either of these risk factors with your child's doctor so he or she can decide whether or not your child's cholesterol levels should be tested. Your child should probably be tested if he or she has high blood pressure, smokes cigarettes, is overweight, or eats a diet high in saturated fats (those found in red meat, butter, cheese, whole milk, and other whole-fat dairy products).

Lead screening A buildup of lead in the bloodstream can retard a child's physical and mental development. Screening of all children for lead is recommended at 6 months and 6 years of age—more frequently depending on a child's risk factors. Many schools require a lead screening before the child starts attending school. Any amount of lead can be harmful, but the more lead found in the child's bloodstream, the greater the damage. For more about lead poisoning and treatments, see page 550. Lead is measured in units called micrograms per deciliter (µg/dL) and blood lead levels are interpreted in the following way:

- **Less than 10 µg/dL** These levels are considered to be relatively harmless.
- **Between 10 and 19 µg/dL** These levels indicate mild lead exposure. The doctor will ask about the potential for lead exposure in the home. Is there chipping paint? Is the home undergoing remodeling? The doctor will repeat the test in 2 to 3 months.
- **Between 20 and 39 µg/dL** These levels require medical treatment and removal of the child from the source of the lead.
- **40 µg/dL or higher** These levels require treatment with an agent that removes the lead from the blood.

URINALYSIS

A urinalysis is a battery of tests performed on a sample of a child's urine to detect potentially serious conditions such as urinary tract infections (see page 657), kidney disorders, or diabetes. The test can also check normal kidney function. At the doctor's office, you can help your child collect a sample of his or her urine. A strip of paper will be dipped into the urine and used to detect the presence of certain substances, such as protein, white blood cells, blood, glucose (sugar), or other elements. The doctor or a technician will also check the urine's physical characteristics, such as color, cloudiness, and concentration. If the screening is abnormal, a urine sample will be examined more thoroughly under a microscope. Based on the results, the doctor will decide what treatment your child needs.

Well-child visits to the doctor

Although you will see your child's doctor more frequently during your child's first year than at any other time, regular checkups will continue to be an essential part of keeping your child healthy throughout childhood and adolescence. These regular checkups–called well-child visits–give you a chance to get to know your doctor so you can work together more effectively to care for your child.

At each well-child visit during your child's first 5 years, your doctor will make sure your child is growing and developing properly, that he or she has no serious abnormalities or health problems, and that he or she has all the recommended vaccinations. The doctor will keep a record of all the vaccinations and any illnesses your child has. Both parents should try to attend these early visits.

THE FIRST VISIT

The first well-child checkup at 2 to 4 weeks (at 2 to 4 days if your baby was discharged from the hospital within 48 hours of birth or at 1 to 2 weeks if you are breast-feeding) will be a little different from the ones that follow, especially if it's the first meeting between you, the doctor, and your baby. If another doctor performed your baby's examination in the first 2 to 4 days after birth, make sure that your child's doctor has the medical records from that examination before your child's first visit.

At this visit, the doctor will ask about your pregnancy, your labor and delivery, and any complications you may have had. He or she will also want to know your baby's birthweight, the estimated length of your pregnancy, and about any problems the baby had after delivery. The first visit is a good time to ask the doctor about your baby's development, feeding, sleeping, or general care, and to discuss any concerns you have. Be open with your doctor if you are experiencing excessive stress or fatigue or are finding the baby extremely disruptive to your or your family's sleep patterns. It is important to safeguard your own health as well as your new baby's.

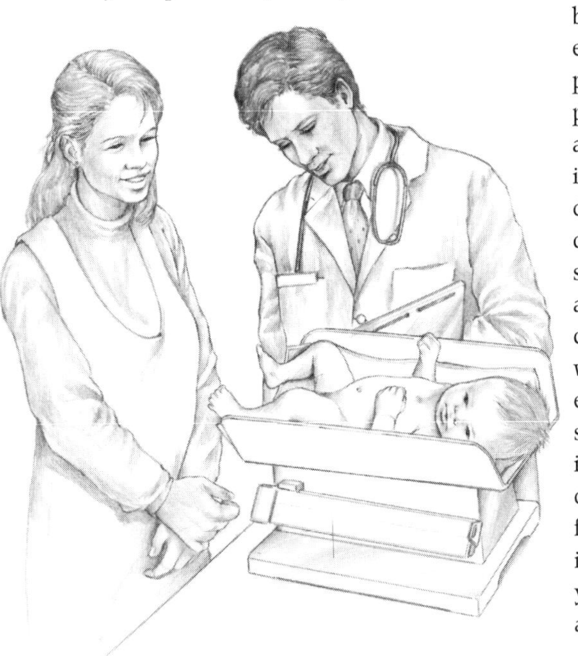

Measuring your child's weight

One of the most important indications that an infant is healthy and thriving is a steady weight gain from one checkup to the next. At the first checkup, the doctor will weigh your baby to make sure his or her weight is at or above the weight at birth. Remember that most babies lose weight during the first 7 to 10 days of life.

The doctor may ask about the following topics:

- Your baby's sleep pattern
- Whether or not you put your baby to sleep on his or her back or side (see SIDS; page 626)
- How well the baby feeds
- Your baby's urination and bowel movement habits
- Whether the baby seems alert
- Whether the baby moves all of his or her limbs
- Whether the baby responds to noise
- Whether or not you use a car seat

The doctor will examine your baby's umbilical cord (the cord should have fallen off by 2 weeks). If your child is a boy, the doctor will examine his genitals to make sure that both testicles have descended into the scrotum (the pouch of skin containing the testicles). If your son has been circumcised (see page 32), the doctor will examine his penis. Your child's skin will be examined for signs of jaundice (see page 540) or newborn rashes (see page 604).

Schedule of well-child visits

Well-child visits are generally recommended at the following ages. If your child has a chronic or recurring health problem, visits to the doctor will be more frequent.

2 to 4 weeks	9 months	24 months
2 months	12 months	Once a year between ages 3 and 18
4 months	15 months	
6 months	18 months	

At each visit

At the first visit and at subsequent ones, checkups focus on the issues that are most important at a child's particular age. The doctor will evaluate your child's growth and development (physical, emotional, and social) and educate you about ways to protect your child from injury. Most well-child visits throughout childhood include the following examinations.

Growth Growth is one of the most important indicators of the

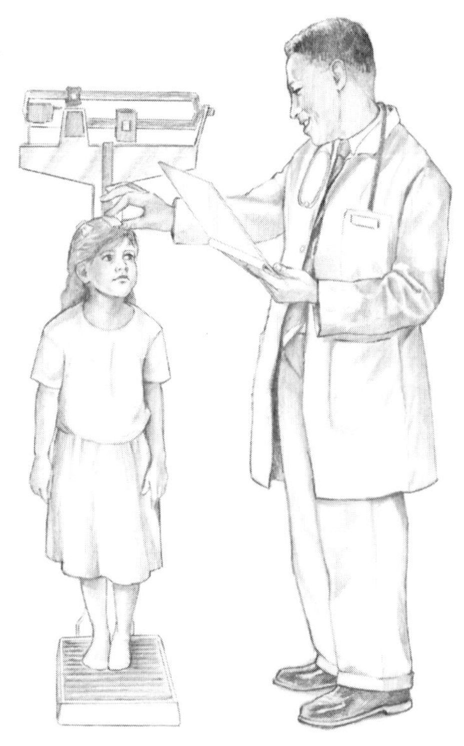

Measuring your child's growth
To make sure that your child is healthy and growing properly, the doctor will measure his or her height at each visit and compare it with the measurement from previous visits.

Physical Growth of Girls From Birth to 36 Months

This chart shows the normal ranges in weight and length for girls from birth to 36 months of age. The numbers 5 through 95 on the right side of the chart show the percentile of growth. For example, if your daughter is about 32 inches long at 18 months of age, she is in the 50th percentile of girls her age for length. That means that about half of all girls her age are longer than she is and half are shorter.

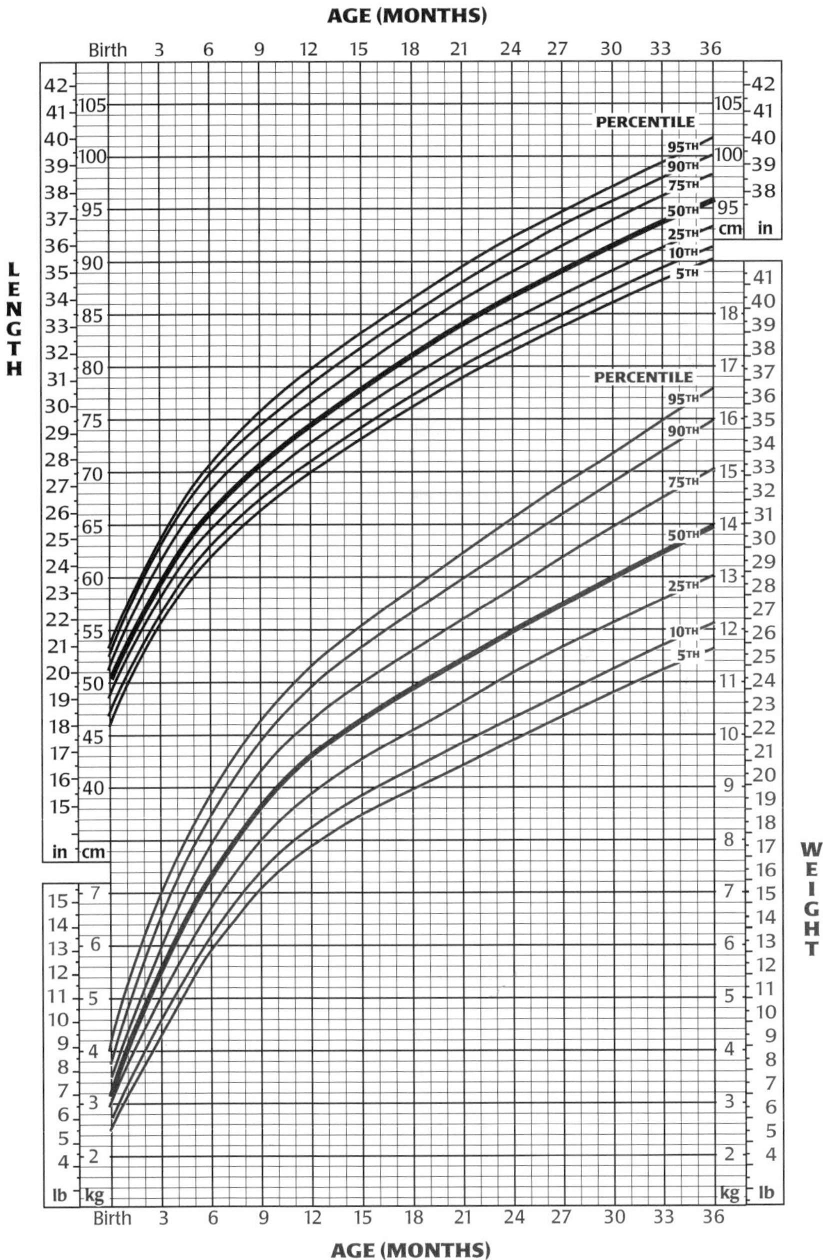

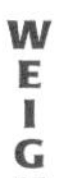

Physical Growth of Boys From Birth to 36 Months

This chart shows the normal ranges in weight and length for boys from birth to 36 months of age. The numbers 5 through 95 on the right side of the chart show the percentile of growth. For example, if your son is about 32 inches long at 18 months of age, he is in the 50th percentile of boys his age for length. That means that about half of all boys his age are longer than he is and half are shorter.

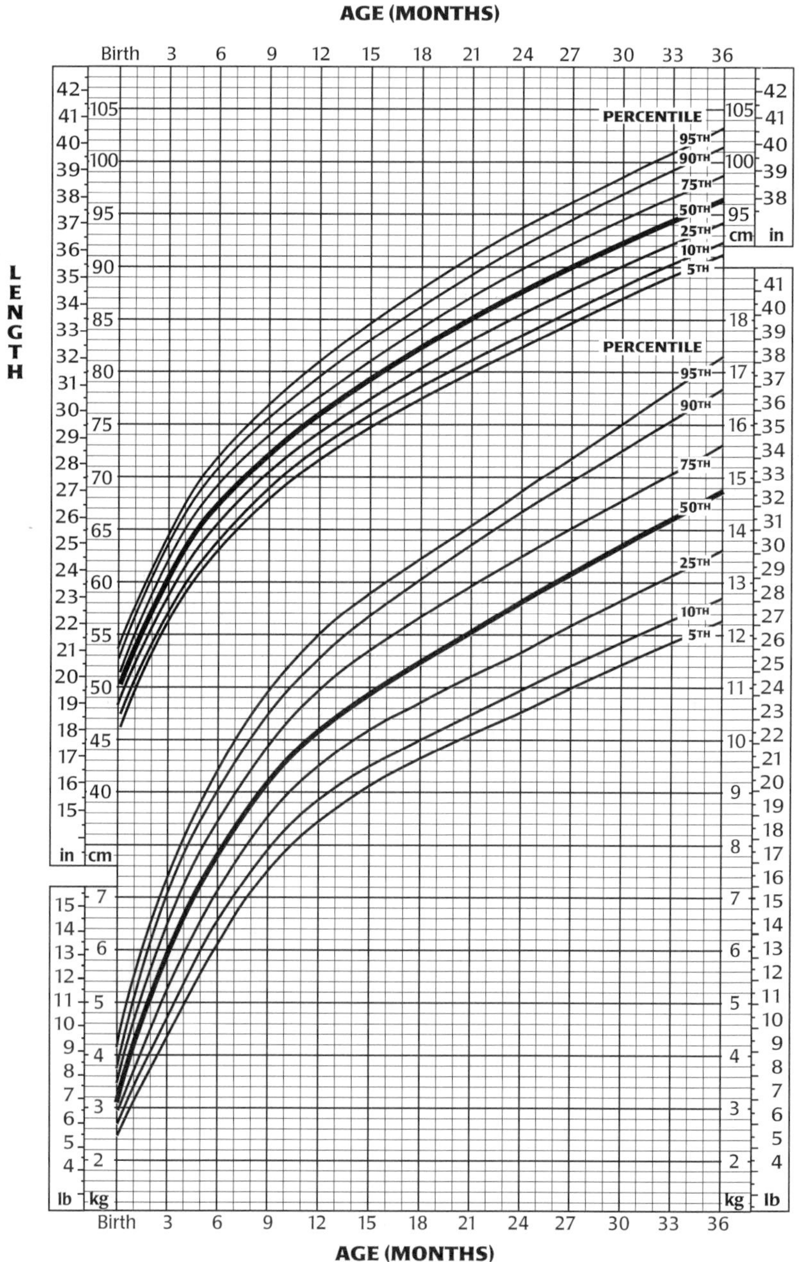

Physical Growth of Girls From 2 to 18 Years

This chart shows the normal ranges in weight and height for girls aged 2 to 18 years. The numbers 5 through 95 on the right side of the chart show the percentile of growth. For example, if your daughter is about 4 feet 5 inches tall at age 9½, she is in the 50th percentile of girls her age for height. That means about half of all girls her age are taller than she is and half are shorter.

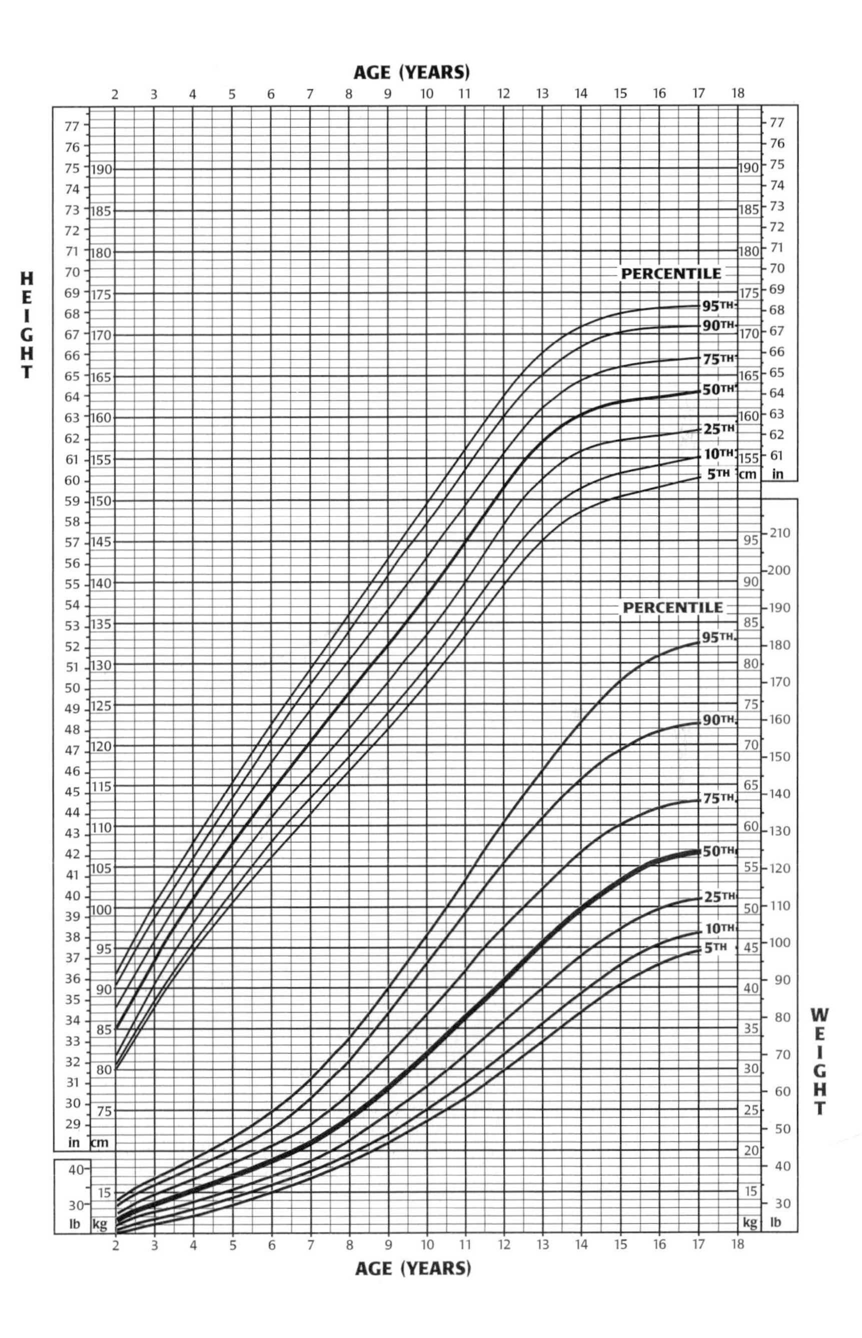

Physical Growth of Boys From 2 to 18 Years

This chart shows the normal ranges in weight and height for boys aged 2 to 18 years. The numbers 5 through 95 on the right side of the chart show the percentile of growth. For example, if your son is about 4 feet 9 inches tall at age 11, he is in the 50th percentile of boys his age for height. That means about half of all boys his age are taller than he is and half are shorter.

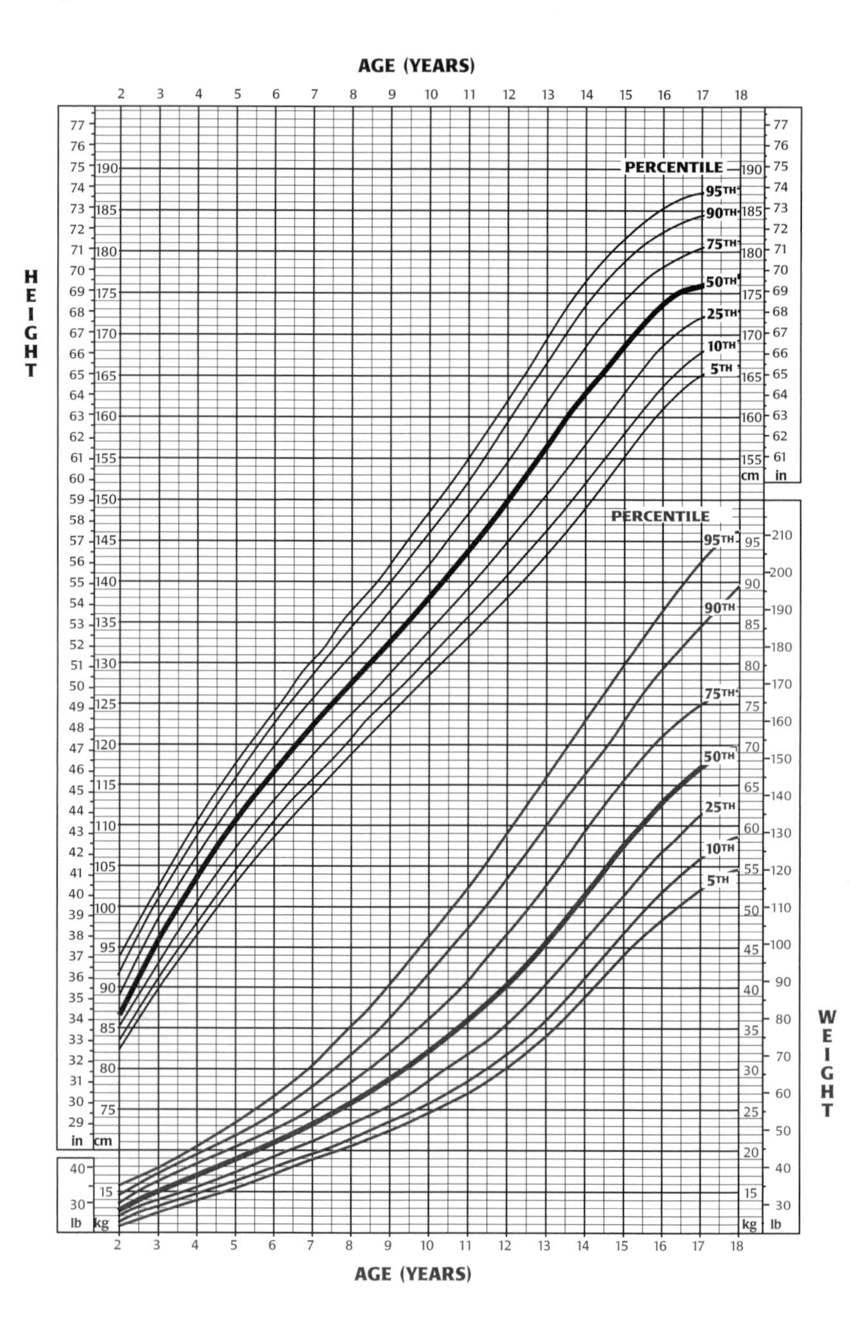

Head Circumference for Girls From Birth to 36 Months

This chart shows the normal range in head circumference for girls from birth to 36 months of age. If your daughter's head circumference is about 18½ inches at 18 months of age, she is in the 50th percentile of girls her age. That means that about half of all girls her age have a smaller head circumference and half have a larger one.

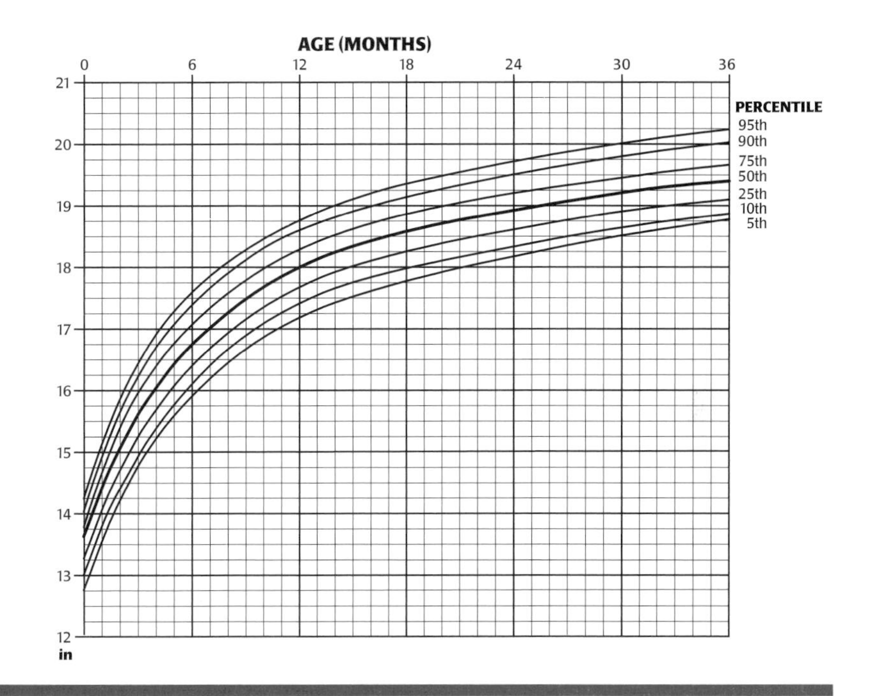

Head Circumference for Boys From Birth to 36 Months

This chart shows the normal range in head circumference for boys from birth to 36 months of age. If your son's head circumference is about 19 inches at 18 months of age, he is in the 50th percentile of boys his age. That means that about half of all boys his age have a smaller head circumference and half have a larger one.

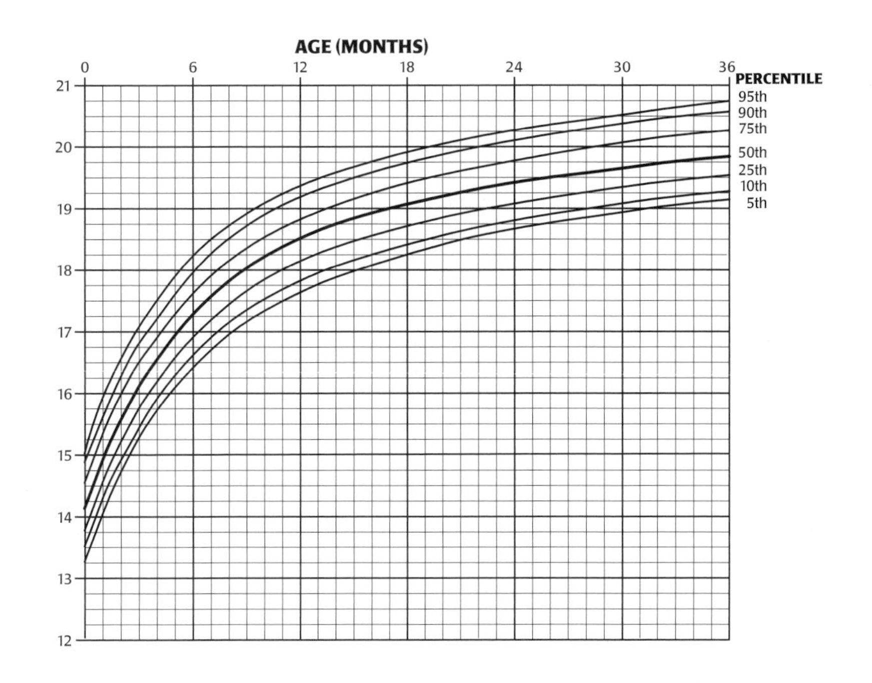

general state of a child's health, especially during the early months and years. At each visit, the doctor will weigh your child, measure his or her length or height, and measure the head circumference (until age 2). Your doctor will plot these numbers on a graph. At subsequent visits, he or she will compare these numbers with your child's measurements at the last visit to make sure your child is growing properly.

To check your child's growth against the average growth of children comparable in age and sex, refer to the charts on pages 239 to 242. But keep in mind that your child's own rate of growth is most important, not the way it compares to other children's. Your child's graph should show that he or she is growing at a steady rate and that there is no unusual speeding up or slowing down of growth that could indicate a problem.

Another way the doctor will make sure your child is growing properly is by measuring his or her head circumference. The doctor will check your child's head circumference against a chart like those on page 243, which show the normal range of head circumference growth for age in girls and boys.

Development The doctor will ask about your child's general development—when he or she started to smile, crawl, walk, or talk. Your doctor will also test the child's reflexes and muscle tone and check fine motor skills (use of the hands and fingers) and gross motor skills (use of the arms and legs). To evaluate your child's social development, the doctor will look for a responsive smile and will observe the way your child interacts with you and siblings. As a sign of your child's language development, the progression from cooing to babbling to words will be tracked.

Head and neck The doctor will measure the size of your child's head with a tape measure and note the shape of the head during the first few visits. Passage through the birth canal during delivery sometimes causes an infant's head to have an abnormal shape. The head usually returns to normal within a few days or weeks. The doctor will also monitor the child's two soft spots (fontanelles; see page 270), checking their size and making sure they are closing properly. The soft spot at the back of the head is closed at birth in most children (otherwise, it closes by about 4 months); the spot on the top of the head usually closes by age 2. The doctor will examine your child's neck to make sure that both sides are symmetrical and to confirm that the neck moves easily.

Hearing An inability to hear interferes with the development of language skills, affecting the child's ability to communicate. At each checkup, the doctor will look inside both of your child's ears with an instrument called an otoscope to detect any abnor-

Could your child have a hearing problem?

If your child does not respond to your voice or to loud noises, he or she could have a hearing problem. Call your doctor if your child does not respond to the following stimuli at home:

- His or her name
- Noise-making toys that are out of the child's range of vision
- Loud noises

malities, such as fluid behind the eardrum or signs of infection, that could affect hearing. This examination can be upsetting to a child because he or she may have to be restrained to enable the doctor to look inside the ear.

If your child is younger than 4, the doctor will evaluate hearing by observing responses to noises, such as clicking or rattling. Parents are often the first to notice that their child is having difficulty hearing so the doctor will also ask about your child's response to noise at home. Most children have a standard screening test for hearing when they are 4 or 5 years old when they enter preschool (sooner if they have a noticeable speech or hearing problem). If your child is at risk for a hearing problem, the doctor will refer you to a hearing specialist (audiologist).

Vision At routine checkups, the doctor will perform different eye examinations, depending on your child's age and abilities. The doctor will check both the outside and inside of the eyes. He or she may look inside the child's eyes with a lighted instrument called an ophthalmoscope to detect anatomical abnormalities such as a cataract (clouding of the lens). The doctor will move a bright-colored

Could your child have an eye problem?

Most eye problems in children are detected during routine well-child examinations, but parents often notice that their child is having difficulty seeing or that his or her eyes are not normal. Call the doctor if your child has any of the following signs of eye problems:

- No steady eye contact, or apparent inability to see by 2 months of age
- Frequent eye rubbing
- Shutting or covering of one eye
- Redness, swelling, crusting, or discharge in the eyes or on the eyelids that lasts longer than 24 hours
- White, grayish-white, or yellowish material in the pupil
- Sensitivity to light
- Inability to see distant objects clearly
- Tendency to bump into objects
- Eyes that don't move together, or look crooked or crossed
- Excessive tearing
- Frequent tilting or turning of the head
- Frequent squinting
- Drooping eyelids
- Pupils of unequal size
- Eyes that "bounce" or "dance"
- Tendency to hold objects close to see
- Injury to the eye
- Cloudy cornea (the transparent layer over the front of the eye)
- Inability to see well at a distance
- Seeing double
- Inability to see clearly
- Frequent headaches
- Dizziness
- Feeling nauseous after reading or watching television
- Itchy, scratchy, or burning eyes
- Difficulty identifying colors after age 3

toy or flashlight in front of your child and observe his or her eyes as they follow it to check movement in each eye. If the child has any eye problems, your doctor will refer you to an ophthalmologist (a doctor who specializes in eye care).

Nose, mouth, and throat The doctor will examine your child's nose, mouth, and throat for signs of infection or other problems. He or she will examine the gums to see how the teeth are coming in. If your child develops a tooth problem, such as discoloration or early decay, your doctor will refer you to a dentist, probably a pediatric dentist, who specializes in dental care of children through the teenage years. You should start bringing your children to the dentist for regular checkups (see page 262) at age 3.

Heart and lungs The doctor will hold a stethoscope to your child's chest and back to listen for breath sounds and heart sounds. The doctor notes the child's breathing pattern and rate, and the heart rate and rhythm for any irregularities or murmurs.

Abdomen The doctor will observe the size and shape of your child's abdomen and then gently press on the abdomen to check the internal organs for tenderness, swelling, enlargement, or abdominal masses.

Genitals The doctor will examine your child's genitals at each visit for signs of infection or rashes. He or she will also evaluate the anatomy of the genitals and the stage of sexual development. The doctor checks a boy's testicles to make sure they have descended into the scrotum.

Hips and legs During the first 18 months to 2 years, the doctor will move your baby's legs to check for any problems in the hip joints (see page 522), such as dislocation. After the child has started walking, the doctor will watch him or her take a few steps to make sure the legs and feet are aligned properly, of equal length, and moving normally. The doctor will also evaluate the shape and strength of the feet and legs.

Skin The doctor will examine your child's skin for any rashes, birthmarks, infantile acne (see page 65), abnormal bruising, infection, or cradle cap (see page 23). If the child has a mole, the doctor will measure it and check it at each visit for any abnormal changes.

Brain and spinal cord To check the functioning of your child's brain and spinal cord, the doctor will check the child's reflexes, sensations, and muscle strength and tone. The doctor will make sure your child has grown out of the infantile reflexes, a sign of proper brain and spinal cord development.

Rectum The doctor will examine your child's rectum to look for any abnormalities. If the child is having abdominal pain or problems with bowel movements, the doctor may need to perform a finger examination of the rectum to check the anus, the sphincter (the muscle that opens and closes during a bowel movement) for tone, and the end of the colon for masses or abnormal narrowing. He or she will also check the stool for blood and firmness.

Vaccinations The doctor will tell you the vaccinations (see page 226) that your child needs at each visit and describe any potential side effects. For the recommended schedule of childhood vaccinations, see page 227. To find out about specific vaccinations and their side effects, see page 228.

Screening tests Your child will be given any screening tests (see page 232) that are recommended at his or her age. These tests can help detect many treatable disorders early, before they become serious.

Eating and sleeping evaluation At each visit, the doctor will ask you about your child's eating and sleeping habits. He or she will inquire about your infant's frequency of feeding and, if you are bottle-feeding, which formula you are using. As your child gets older, the doctor will tell you when and how to introduce solid foods and how to provide a nutritious diet. He or she will give you tips for helping your child develop healthy eating habits.

The doctor will also ask about the child's nighttime sleeping habits and daytime naps. Waking at night and nightmares are very common in children. Developing a healthy sleeping routine helps keep children of all ages well rested.

Safety During each new stage of development, your child will become more mobile—and more at risk of injury. At each visit, your child's doctor will describe the safety issues you should consider in the coming weeks or months. For more information about safety, see chapter 11.

THE SCHOOL-READINESS CHECKUP

When your child is about 4 or 5 years old, the annual well-child visit will focus on the child's readiness to begin school. The doctor will evaluate your child's development, attention span, social skills, and ability to conform to a structured environment. He or she will also look for any vision, hearing, speech, or development problems that could affect school performance. If the doctor suspects that your child has any problems in these areas, he or she may recommend that your child have a standardized developmental test administered by qualified professionals who have experience working with children. Such professionals may include child psychologists, speech and language pathologists, special education experts, and pediatricians who have expertise in early childhood development. During this checkup, the doctor will also update your child's vaccinations, especially those for diphtheria, tetanus, pertussis; polio; and measles, mumps, rubella. A school-readiness examination will usually include the following tests.

Vision As many as 10 percent of preschool children have some kind of vision impairment. If your child did not have a formal vision test at a routine well-child checkup at age 3 or 4, he or she should have one now to take care of any vision problems before they interfere with learning. If your child's vision is worse than 20/40, the doctor will refer you to an ophthalmologist (eye specialist) for diagnosis and treatment or correction.

Hearing Severe hearing loss in children is usually detected at a young age, long before a child is ready to enter school. But to make sure your child's hearing is normal, the doctor will test his or her ability to hear as part of the school-readiness examination. Through headphones, your child will hear words said at different volumes of sound. When the child hears the name of a familiar object, such as a sandbox, he or she points to a corresponding picture. Normal hearing detects sounds as low as 15 decibels. If your child can only hear sounds above 30 decibels, he or she probably has a hearing deficit.

Speech Like hearing loss, speech impairment can affect school performance. Some speech difficulties reveal a learning problem that interferes with a child's ability to understand words. Your doctor will ask about your child's speech development and listen to his or her speech. If the doctor detects a speech problem, he or she will refer you to a speech pathologist, who can diagnose the problem and recommend therapy. Your child should begin this therapy before entering school. A child with speech difficulties also needs a hearing evaluation because hearing deficits are the major cause of speech problems.

Emotional development and behavior Children vary greatly in their emotional development. Some children are ready for school long before age 5; others may not be ready at this age. Your child's doctor will help evaluate whether or not your child has the maturity and social skills needed for success at school. If you have concerns about your child's readiness, discuss them fully with your doctor.

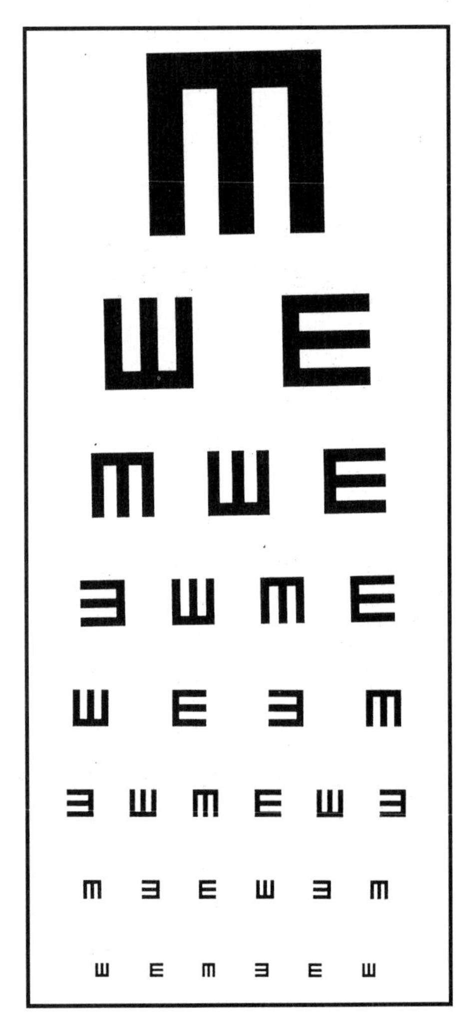

Vision test chart

A doctor evaluates your child's vision by asking the child to look at a chart containing rows of letters in increasingly smaller sizes. The child tells the doctor in which row the letters become too small to see clearly.

Vaccinations At the school-readiness checkup, your doctor will make sure that all of your child's vaccinations are up to date. Ask for the proper documentation so you can give it to school officials. For information about specific vaccinations, see page 228. For the recommended schedule of vaccinations, see page 227.

Screening tests Depending on your child's risk factors for tuberculosis, your pediatrician may recommend that your child have a tuberculin skin test (see page 234). The doctor may recommend a urinalysis (see page 236) at this visit to screen for kidney problems, a urinary tract infection, or type I diabetes (see page 471). Many schools require lead screening (see page 236) and a hematocrit test (see page 235) before enrollment.

CHECKUPS FOR THE SCHOOL-AGE CHILD

Regular visits to the doctor continue throughout the school years. At each visit the doctor will perform a routine physical examination and evaluate your child's growth and development (see page 238). The doctor will also want to know how well your child is doing in school both academically and socially. School-age checkups give you the chance to ask your doctor about any concerns you may have about your child's progress or behavior. During these regular checkups, your doctor will probably cover the following topics:

School The doctor will discuss the importance of encouraging your child to do homework and of helping the child whenever necessary. Ask your doctor how you can give your child the emotional support he or she needs to have a positive attitude toward school and after-school activities.

Behavior The doctor will ask if your child has any behavior problems. He or she will want to know how your child interacts with friends and how much television the child watches. The doctor will also talk about the benefits of involvement in a sport or a group activity to foster responsibility, self-discipline, and teamwork. Discipline is a concern at all ages and you should feel free to ask your doctor for advice about handling it.

By about age 10, some children start experimenting with risky behaviors, such as smoking or chewing tobacco, and drug and alcohol use. Your child's doctor can give advice about ways to help your child resist peer pressure to take up these unhealthy habits. Setting a good parental example at home helps instill the self-control needed to avoid such risky behaviors.

Sex education At the 10-year checkup or before your child enters junior high, the doctor will discuss with you and your child the changes brought on by puberty. He or she can offer advice about ways to handle sex education at home. The doctor may want to talk to your child alone to nurture confidentiality and instill a sense of responsibility for his or her own body.

Safety Your child's doctor will discuss the safety issues that are most important at your child's age, including bicycle safety, water safety, fire safety, and gun safety. The doctor will want to make sure that your child knows his or her phone number and address (by age 4 or 5), and how to avoid strangers. For more information about safety, see chapter 11.

CHECKUP FOR SPORTS PARTICIPATION

More than 5 million American teenagers compete in high school athletics each year and as many as a third of them experience sports-related injuries. Twice as many boys are injured as girls. The sports most likely to cause injury are football, basketball, soccer, wrestling, gymnastics, and track.

Before teen athletes can participate in school sports, most schools require a medical checkup, called the preparticipation athletic examination. Some schools provide free physicals. Certain states require examinations every year; others require them every 3 years. The examinations determine an athlete's fitness to play, detect conditions that might put the child at risk of injury, evaluate the child's general health, and teach the best way to train for the sport and avoid injuries. If your child is not required to have an athletic examination, he or she should get one from his or her own doctor.

Children who have a known injury or chronic underlying disease will need further evaluation before being allowed to participate in a sport. A child may need to limit or delay sports participation if he or she:

- Has experienced light-headedness or become unconscious while exercising
- Has a heart murmur or a disturbance of heart rhythm
- Uses potentially harmful drugs, such as tobacco or alcohol, or illegal drugs, such as anabolic steroids (that mimic the male hormone testosterone used to build muscle) or cocaine

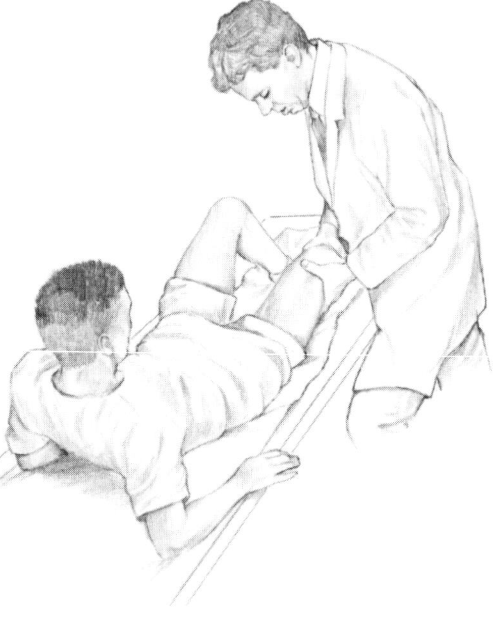

The athletic checkup
Preparticipation athletic examinations can help doctors detect problems that could become worse during sports activity. For example, to make sure that a child can safely play a running sport such as soccer, the doctor will carefully check the child's knees, which bear most of the stress in that sport.

- Has high blood pressure
- Is very overweight
- Has any respiratory disease

The doctor conducts a comprehensive physical examination, paying special attention to the areas of the body used in the particular sport. Examination of the bones, muscles, and joints is especially important.

The preparticipation athletic examination includes the measurement of height, weight, blood pressure, pulse, and breathing rate. The doctor will also examine the child's head, eyes, ears, nose, throat, abdomen, and external genitals. A child who is not as physically mature as peers competing in the same sport—especially a collision sport such as football or a contact sport such as basketball—is at increased risk of injury.

The doctor listens to the child's heart to rule out a murmur or abnormal rhythm. The lungs are checked for wheezing or other signs of disease (see page 605), which need to be controlled before a child can participate in a sport. If the child has any open sores, he or she may not be allowed to compete in a contact sport until they have healed.

CHECKUPS DURING ADOLESCENCE

Adolescence is the bridge between childhood and adulthood. Adolescents typically struggle for independence from their parents and begin to cherish their privacy. When interacting with your adolescent, a good doctor will be sensitive to these feelings.

By age 13, checkups will generally involve only the child and doctor. This arrangement gives the child a sense of privacy and helps establish a trusting relationship with the doctor. The only time the doctor may break this confidentiality is if your child is in danger of hurting him- or herself or others. Your doctor can provide counseling to your adolescent and help him or her learn to solve problems and negotiate the difficult transition to adulthood.

These are the years when young people challenge parental authority and seek approval from their peers, often through unconventional or risk-taking behavior. Adolescents who are not skilled at handling anger and frustration may become severely depressed and withdrawn. Some teenagers who feel unimportant may drift into a downward spiral of school absenteeism, substance abuse, conflict with peers, high-risk sex, or petty crimes such as shoplifting. Adolescents are twice as likely as people in other age groups to be victims of violent crimes. For all of these reasons, your child's visits to the doctor will usually involve much more than a physical examination.

Interviewing your child Some common adolescent problems, such as depression and drug use, are not always obvious, so the doctor may need to ask probing questions. Your child's doctor will conduct a confidential interview with the adolescent to discuss self-esteem, nutrition, sexuality, peer relationships, body image, and school. These discussions give the doctor a chance to reinforce behaviors that promote good health and discourage behaviors that may be harmful.

The doctor may decide to perform medical tests for specific problems, such as sexually transmitted diseases, or refer the adolescent to another doctor or other health care professional for further evaluation. Doctors look for the following common problems during these routine checkups:

Tobacco use Cigarette smoking and chewing tobacco are increasing among adolescents, despite all the health warnings. Adolescent smoking is important because most adult smokers became addicted to cigarettes before they were 17. At each annual adolescent checkup, the doctor will ask if the child smokes or chews tobacco and how much. The doctor will warn the child of the dangers of these unhealthy habits, encourage him or her to quit, and recommend a stop-smoking program.

Use of alcohol and other drugs At each annual checkup, the doctor will question the child about the use of alcohol and other drugs, including illegal drugs and over-the-counter or prescription medications used for nonmedical purposes. If the doctor suspects that drug use is affecting your child's mental or physical health, he or she may order a urine test to screen for drug use. The doctor may refer your child to a substance abuse program or to a mental health professional for counseling.

School problems Repeated absences from school or poor grades may signal a learning disability (see page 551), an attention disorder (see page 425), a medical problem, a mental disorder such as depression, family dysfunction, use of alcohol or other drugs, or physical or sexual abuse. The doctor will work together with you, your son or daughter, and school personnel to find the

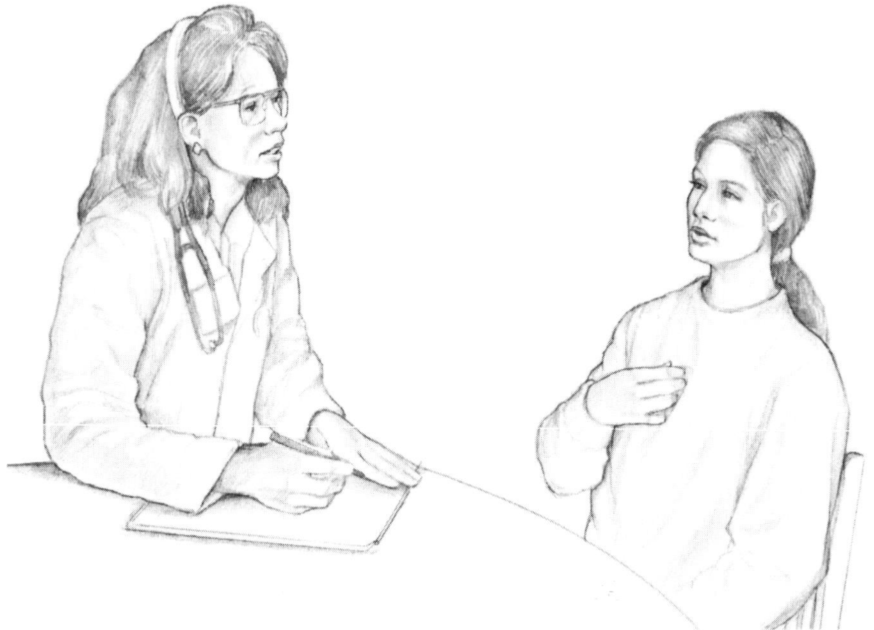

Gathering information

One of the most important parts of the adolescent checkup is a give-and-take discussion between the doctor and teenager. By learning about an adolescent's concerns and potential health risks, the doctor can teach the child how to reduce those risks.

cause of the problem and to develop a treatment plan that will help your child overcome it.

SEXUAL ACTIVITY At routine checkups, doctors ask adolescents if they are sexually active and whether they use latex condoms every time they have sex to prevent sexually transmitted diseases (STDs) and contraceptives to prevent unintended pregnancy. Teens receive education about prevention of STDs and pregnancy and may be tested for the most common STDs (see page 183). Sexually active girls will be given a Pap smear (see page 255) to test for cervical cancer, which is usually caused by a sexually transmitted virus. Girls at risk of pregnancy may also be given a pregnancy test (see page 255). Be aware that a doctor can prescribe birth-control pills or other contraceptive devices for your teenage daughter without your consent.

DEPRESSION Depression among adolescents is common and should always be a cause for concern. Suicide is the third leading cause of death among teenagers. Signs of depression can include falling grades in school, fatigue, persistent feelings of sadness, sleep disturbances, dropping out of activities, use of alcohol or other drugs, running away, withdrawing, stealing, lying, or attempting suicide. If the depression is severe, the doctor will refer the child to a psychiatrist or other mental health professional or admit the child to a hospital for treatment.

EMOTIONAL, PHYSICAL, AND SEXUAL ABUSE Teenagers are often victims of adults who abuse them emotionally and sexually. If the doctor suspects an adolescent has been abused, he or she will try to find out the circumstances of the abuse, notify legal authorities, and determine whether or not the child shows any physical, emotional, or mental effects. The doctor may refer the child to a psychiatrist or other mental health professional for evaluation and treatment.

Physical examination Adolescents should have a complete physical examination every year. Teenagers have many concerns about their changing bodies and, during these examinations, the doctor can reassure them that they are developing normally.

WEIGHT Being severely overweight or underweight during adolescence can have serious effects on a child's health. Obesity (being more than 20 percent over ideal weight, see page 580) can increase a child's future risk of developing heart disease, high blood pressure, and type II diabetes. Teenagers who are overweight often experience social and emotional difficulties as well.

If your adolescent's weight is higher than the 95th percentile compared with his or her height, age, and sex (see pages 239-242), he or she will receive a more thorough examination including a thyroid and cholesterol test. The doctor will provide general guidelines about diet and exercise and may refer the child to a dietitian.

Severe underweight can signal the presence of an eating disorder (see page 478), which can cause life-threatening health problems, such as an abnormal heart rhythm. The doctor may suspect an eating disorder if your child's weight percentile for his or her age and sex (see pages 239-242) begins to level off or drops.

BLOOD PRESSURE If an adolescent's blood pressure reading is at or above the 90th percentile for his or her sex and age, the doctor will want to retake the blood pressure measurement three more times within a month to confirm it. Should the blood pressure remain elevated, the doctor will evaluate the cause and decide on appropriate treatment.

SCOLIOSIS SCREENING Scoliosis (see page 618) frequently begins during the growth spurt of puberty between ages 10 and 13. The condition affects four times as many girls as boys but both male and female adolescents receive a screening test (see page 233).

SKIN-CANCER CHECK Doctors always examine an adolescent's skin for abnormal changes and teach self-examinations of the skin. Teens should learn how to check for changes in any moles or birthmarks that could indicate early skin cancer. The incidence of the deadliest form of skin cancer, malignant melanoma, is rising faster than any other cancer and is occurring earlier in adulthood.

HEARING Teenagers like to listen to loud music, often through headphones, and increasing numbers of them are experiencing hearing loss, so doctors test hearing in both ears every few years during adolescence. If a teen seems to have incurred some hearing loss, the doctor will explain to the child how to reduce the risk of further loss by wearing ear plugs at loud concerts and lowering the volume on the television, stereo, and radio.

VISION The growth spurt of puberty can sometimes change the structure of the eye, causing nearsightedness (the inability to see well at a distance). Schools often conduct adolescent vision screening and doctors generally perform vision tests every few years. The doctor will refer a child with a vision problem to an ophthalmologist (a doctor who specializes in eye care), who can evaluate it further and recommend treatment.

VACCINATIONS Between ages 10 and 14, your child should get caught up on any outstanding vaccinations (see page 227). He or she may need a second dose of the combined measles, mumps, and rubella vaccination. If your child has not previously had the hepatitis B vaccination, the doctor will recommend it now. The child should also have the tetanus and diphtheria booster, which is effective for 10 years. He or she will need to have one every 10 years throughout life. If your child has not had either chickenpox or the chickenpox vaccination, the doctor will recommend that your child get the vaccination now.

SCREENING TESTS The doctor may order certain laboratory tests, depending on a child's risk factors for specific problems. A screening hematocrit or hemoglobin test to detect anemia (see page 412) is recommended every few years during adolescence, especially for girls who are menstruating. Blood loss is a common cause of iron-deficiency anemia among adolescent girls. For information about individual tests, see pages 232 to 236.

Female reproductive system examination Most girls do not begin having routine gynecologic examinations until they are 18 years old. But if your daughter has a menstrual irregularity or abnormal vaginal discharge, or if she is sexually active, the doctor will perform a gynecologic examination (see page

172), including a Pap smear (see page 173). The first pelvic examination can be scary and embarrassing for a teenager, so doctors try to make the experience as comfortable as possible. Talk to your daughter about the exam ahead of time so she will know what to expect.

Your daughter should feel free to discuss any concerns with the doctor without you being present. You may feel left out but confidentiality is in the best interest of your child's health. A nurse or other health care professional will be present at the examination to give her encouragement and support. Tell your child to ask the doctor to explain each step so she understands what is going on. The first part of a gynecologic checkup is usually a breast examination.

BREAST EXAMINATION Yearly breast examinations enable the doctor to evaluate a girl's sexual development and provide reassurance that everything is normal. Some girls worry if their development seems to be slower or faster than that of their friends, or that their breasts are not the same size. The doctor can reassure them that these are normal variations.

The doctor looks for signs of lumps and then feels each breast for any abnormal growths. The doctor feels under each arm to try to detect enlarged lymph nodes, which can be a sign of infection or breast cancer. He or she checks each nipple for any discharge.

At the initial breast examination, the doctor will teach the girl how to examine her own breasts (see page 173) and encourage her to develop the habit of doing it once a month as she gets older and her risk of breast cancer increases.

PELVIC EXAMINATION The pelvic examination (see page 172) usually follows the breast examination. The doctor will look for any abnormalities, including changes in the skin, signs of irritation, swelling, or bumps on the outer genital area, and for any unusual vaginal discharge. The doctor will then do an internal pelvic examination by hand and with an instrument called a speculum.

PAP SMEAR A Pap smear (see page 173) is a test for cancer of the cervix (the opening into the uterus from the vagina). Pap smears can also detect some sexually transmitted diseases such as genital warts (see page 500). Annual Pap smears are recommended for all girls who are or have ever been sexually active and for women over the age of 18.

PREGNANCY TEST Many teenagers are reluctant to see a doctor to obtain a reliable contraceptive and may not see a doctor until they suspect they are pregnant. When a doctor finds out during a routine checkup that a girl is sexually active, the doctor may recommend a pregnancy test. Pregnancy can be detected by testing a sample of urine for the presence of a pregnancy-related hormone. If the test results show that the girl is pregnant, the doctor will refer her to an obstetrician/gynecologist (doctor who specializes in the care of a woman's reproductive system, pregnancy, and childbirth) for further evaluation and treatment.

Testicle examination Adolescent boys receive a testicle examination at puberty and at each subsequent visit. The doctor will also teach a boy how to perform a self-examination of the testicles (see page 175) to help detect cancer of the testicle (see page 645), the most common cancer in young men between ages 15 and 35.

Tests for sexually transmitted diseases Adolescents have a higher rate of sexually transmitted diseases (STDs) than any other age group. Many of these diseases have no noticeable symptoms, especially in women. Untreated, some of these infections can cause infertility in both men and women. Doctors recommend testing all sexually active adolescents for the most common STDs–chlamydia (see page 452), gonorrhea (see page 503), and genital warts (see page 500). They may also offer other tests, such as for syphilis and HIV (human immunodeficiency virus), the virus that causes AIDS (see page 404), depending on the adolescent's risk factors.

CHAPTER • 9

Dental care

A healthy, pain-free mouth and teeth are indispensable for your child's overall health and well-being. Strong teeth enable your child to chew easily, speak clearly, and produce that smile you so much love to see. You are responsible for your child's oral hygiene in the early years. You also need to teach the basics of brushing and flossing, take your child to the dentist regularly for checkups and cleanings, and make sure that he or she is eating right.

Your child's teeth

Primary teeth, or baby teeth, are just as important as permanent teeth. The primary teeth preserve space for the permanent teeth and guide them into position. Primary teeth also encourage normal development of the jawbones and muscles. Baby teeth that become infected or decayed or are lost too early can cause pain, poor eating habits, speech problems, or crooked or damaged permanent teeth. The rate at which children get their first teeth varies greatly, but baby teeth usually start coming in when a child is between 5 and 9 months old and continue until about age 2½, when all 20 baby teeth are present.

Your baby's first teeth
The first teeth to appear are usually the two lower center front teeth (the numbers next to teeth indicate order of appearance) and then the four upper front teeth. Between 1 and 2 years of age, the remaining two bottom front teeth, the first four molars (large, chewing teeth), and the pointed (canine) teeth on the top and bottom come in. The last four molars appear between 2 and 3 years of age.

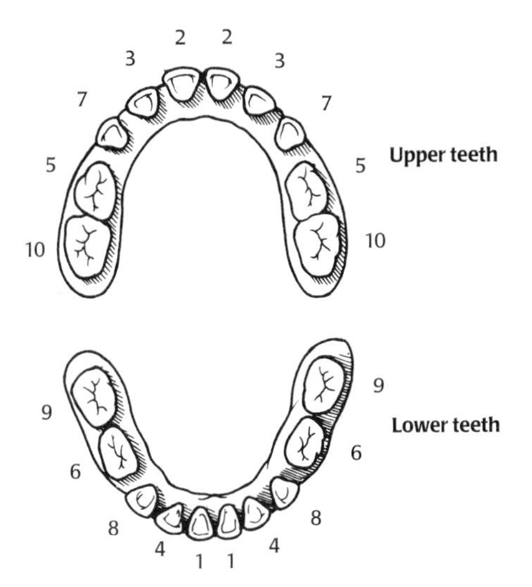

TEETHING

Just before a primary tooth starts coming in, the gum above the tooth may become swollen or sore. If you rub your finger along the gum, you may feel a bump in the gum over the new tooth or the tip of the tooth itself. A teething child may be fussier than usual and may pull on his or her ears, have a poor appetite, and drool.

To help reduce the discomfort, try giving your child a one-piece teething ring or pacifier. (Teething rings and pacifiers made of more than one piece can break apart and cause choking.) Some are made to be chilled in the refrigerator; the cold can be very soothing. Never dip a teething ring or pacifier in sugar or honey because the sugar can cause tooth decay. Some parents find it helpful to apply a cold, wet washcloth to their child's gums or to rub the gums with their finger. If your child experiences a lot of discomfort, your doctor may recommend giving the over-the-counter pain reliever acetaminophen. Use numbing medicines with caution because they can numb the back of the child's throat and inhibit swallowing.

When they are 3 to 4 months old, babies start producing more saliva than they can swallow, so they often begin to drool. They also begin to put objects in their mouth and bite or chew on them. Drooling and chewing on objects (or

When teeth come in

Incisors appear at 6 to 9 years.

Canines appear at 9 to 12 years.

Premolars appear at 10 to 12 years.

First molars appear at 6 to 7 years.

Second molars appear at 11 to 13 years.

Third molars appear at 17 to 21 years.

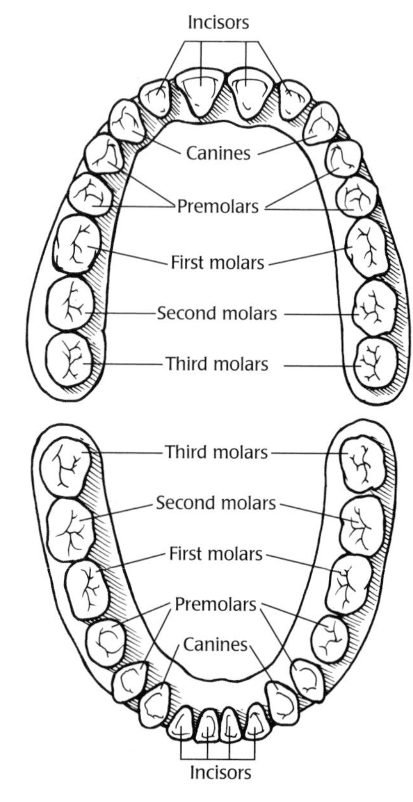

The permanent teeth
Although permanent teeth do not come in until a child is 6 or 7, their development begins in the first few months of life. The permanent teeth appear in about the same order as the primary teeth but, instead of 20 teeth, there are 32. Permanent teeth continue coming in until a person is in his or her 20s, when the four back molars, usually referred to as wisdom teeth, erupt.

rubbing them against the gum) are normal parts of infant development and may not always be a sign of teething. Teething does not cause fever, rash, diarrhea, or other illnesses. If your child has these symptoms, talk to your doctor; they are probably from something other than teething.

PREVENTING TOOTH DECAY

Tooth decay is the leading dental problem in children. Decay occurs when bacteria normally present on the teeth (in a sticky film called plaque) interact with sugars and starches from foods. The bacteria use the starches to produce acid, which softens the enamel on the teeth, causing a cavity.

Teeth cleaning By age 1, many children already have decaying teeth from exposure to sugary liquids for long periods. Care of the mouth and teeth is essential to prevent tooth decay. You need to thoroughly wipe your baby's gums after each feeding with a damp cloth or piece of gauze to loosen the bacteria that cause cavities. Later, as your child's primary teeth come in (usually between 5 and 9 months of age), brush them at least twice during the day and at bedtime with a small, soft-bristle toothbrush dipped in warm water. The bristles should be made of polished nylon and have a flat brushing surface. Don't use toothpaste until your child is able to rinse and spit it out (at about age 2 or 3). Even then, use only a small, pea-sized amount.

By the time your child is about 2 or 3 years old, you should begin teaching the child how to brush his or her own teeth at least twice a day. Until the child

Symptoms of tooth decay

Take your child to the dentist if he or she has any of these symptoms of tooth decay:

- Discoloration
- Pain
- Sensitivity to hot or cold foods or liquids

Preventing baby-bottle tooth decay

Never let your baby sleep with a bottle of formula, milk, or juice in his or her mouth because the prolonged exposure to the sugars in these foods can cause your baby's teeth to decay. Baby-bottle tooth decay is the main dental problem in children under 3 years old and can prevent them from developing healthy primary teeth.

When a child is awake, saliva in the mouth helps wash away sugars from food. But during sleep, the baby swallows less often so the sugary liquids remain on the teeth, especially the upper front ones, quickly leading to decay. It's all right to let your baby fall asleep while feeding, but take the bottle away once you put the baby in the crib. You can also try these other soothing ways of helping your baby get to sleep:

- Rub your child's head or back.
- Read or tell a story.
- Sing or play soft music.
- Hold or rock your baby.
- Put a musical toy or mobile near the bed.
- Offer a blanket, soft toy, or pacifier.
- If your child insists on sucking on a bottle, fill it with water only.

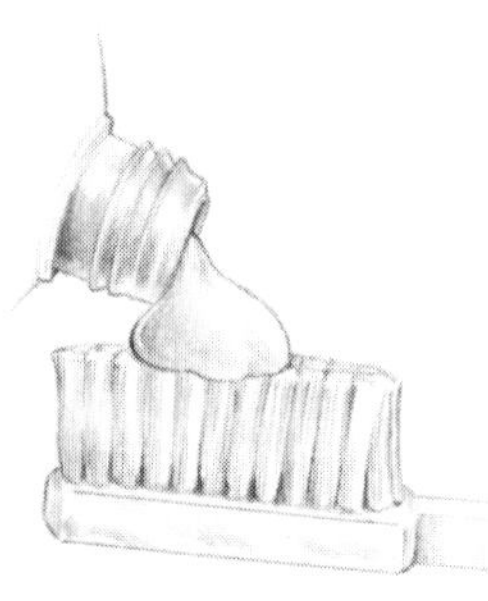

How much toothpaste?

For a young child, use only a pea-sized amount of toothpaste on the brush.

is about age 6, it's a good idea for you to do the brushing at least once a day. When your child brushes, check such hard-to-reach areas as the inner surfaces of the teeth and the back teeth and do a follow-up brushing when needed. A worn-out toothbrush will not clean your child's teeth; replace the brush about every 3 months. Here are some more toothbrushing tips:

- Use only a pea-sized amount of fluoride toothpaste on the brush.
- Change the position of the toothbrush frequently; it will only clean one or two teeth at a time.
- Brush gently with very short back-and-forth or circular strokes but with enough pressure to feel the bristles against the gum.
- Brushing after every meal is ideal, so try to instill this habit early. But your child should brush thoroughly at least twice every day. Supervise bedtime brushing until the child is competent enough to do it alone.
- If your child has any discomfort or bleeding during toothbrushing, tell your dentist.

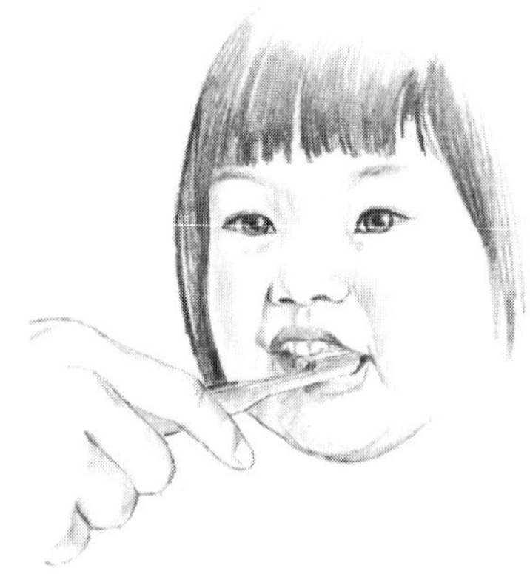

Toothbrushing

Holding the toothbrush at an angle, gently move it back and forth along the teeth.

Begin gently flossing your child's teeth when the permanent ones start coming in. By age 7 or 8, children usually have enough dexterity to do all of their own brushing and flossing. Ask your dentist or dental hygienist to show you how to properly floss your child's teeth. Here are the basic steps:

1. Break off about 18 inches of floss and wind most of it around one of your middle fingers.
2. Wind the rest around the middle finger of the opposite hand; this finger can take up the floss as you use it.
3. With an inch of floss between your thumbs and forefingers, guide the floss between the teeth.
4. Holding the floss tightly, use a gentle sawing motion to insert the floss between the teeth (see illustration). Don't snap the floss into the gums or you could cut them. When the floss reaches the gum line, curve it into a c-shape against one tooth and gently slide it into the space between the gum and the tooth until you feel resistance.
5. While holding the floss tightly against the tooth, move the floss away from the gum by scraping it up and down against the side of the tooth.
6. Repeat the above steps on the rest of the teeth.

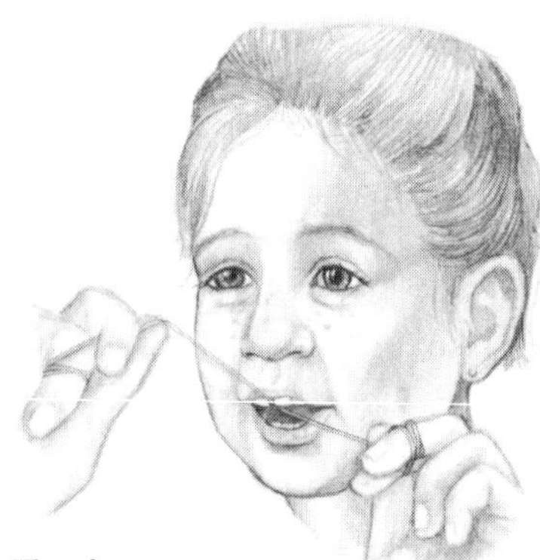

Flossing

Hold the floss firmly and gently slide it between the teeth, using a sawing motion.

A healthy diet For healthy teeth, children need to eat a nutritious, well-balanced diet (see page 111) that includes lots of whole-grain breads and cereals, vegetables, and fruits. Your child also needs to consume all the essential vitamins and minerals. Calcium is especially important for building strong teeth. Dairy products, such as milk and yogurt, are excellent sources of calcium. After your child is 3 years old, you can begin giving

Preventing tooth problems

Most cavities and tooth injuries can be prevented with a few simple measures. Here are some tips for keeping your child's teeth strong and healthy:

- Find out the level of fluoride in your water supply. If the water is not fluoridated, ask your pediatrician or dentist about fluoride supplements.
- Clean your infant's gums with a wet cloth or gauze after feedings and at bedtime, even before the baby teeth come in.
- If your child uses a pacifier, make sure it's a type recommended by your doctor (see page 41); never dip the pacifier in anything sweet before giving it to your child.
- Once your baby's teeth start coming in, brush them gently with a small, soft-bristled brush and water only at least twice daily and at bedtime. When your child is 2 years of age, use a small (pea-size) amount of fluoride toothpaste on the brush.
- Teach your child to drink from a cup as soon as he or she can sit up alone, usually between 6 months and a year.
- Wean your child from the bottle by age 1.
- Instill the habit of brushing with fluoride toothpaste twice a day and flossing once a day.
- If you give your child gum and soda pop, make sure they are sugarless.
- Encourage your child to stop thumb-sucking by age 2. By age 5, thumb-sucking can cause tooth misalignment and malformation of the roof of the mouth.
- Make sure your child wears protective equipment such as a mouth guard and helmet when playing sports.
- Discourage your child from smoking cigarettes or using chewing tobacco.
- Don't let your child chew on pens and pencils; the teeth can chip and crack. Chewing on ice can cause a tooth to fracture.
- If your child grinds his or her teeth (usually while sleeping), ask your dentist about a protective mouth guard (called a bite guard) to wear during sleep.

Here are some things you shouldn't do:

- Don't let your child sleep with a bottle of formula, milk, juice, or any other drink containing sugar. If you must give your baby a bottle for comfort, fill it with water.
- Don't use a bottle of milk or juice as a pacifier during the day.
- Don't let your toddler carry around and suck on a bottle filled with milk, juice, or other sugary liquids.
- Don't allow your child to snack on sweets excessively.
- Don't give your child starchy foods such as crackers, sticky foods such as raisins or jelly beans, or fruit or fruit juices before bedtime. These foods stay on the teeth and promote tooth decay.

him or her low-fat or fat-free dairy products, such as skim milk, so he or she gets the calcium without excessive calories from fat.

The sugar in sweet foods, such as candy or cookies, can cause tooth decay. Starchy foods, such as crackers, and sticky foods, such as raisins and other dried fruits, promote tooth decay because they don't dissolve in saliva and collect on the teeth microscopically. But starches and fruits are an essential part of a healthy diet so you shouldn't avoid them. Just give them to your child only at mealtime—not at bedtime—to help reduce the risk of cavities. Avoid letting your child have sugary soft drinks—they are the primary source of sugar in most American children's diets. One can of soda pop contains about 9 teaspoons of sugar. Soft candies—such as licorice or jelly beans—can stick to the teeth and promote tooth decay. Children need to snack to consume enough calories for growth, so stock up on snacks that don't contain a lot of sugar.

Dental checkups and procedures

Your doctor will check your infant's teeth for any signs of decay during regular checkups. You can begin taking your child to the dentist when he or she is about 3 years old for regular teeth cleanings, after the primary teeth have come in. From then on, your child should see the dentist twice a year. You may want to ask your doctor to recommend a pediatric dentist, who has 2 to 3 years of additional training in children's dental care, health, and development.

AT THE DENTIST'S OFFICE

The major dental problem in children is tooth decay, but some children have abnormalities in their bite or jaw that require correction. Many children have misaligned teeth that will require braces or other orthodontic treatments (see page 265).

After checking for dental problems, the dentist will instruct you about your child's diet, the use of bottles, and toothbrushing, and will discuss the importance of fluoride (see below). These early dental visits will help your child get accustomed to regular checkups; he or she will come to view visits to the dentist as routine–not scary or painful. Most dentists are sensitive to children's fear as well as their dental care. Try "playing dentist" with your child to make the process more familiar, but avoid using frightening words such as drill, shot, or hurt.

To help diagnose tooth decay or other abnormalities, the dentist may sometimes take X-rays of your child's teeth. The need for X-rays varies from child to child. Children who are susceptible to tooth decay may need to have X-rays at every 6-month checkup; others may need them less frequently. X-rays can detect more than cavities. They can also show erupting teeth, diagnose bone diseases, or evaluate an injury. The dentist will recommend X-rays only after he or she performs a complete examination of your child's teeth and suspects a problem that may not be easily visible.

The equipment used today for dental X-rays minimizes exposure to radiation. To be extra careful, the dentist will place a protective lead apron or shield over your child's neck and torso before taking the X-rays.

Fluoride Fluoride, a mineral that occurs naturally in many foods and in water, is the most effective agent known to reduce tooth decay. Many municipalities in the United States add fluoride to their water supply, a measure that has greatly reduced tooth decay in both children and adults over the past few decades. The use of fluoride-containing toothpastes has also contributed to a reduction in cavities.

Fluoride provides anticavity protection in a number of ways. It makes teeth harder and more resistant to the corroding effects of acid in the mouth. It can also repair areas of the teeth that have already been damaged, reversing the early decay process. Ask your dentist or doctor if your local drinking water is fluoridated. If not, your dentist may recommend fluoride supplements.

FLUORIDE SUPPLEMENTS Your doctor or dentist may recommend giving daily fluoride supplements to your child in drops, tablets, or lozenges, beginning at about 6 months of age. Your child should take these supplements until age 16 as long as the water supply in your area is not fluoridated. If you move, check with the dentist in your new area to find out if your child needs to continue taking the supplements. A child older than 6 months needs fluoride supplements if breast milk is his or her only source of nourishment. If you are breastfeeding, talk to your doctor.

Follow your dentist's instructions carefully when giving your child fluoride supplements; give only the dose prescribed. Too much fluoride can cause developing teeth to become discolored, a condition called enamel fluorosis. Fluorosis can cause brown marks on the teeth and may make them pitted, rough, and hard to clean. Mild fluorosis causes tiny, barely visible white specks or streaks on the teeth.

FLUORIDE TOOTHPASTES AND MOUTH RINSES Because of the risk of fluorosis, you should not give children fluoride-containing toothpaste or mouth rinse until they can spit it out (usually at about age 2 or 3), or they may swallow too much fluoride. When your children are old enough to use toothpaste and mouth rinse, make sure they don't swallow any. Remember to use only a small, pea-sized amount of fluoride toothpaste on your child's brush.

FLUORIDE TREATMENTS Many dentists recommend topical fluoride treatments for children beginning at about age 3, as part of a child's regular checkups. The dentist or dental hygienist applies concentrated fluoride in a gel or foam to the teeth and keeps it there for 1 minute with a disposable mouth guard. After the guard is removed, the child should not eat or drink anything for 30 minutes to allow the teeth to absorb the fluoride.

Sealants The surfaces of the molars have tiny pits and grooves that can trap food particles and bacteria, making the molars especially prone to decay. Many dentists apply a clear, plastic coating called a sealant to the biting surfaces of the permanent molars to prevent decay. It is best to apply a sealant as soon as the permanent molars come in, before they have a chance to decay. The dentist may sometimes recommend sealants on baby molars in young children whose baby teeth are susceptible to cavities.

The procedure for applying a sealant is simple and painless. The dentist "paints" the liquid sealant on the chewing surface of the tooth and then points a light wand at the sealant to harden and attach it to the tooth, forming a protective shield. As long as a sealant remains intact, it is almost 100 percent effective in preventing cavities for up to 5 years. But even if your child has sealants, he or she still needs to see the dentist regularly for checkups and cleanings. The dentist can examine the sealants for chipping and add any more sealant material, if necessary. Sealants do not protect the areas between the teeth from decay.

Tooth injuries

Baby teeth usually stay in place until the permanent teeth push them out and take their place. Permanent teeth are made to last a lifetime, but falls can injure permanent teeth. Tooth loss can often be avoided if you see a dentist promptly any time your child injures a tooth, even if you don't notice anything unusual. Many injuries in the mouth are easy to see, but some can be hidden beneath the gums.

Injuries from a blow Injury to a baby tooth from a sharp blow can damage the nerve and cause the tooth to bleed inside and become discolored. Unless a discolored baby tooth develops a serious infection, it is best to leave it in place to maintain the space for the permanent tooth. If the nerve dies in a permanent tooth, the dentist must perform a root canal treatment to save the tooth. A dead nerve left in a permanent tooth will eventually cause an abscess, a pus-filled sac that causes severe pain, swelling, and infection. If an abscess develops, a root canal may save the tooth; otherwise, the tooth will need to be extracted.

If your child receives a blow that pushes a permanent tooth up into the gum, take him or her to the dentist right away. The dentist will pull the tooth back down into position. Leave a tooth that is jammed only a short way into the gum; it will gradually return to its normal position. Immediately retrieve a permanent tooth that has been knocked completely out of the socket. Rinse the tooth in cool water (don't use soap), and put it in a clean container with some milk or saliva, which will keep the tooth alive until the dentist can reimplant it. If your child is old enough to follow instructions, he or she can hold the dislodged tooth in its socket with a clean washcloth or piece of gauze until you get to the dentist. (Call the dentist's emergency number if the accident occurs after office hours.) The dentist can then reimplant the tooth and save it. A tooth can be most successfully reimplanted within 30 minutes after it has been knocked out. If your child loses a baby tooth, it will not be reimplanted.

Chipped or extracted teeth Prompt treatment can also save a tooth that is chipped, reducing the risk of infection and the need for extensive dental treatment. Should your child chip a tooth, call your dentist right away. Rinse the child's mouth with water and apply cold compresses to the gum around the tooth to reduce swelling. If you have the chipped piece of tooth, bring it with you to the dentist. Sometimes the dentist can bond the chip back onto the tooth. If the child is in pain, you can give him or her acetaminophen or ibuprofen.

If your child has a baby tooth extracted early, your dentist may need to insert a metal or plastic device called a space maintainer to prevent the child's adjacent teeth from shifting into the empty space. Without a space maintainer, the permanent teeth could grow in crooked and crowded and eventually require orthodontic treatment (see page 265). Space maintainers may be temporary or permanent, are custom-made to fit the child's mouth, and are hardly noticeable. Most children adjust to them within a few days.

ORTHODONTIC TREATMENTS

The dentist will routinely look for abnormalities in the position of your child's teeth. If the dentist notices any spacing problems, he or she will refer you to an orthodontist, a dentist who specializes in the treatment of misaligned teeth.

Poor alignment between the upper and lower teeth is known as malocclusion. One type of malocclusion, commonly known as an overbite, occurs when the upper teeth project too far in front of the lower teeth and is often inherited. Orthodontic problems (see page 641) can also result from dental injuries, thumb-sucking, fingernail or lip biting, or overuse of a pacifier.

To diagnose the problem, the orthodontist may take X-rays of the child's head and jaws or make a quick-setting mold of the teeth and gums. This impression enables the orthodontist to study the position of the teeth and structure of the mouth and to design an orthodontic appliance to correct the problem. Some malocclusions are best treated early, at about age 7, while the permanent teeth are coming in and the bones of the jaw are still developing. Early treatment can often forestall more extensive later treatment.

Braces put sustained pressure on the teeth and guide them so they grow into the proper position. Dentists use braces to straighten crooked teeth, guide erupting teeth into position, correct bite problems, and prevent the need for tooth extractions. Some overly crowded teeth may have to be extracted before the braces are put on. Your orthodontist will explain which type of appliance is best for your child, what the treatment can do, and how long it will take.

There are two types of braces—fixed and removable. Fixed braces exert continuous pressure on the teeth

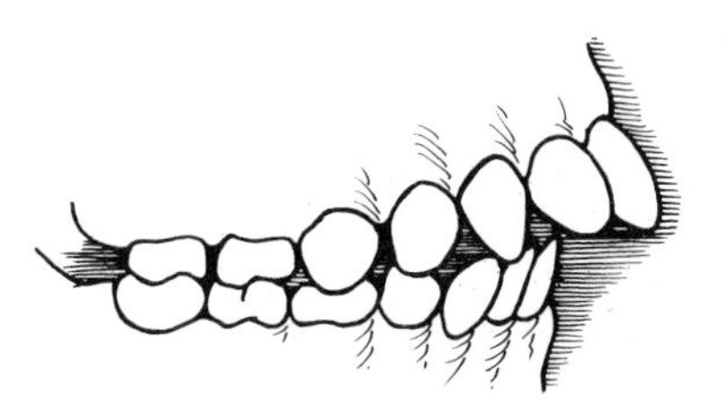

Overbite

When a child has an overbite, the most common type of tooth misalignment, either the upper jaw has grown too far forward in relation to the lower jaw, or the lower jaw has not grown forward enough.

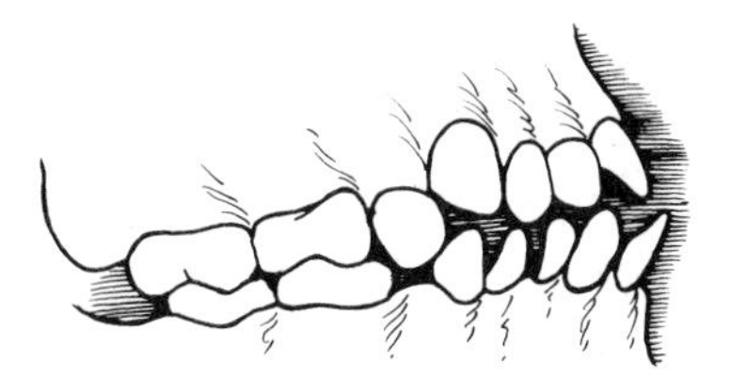

Underbite

The lower jaw of a child with an underbite has grown too far forward in relation to the upper jaw. This type of tooth misalignment is less common than an overbite.

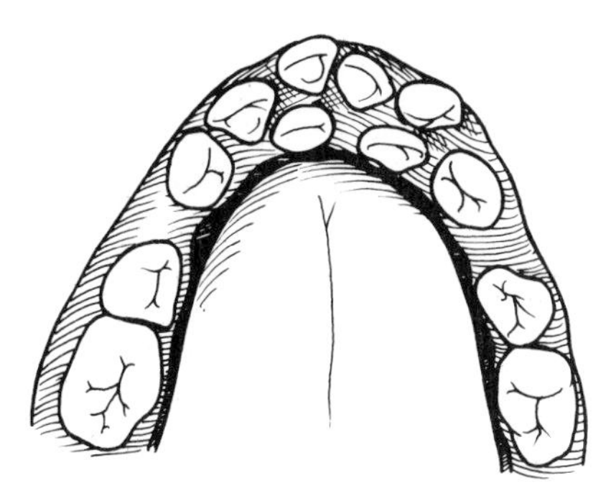

Severe crowding

The top front teeth shown here are crowded because the molars on each side have grown too far forward.

and remain in the mouth until the teeth have moved into the correct position. They are fitted to all upper or lower teeth (or both) when many teeth need to be repositioned. Realignment can take a year or longer. Some braces temporarily affect speech, but most children adapt quickly. Fixed braces control tooth movement better than removable braces, but are more expensive and take longer to fit and adjust. They also make cleaning the teeth more difficult.

Removable appliances are used to guide the growth of the upper or lower jaw or for less serious misalignments. There are many types of removable appliances. One type consists of a plastic plate that covers the roof of the mouth and attachments that anchor it over the back teeth. Force is applied to the teeth with springs, wires, screws, or rubber bands fitted to the plate, sometimes combined with headgear. Removable appliances have some disadvantages; they are bulky and can interfere with speech and the child can remove them so often that they are not effective.

Careful brushing and flossing are essential for keeping the braces and teeth in good condition. Removable appliances should be brushed each time the child brushes his or her teeth.

A child who has braces can continue to eat a normal diet—with the exception of sticky foods (such as gum or caramels) and large, hard foods (such as peanuts, whole apples, ice chips, or unpopped popcorn kernels). Dentists prescribe a daily fluoride rinse for most children undergoing orthodontic therapy.

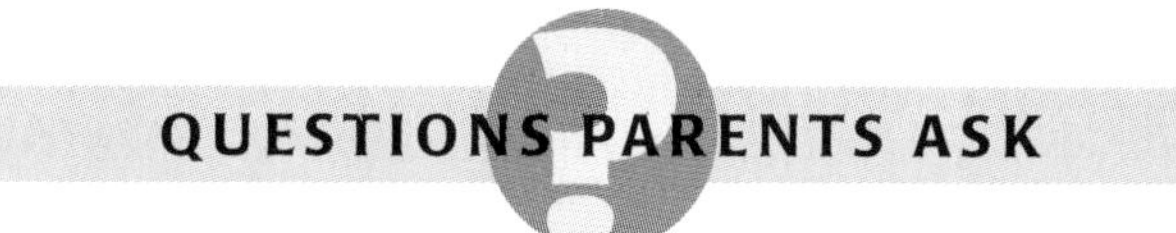

Dental care

Q Is thumb-sucking bad for my daughter's teeth?

A It is normal for children to suck their thumb, fingers, or a pacifier. Most children give up the habit on their own between ages 2 and 4. Thumb-sucking always has the potential to distort the tooth alignment in the upper jaw, but if the child stops the habit before age 5, the chances are usually minimal. If your daughter's thumb-sucking concerns you, talk to your dentist and ask for tips about helping her stop the habit, especially if she is still sucking her thumb at age 5.

Q My 4-year-old son grinds his teeth in his sleep. Does he need a mouth guard?

A Grinding of the teeth, known as bruxism, is normal between the ages of 3 and 6 years—when the baby teeth have erupted—so your son does not need a bite guard right now. Most children stop grinding their teeth on their own. If your son continues the habit when his permanent teeth come in, see your dentist, who can decide whether or not to treat the problem.

CHAPTER • 10

When your child is sick or injured

When your child is sick, he or she will look to you for comfort and, naturally, you will want to do everything you can to make him or her feel better. It's all right to pamper a sick child because your child needs your affectionate care and concern as much as he or she needs medicines or bandages.

Recognizing symptoms

A sick child's symptoms sometimes–but not always–indicate how severe the illness is. When your child is sick, ask the child exactly how he or she feels. If your child is too young to tell you, you will have to judge the seriousness of the child's condition the best you can by observing his or her behavior and by taking his or her temperature.

If you recognize the symptoms of a minor condition that your child has had before, you will probably feel confident enough to take care of the problem yourself. But if your child has unfamiliar symptoms and you are unsure of the cause, call your doctor and describe the symptoms as specifically as you can. Tell the doctor when the symptoms began and whether they come and go. Think about what your child last ate before he or she got sick and if anyone else who is in contact with your child is sick.

TAKING YOUR CHILD'S TEMPERATURE

Some parents can tell that their children have a fever just by looking at them or by feeling their forehead with the back of their hand. But the only way to obtain an accurate temperature measurement is with a thermometer. Several different types of thermometers are available and each is used a different way.

Digital thermometers are easy to use and record a temperature quickly and accurately. This type of thermometer runs on a button battery and registers a temperature reading in less than 30 seconds. The thermometer beeps when it records the reading, which is displayed on a small screen. Digital thermometers are just as accurate as glass thermometers but are slightly more expensive.

Glass thermometers are the least expensive type, but they take a temperature slowly (in about 3 to 4 minutes) and are often difficult to read. When the mercury-filled bulb end is placed in a child's rectum, armpit, or mouth, the mercury travels up the glass rod and stops at a mark that indicates the child's temperature.

Before using a glass thermometer, always check to make sure that the mercury bulb is not broken or cracked and that the mercury band has stopped below 98.6°F. If the band has not fallen below 98.6°F, hold the thermometer at the nonbulb end and shake it by snapping your wrist sharply to force the mercury back toward the bulb.

To read a glass thermometer, hold it at eye level and turn the rod until you see the degree marks and numbers. Look for the silver band of mercury and make note of the number at the end of the band, farthest away from the bulb. This number indicates the temperature degree.

Avoid putting a glass thermometer in hot water; the mercury could get stuck in the top of the thermometer. Always store a glass thermometer in its protective case, out of a child's reach.

Ear thermometers measure the amount of infrared radiation in the eardrum. They do not record accurate temperatures, especially in infants, so doctors discourage their use. Doctors also advise against the use of liquid crystal strips applied to the forehead and temperature-reading pacifiers because they fail to detect an elevated temperature in most children.

How to take a temperature You can take a temperature by placing a thermometer in your child's rectum, armpit, or mouth. Many doctors recommend that parents take their child's temperature rectally for the first 3 years because it gives the most accurate reading. Your child won't be able to keep a thermometer under his or her tongue with a closed mouth until about age 4 or 5. Wipe a digital or glass thermometer before and after use with a tissue soaked in rubbing (isopropyl) alcohol or soap and water and rinse it well with cool water.

HOW TO TAKE A RECTAL TEMPERATURE A rectal temperature can register one or more degrees higher than a temperature taken in the mouth or armpit. To take a child's temperature rectally:

1. Lubricate the bulb end of the thermometer and the opening of your child's anus with petroleum jelly to reduce discomfort.

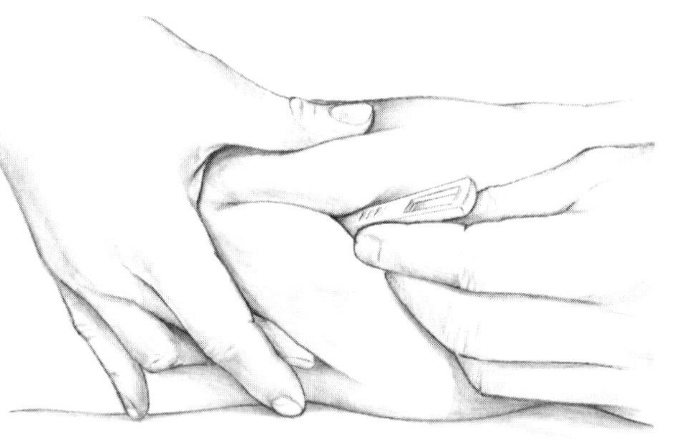

Taking a rectal temperature
To take a child's temperature rectally, insert the thermometer ½ to 1 inch into the anus and pinch the child's buttocks together.

2. Lay the baby across your lap, stomach down. Ask an older or highly active child to lie on the floor or bed.
3. Press the palm of one hand against the child's lower back just above the buttocks. With your other hand, carefully

insert the thermometer ½ to 1 inch into the anus. Pinch the buttocks together (see illustration on page 268). Never force a thermometer in because you could injure the delicate tissues inside the rectum. Be aware that inserting a thermometer into your child's rectum can sometimes stimulate your child to have a bowel movement.

4. Hold the thermometer in place for 30 seconds (or when you hear the beep) for a digital thermometer or for a full 2 to 3 minutes for a glass thermometer.
5. Gently pull the thermometer out and read the recorded temperature. Your child has a fever if the thermometer shows that the rectal temperature is higher than 101.5°F.

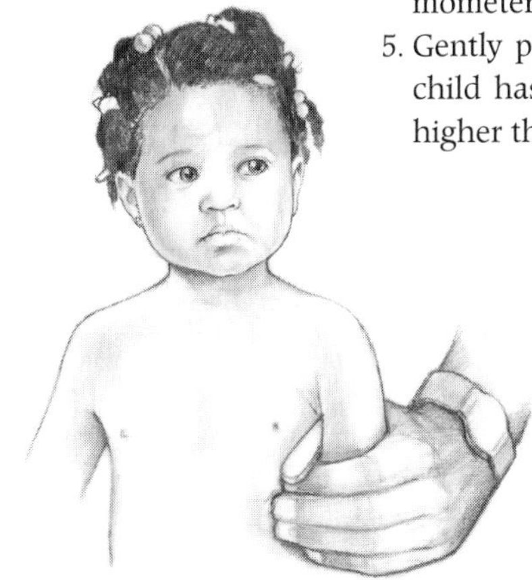

Taking an armpit temperature
To take an armpit temperature, place the thermometer in your child's armpit and hold his or her arm down for the proper amount of time, according to his or her age.

HOW TO TAKE AN ARMPIT TEMPERATURE An armpit recording is the least reliable temperature measurement, but it may be the safest way to take a temperature in a restless or active child. To take an armpit temperature:

1. Raise your child's arm and let the armpit cool and dry out for a few minutes because moisture can lower a temperature. The wearing of heavy clothes can falsely elevate the armpit temperature.
2. Sit your child on your lap or next to you.
3. Place the tip of the thermometer in your child's armpit.
4. Hold your child's elbow against his or her side for 4 minutes if your child is under age 2; 5 or 6 minutes if your child is over 2 (see illustration, left).
5. An armpit temperature higher than 100.5°F may indicate a fever. If in doubt, take the temperature rectally for a more accurate reading.

HOW TO TAKE A TEMPERATURE BY MOUTH If your child has had anything cold or hot to drink within the last 10 minutes, wait another 10 minutes before taking the temperature. To take a temperature by mouth:

1. Place the tip of the digital or glass thermometer under one side of your child's tongue toward the back of his or her mouth (see illustration, left). If you're not sure exactly where to place the thermometer, ask your child's doctor to show you.
2. Tell your child to hold the thermometer in place with his or her lips and fingers, not with the teeth. Clenching the teeth could break the thermometer.
3. Ask your child to keep his or her mouth closed and breathe through the nose.
4. Hold the thermometer in the child's mouth until you hear the beep on a digital thermometer. If you are using a glass thermometer, keep it in your child's mouth for 3 minutes.
5. Remove the thermometer and read the recorded temperature. Your child has a fever if the oral temperature is over 100.5°F.

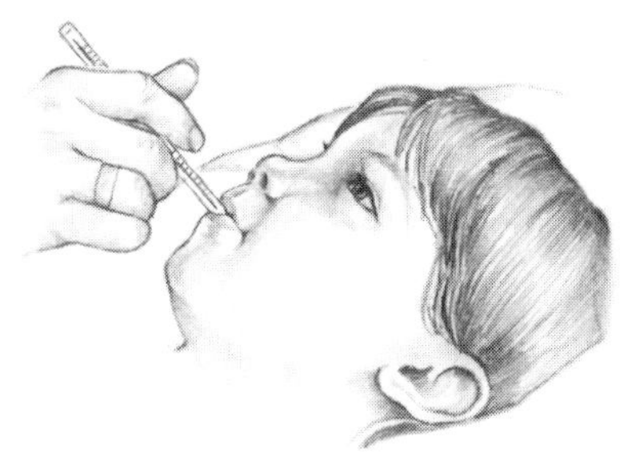

Taking a temperature by mouth
To take a child's temperature orally, place the tip of the thermometer under one side of his or her tongue, toward the back.

WHEN TO CALL THE DOCTOR

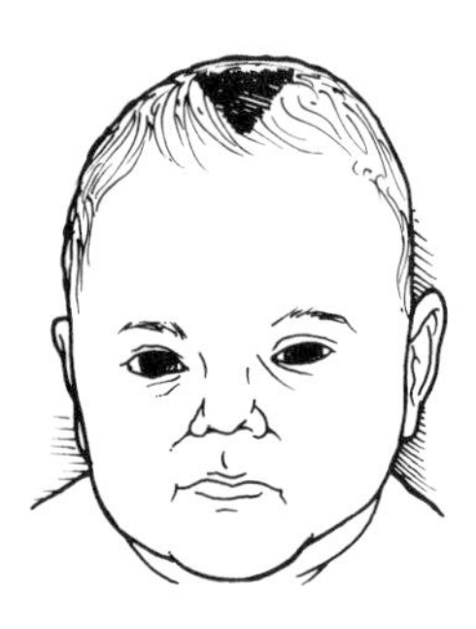

The soft spot
Babies have a soft area (fontanelle) on the top of their heads because the skull bones have not yet joined. If your child's soft spot is sunken in, it may be a sign of dehydration.

Serious symptoms–severe burns, heavy bleeding, choking, or convulsions–are easy to identify. But symptoms of some potentially dangerous conditions are harder to recognize. If you have any doubts at all about your child's health, don't hesitate to call your doctor. Always call your doctor immediately if your sick baby is less than 2 months old. At this age, seemingly mild symptoms can signal a serious disorder. The following symptoms can indicate life-threatening problems that require immediate medical attention.

- **Severe fatigue** If your child stares into space, won't smile, won't play, is too weak to cry, is floppy, or is hard to awaken, he or she could be seriously ill.
- **Severe pain** If your child cries at your touch, does not want to be held, screams constantly, or cannot sleep, he or she could be in severe pain, indicating a dangerous condition such as meningitis (see page 564).
- **Bluish lips** Bluish lips can be a sign of reduced oxygen in the bloodstream, possibly from a lung or heart problem or poisoning.
- **Drooling** Sudden onset of drooling or spitting, especially with difficulty swallowing, can indicate a serious infection of the tonsils, throat, or top of the windpipe (epiglottis).
- **Dehydration** Signs of dehydration (see page 283) include a dry mouth; cool, dry, pale skin; crying that produces no tears; thirst; listlessness; rapid pulse; sunken eyes; no urination for about 8 to 12 hours; or, in infants, sinking of the soft spot on top of the head.
- **Bulging soft spot** If the soft spot is firm and bulging when your child is quiet and in an upright position, the child's brain could be under pressure from fluid accumulation, infection, or a tumor. (The soft spot normally bulges when a child cries.)
- **Stiff neck** To check for a stiff neck, have your child lie down and lift his or her head from the back of the neck to see if the chin can touch the middle of the chest. A stiff neck can be an early sign of meningitis (see page 564).
- **Injured neck** Call your doctor any time your child injures his or her neck, even if it doesn't appear to be serious. A neck injury could cause damage to the spinal cord. Don't manipulate the child's head or neck if you suspect an injury.
- **Difficulty breathing** If your child has trouble breathing after you have cleaned out his or her nose, or if he or she has a deep cough or wheezing, the child needs immediate medical attention. Other signs of a serious breathing problem include rapid breathing (more than 60 breaths per minute), pulling in of the skin between the ribs with each breath, a change in skin color, or sucking in of the abdomen with each breath.
- **Tender abdomen** You should be able to press an inch or so in on all parts of your child's abdomen without any resistance. If your child repeatedly pushes your hand away or screams, or if the abdomen is bloated and hard, he or she could have appendicitis (see page 418) or an obstruction in the digestive tract.

• **Tender testicle or scrotum** Sudden pain in the groin can result from twisting (torsion) of a testicle (see page 644). Surgery is needed within 8 hours to save the testicle.
• **Inability to walk** If, after learning to walk, your child has trouble standing or walking, he or she could have an infection or injury in the hips or legs. A problem with balance could indicate a viral infection, an ear infection, or a brain disorder. If your child walks bent over, holding his or her abdomen in pain, he or she could have appendicitis (see page 418).
• **Purple spots on skin** Purple spots on the skin (other than bruises) can indicate abnormal clotting from infection, cancer, or blood disorders.

WHEN TO KEEP YOUR CHILD HOME

When deciding whether or not to keep a sick child home, consider the child's symptoms and how ill he or she appears to be. Even a child with a contagious infection may not always need to be isolated. By the time you realize that your child has a cold, other people have already been exposed to the germs.
• **Fever** Doctors and most day-care centers allow a child with a temperature under 101°F who otherwise seems OK to go to school or day care. But if your child has a fever and is lethargic or irritable, keep the child home.
• **Colds** Mild symptoms of a cold should not keep a child home from day care or school. But, if your child has a persistent cough or an excessively runny nose, keep him or her home.
• **Ear infections** Keep your child home if the ear is painful or draining, or if the child has not yet been taking antibiotics for 24 hours since it started draining.
• **Strep throat** Children with a strep infection (see page 635) of the throat should stay home while they are contagious–from the start of their symptoms until they have been on antibiotics for 24 hours.
• **Chickenpox** Keep a child with chickenpox home when he or she is contagious–from the time the rash appears until all the sores have crusted over, usually after about 7 to 10 days.
• **Digestive tract infection** If your child has diarrhea and a fever, keep the child home until the symptoms subside and he or she can tolerate food again. If your child is vomiting, keep him or her home for 24 hours after the vomiting stops.
• **Conjunctivitis** A child with the highly contagious eye infection conjunctivitis ("pinkeye") should stay home as long as pus is draining from the eye.

Home-care basics

As you gain experience, you will become an expert at giving your child medicine, taking his or her temperature, and treating cuts and scrapes. But it's always best to prevent colds and upset stomachs before they happen. Minimizing the spread of infection helps keep your child healthy and active.

Reducing the spread of infection

Most childhood illnesses are caused by viruses and bacteria that infect either the airways–causing coughs, colds, and sore throats–or the digestive system–causing nausea, vomiting, and diarrhea. A child's immune system continually encounters, fights, and develops resistance to organisms that cause disease, so that, by adulthood, the immune system has built up protection against a wide range of infectious diseases. But you can help reduce your child's exposure to disease-causing germs if you understand how they spread from person to person.

- Colds are usually transmitted in nasal secretions or saliva when a person who has a cold touches or kisses another person. Cold viruses can also be spread through the air from coughs and sneezes. Toddlers are especially susceptible because they put so many things into their mouths.
- Bacteria, viruses, or parasites from feces can travel from contaminated hands to food or other objects that end up in a child's mouth. This mode of transmission accounts for most cases of diarrhea and hepatitis A (see page 517).
- Food poisoning (see page 488) often occurs after eating raw or undercooked poultry, fish, meat, or eggs, or even unwashed fruit.
- Respiratory or intestinal infections can be transmitted by sharing contaminated silverware, glasses, bottles, and dishes.
- Parasites, such as lice, are spread by sharing combs, brushes, and hats.
- Skin infections such as ringworm, cold sores, chickenpox, and impetigo can be spread through skin-to-skin contact.

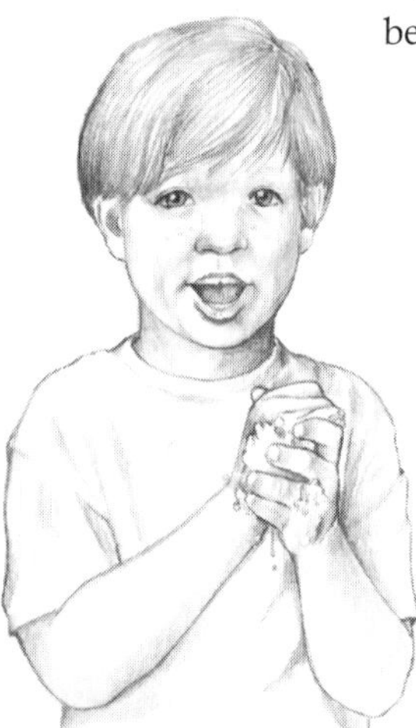

Reducing the spread of germs

Hand washing is the best way to prevent the spread of infection. Make sure your children always wash their hands after using the toilet and before they eat.

It's impossible to completely eliminate the risk of infection within your household, but you can reduce the risk by taking the following precautions:

- Encourage hand washing. Hand washing is especially important after changing diapers, using the toilet, blowing or wiping the nose during a cold, or touching aquarium water or reptiles, such as pet turtles and iguanas (which can spread salmonella bacteria). Adults and children who clean cat litter should wash their hands and face afterward or use gloves. (Pregnant women should never clean litter boxes because of the risk of developing toxoplasmosis, a disease that can harm the fetus.)
- Supervise your children when they use the toilet until they learn to wash their hands on their own, without you reminding them. Make sure the staff at your child's day-care center wash their hands after they change diapers and that they supervise young children when the children use the toilet.
- Encourage face washing. Wash your child's face at least once a day–more often if he or she has a cold.
- Discourage your children from touching their mouths and noses. Also keep them from touching their eyes after they touch their noses, to avoid spreading infection from the nose to the eyes.

Preventing urinary tract infections

Both boys and girls get urinary tract infections but the structure of the female anatomy makes girls more susceptible. The opening to a girl's urinary tract is close to the rectum, making it easily accessible to intestinal bacteria. You can help your children avoid urinary tract infections by following these basic guidelines:

- When changing a diaper, always wipe the diaper area from the vagina or penis to the rectum (front to back) to avoid wiping bacteria into the urinary opening.
- Teach your children to always wipe from front to back when using the toilet and to wash their hands afterward.
- When they are old enough, teach your children to wash their genital area daily with soap and water, always wiping from front to back.
- Encourage your children to drink plenty of fluids and to urinate when they have the urge. Urinating frequently helps keep urine (an ideal environment for the growth of bacteria) out of the bladder.

Urinary tract infection

Call your doctor if your child has any of the following symptoms of a urinary tract infection:

- Red or dark-colored urine
- Painful or difficult urination
- Strong urge to urinate even when the bladder is empty
- Pain in the lower back just below the ribs, and a fever over 101°F (signs of a kidney infection, which is serious)
- Frequent urination

- Keep toys clean and minimize sharing of cups and utensils. Wash toys in hot, soapy water. If your child is in some form of day care, make sure your child's day-care provider takes the same precautions.
- Don't expose your child to others who are sick. Keep your own children home when they aren't feeling well.
- Get your child immunized. Make sure that your children have all the recommended vaccinations (see page 227).
- Don't smoke around your children. Children who live with smokers are at increased risk of respiratory, ear, and sinus infections, as well as asthma, throughout childhood. They also have an increased cancer risk as an adult.
- Discourage your children from kissing pets. Pets (especially puppies) can transmit worms and germs that cause bloody diarrhea and other illnesses. Pets can also transmit fleas and cause skin infections. Make sure that your pet is healthy and that you get immediate treatment for your pet's health problems.
- Choose a small day-care home instead of a day-care center, if possible. Children in a private day-care home with fewer children get fewer infections than children in a larger day-care center. Those cared for in their own home by a baby-sitter have the fewest infections. Colds cause more complications in infants than in older children, so try to arrange for home-based day care during your child's first year.
- Breast-feed your baby. Breast milk provides infection-fighting substances not present in formulas or cow's milk that strengthen the immune system and reduce the risk of developing respiratory and intestinal infections.
- Call the doctor if your child is exposed to meningitis or hepatitis. If you learn that someone with whom your child has had recent contact has developed either of these serious infections, tell your child's doctor immediately.
- Handle food safely. Food contaminated with bacteria and other germs is a common cause of food poisoning (see page 488). Follow the food safety guidelines on page 489.

Essential supplies for care at home

Helping a sick child feel better is easier if you have the right supplies on hand. Following is a list of basic equipment and supplies:

- **Thermometer** Glass or digital.
- **Acetaminophen** To reduce pain and fever; available in drops, liquid, chewable tablets, and caplets; also available in infant and child suppositories.
- **Ibuprofen** To reduce fever, pain, and muscle and joint inflammation; comes as liquid or tablets.
- **Bandages** Adhesive bandages for minor cuts and scrapes; gauze pads and surgical tape for larger wounds.
- **Topical antibiotic** To treat minor scrapes and cuts; can also be used for minor burns.
- **Hydrogen peroxide (3 percent)** To help eliminate dirt and debris from wounds; dilute it in half with water, then rinse the wound with clean water.
- **Syrup of ipecac** To induce vomiting in a person who has swallowed something poisonous; never give ipecac until you first call your doctor or the local poison control center–some poisons can cause more harm when they are vomited back up.
- **Petroleum jelly** To lubricate a rectal thermometer, protect a healing circumcision or your child's diaper area, or moisturize dry skin.
- **Diaper cream** Use one containing zinc oxide, which protects against moisture and heals irritated skin.
- **Rubber bulb syringe** To clear out an infant's stuffy nose; squeeze the bulb before you place the tip in your child's nostril, then release the bulb slowly.
- **Saline nose drops** To loosen nasal secretions, making them easier to remove with a rubber bulb syringe. To make your own saline solution, dissolve ¼ teaspoon of salt in 1 cup of warm water.
- **Oral rehydration solution** Oral electrolyte maintenance solution containing water, sugar, chloride, sodium, and potassium, which are lost when a child is dehydrated (see page 283).
- **Tweezers** To remove splinters or ticks.
- **Ice packs** To reduce swelling; don't use chemical ice packs around your child's eyes; make an ice pack at home by filling a sealable plastic bag with ice cubes, squeezing out the excess air and sealing it tightly; wrap in a clean towel before using.
- **Ice pops** To reduce swelling of the lips or tongue and for relieving the pain of sores in the mouth.
- **Hydrocortisone cream** To reduce inflammation and swelling from skin irritations and allergies such as poison ivy, atopic dermatitis (see page 424), and insect bites; don't use unless your doctor recommends it; overuse can cause skin thinning and sensitivity; do not apply hydrocortisone cream to infected skin.

Acetaminophen and ibuprofen

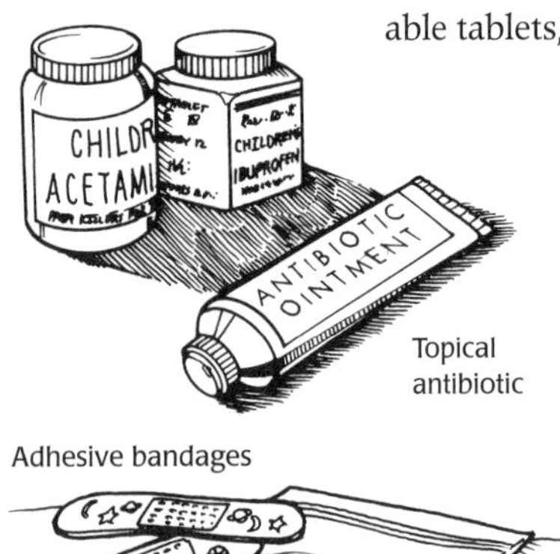

Topical antibiotic

Adhesive bandages

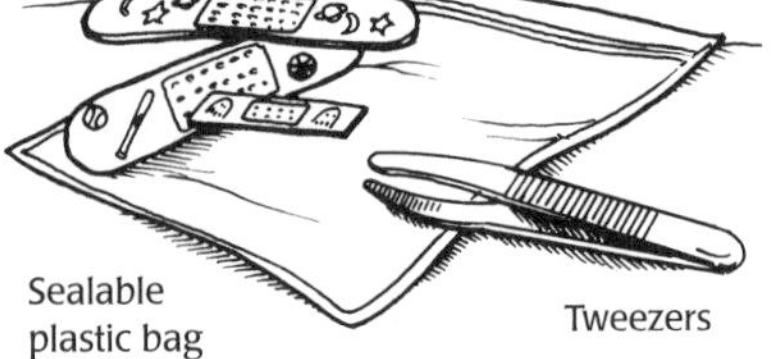

Sealable plastic bag

Tweezers

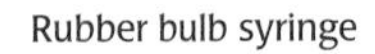
Rubber bulb syringe

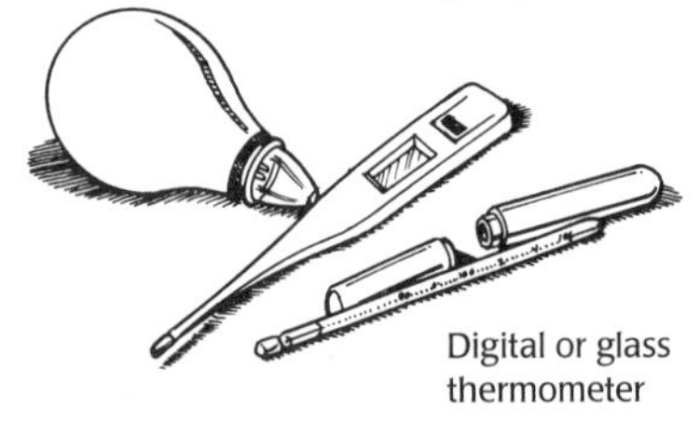

Digital or glass thermometer

Keep these supplies on hand

Every home with children should have some basic supplies on hand to take care of the common problems that all children have from time to time. Make sure that all medications have child-proof caps.

• **Diphenhydramine** An antihistamine that relieves the symptoms of allergic reactions and itching from insect bites or chickenpox; comes in liquid and tablets; don't give it to your child without asking the doctor first.
• **Calamine lotion** To relieve itching caused by chickenpox, insect bites, or contact dermatitis (see page 460).
• **Eyewash** To flush out your child's eye when something gets in it, although a gentle stream of tap water poured from a glass works just as well as a commercially prepared solution.

GIVING YOUR CHILD MEDICINE

Giving medicine to children, especially infants and toddlers, can be difficult. Children will squirm, spit, clench their teeth, and even vomit to avoid taking medicine. If you are having trouble getting your child to take medicine, talk to your doctor. He or she can suggest a helpful way to administer it or might prescribe the medication in a form that your child accepts more readily. Tell your doctor if your child vomits after taking medicine because the child may not have gotten the right dose.

Always dispense a medication in the exact dose your doctor prescribes. Giving too much medication or not enough can be harmful. If you don't understand something about a medicine that has been prescribed for your child, ask your doctor or pharmacist for an explanation. Ask your pharmacist to give you an information sheet with the medicine.

Make sure the doctor knows about any medications your child is already taking–both prescription and over the counter. Tell the doctor about any allergies you know your child has. Be sure to find out these important points about any new medication:
• The exact name of the medication and its strength.
• What the medication is supposed to do.
• The exact dose to give.
• The number of times a day it should be given and when during the day or night. For example, does "four times a day" mean every 6 hours around the clock or at breakfast, lunch, dinner, and bedtime? You don't usually need to wake up a child in the middle of the night to give medication.
• Whether or not to give the medication with food.
• Any special instructions, such as shaking a liquid medicine before giving it.
• How to tell if the medicine is working.
• The most common and serious side effects.
• Any special storage instructions, such as refrigeration.
• Whether the benefits outweigh any known risks.
• If a generic form of the drug can be used.
• If the medicine interacts with any other medicines.

Here are some general guidelines for handling medications:
• Make sure that all labels are clearly marked so you won't give medication prescribed for one child to another.

Teaching your child to swallow a pill

Many children have difficulty swallowing pills. In fact, most children can't swallow pills until they are at least 4 or 5 years old. The best way to teach your child how to swallow a tablet is by showing him or her how you do it. When giving your child a pill, tell the child to place the pill on the back of his or her tongue. Keeping the tongue flat, the child should then sip a small amount of liquid and hold it in his or her mouth. While tilting the head back slightly, the child can then swallow both the pill and the liquid.

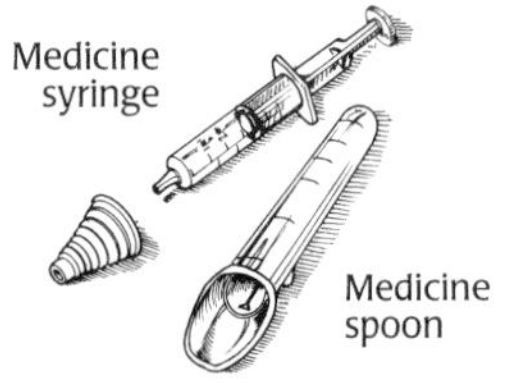

Measuring liquid medicines

You can use either a syringe-type measuring device or a medicine spoon with measurements marked along the side. The syringe may make it easier to get medicine into the mouth of a squirmy infant and usually causes less spilling.

- Don't give more medicine than is prescribed.
- Give the entire amount your doctor has prescribed or the illness could worsen or recur, even if your child starts to feel better before finishing the prescribed amount.
- Use a medicine syringe or medicine spoon available from your pharmacist. Ordinary kitchen spoons may not measure the correct amount of medicine.
- Before you first use a syringe-type measuring device to give liquid medicine to your child, throw away the cap to the syringe. A child can choke on it.
- If your child has a bad reaction or is allergic to a medicine, tell your doctor immediately. Keep a record at home of the name of the medicine that caused the reaction.
- If a prescription drug is more than 1 year old or if you're not sure of the expiration date of a medicine, rinse it down the sink or flush it down the toilet.
- Store all medications in a cool, dry, dark place–not the medicine cabinet–locked away from small children.
- Never give your child medication prescribed for another person.

Giving liquid medication Doctors usually prescribe liquid medication for young children because it is easier to take. But many liquid medications leave a bitter aftertaste that children dislike. A syringe can make giving liquid medicines easier and more precise. Your doctor or pharmacist can show you how to use one, but here are the basic steps:

1. Dip the open end into the medicine and pull the plunger up.
2. Holding the tip straight up, remove any large air bubbles by gently tapping the syringe.
3. Push the plunger in slowly to force air out, checking to make sure you still have the correct amount of medicine in the syringe.
4. Open your infant's or toddler's mouth by gently pulling down on the chin or by pinching a cheek. Insert the open end of the syringe into the mouth, placing the tip to the side of the tongue, inside the cheek (see illustration, left).
5. Slowly push the plunger in to allow a small amount of the medicine into your child's mouth. Giving too much medicine at once can cause it to run out of the mouth or the child to vomit.
6. Remove the syringe and allow the child to swallow the medicine before giving more.
7. After giving the full dose of medication, wash the syringe and tightly close and store the medicine bottle.

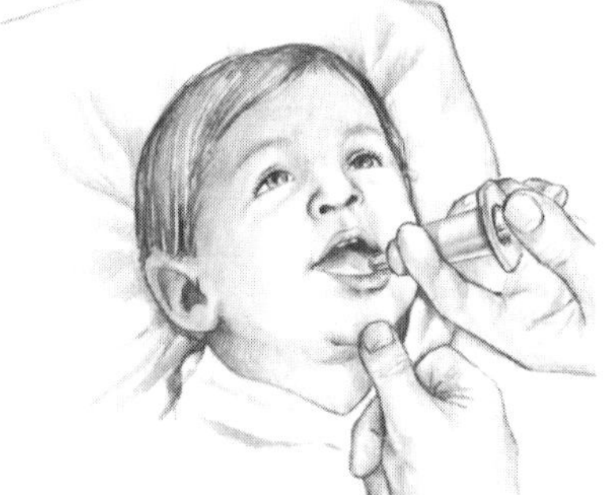

Using a syringe

Gently pull down on the infant's chin or pinch a cheek. Insert the syringe in the mouth with the tip to the side of the tongue, inside the cheek.

A school-age child may prefer taking medicine out of a small cup. Measure out the correct dose from the medicine bottle, pour it into a cup, and give the cup to your child. Watch your child to make sure he or she finishes each dose.

Giving nose drops A stuffy nose can make nursing on a bottle or breast extremely difficult. If your child has a stuffy nose, your doctor may recommend using saline (salt water) nose drops to provide some relief. Don't use medicated nose drops that contain decongestants unless your doctor recommends them and then for no longer than a day or two because they could make a stuffy nose worse. Give the drops right before you feed your baby or before a nap or bedtime. Infants can't clear their nose, so you will need to suction out your baby's nostrils with a rubber bulb syringe (see page 274) after giving the nose drops. Here's how to give nose drops to your child:

1. Warm the drops slightly by putting the container in a cup of warm (not hot) water for a few minutes. Test on your own skin before using.
2. Lay your baby face up over your lap or ask an older child to lie on the bed with the child's head back slightly.
3. Draw the correct amount of medicine into the dropper.
4. Hold your child's head with one hand and use the other to place the drops into one nostril. Don't touch the tip of the dropper to the skin.
5. Hold the child still for a moment and repeat the steps with the other nostril. Keep an older child from sitting up too quickly because the bitter-tasting medicine may run into his or her throat.

Giving eardrops Doctors prescribe eardrops for swimmer's ear (see page 638) and severe ear infections in which the eardrum has perforated and is draining pus. Here's how to give eardrops:

1. Warm the bottle of eardrops in a cup of warm (not hot) water for a few minutes. Test on your own skin before using to ensure that the temperature is comfortable.
2. Ask your child to lie down or hold your infant on your lap with his or her head turned to one side and the affected ear facing up.
3. Draw up the correct amount of medicine into the dropper and apply the drops into the outer part of the ear canal. Let the medication flow down into the ear. Don't touch the tip of the dropper to the skin or bacteria could be transmitted into the dropper.
4. Keep your child still for a few minutes to allow the medicine to enter the inner part of the ear.
5. Place a cottonball in the ear canal to keep the medicine from draining out.

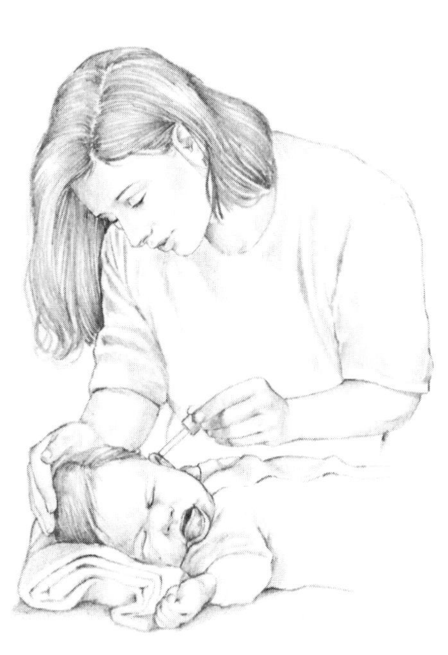

Giving your child eardrops
When placing eardrops in your child's ear, don't touch the dropper to the skin or you could transmit bacteria into the dropper.

Giving eye drops Many children develop the eye infection called conjunctivitis or "pinkeye." Caused by either viruses or bacteria, conjunctivitis is very contagious. Your doctor may prescribe antibiotic eyedrops to treat the infection. Eye medications expire quickly and can easily become contaminated, so use the medicine to treat one eye infection only and then discard the medication. Using an eye medication on more than one person can spread an infection.

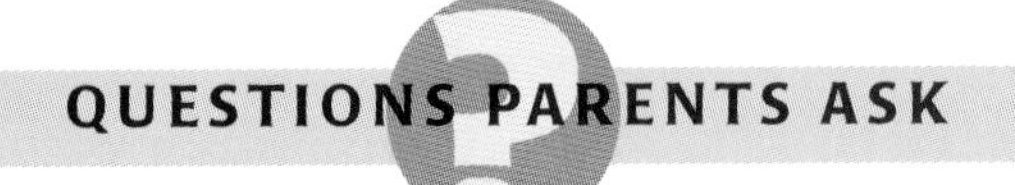

Antibiotics

Q Why do some antibiotics work in 3 days while others take 10? And why do some work in only one dose while others require many more?

A The number of doses and the length of time your child needs to take an antibiotic depend on his or her illness, the antibiotic prescribed, and the way it needs to be taken—by mouth, by injection, or intravenously (through a tube inserted into a vein). In general, your child's doctor will prescribe the antibiotic that works best against the specific type of bacteria causing your child's infection. Children and adults usually need at least 7 to 10 days of antibiotic treatment for common bacterial infections such as strep throat, ear infections, pneumonia, or skin infections. Some diseases require even longer treatment. The type of antibiotic the doctor prescribes determines the number of times a day your child needs to take it. For example, the penicillin family of drugs usually needs to be taken three to four times per day. The dosage also depends on your child's weight and how his or her body absorbs and uses the drug.

Q Why did my son's doctor tell me to make sure my son takes the whole prescribed amount of antibiotic for his strep throat? He's already feeling better. Can't he stop taking the drug?

A Your son needs to take the entire prescribed amount of antibiotic because the drug has to stay in his bloodstream long enough to kill the bacteria causing his strep throat. If he stops taking the drug too soon or doesn't take enough of it, the infection in his throat could come back. Remember that, improperly treated, strep throat can lead to rheumatic fever, which can permanently damage the heart.

Q Do antibiotics have any side effects?

A Antibiotics can cause diarrhea because they alter the balance of the bacteria that naturally reside in your intestines. Some antibiotics can also irritate the stomach and cause vomiting. The antibiotic tetracycline can stain the teeth. Antibiotics can also interact with other drugs to produce unwanted side effects. For example, the antibiotic erythromycin can increase the effect of the asthma drug theophylline, causing vomiting, rapid heartbeat, and seizures.

Q I've heard that antibiotics are overprescribed and that they are causing antibiotic-resistant strains of bacteria to appear. Does that mean that my daughter shouldn't take an antibiotic when she has an ear infection?

A It is true that strains of bacteria have appeared that are resistant to antibiotics. But that does not mean that you should avoid giving your daughter antibiotics when her doctor has prescribed them for an ear infection. Ear infections need treatment because they can have serious complications. Pressure behind the eardrum could cause the eardrum to burst. The infection could extend into the bone behind the ear or into the membranes surrounding the brain. Your doctor will only prescribe an antibiotic when it is needed. When your daughter has an ear infection, your doctor will probably prescribe an antibiotic that kills the specific type of bacteria causing the infection, not a "broad-spectrum" antibiotic used to fight many different types of bacteria unrelated to her infection. Whenever your doctor prescribes an antibiotic, don't be afraid to ask questions. Find out exactly what the antibiotic is for and why your daughter needs to take the prescribed amount. But don't ask your doctor for an antibiotic every time your daughter has a cough or cold. Antibiotics do not cure colds, vomiting, or diarrhea because these problems are mainly caused by viruses, which can't be killed by antibiotics.

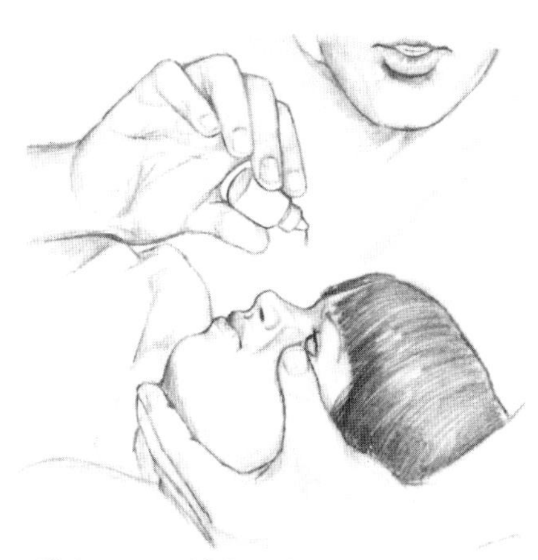

Giving your child eyedrops
Apply the drops when your child blinks so the medication will land in the eye when it opens between blinks.

Here's how to apply eyedrops:

1. Place the child on his or her back. If your child is an infant or will not cooperate, ask a helper to hold the child down while you apply the drops.
2. Draw the proper amount of medicine into the eyedropper.
3. Gently hold your child's top and bottom eyelids apart with the thumb and forefinger of one hand. Your child will automatically blink when you do this. Apply the drops into the inner corner of the eye just as your child blinks so that the medication will land in the eye when the eye opens between blinks. Don't touch the tip of the dropper to the eye.
4. Keep your child still for a few seconds to allow the drops to spread across the eye.

Doctors often prescribe eye ointments for infants. To apply an eye ointment, place it carefully in the corner of the child's eye or along the lower eyelid. When the child blinks, the medicine spreads across the eye.

Taking care of minor illnesses and injuries

Like all children, your child will get a number of colds, cuts, and scrapes. Over time, you will become skilled at treating these common problems–in many cases, without having to consult your doctor. But keep in mind that, no matter how experienced you are, your child is bound to have an occasional severe illness that requires a doctor's attention. Whenever you are in doubt, call your doctor.

FEVER

A fever is an abnormally high body temperature, usually over 101.5°F. Fever is one of the ways the body fights infection. It stimulates the immune system to send out germ-fighting cells to prevent an infection from spreading. Most fevers are caused by viruses, range from 101°F to 104°F, and last 2 to 3 days. Some noninfectious childhood diseases and certain medications or poisons can also cause a fever.

The degree of a fever does not necessarily indicate the seriousness of an illness. Normal temperatures can range from 97°F to 100.5°F (98.6°F is the midpoint of this range). On any given day, your child's body temperature can vary by a degree or two, with the lowest reading between 3 AM and 6 AM and the highest reading between 5 PM and 7 PM. Physical activity can cause body temperature to rise, as can the weather, wearing excess clothing, drinking warm liquids, or taking a hot bath. If your child's temperature is between 100°F and 101°F, take it again an hour later to see if it is still high.

Infants and young children develop fevers more often than older children. Infants and young children also develop fevers more quickly than older children because their body's natural cooling system–perspiration–does not yet

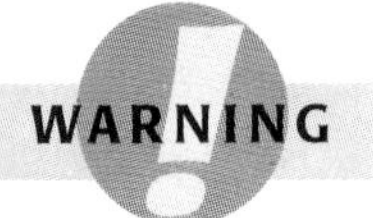

If your child has a seizure from a fever

Children who are between 6 months and 5 years of age can have seizures when they have a high fever or a fever that comes on quickly. Called febrile seizures (see page 486), these seizures can vary in severity. During the seizure, the child may roll his or her eyes or twitch and jerk the whole body. The child may also vomit. Seizures usually last only a few minutes and the child quickly returns to normal. While the episode may be very frightening, in most cases, the seizure causes no problems. The best way to handle a febrile seizure is to place the child on the floor or bed on his or her back and turn the child's head to the side to allow saliva or vomit to drain out of the mouth. Don't put anything into your child's mouth.

If this is your child's first seizure, call your doctor immediately. If the seizure lasts for more than 2 or 3 minutes or is especially severe (if your child seems to have difficulty breathing, is choking, or has bluish skin) or if your child has several seizures in a row, call 911 or your local emergency number for immediate medical help.

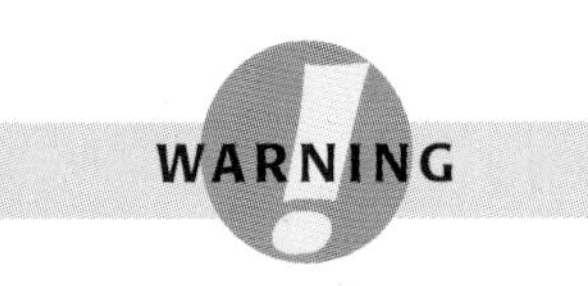

Don't give a child aspirin

Never give aspirin or other medications that contain salicylates to a child under 18 years old because these drugs have been linked to a life-threatening condition called Reye's syndrome, which affects the brain and liver. Salicylates are present in many over-the-counter medications, so check all labels carefully.

work as well. For this reason, you should avoid over-dressing your infant or toddler or putting on heavy blankets, especially if the child has a fever. The extra warmth can make a fever worse.

When to call the doctor As you get to know your child, you will become a good judge of whether or not a fever requires a call to the doctor. You should definitely call the doctor about a feverish child if he or she:

- Has a temperature of 104°F or higher.
- Is less than 3 months old and has a temperature of 100.2°F or higher.
- Is irritable or crying continuously and inconsolably.
- Will not wake up or is unusually drowsy.
- Has a stiff neck, a possible sign of meningitis (see page 564).
- Has purple spots on the skin, a possible sign of infection in the blood.
- Has trouble breathing after you have cleared the child's nose.
- Is drooling and can't swallow anything, a possible sign of an infection of the trachea (windpipe) or the opening into the windpipe (epiglottis).
- Looks and acts very sick, even 1 hour after you have given fever-reducing medication.
- Has burning or pain during urination.
- Has had a fever longer than 72 hours, or longer than 24 hours if the cause is unknown.
- Has a seizure or has previously had seizures with a fever (see page 486).
- Has persistent vomiting or diarrhea.
- Urinates less frequently than usual.
- Shows signs of pain, such as pulling at his or her ears, a possible sign of an ear infection.
- Cries when you move or touch him or her.
- Refuses to drink liquids for several hours.
- Had a fever that subsided for more than 24 hours and then returned.

Treating a fever If your child has a slight fever but seems comfortable and is eating well, you don't need to treat the fever. When deciding what to do about a fever, consider any other symptoms and how sick your child seems. If your child's temperature is over

100°F and he or she is uncomfortable, give the proper dose of acetaminophen or ibuprofen. Never give a child under 18 years old aspirin because of its link to Reye's syndrome (see page 609) and don't give ibuprofen to a child less than 6 months old. Monitor your child's temperature closely to see if it goes up.

Fever can cause fluid loss from sweating, so offer your child liquids frequently to prevent dehydration (see page 283). Keep your child's room comfortably cool and dress him or her lightly because most heat is lost through the skin. Bundling infants can be dangerous because they can't remove clothes or bedding when they become overheated. Sponging a feverish child with room-temperature water is usually not necessary unless the child is very uncomfortable or listless, the child has a temperature higher than 104°F, the fever was caused by heat stroke (see page 679), or acetaminophen or ibuprofen has not helped. Never use alcohol for sponging because it can be absorbed into the skin and cause seizures.

COLDS

Colds are caused by viruses that spread through the air in sneezes or coughs. A virus can also be transmitted by direct contact with someone who has a cold, or by sharing toys or utensils. Common symptoms include a runny nose, sneezing, mild fever (101°F to 102°F), decreased appetite, red eyes, sore throat, cough, irritability, or slightly swollen glands.

Children may have 5 to 10 colds each year. Children who are in day care and those with older siblings who bring germs home from school are most susceptible. A child gets fewer and fewer colds as he or she gets older because the immune system builds up protection against different cold viruses.

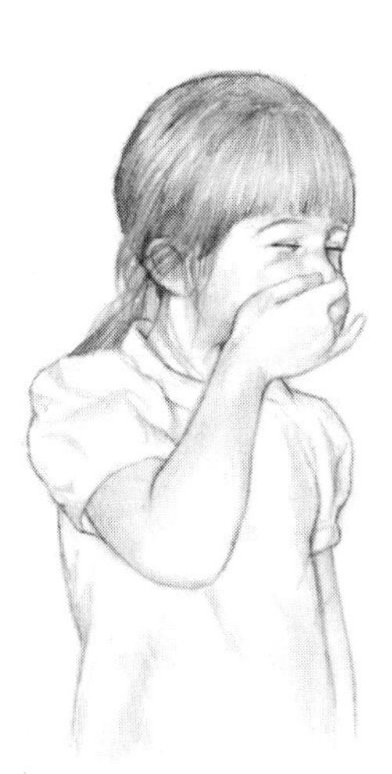

Preventing colds from spreading

To help prevent colds from spreading, teach your children to cover their mouths with their hands whenever they sneeze or cough. Better still, tell them to cover their mouths with a tissue when they sneeze or cough, throw the tissue away, and then wash their hands.

When to call the doctor Most colds go away on their own within 7 to 10 days. Colds in infants can develop into more serious respiratory conditions such as bronchiolitis (see page 440) or pneumonia (see page 595), so try to keep your infant away from people who have colds.

Call your doctor if your child has:

- Noisy breathing or difficulty breathing in and out
- Blue lips, skin, or nails
- A cough that produces green or gray mucus
- Pus on the tonsils, a possible sign of a strep infection (see page 635) of the throat
- Green mucus from the nose
- A cough that lasts longer than a week
- Pain in the ear
- Temperature over 101.5°F or one that lasts longer than 48 hours
- Excessive sleepiness or crankiness
- Shaking chills
- Chest pain or shortness of breath
- Discharge or crusting of the eyes
- Waking at night from a cough, congestion, or discomfort

- Raw or cracked skin under the nostrils
- Difficulty swallowing
- A poor appetite or irritability (in infants)

Treating the common cold Colds are caused by viruses and there are no medications that can prevent or cure them. Your doctor probably will not prescribe an antibiotic for a cold because antibiotics work only against bacterial infections, so don't insist on a prescription. The best thing you can do is to make your child comfortable by relieving the symptoms and encouraging him or her to rest and drink plenty of fluids (juice, water, or carbonated beverages).

If your child has a sore throat or a headache, give acetaminophen or ibuprofen to help reduce the pain. Do not give aspirin. You should not give your child an over-the-counter or prescription cold remedy unless your doctor recommends one. Cold medications can worsen symptoms in children. Don't give cough medicine to a child under 3 years old unless your doctor prescribes it. Coughing is beneficial because it clears mucus from the lower part of the respiratory tract.

If your infant is less than 6 months old and a stuffy nose is making it difficult for him or her to feed, clear the baby's nose with a rubber bulb syringe (see page 274) before each feeding. You can treat older children with saline (salted water) nose drops (see page 276) to help thin out nasal secretions and make it easier to suction them out. Teach and encourage your older children to blow their nose frequently during a cold and to wash their hands with soap and water afterward.

Moist air helps loosen nasal mucus so a cool-mist humidifier in your child's room can help relieve nasal congestion. But make sure you follow the manufacturer's instructions for keeping the humidifier clean. Hot-water vaporizers work just as well as cool-air humidifiers to relieve nasal congestion and work even better to relieve the symptoms of croup (see page 463). But hot-water vaporizers can cause scalding. If you use a hot-air vaporizer, keep it out of the reach of children.

Diarrhea

A child's bowel movements vary and an occasional loose stool is no cause for alarm. But if your child's bowel movements suddenly change to loose and watery and they occur more frequently than usual, your child has diarrhea. Diarrhea usually lasts from 3 to 7 days and then goes away with no complications. But severe or prolonged diarrhea can cause the body to lose an excessive amount of fluid, resulting in dehydration (see page 283), which can have serious health consequences. To prevent dehydration, give your child electrolyte rehydration fluids. Avoid giving your child milk and juices because they can make the diarrhea worse. If you are breast-feeding and your child develops diarrhea, you can usually continue breast-feeding, but talk to your doctor. Certain substances (caffeine, herbal teas, antibiotics, and some laxatives) that a woman consumes can pass through her breast milk to a nursing child and cause diarrhea.

Signs of dehydration

A dehydrated child has a dry mouth; cool, dry, pale skin; crying that produces little or no tears; excessive thirst; listlessness; rapid pulse; sunken eyes; less frequent urination (less often than every 8 hours); or, in infants, sinking in of the soft spot on top of the head.

When to call the doctor A severely dehydrated child may need to be hospitalized and given fluids intravenously (through a vein), the fastest way to replace lost fluids. Call your doctor immediately when your child has diarrhea under any of the following circumstances:

- Your child is less than 6 months old.
- Your child has signs of dehydration.
- Your child has abdominal pain for longer than 2 hours.
- Your child has a watery bowel movement every 1 to 2 hours or more, or the diarrhea has blood in it.
- The diarrhea gets worse instead of better.
- Your child has a fever that lasts longer than 48 hours.
- Your child has been vomiting for longer than 12 hours.
- Your child refuses to eat or drink.
- Your child has a rash or jaundice (yellowing of the skin and the whites of the eyes).

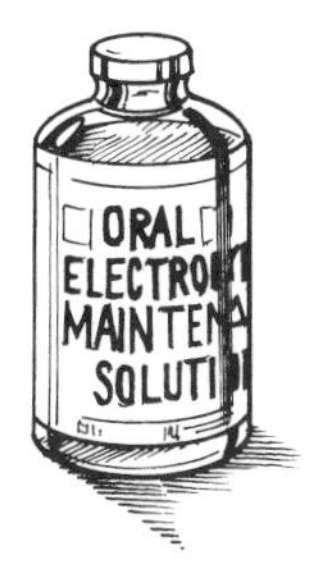

Rehydration solution
A child with diarrhea or who is vomiting can lose so much fluid that he or she becomes dehydrated. Your doctor will recommend a specially formulated drink made of water, sugar, and electrolytes (body salts) that you can buy at the grocery store or drugstore and keep on hand to prevent or treat dehydration.

Treating diarrhea Most children with diarrhea get better without antidiarrheal medication. Some over-the-counter antidiarrheal drugs can actually be harmful, so don't give your child any medicine for diarrhea unless your doctor recommends it. The most important treatment is fluids. Give your child at least twice as much fluid as he or she usually drinks. Your doctor may recommend a commercial rehydration solution, called an oral electrolyte maintenance solution. The doctor will tell you how frequently to give it to your child.

Let your child drink as much of the solution as he or she wants, but make sure that the child is getting enough. Increase the amount slowly to avoid vomiting. Give a 1-year-old child at least 4 ounces of the solution each hour (or 1 ounce every 15 minutes), an older child a little more, and a younger child a little less. Keep giving the solution for about 24 hours. If your child won't take the solution, give him or her a sports drink, flavored gelatin water (made from one packet of dry gelatin mixed with 1 quart of water), or a weak broth.

Do not give your child drinks that are high in sugar or artificially sweetened (soft drinks, undiluted fruit juices, or fruit punch) because they can make diarrhea worse. Don't give your child fried or high-fat foods or dairy products. You can continue breast-feeding.

After your child has been taking the rehydration solution for 24 to 48 hours and the diarrhea has begun to subside, gradually add "binding" foods, such as applesauce, apples, bananas, flavored gelatin, noodles, crackers, oatmeal, rice, rice cereal, and potatoes. If your child has not taken anything but the electrolyte solution for more than 2 days, talk to your doctor.

VOMITING

Vomiting is different from the spitting up that infants frequently do after a feeding. Spitting up is not serious and usually stops by the end of the first year.

Vomiting has various causes, depending on a child's age. After a child is a few months old, most vomiting is caused by viruses that infect the stomach or intestines. Vomiting can also be caused by infections in the ear, respiratory system, central nervous system, or urinary tract. Food poisoning and intestinal parasites can also bring about vomiting, along with fever and diarrhea.

When to call the doctor Certain serious conditions, such as meningitis (see page 564) or appendicitis (see page 418), can cause vomiting. If your child is vomiting, call your doctor right away if the child also:

- Is younger than 1 month and vomits more than once.
- Has diarrhea and vomits clear fluids three or more times.
- Becomes difficult to awaken or is confused after vomiting.
- Is producing bloody, green, or dark brown vomit.
- Has severe abdominal pain for more than 2 hours or has a swollen abdomen.
- Is lethargic and very irritable.
- Has convulsions.
- Has symptoms of dehydration (see page 283).
- Has not urinated in 8 hours or more.
- May have ingested a poisonous plant, spoiled food, medicine, or chemicals.
- Has a fever over 101.5°F.

Preventing constipation

Doctors define constipation as hard, infrequent stools. A constipated child may move his or her bowels once every 2 to 3 days or once every 5 to 7 days, depending on the child's age. Constipation is unusual in infants, but some children develop bowel problems during the toilet-training period–usually between the ages of 2 and 4. A child may be reluctant to move his or her bowels on the potty chair or toilet and may hold the stool in for so long that it hardens, making the next bowel movement painful. Do not use enemas, laxatives, stool softeners, or any other medication for constipation without talking to your doctor first. Feed your child a high-fiber diet and put some sugar in your child's water to treat the constipation. Taking a baby's temperature rectally will sometimes stimulate a bowel movement.

When it comes to constipation, prevention is the best medicine. Become familiar with your child's bowel habits so you can recognize any changes before they become a problem. Here are some simple measures for preventing constipation:

- Encourage your child to drink plenty of fluids, especially water.
- Provide fiber-rich foods such as fruits, vegetables, whole-grain cereals and breads, and dried peas and beans (legumes).
- Teach your child to use the toilet as quickly as possible whenever he or she has the urge to have a bowel movement.
- Encourage daily exercise–taking walks, going to the park or playground, riding a bike, getting involved in a sport.

- Cannot keep down fluids or has been vomiting longer than 12 hours.
- Has breathing problems after vomiting.
- Has recently had a head or abdominal injury.

Treating vomiting Vomiting usually stops in 12 to 24 hours with no treatment. Temporarily changing your child's diet often speeds up the process. Make sure your child gets enough fluids to replace those that have been lost. Never use over-the-counter or prescription medications for vomiting unless your doctor has recommended one. If the child has a fever of 101.5°F or higher, call your doctor. You may be told to give your child an acetaminophen suppository to bring down his or her temperature.

Doctors recommend these guidelines for a child who is vomiting:

- Keep an infant or young child lying on his or her side to prevent vomit from being inhaled.
- Don't give the child solid foods for the first 24 hours.
- Give your child an oral rehydration solution (see page 283) or clear fluids such as sugar water (mix ½ teaspoon of sugar in 4 ounces of water), a sports drink, or gelatin water (mix 1 teaspoon of flavored gelatin in 4 ounces of water) to drink or ice cubes or ice pops to suck on.
- Give an older child half-strength soft drinks, but stir them until all the fizz is gone; carbonation can inflate the stomach and cause more vomiting.
- Give the child one small sip of liquid at a time to see if it stays down and then gradually increase the amount.
- After your child has stopped vomiting for 12 to 24 hours, begin giving bland foods, such as saltines, bread, chicken soup with rice or noodles, rice, or mashed potatoes.
- If a child of any age cannot retain clear liquids or if his or her symptoms worsen after 12 to 24 hours, call your doctor. The child may have a more serious problem.

CUTS AND SCRAPES

Children can't get through childhood without a few cuts and scrapes. Most are superficial injuries that need only cleaning with soap and water and loving reassurance.

You can help your child avoid cuts and scrapes by keeping dangerous objects, such as sharp knives and breakable glass objects, out of reach. Periodically check your house, garage, and yard for hazards. Encourage your child to wear appropriate clothing and protective gear during sports and other outdoor activities.

When to call the doctor Most cuts and scrapes can be treated at home. But sometimes a minor scrape can become infected. Call your doctor if the injury is difficult to clean, gets increasingly tender or red, or begins draining pus, or if reddish streaks leading away from the cut appear in the skin. The doctor may need to clean out the wound and may prescribe an antibiotic to be taken by mouth or as an ointment or cream applied to the skin.

Long or deep cuts should be seen by your doctor. An injury that breaks through the skin and into the tissue beneath can cause damage to nerves and tendons. If your child has a long or deep cut, stop the bleeding by firmly holding a clean piece of gauze or cloth over the cut for 5 minutes. If the bleeding starts again after the 5 minutes, reapply pressure. Call your doctor immediately if the bleeding is severe.

If you are not sure whether an injury requires stitches, call your doctor. If a plastic surgeon is available, you can request that he or she stitch your child's cut. Cuts through the lip should always be stitched by a plastic surgeon. Wounds need to be stitched within 8 hours of injury. Sometimes, instead of stitches, doctors use a bandage that pulls the ends of the cut together so it can heal without scarring. Many deep cuts prompt the doctor to give a precautionary tetanus vaccination. Always bring your child's vaccination record along when your child needs to go to the hospital emergency department.

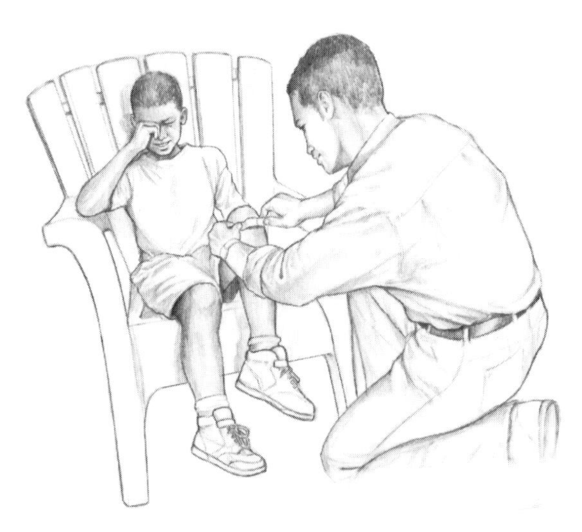

Cover an injury
When your child gets a cut or scrape, wash the wound with soap and water and then cover the injury with an adhesive bandage or gauze pad.

Treating cuts and scrapes at home

Tending to cuts and scrapes will be one of your most frequent first-aid duties. Here are some basic guidelines:

- Rinse the area with water to flush away dirt.
- Wash the wound with soap and warm water to prevent infection.
- If the scrape is large and oozing, apply an antibiotic cream (such as bacitracin) and cover the injury with a bandage or a gauze pad fastened with adhesive tape. Don't apply a dressing too tightly, especially on the fingers or toes, or it could interfere with circulation. Iodine, alcohol, and other antiseptic solutions can cause further damage and they sting and burn. You can take the bandage off after the wound begins to heal, unless the cut has been stitched. Always cover a cut when your child is playing outside.
- Check the injury daily and change the dressing when it gets dirty or wet. If a bandage sticks to the skin, soak it off with warm water.

Burns

Doctors categorize burns–from hot water, fire, electrical contact, chemicals, and the sun–according to their severity: first degree, second degree, and third degree. First-degree burns are the least serious, causing redness and sometimes swelling. Second-degree burns also produce blistering. Third-degree burns may look white or charred and can cause serious injury to deep layers of the skin or muscle. Third-degree burns and extensive burns require emergency medical treatment.

When to call the doctor You can usually treat superficial burns at home. But if a burn goes through all layers of the skin or blisters, or if redness and pain continue for more than a few hours, take your child to the doctor. Always see the doctor if your child has:

- An electrical burn
- A burn on the hands, feet, face, or genitals, or over a joint
- A burn larger than the palm of the child's hand
- A charred, deep white burn (signs of a third-degree burn)
- A burn near the eyes
- A burn with more than 10 blisters or an open blister
- Multiple burns or burns covering large areas of the body

Treating burns at home You need to act quickly when your child is burned to minimize pain, discomfort, and possible complications. Follow these general guidelines for treating burns:

- If the burn is on an arm or leg, place the affected area under cold water immediately and hold it there for several minutes. Apply cold, wet cloths to burns on other areas of the body for several minutes. Don't apply ice to a burn; it can cause more damage.
- Remove clothing from around the burned area.
- If the burn is not oozing, cover it with a sterile gauze pad.
- Never use butter, grease, petroleum jelly, or other oily substances on a burn because they can trap heat in the skin and worsen the burn. Do not use first-aid creams or sprays that contain benzocaine because they can cause an allergic rash.
- If the burn is oozing, leave it open or cover it lightly with sterile gauze and take your child to the doctor's office immediately.
- Watch for redness, swelling, a bad odor, or discharge, which can signal infection. Infection needs to be treated by a doctor.
- If the burn is painful, give your child a pain reliever such as acetaminophen or ibuprofen (never aspirin) and carefully apply cold, wet cloths to the site of the burn.

Sunburn Sunburn is one of the easiest injuries to prevent. One bad sunburn during childhood can increase a person's risk of malignant melanoma, a deadly form of skin cancer, later in life. Frequent overexposure to the sun also predisposes a child to less serious forms of skin cancer. Sun exposure is especially dangerous for children with fair skin.

You can reduce your child's future risk of skin cancer by limiting exposure to the sun, using sunscreen after 6 months of age, and dressing the child in clothing that covers the arms and legs. Include a hat to protect the head.

Take these additional precautions:

• Keep a child under 6 months of age out of the sun as much as possible.

• Avoid excessive sun exposure between the hours of 10 AM and 3 PM, when the sun is most intense, even on an overcast day.

• If your child will be in the sun for 30 minutes or longer, apply a sunscreen with a sun protection factor (SPF) of at least 30 (the SPF is indicated on the label). An SPF of 30 means that your child can stay in the sun 30 times longer with the lotion than he or she could without it before getting a sunburn. Read labels carefully and make sure the sunscreen protects against both types of rays—ultraviolet A (UVA) and ultraviolet B (UVB)—and that it is waterproof. Don't use a sunscreen that contains para-aminobenzoic acid (PABA) because it can irritate the skin and can cause an allergic skin reaction in a child taking penicillin. Apply sunscreen at least 20 minutes before your child goes outdoors to give it time to penetrate the skin.

• Reapply sunscreen that has been washed off according to package directions or every 3 to 4 hours.

• Have your child wear sunglasses. Even young children should wear them, but not all sunglasses provide equal protection. The darkness of the lens does not determine the level of protection. Buy only those glasses labeled "UV absorption up to 400 nm," "maximum or 99 percent UV protection or blockage," "special purpose," or "meets ANSI UV requirements." Also, hats reduce eye exposure to sunlight by up to 50 percent.

If your child has a sunburn that causes blistering, you should call your doctor. For a less severe sunburn:

• Dress your child in loose clothing to maintain his or her body temperature.

• To reduce pain and inflammation, give the child ibuprofen according to package directions.

• Apply a nonperfumed moisturizing cream, not a lotion, which can contain alcohol.

• Give your child a cool bath or apply cool, wet compresses to sunburned areas several times a day.

• Discourage your child from picking at blisters or peeling skin; it could interfere with healing.

INSECT BITES AND BEE STINGS

Bee stings and insect bites usually cause only mild discomfort. But some children can have a severe, life-threatening allergic reaction that requires emergency medical treatment (see page 289). The best way to avoid insect bites is to dress your children in long pants, long sleeves, and a hat and to use insect repellent.

Insect bites The bites of mosquitoes, chiggers, fleas, and bedbugs usually cause itchy red bumps but few other problems. Relieve the itching by applying calamine lotion, except around the eyes and genitals. If the itching is severe, your doctor may prescribe hydrocortisone cream or ointment or an oral antihistamine to reduce the itching. Giving your child an oatmeal bath can also relieve itching.

Insect repellents are effective against mosquitoes, ticks, fleas, chiggers, and biting flies, but do not repel stinging insects such as bees, hornets, and wasps. When using insect repellent, apply it mainly to clothing and shoes; do not apply repellent to your child's hands because the child can transfer it to his or her mouth or eyes. The most effective insect repellent is a chemical called diethyltoluamide (known as DEET), but make sure you buy a repellent with no more than 10 percent DEET (check the label). DEET can be absorbed into the skin and cause serious harm.

If your child is bitten by a tick, he or she could be exposed to such diseases as Rocky Mountain spotted fever (see page 613) or Lyme disease (see page 557). To remove a tick, use tweezers to grasp it where its claws enter the skin, gripping it by its head. Pull upward, away from the skin, until the tick comes out. Make sure you have removed the whole tick, including its mouth. Try to save the tick so your doctor or a laboratory can evaluate and identify it. If the tick's head remains in your child's skin, take the child to the doctor to have the head removed. Wash the bite area with soap and water. Never remove a tick with your fingers and don't crush a tick with your hands because you could get infected yourself.

Bee stings When a bee stings, it injects a poison into the skin. Bee stings immediately cause a painful red bump to appear that may swell. The pain usually subsides within 2 hours but the swelling could increase for several hours.

If your child has been stung by a bee, look at the center of the raised red area for the stinger. Remove the stinger quickly by pinching it with your fingernails or a tweezers or by scraping it with your fingernails. The more quickly you remove the stinger, the less severe a reaction your child will have. After removing the stinger, press a cold, wet cloth or an ice cube over the sting to reduce pain and swelling. Rubbing the area for 15 minutes with meat tenderizer can also relieve the pain. Apply calamine lotion or a paste made of baking soda and water to alleviate itching.

Most bee stings are harmless but multiple stings can cause vomiting, diarrhea, a headache, and fever. A sting on the tongue or in the throat can cause swelling that could interfere with breathing. Some children are allergic to the venom of bees and can have a severe reaction called anaphylactic shock that can be fatal. Call your doctor immediately if, after being stung by a bee, your child has difficulty breathing or swallowing; tightness in the chest or throat; a fever; hives; dizziness or light-headedness; swelling near the eyes, lips, or genitals; severe headache; nausea; abdominal cramps; or diarrhea or is coughing or faints within a few hours of the sting. Take your child to the doctor or call 911 if he or she has been stung inside the mouth or has a known allergy to bee stings. Children known to have an allergy to bee venom should wear a medical identification tag and carry the drug epinephrine, which counteracts shock.

If your child needs to be hospitalized

Going to the hospital can be a frightening experience for a child. But you can minimize your child's fears by preparing him or her for the visit ahead of time. The more your child knows about what is going to happen, the less scared he or she will be. Tell your child what to expect in language he or she can understand. Remember that your presence will be the most reassuring thing to your child.

PREPARING YOUR CHILD

If your child is scheduled to have a nonemergency procedure, ask your doctor if the hospital has a program designed to educate parents and children about what to expect. You may be able to visit the hospital, see the ward where your child will be, and meet the people who will care for your child. Ask if you can stay with your child during the procedure or overnight. If the hospital does not allow this and it is important to you, talk to your doctor, who may be able to refer you to a specialist at a different hospital.

Many children have misconceptions about hospitals based on what their friends have told them or from television or the movies. Try to clear up these misconceptions before they become exaggerated. Don't wait for the child to ask questions because he or she probably doesn't know what to ask. Explain the following points before your child goes into the hospital:

- **Why he or she needs to go to the hospital** Make sure your child understands that entering the hospital is not some form of punishment.
- **What will be done** Describe exactly which body part is going to be fixed by pointing it out on the child's body.
- **How the procedure is done** Explain the procedure itself as clearly as you can. But choose your words carefully. For example, when talking about anesthesia, don't use the phrase "put to sleep." Your child may recall what happened to the family pet.
- **When you will be there** Knowing when to expect you at the hospital will help make your child less disappointed if you are not there at a particular time.
- **What to expect after the procedure** Tell your child if he or she is going to be in pain after the procedure but explain that medicine will make it hurt less.
- **When the child can expect to go home** Your child will be reassured by the reminder that he or she can return home soon.

YOUR ROLE AS A PARENT

Your child depends on you, so you need to do everything possible to stay with him or her at the hospital and provide comforting reassurance. Some hospitals have special rooms for the child and parent or a ward with cubicles that have both adult beds and cribs. Others can provide only a folding bed or chair for

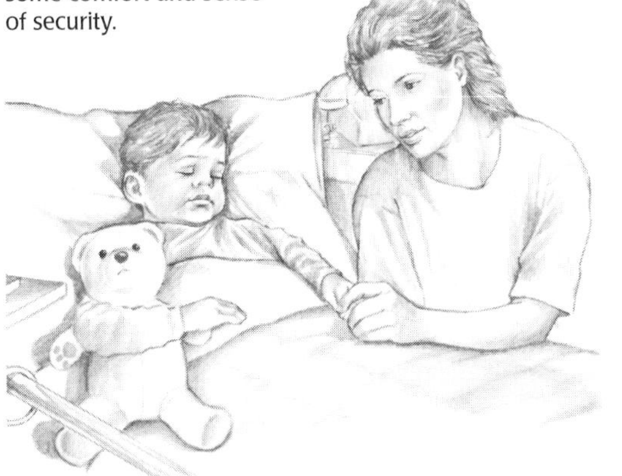

At the hospital
A hospital stay can be especially frightening for young children, who may be away from home overnight for the first time. A few familiar toys can give your child some comfort and sense of security.

sleeping. If you can't stay overnight with your child, the hospital may make special arrangements so you are able to see your child whenever you can, not just during visiting hours.

If your child is admitted to the hospital on an emergency basis, stay with him or her throughout the experience. Accompany your child through the examinations performed in the emergency department and during the transfer to a room. Find out everything you can about your child's condition and ask the doctor and nurse who will be caring for your child what tests or additional treatments will be given. Don't leave your child until you have passed this information on to him or her. During an emergency, your most important task is to nurture and reassure your child, so try to stay as calm and composed as possible.

Adolescents in the Hospital

Some hospitals have units designed specifically for adolescents but most do not. An adolescent may feel uncomfortable in a ward with very young children. Ask the nurses if your teenager could be placed in a room with a person of the same sex and age to ensure a more comfortable stay. One of the biggest concerns of adolescents in the hospital is the invasion of their privacy. To reduce your child's embarrassment and discomfort, provide nightclothes and a bathrobe.

Adolescents may prefer to face unpleasant procedures on their own, especially if they want to appear brave for a parent's benefit. Ask your older child how much time he or she wants you to spend at the hospital. Your adolescent needs autonomy, so allow him or her to make as many decisions as possible about care and treatment. Encourage the doctors to discuss the diagnosis and treatment program with your teenager in your presence.

If Your Child Needs Surgery

If your child is scheduled to have surgery, begin preparing him or her as soon as possible. Try to find out as much as you can about the procedure, the type of anesthesia that will be used, and how it will be administered. Ask whether any medication will be given for pain relief after the operation, and how long your child will be in the recovery room. The more informed you are, the more you can calm his or her fears. Be honest with your child—without giving details that might be frightening. Use words such as "pressure," "prick," or "sting" instead of "pain." Tell your child that he or she will not feel anything during the operation but may experience some discomfort afterward. Some hospitals allow families to tour the surgical area to familiarize the child and alleviate his or her fears.

Let your child know that you won't be with him or her in the operating room, but that you will be waiting nearby and that you can be together before and after the procedure. Tell your child whether or not you will be staying overnight with him or her.

A few days before the scheduled surgery, your doctor will probably ask you to bring your child in for routine preoperative procedures, such as having a physical examination and giving samples of blood and urine. You will be given written instructions about things you need to do to get your child ready for surgery, such as restricting his or her intake of food and liquids for a certain time before the operation. It is extremely important to follow these instructions exactly.

Anesthesia Many parents are concerned about general anesthesia, the use of medication to induce loss of sensation (which blocks feelings of pain) and to induce unconsciousness (which blocks memories of the operation). These medications are administered by a doctor called an anesthesiologist, who closely monitors a patient's vital signs–breathing, blood pressure, heart rate, and oxygen level–throughout the operation. Surgeons, anesthesiologists, and other operating-room personnel work together to make the experience as comfortable as possible for children.

Unless the surgery is complicated, you probably won't meet the anesthesiologist until the day of the operation. The anesthesiologist will give your child a brief physical examination. He or she will ask if your child has any allergies to medications or chronic illnesses, such as asthma, that might influence the type or amount of anesthesia used. He or she will also want to know if your child was premature or if he or she had any problems after delivery, if anyone in the family has had an allergic reaction to anesthesia, or if your child has any previous experience with anesthesia. Be sure to ask the anesthesiologist any questions you might have.

If your child takes any medications regularly, bring a list of them to give to the doctor. If your child has a cough from a cold or the flu, the doctor may recommend postponing the operation until the problem clears up, depending on the type of surgery and anesthesia to be used, because irritation in the airways can sometimes cause problems during anesthesia.

After your child's surgery, you will probably be allowed to be with him or her in the recovery room as soon as he or she is awake. In the recovery room, a nurse will monitor your child's vital signs and make sure he or she is comfortable and in as little pain as possible. When your child is allowed to go home, you will be given written instructions about how to care for the incision, how and when to give pain relief medication, and possible complications to watch for. Make sure all your questions and concerns are cleared up before you leave the hospital.

CHAPTER • 11

Keeping your child safe

Each year, more children in the United States die of injuries than of all childhood illnesses combined. But many common injuries can be prevented. You can do a lot to protect your children from injuries, especially when they are young and have little sense of danger or self-preservation. Children are more susceptible to certain types of injuries at certain ages. For example, from birth to age 5, children are most at risk for falls. Between ages 6 and 10, a child's biggest risk is being hit by a car as a pedestrian, while a preteen is most likely to be injured while riding a bicycle. Many adolescents engage in risk-taking behaviors that can threaten their health and safety; they are most at risk of being injured in a car collision or by a gun.

Preventing injuries

As children develop, they acquire new skills that enable them to explore their surroundings. This exploration is necessary for a child's development. But you need to be aware of the new risks that each stage of development brings so you can protect your child. Many everyday circumstances can pose threats to your young child's safety. For guidelines on how to safeguard your home, see "A Parent's Guide to Childproofing Your Home," page 76. If your child does get injured, see pages 666 to 680 for emergency and first-aid information.

MOTOR VEHICLE SAFETY

Motor vehicle collisions are the single greatest threat to the lives of children over 3 months of age. By using child safety seats and seat belts, you can protect your child from serious injury or death. A child who is thrown from a vehicle is 25 times more likely to die than one who is restrained by a safety seat or seat belt. Children need to ride in a safety seat until they weigh 60 pounds. Then they can use a regular seat belt with a lap and shoulder strap. Don't strap a small child weighing under 60 pounds into a seat belt unless you have no choice. Using a seat belt is better than leaving your child unrestrained. For information about the best kind of child safety seats for children at different ages, see page 294.

CAR SAFETY SEATS

You probably won't be able to leave the hospital with your newborn unless you have a child safety seat installed in your car. When buying a safety seat, choose one that is right for your child's age and weight. You also need to make sure that the car seat you buy fits your car. Check to see that the seat carries a label showing that the product meets Federal Motor Vehicle Safety Standard 213 (FMVSS 213). To find out if the seat you have chosen has been subject to any recalls, call the National Highway Traffic Safety Administration Auto Safety Hotline at 1-800-424-9393.

Correct installation is a must

A car safety seat can save your child's life in a collision—but only if you install the seat properly and use it every time your child is in the car. Read the installation instructions before buying a seat because not all seats fit easily in all cars. If it looks like a certain type of seat will not work in your car, buy a different one. Practice installing and removing the seat. Follow the manufacturer's directions and refer to your car owner's manual to see how to secure the safety seat. Always install the seat in the middle of the back seat, where it is most protected on all sides. To make sure the seat is properly installed, pull on it as hard as you can—you should not be able to move it. If you have read the instructions and your car owner's manual and you still can't install the seat correctly, call your car seat manufacturer or your car dealership.

Infant seats

The best child safety seats for infants under 20 pounds and 1 year of age are those designed for infants only. Infant safety seats must face the rear of the car to protect an infant's head, neck, and back. When your child reaches 28 inches in length, he or she can sit facing forward. Never put an infant seat in the front seat of the car—especially if you have a passenger side air bag—because an inflating air bag can severely injure a small child (see page 298). Infant-only seats are easier to use for babies because the seats are smaller, more comfortable, more secure, and more portable. But remember that most babies will outgrow them in the first year and will require a larger child safety seat.

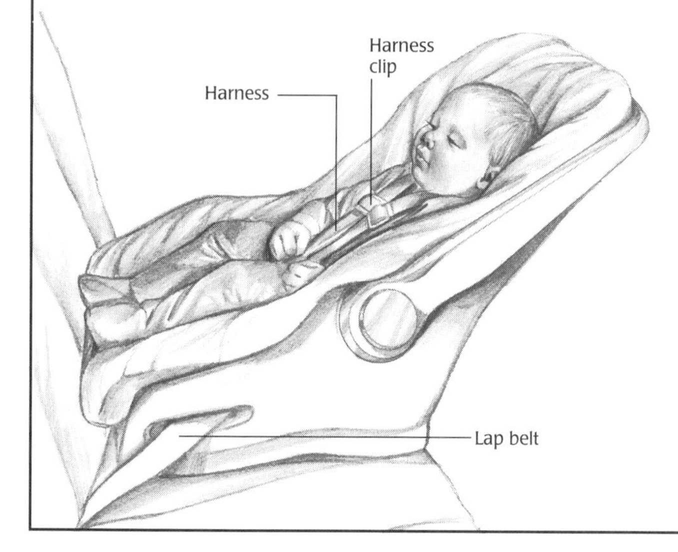

Infant-only safety seats

Infant-only seats usually have straps that go over the child's shoulder and form a V when buckled between his or her legs. Use a plastic or fabric harness retainer clip to keep the straps on the baby's shoulders and away from his or her neck. If your baby's head falls forward when he or she is in the seat, put a tightly rolled bath towel or diaper under the front edge of the safety seat to tilt it back. If the baby's head falls to the side, put a rolled towel or a cushioned head support on either side of his or her head. Always dress your child in clothes that let you buckle the strap between his or her legs.

Child safety restraints on airplanes

Flying isn't always a smooth ride. Airplanes can pass through turbulence caused by jet streams, cold or warm fronts, or thunderstorms. Although air turbulence is rare, it can cause serious injury to unrestrained passengers, especially children under 2 who are sitting on a parent's lap. Because of the risk of injury, the Federal Aviation Administration (FAA) recommends that all children, regardless of age, be restrained on airplanes. Airlines have traditionally allowed parents to fly a child under 2 for free and hold him or her on their lap, or pay full fare to reserve a seat for the child. But now, in response to safety concerns, most major airlines offer discounts of up to 50 percent for children under 2 who travel in a child safety seat. On flights that are not full, airlines often allow parents to use an empty seat for a child in a safety restraint, but the only way to guarantee that your child will have a seat is to buy a ticket (make sure you reserve an adjoining seat for yourself). A child safety restraint must be placed in a window seat so it won't block the escape path in an emergency.

The FAA regulations for child safety restraints on airplanes are based on a child's weight and size and are similar to the rules for safety restraints in motor vehicles. Children who weigh 20 pounds or less should be placed in a rear-facing child safety seat; those weighing between 20 and 40 pounds should ride in a forward-facing safety seat. Children weighing more than 40 pounds need to use an aircraft seat belt, just like adults. Check your car safety seat for a label that says it is certified for use in motor vehicles and aircraft; most newer models can be used for both. Measure the width of your safety seat—it must be no more than 16 inches wide to fit in a standard coach seat on an airplane. Booster seats can cause abdominal and head injuries in airplane emergencies and are not allowed on aircraft. If you want to take your booster seat on the trip, you will have to check it as baggage.

Convertible seats

You can use a convertible infant-toddler safety seat for both infants under 20 pounds who are 1 year old or younger and for children under 40 pounds who are under age 4. Convertible car seats are not as easy to use as infant-only seats because they are more cumbersome and less portable. When using a convertible safety seat for an infant, install it so that it faces the back of the car.

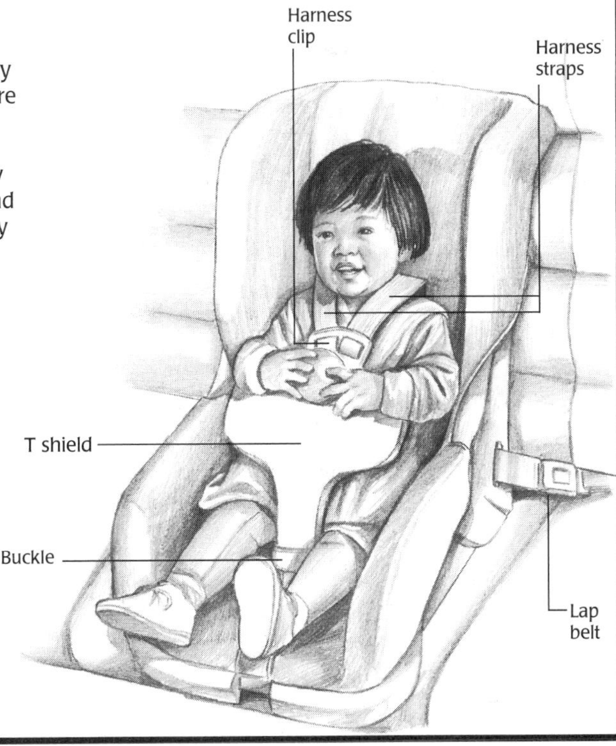

Convertible infant-toddler safety seats

You can use a convertible infant-toddler safety seat for any child under age 4 or who weighs less than 40 pounds—including an infant. These seats have different types of harnesses; one type has a padded T shield like the one shown here. The shield attaches to the shoulder straps and buckles into the seat between the legs. Harnesses without shields are usually better for infants because the shields are often positioned too high and too far from an infant's body to fit snugly.

Safe driving tips

Although using child restraints and seat belts can greatly reduce the risk of injury during a collision, the best prevention is to avoid collisions by driving safely.

- Always drive within the speed limit. Drive slower in bad weather or when road conditions are unsafe.
- Never drive after drinking alcohol or using other drugs that might impair your perception, responses, and judgment.
- Drive defensively—many other drivers don't drive safely. Stay far enough away from the car in front of you to be able to stop suddenly and stay well behind a reckless driver.
- Whenever possible, refrain from driving when conditions are unsafe (such as in heavy rain or snow) or very late at night (when people tend to be more tired and careless).
- Avoid driving when you are emotionally upset; you may be too distracted to drive safely.

Booster seats

Use a booster seat for children who have outgrown a child safety seat but are not yet big enough (who weigh at least 60 pounds and are between ages 4 and 8) to use just the car's lap and shoulder belt. Many booster seats do not provide adequate protection during a collision, especially those that have only a bar or shield in front of the child's abdomen. The shield may not restrain the child as well as do the harness straps on a standard car seat or a car shoulder strap, so doctors recommend keeping a child in a regular child safety seat as long as possible. If you use a booster seat, find one that lets you use the car lap and shoulder belt for more protection.

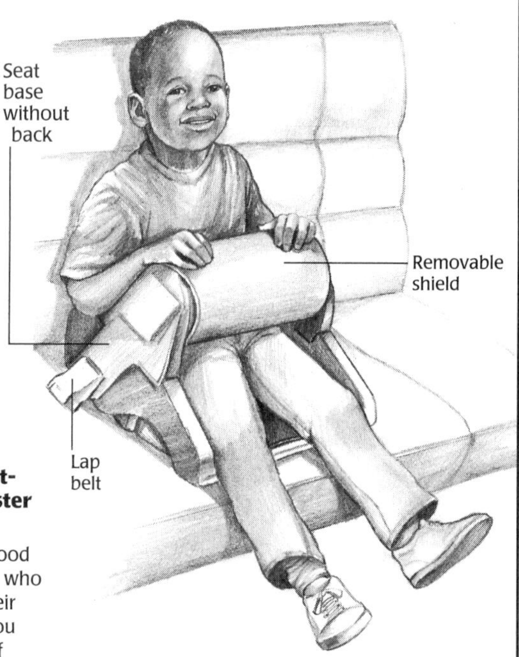

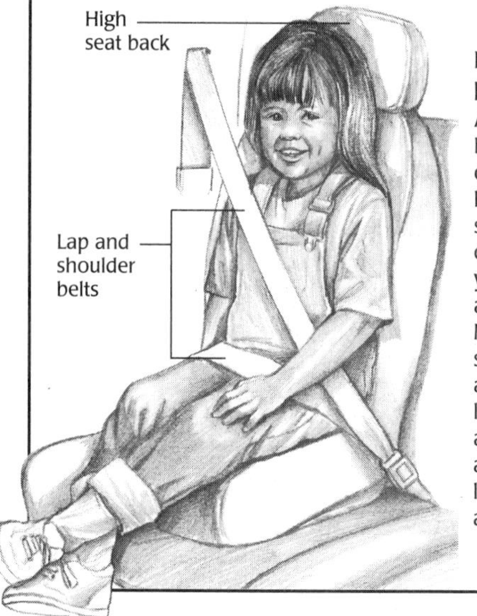

High-backed belt-positioning booster
A belt-positioning booster seat is a good choice for children who have outgrown their safety seats. But you can only use one if your car has both lap and shoulder belts. Make sure that the shoulder belt lies flat across your child's collarbone and shoulder, away from the neck and face, and that the lap belt is tight and low across his or her hips.

Shield booster
If your car has only lap belts, you need to use a booster seat with a shield. This type of seat does not protect the child's head and upper body as well as the belt-positioning booster, but it is better than using a lap belt alone. Some models have a removable shield that converts the seat into a belt-positioning booster in cars with lap and shoulder belts. Never use a booster seat with a shield for a child who weighs less than 40 pounds.

Seat belts

Children who weigh more than 60 pounds are usually big enough to use the car lap and shoulder belt. If your child weighs more than 60 pounds but is too small to wear a lap and shoulder belt, use a belt-positioning booster seat like the one shown on page 296, which allows you to correctly position the seat belt. You can buy a shoulder-belt adjuster that repositions the strap so it won't cross your child's throat.

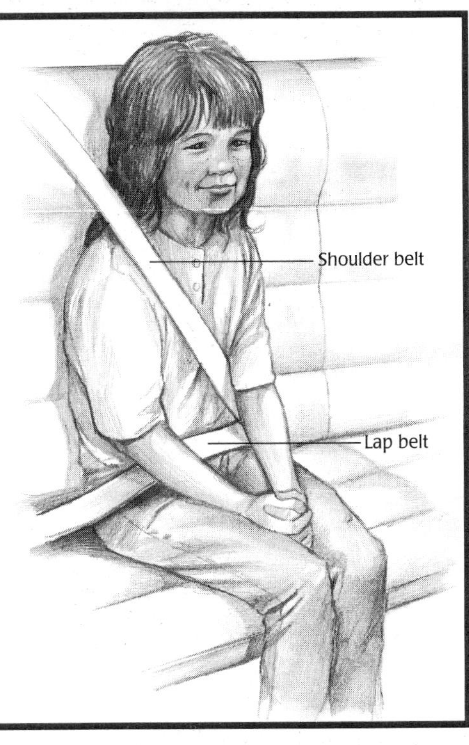

Make sure your child's seat belt fits

A seat belt cannot protect your child in a crash if it fits improperly. The lap part of the belt should fit snugly across your child's hips (not the abdomen) and the shoulder belt should cross his or her shoulder and chest. If your child is still so short that the shoulder strap crosses his or her throat, he or she is too small for a seat belt and should stay in a booster seat. Never put a shoulder strap under a child's arm.

Make seat belts a habit

Set a good safety example. Always wear your own seat belt and insist that all passengers buckle up. Praise your children often for riding in the safety seat or wearing a seat belt. They will eventually make it a habit and automatically climb into their safety seat or put on their seat belt whenever they get into a car—without reminders.

WARNING

Air bags

The powerful force of an air bag deploying in a collision can kill a child sitting in the front passenger seat. Safety experts recommend that all children under 12, or who are short or petite, sit in the back seat in cars that have air bags.

Built-in seats

More and more cars and vans now have built-in safety seats for toddlers. Be sure to follow the manufacturer's specifications for weight and age of the child. As with booster seats, the seat belts and harness straps should always fit your child snugly.

Use car seat at all times

Never take your child out of his or her car seat while the car is moving. Even a slow-speed collision is enough to wrench a child from your arms. If you need to remove your child from the car seat, tell the driver to pull over and stop the car first.

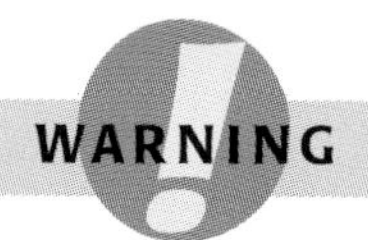

Air bags—a potential hazard to children

Air bags are becoming a standard safety feature in American cars. Although an inflating air bag can save a life during a collision, it creates a force powerful enough to kill a child (or small adult) riding in the front passenger seat. Children are especially vulnerable to injury from an air bag if they are in a safety seat. Always place child safety seats—both front-facing and back-facing ones—in the back seat of your car. A child should be close to adult size before being allowed to sit in the front seat. Air bags cause less severe injury when the child or adult is wearing seat belts properly.

Taking the following precautions every time your child rides in a car or van could save your child's life:

• On every trip, make sure that all children in the car wear seat belts or are fastened into a correctly installed safety seat. Doctors recommend that children use safety seats until they weigh 60 pounds.

• Always place child safety seats in the back seat. Never place a safety seat (facing either backwards or forwards) in the front seat of a car.

• When your child is old enough to use a seat belt, teach him or her to use it correctly. Make sure it fits properly. The lap belt should cross the upper thighs (not the abdomen) and the shoulder belt should cross the shoulder and chest (not the neck). You can buy a safety attachment that adjusts the lap and shoulder straps to fit a child. A lap or shoulder belt alone will not protect a child as well as both used together. Never place a shoulder belt under a child's arm, or belt two children with one belt.

• Do not allow a child younger than 12 years old to sit in the front seat. Sitting in the back seat can significantly improve his or her chances of surviving a crash and avoiding serious injury.

• Set a good example for your children by always wearing your own seat belt. Ask your children to remind you to wear it so they will be motivated to be responsible for their own.

Electric garage door openers can be dangerous

Electric garage door openers can entrap children under a closing garage door, causing serious injury or death. To prevent such accidents, electric door openers now have an automatic reversing device triggered by an electric eye or a sensor at the base of the garage door. But some sensor-reversing mechanisms do not reverse quickly enough to prevent serious injury. If you have a garage door opener triggered by a sensor at the bottom of the door, test it by placing a roll of paper towels under the door. If the door does not reverse when it hits the paper towels, disconnect the electric door opener and operate the garage door by hand until you can replace the opener with one triggered by an electric eye. Make sure the activating button is out of the reach of children. Teach your child never to run under a closing door and never run under one yourself—your child will quickly imitate your behavior.

• Never hold an infant or child in your lap or allow anyone else in your car to do so. Your arms are not strong enough to hold a child against the force of a collision and the weight of your body could crush the child against the dashboard or the back of a seat.
• Never let a fussy child get out of a safety seat or seat belt while the car is moving. Stop the car if you need to calm the child down or take a break.
• Do not allow your children to play in the car while it is parked.
• If the windows and doors of your car have childproof locks, use them. Never allow young children to open or close power windows because they could get their hand or head caught in a rising window.

PREVENTING FALLS

Falls are the leading cause of emergency department visits and hospitalizations among children under 5 years old. If your child falls and you suspect he or she has an injury, especially if there was a blow to the child's head or a broken bone, call your doctor immediately. Here are some steps you can take to help prevent your children from injuring themselves in a fall:
• Never leave your infant alone on a bed, changing table, couch, or chair. If you cannot hold your baby for some reason, put him or her in a safe place such as a crib or playpen.
• Never use a walker—your child could tip it over and get a serious head injury.
• Always strap your child into a high chair or stroller. When purchasing these items, choose those with straps that are easy for you to fasten and unfasten (see page 300), so you will be more likely to use them properly each time.
• When your baby starts to crawl, install gates at the top and bottom of your stairways and close the doors to rooms in which your child could get hurt. Use only mesh gates that have very small openings or gates with horizontal slats that are spaced no more than 2⅜ inches apart. Avoid the older accordion gates with large openings, which can trap a child's neck or fingers.
• In the tub or shower, use a rubber mat or apply adhesive strips to the bottom.
• Install window guards on all windows above the first floor. An unguarded window that is open only 5 inches can pose a danger to children under 10 years of age. Don't rely on screens to prevent falls. Screens are designed for keeping insects out—not for keeping active children in.
• Keep stairways well lighted and free of clutter. Don't let children play on stairs or play alone on a fire escape, high porch, or balcony. Fix all loose railings or boards. If you rent, ask your landlord to make these repairs.
• Move chairs and other furniture away from windows, kitchen counters, and other high places that are tempting to curious young climbers.
• Remove furniture with hard or sharp edges from areas where your child plays, or cover the edges with specially made cushioning.
• If you allow your child to ride in a shopping cart at the grocery store, always use the restraining belts in the cart. Don't let an older child climb into a shopping cart or hang onto the side or front of the cart.

Are your child's crib and high chair safe?

New cribs and high chairs must meet certain standards for safety. But many parents buy or borrow used baby furniture manufactured before such standards were set. When a friend or relative offers you a used crib or high chair, or when you find these items at a garage sale, check them out carefully before you accept or buy them. Older furniture and equipment for children may not have had to pass the rigorous safety standards that are required today. Avoid buying an old crib or high chair that looks as though it has been painted; the paint could contain lead. When shopping for a crib and high chair for your child, make sure they have the safety features shown here.

When making up your baby's crib, don't cover the mattress with a plastic cover that comes in direct contact with your baby because the plastic could cause suffocation. Never use a water-bed mattress in a crib because your baby isn't strong enough to lift his or her head up off of it and could suffocate. For the same reason, keep pillows and stuffed animals out of the crib. Avoid bumper pads, which could trap your baby's head between the pad and the side of the crib. If you choose to use pads, attach them securely and tuck them down between the mattress and the side of the crib. The crib should be adjustable so you can lower the mattress as your child grows taller and begins to stand in the crib to prevent him or her from falling or climbing out.

Features to look for in a safe crib

- Slats that are no more than 2⅜ inches apart
- If painted, surfaces covered with lead-free paint
- End panels with appropriately spaced (2⅜ inches apart) slats or ones that are solid (without any cutout areas)
- Corner posts that are flush with the end panels or as tall as the posts on a canopy bed
- A firm, flat mattress that fits the bed frame snugly (you should not be able to fit two fingers between the mattress and the side of the crib)
- Drop sides with a locking, hand-operated latch that will not release accidentally
- Spring-loaded pins that allow the mattress to be lowered as the child grows to minimize risk of the child climbing or falling out

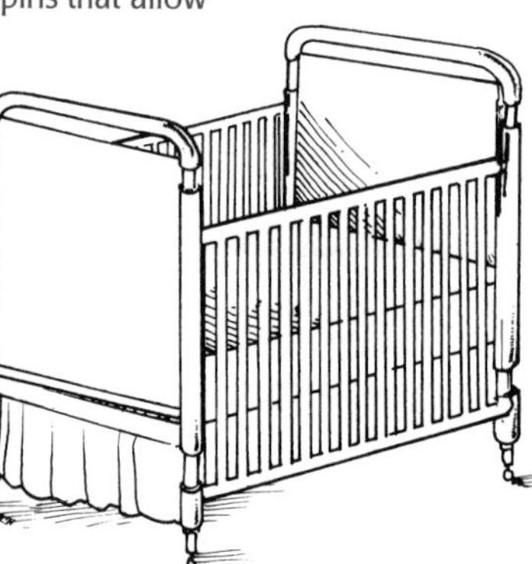

Features to look for in a safe high chair

- Waist and crotch restraining straps that are not connected to the tray
- Waist buckle that is easy to use
- Tray that locks securely
- Wide and stable base
- Parts that are firmly attached and cannot be pulled off
- Locking device on a folding high chair that keeps the chair from collapsing when the child is inside
- Rounded edges

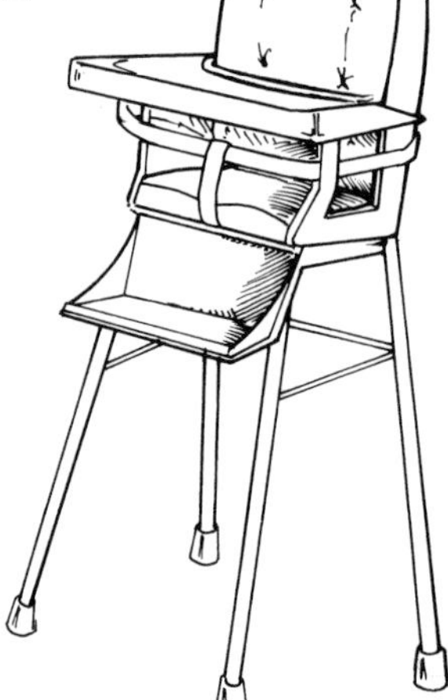

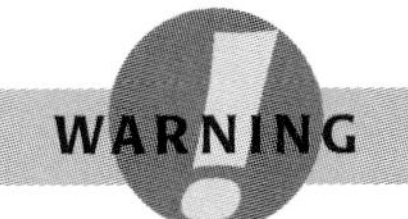

Head injuries can cause a concussion

A head injury that causes a temporary loss of or change in consciousness without permanent damage to the brain is called a concussion. If your child sustains a head injury, you should observe him or her closely for evidence of a concussion. Check your child every 3 to 4 hours for the first 24 to 36 hours. When your child is asleep, wake him or her and ask questions such as "What's your name?" A child with a concussion may look pale, have amnesia, or vomit several times. Call your doctor right away if your child has any of the following warning signs of a severe head injury:

- Persistent nausea, or two or more episodes of vomiting
- A large or deep cut or severe bruising
- Inability to walk normally
- Pupils that are larger than usual or of different sizes
- Seizures
- Increasingly severe headache
- Changes in levels of alertness
- Inability to wake up from sleep
- Behavior changes, such as irritability, confusion, or combativeness

PREVENTING POISONING

Although poisoning can occur at any age, children between ages 1 and 3 are especially prone to poisoning accidents because they are old enough to move throughout the home independently and young enough to be exploring their world by constantly putting things in their mouths. You might be surprised at how many ordinary household items you have throughout your home that could poison a young child.

Your medicine cabinet contains many common drugs and medications that, taken in sufficient quantity by a small child, can cause poisoning, including acetaminophen, ibuprofen, aspirin, tranquilizers, sleeping pills, and iron pills. If your child has seen you take these medications, he or she may be tempted to imitate you. Certain household products–bleach, mothballs, furniture polish, drain cleaners, weed killers, insecticides, rat poisons, lye, paint thinners, and cosmetics (such as fingernail polish and permanent wave neutralizers)–are poisoning hazards. These items are commonly stored throughout the home and garage. Some plants–including philodendron, dieffenbachia, poinsettia, jade plant, holly

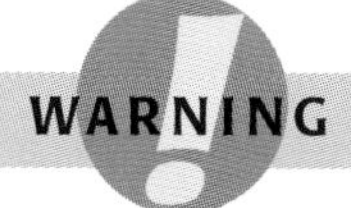

Prevent carbon monoxide poisoning

Carbon monoxide (CO) is an odorless, colorless gas that can escape from defective or improperly vented home heating systems. Inhaling carbon monoxide can cause a loss of consciousness and death. In fact, entire families have died in their sleep from carbon monoxide poisoning caused by a faulty heating system. To prevent carbon monoxide poisoning in your home, have your furnace or boiler inspected and cleaned every year and install a carbon monoxide detector on each floor of your home. If you rent your home or apartment, ask your landlord to install a CO detector for you. If your detector alarm goes off, evacuate your family from your home immediately and call a home heating repair service to correct the problem.

berry, schefflera, pokeweed root, pepper plant, yew, pyracantha, azalea, and oleander—are also poisonous. Follow these guidelines at home to protect your child from getting poisoned:

- Buy medicine and household products in childproof packages. Always replace the safety caps immediately after use.
- Keep household products in their original containers. Never store inedible products (such as bleach) in food or drink containers and don't store food and cleaning products together in the same cabinet.
- Read labels carefully before using any product and observe warnings and precautions.
- Never use medicine from an unlabeled container or one with a label you can't read.
- Teach your children not to drink or eat anything unless an adult gives it to them.
- Do not take medicine in front of small children because they tend to copy adult behavior.
- Check your home often for old or expired medications or household products and discard them. Flush old medicines and other substances down the toilet, rinse the containers out well, and discard them.
- Be alert for repeated poisonings; a child who swallows a poison is likely to try again within a year.
- Never leave bottles of alcohol, alcohol-containing products such as mouthwash or aftershave lotion, or alcoholic beverages within a child's reach.
- Identify all the plants, trees, and bushes in your house and yard. Keep only nonpoisonous plants in your home. If you are not sure whether a particular plant is poisonous, take it to a local nursery for identification.
- Keep a 1-ounce bottle of syrup of ipecac in your home. Syrup of ipecac induces vomiting in a person who has consumed a poison. But don't give the syrup to your child unless you have been told to do so by the local poison control center or your doctor. Replace the syrup every 2 years; check the label for an expiration date.
- Store potentially poisonous chemicals and medicines in a locked cabinet that is out of your child's reach.

If your child swallows anything other than food, get help immediately. Call the poison control center in your area or your doctor. Keep the telephone numbers of your doctor, the poison control center, and a local hospital near your phone.

No sips of beer for baby

Some adults think it's harmless to give a child an occasional sip of beer or another alcoholic beverage, but alcohol is a potential poison for an infant or toddler. A small sip or two is insignificant to an adult but has a much greater effect on a child's small body. Never give your child beer, wine, or anything else to drink that contains alcohol.

Preventing lead poisoning One out of every six children has a high level of lead in his or her blood. Children between the ages of 6 months and 6 years are most at risk. Before the dangers of lead exposure were known, the metal was used in paints, gasoline, water pipes, and many other products. Lead-based paint is the most common source of lead poisoning in children. You cannot see, taste, or smell lead, and children who have lead poisoning do not always act or look sick. The only way to know for sure if a child has been exposed to lead is by giving the child a blood test (see page 236) that detects the metal. Ask your doctor about having your child tested. The long-term effects of exposure to lead–learning disabilities, decreased growth, hyperactivity, impaired hearing, seizures, and brain damage–can be severe and irreversible. You can limit your child's exposure to lead by taking the following simple steps:

- Keep your home clean. Children can swallow lead if they play in dust or dirt and then put their fingers or toys in their mouths, or if they eat without washing their hands first. Keep the areas where your children play–especially around windowsills and stairwells–as dust-free and clean as possible. Wash toys, pacifiers, bottles, and stuffed animals regularly.
- Reduce exposure to lead-based paint. Almost all homes built before 1978 contain lead-based paint on the walls, window frames, and exterior of the house. Tiny pieces of peeling or chipping lead paint can cause lead poisoning if eaten. If the paint in your home is chipping or peeling, ask your local health department to test it for lead. If you rent, tell your landlord about any peeling or chipping paint. Make sure your child does not chew on anything covered

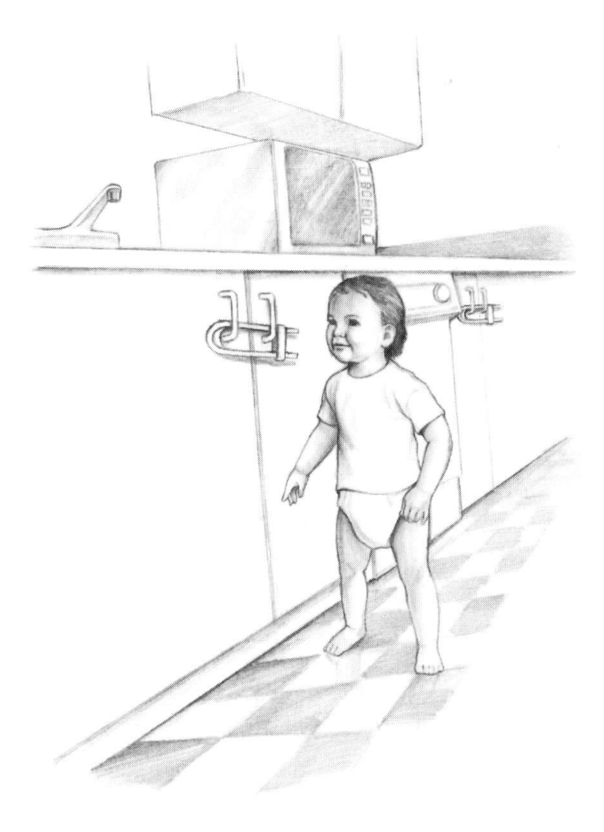

Keeping poisons out of reach

To avoid poisoning accidents, keep harmful products out of your child's sight and reach, preferably in a locked cabinet. But remember that putting a lock on a cabinet is no guarantee that it won't be opened; a persistent child can eventually figure out how to open even a "childproof" lock. Store potentially dangerous products with your child's stage of development in mind. For example, if your child can crawl or walk, store poisonous products above the kitchen or bathroom counter, not under the sink. But it's a good idea to lock up the lower cabinets anyway, to keep your young child out of the garbage and to prevent him or her from pulling out heavy items, such as canned goods, that could fall on his or her toes.

with lead paint, such as painted window sills, cribs, or playpens. Dust from plastic miniblinds has also been shown to contain lead. Do not put cribs, playpens, beds, or high chairs next to areas where paint is chipping or peeling.

• Don't remove lead paint yourself. Scraping or sanding lead paint can expose you and your children to dangerous levels of lead dust that can remain in the building long after the work is finished. Stripping lead paint using heating devices can also release lead into the air. If you need to have lead paint removed from your home, hire a trained lead abatement specialist–someone who knows how to do the work safely and has the proper equipment to clean up thoroughly.

• Get lead out of your drinking water. Tap water doesn't contain lead naturally–it usually picks the metal up from household lead plumbing. Boiling water will not reduce the amount of lead in tap water. (Bathing in water that contains lead is not dangerous because the metal does not enter the body through the skin.) The only way to find out if your water contains lead is to have it tested. Call your local health department or water supplier to find out how. Testing is simple and relatively inexpensive. To reduce your exposure to lead in your tap water, use only cold water for cooking and drinking and always run the tap water at least once a day for 2 or 3 minutes before using it.

Iron supplements can poison toddlers

Many children die each year in the United States after swallowing iron tablets that were left within their reach. Iron supplements often have brightly colored sugar coatings that attract young children. Keep iron tablets and all other vitamin and mineral supplements out of the reach of your small child.

• Limit exposure to lead outdoors. Always wash your child's hands after he or she has played outside to prevent ingestion of lead from soil or sandboxes.

• Don't store beverages in lead containers. The lead in lead crystal and lead-containing pottery glazes can leach out into the liquid inside and cause lead poisoning when you or your child drinks the liquid. Pottery imported from other countries is more likely to be covered with a glaze containing lead.

• Provide the right foods. A child who gets enough iron and calcium from his or her diet will absorb less lead. Foods rich in iron include lean red meat, dried beans and other legumes, fortified cereals, and eggs. Dairy products such as milk, cheese, and yogurt are high in calcium.

• Don't use home or herbal remedies that contain lead. Some traditional ethnic home remedies–such as azarcon and greta, which are used to treat an upset stomach–can contain enough lead to poison a child. Don't give them to your child or any other member of your family.

Preventing choking

Few sounds are more alarming to a parent than those of a child who is choking. Although choking occurs in children of all ages, those under age 4 are most at risk because they put things in their mouths as they explore the world around them. The most common causes of choking in children under age 2 are

Balloons are the top choking threat to children

Latex or rubber balloons cause more choking deaths in children than anything else. A collapsed balloon can lodge in a child's upper airway and block the flow of air into the lungs. Instead of rubber balloons, use the shiny, silver, polyester-film balloons you can purchase in many specialty stores. They are safer than rubber balloons because they are larger and stronger and don't deflate or break as easily. If you see rubber balloons at a party or in someone else's home, watch for and discard any broken or deflated ones.

round or cylindrical foods, such as hot dogs, candy, nuts, raisins, and grapes. Other food culprits include fruit and vegetable pieces, seeds, popcorn, cookies, hard candy, and meat. Nonfood choking threats include rubber balloons, batteries, small toys, beads, pen caps, coins, nails, tacks, bolts, earrings, straight pins, safety pins, and small rocks. Be mindful that any small object can cause choking. Observe your child closely and, if you are unsure whether something might cause your child to choke, play it safe and take the object away from your child. If your child swallows a nonfood item, call the doctor immediately. The following steps can protect your child from choking hazards:

- When introducing new foods to your child, follow your doctor's recommendations. A child's chewing skills are not fully developed until about age 4.
- Cut your children's food into bite-size pieces. Encourage your children to eat small bits of food and to chew all of their food thoroughly.
- Don't allow your children to walk, run, or jump when they have food or other objects in their mouths. Serve them food only when they are seated and never leave them unsupervised while eating.
- Teach your children not to talk with food in their mouths.

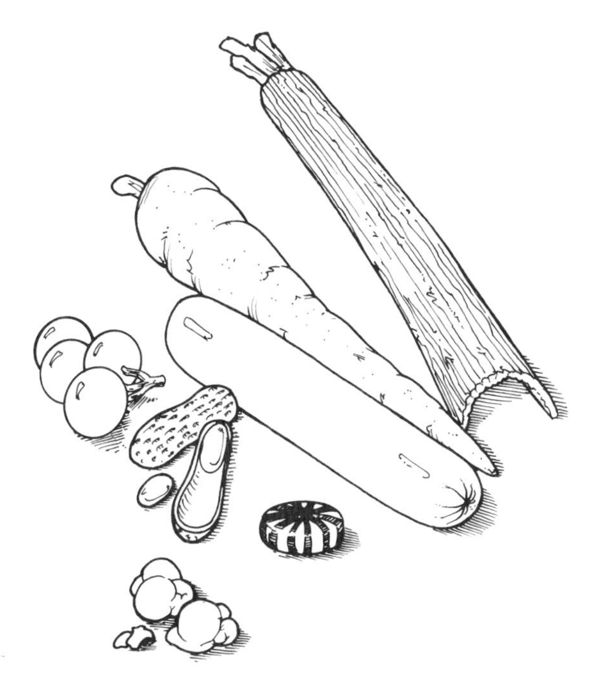

Some foods can cause choking

Take extra care when introducing solid foods to your child because some foods can cause choking when they become lodged in a child's windpipe and block it. Examples include nuts of any kind, popcorn, raw carrots, raw celery, and hard candies. Never give these hard foods to children younger than age 4 because they may not chew them thoroughly enough to swallow them safely. Before you give your child softer foods such as hot dogs or grapes, cut them up into tiny pieces that your child can easily swallow. Otherwise, avoid them altogether.

Preventing suffocation

An infant or small child has no sense of danger and can easily suffocate if his or her nose and mouth become blocked accidentally. Take the following precautions at home to prevent your child from accidentally suffocating:

- Do not put pillows, stuffed animals, or toys near your infant's head in the crib.
- Never use a plastic cover on the mattress of your child's crib.
- Always put your infant to sleep on his or her back in order to prevent the risk of SIDS (sudden infant death syndrome).
- Store plastic grocery and dry cleaning bags out of reach of your children or recycle them promptly to prevent suffocation. Tie them in knots so your child cannot place one over his or her head.
- Don't have beanbag chairs in your home and don't place your child to sleep on a water bed.
- Lock or remove the door from any unused refrigerator or freezer stored in the garage or basement.
- Take a course in infant and child cardiopulmonary resuscitation (CPR) so you can try to revive your child in the event of suffocation. Call your local hospital or Red Cross for information on CPR classes.

- Don't allow your children to eat or chew gum while in a moving car. You may not be able to get to the side of the road quickly enough to do anything if they begin to choke.
- Make sure your home is childproof (see page 76). Constantly be on the lookout for objects that your child could choke on and move them out of reach. Don't forget to check under furniture, especially if you have a crawling child, whose view of the world is close to floor level.
- Keep your older child's toys away from your infant or toddler because they could contain small parts.
- Take a course to learn how to perform the Heimlich maneuver (see page 670) on both children and adults.

SAFE TOYS

Children can be injured by their favorite toys. Some of these injuries are caused by toys that are poorly designed or constructed but most happen when children use toys improperly or play with toys designed for older children. Make sure that your child's toys pose no threat to health or safety. The most

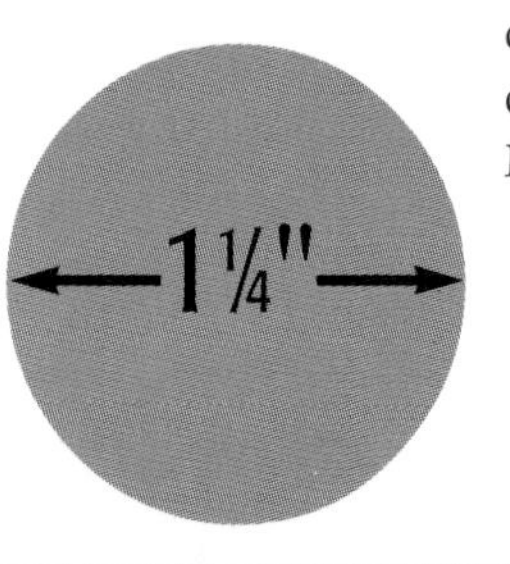

A measure of safety

Your toddler is likely to put just about anything into his or her mouth, so you need to be vigilant about keeping small objects that could cause choking out of reach. Don't allow children under 3 years old to play with items that are smaller than 1¼ inches in diameter (circle shaped) or less than 2¼ inches long (bar shaped). A good rule of thumb is to keep anything that can fit inside the tube of a toilet paper roll away from your child.

Drawstrings on clothing are potential strangling hazards

Children can become entangled in the neck drawstrings of hooded sweatshirts and jackets and be strangled. Don't buy clothing for your child that has drawstrings on the hood or at the waist and remove all drawstrings from clothing your child already has. Instead, purchase hooded shirts or jackets that have safe closures, such as plastic hook and loop fasteners, buttons, or snaps (above right). When putting a scarf on your child during the winter, always tuck the ends into his or her jacket because the scarf can get caught on something and strangle your child.

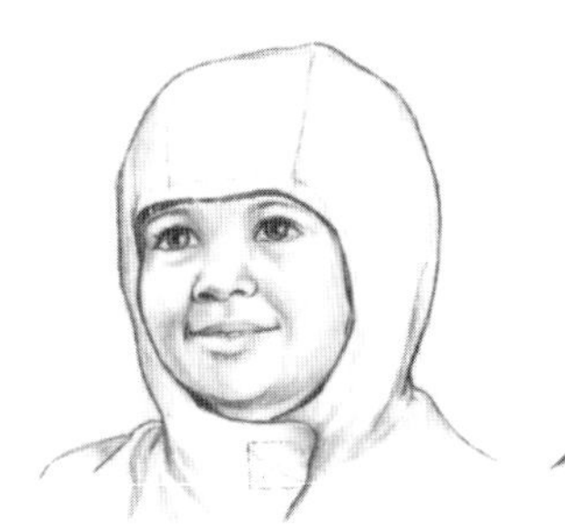

Plastic hook and loop fastener

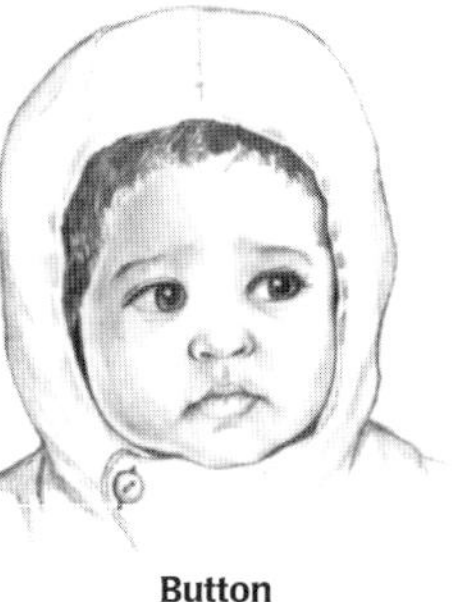

Button

Snap

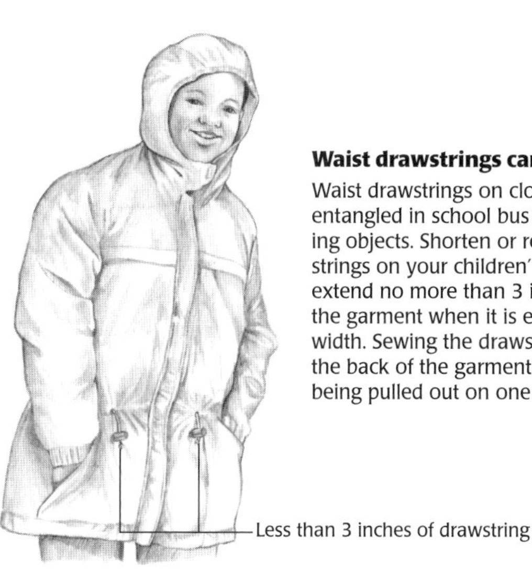

Waist drawstrings can get caught

Waist drawstrings on clothing can become entangled in school bus doors and other moving objects. Shorten or remove all waist drawstrings on your children's clothing so the strings extend no more than 3 inches from the edge of the garment when it is expanded to its fullest width. Sewing the drawstring to the middle of the back of the garment can prevent it from being pulled out on one side.

important consideration when buying toys is to select those that are appropriate for a child's age, skill level, and interests. Although the manufacturer's suggestions listed on the package can serve as a guide, you are the best judge of whether or not your child is mature enough and skilled enough to play with a particular toy safely. Follow these guidelines:

- Look for toys that are well constructed and sturdy enough so that they won't break when your child throws or bangs them.
- Don't buy toys with sharp edges, pointed pieces, or parts made of glass or rigid plastic that could shatter.
- Discard plastic wrappings on new toys as soon as you open them because your child can suffocate on the plastic.
- Make sure that toys do not have parts that your child could detach and choke on, such as the squeakers in squeeze toys and the eyes and nose on stuffed animals or dolls.
- Always keep older children's toys out of the reach of a younger child, especially if the toys have small parts. Make sure your older children understand why they need to put their toys away when they're finished with them.
- Never give a child under age 10 a toy that must be plugged into an electrical

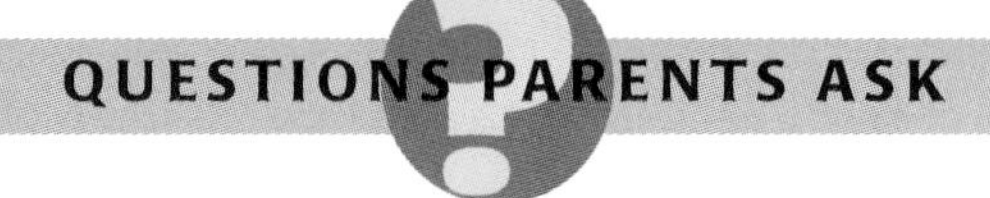

Pet safety

Q We have a cat and a dog and we want them to accept our new baby. How can we make sure the baby interacts with the animals safely?

A Introduce the animals to your child gradually and always be there when the animals are near your baby. Observe how the pets act with your child and give them lots of love and attention so they won't feel neglected. Teach your child how and where to pet the animals and not to pull their fur or tails. If your child learns to respect the animals—for example, by not waking them up when they are sleeping and not teasing them—he or she will establish a playful and loving relationship with your cat and dog that lasts for life. As your child gets older and becomes mobile, he or she will interact with your pets eye to eye, at ground level. This direct contact sometimes unnerves pets, who may react by scratching, biting, or just running away. If you have an especially large, unruly, or unpredictable dog, evaluate the dog's personality to make sure it can get along with children. If not, it may be best to find the dog a new home. Make sure your pets have all their shots and give them good care so they stay healthy. If you set a good example by taking care of your pet, your child will learn to treat animals well.

Q We'd like to get a pet, but want something a little unusual, not just a cat or dog. We're not sure what kind of pet would be most compatible with our children, ages 3 and 7. Are there any pets that could injure our children?

A Avoid large birds because they can bite small, probing fingers badly. Iguanas also bite and the force of their swinging tail can cause eye injuries. Iguanas and turtles also carry the bacterium salmonella, which your children can contract if they don't wash their hands after handling the reptiles. Snakes are not appropriate for younger children. Even hamsters and ferrets can bite small children if the animals are handled improperly; wait until your children reach adolescence before you buy them a hamster or ferret. Whatever pet you buy, follow your veterinarian's recommendations for good care.

outlet; buy only battery-operated toys. Teach older children how to use electric toys properly and cautiously, and supervise them until you feel they can play safely on their own.

- Carefully examine toys that have mechanical parts such as springs, gears, or hinges that could trap a child's hair, clothing, or fingers.
- Don't allow your child to play with very noisy toys, including squeeze toys with unusually loud squeakers. Toy caps, noisemaking guns, and other loud toys can produce sounds loud enough to damage your child's hearing.
- Never give your child a toy gun that fires anything except water. BB guns can

cause disabling and fatal injuries. Don't give your child a gun that looks like a real gun; children have been killed by police who mistakenly thought the children had a real gun.

• Stay away from toys that fly, such as guided missiles, because they can cause serious eye injuries. Don't allow your children to play with adult lawn darts or any other sporting equipment that has sharp points.

• Don't give toys or pacifiers with long cords to an infant or very young child. The cord can become wrapped around the child's neck, causing strangulation. Never put a pacifier on a cord around a child's neck. Don't hang toys with long strings, cords, loops, or ribbons in cribs or playpens where they can entangle children. To avoid strangulation, remove a crib gym from your child's crib as soon as he or she can reach up or get up on his or her hands and knees.

• Make sure battery-operated toys have a secure battery compartment lid. Batteries can cause choking or intestinal injury if swallowed. Be especially wary of the button-sized batteries that operate talking books.

• Buy pacifiers that are made securely. Inspect all pacifiers to make sure that the nipple is made of good quality rubber or latex and that it is attached firmly to the holder. Discard all worn-out pacifiers.

PREVENTING BURNS

Children are at high risk of burns that are serious enough to require medical treatment, but most burns are preventable. A child can be burned by hot liquids, flames, chemicals, or electrical sources. Most fires that kill children under age 5 are started by children playing with matches or by faulty or improperly used space heaters or defective electrical wiring in the home.

Preventing scald burns Scald burns are caused by hot liquids or steam. Here are some steps you can take to reduce your children's risk of being scalded:

• Keep hot food and liquids at least 12 inches from the edge of a counter; it's easy for a small child to reach up and pull something down.

• Don't drink a hot liquid while holding a child on your lap.

• Check the maximum temperature setting on your hot water heater. It should be set at "low," "warm," or 120°F. You can also install antiscald devices in your shower and bathtub fixtures that stop the flow of water when the temperature exceeds 120°F. (If you rent, ask your landlord to take these precautionary measures.)

• Always test bathwater with your hand before placing your baby in the tub to make sure the water is not too hot.

• Always supervise young children in the bathtub to make sure they don't turn on the hot water. Buy faucet covers that prevent the hot water faucet from being turned on.

• Keep small children out of your kitchen while you are cooking.

• Taste hot food and liquids before giving them to your child to avoid burning his or her mouth.

- Avoid using tablecloths when you have toddlers; they can pull the cloth, and anything on it, down on themselves.
- Turn handles on pots and pans toward the back of the stove.
- Remove any stove knobs that are low enough to be within your child's reach.
- Use caution when cooking with the microwave oven. The food may feel cool on the outside but be scalding in the center. Because of this uneven temperature distribution, never heat infant formula or breast milk in the microwave. (Bottles with plastic liners may also burst when heated.) Punch holes in plastic wrap or loosely wrap foods before heating them to prevent steam from building up underneath the plastic. Never hold a child in your arms when removing hot items from the microwave or stove.
- Don't let your child use any kitchen appliance, including a microwave oven, without supervision until he or she is a teenager.

Preventing burns from fires Home fires are a major cause of injury and death in children under 9 years old. More people die from the smoke than from the flames of a fire, and smoke can overwhelm a child or adult in minutes. Take these precautions to prevent burns from fires:

- Never leave small children alone at home, even for a minute.
- Keep matches and cigarette lighters out of the reach of small children, preferably in a locked cabinet or drawer. A child as young as 2 years old can start a fire with a lighter. Buy only child-resistant lighters.
- If you smoke, never smoke in bed or when you're drowsy. Use large, deep ashtrays and carefully dispose of cigarette butts, matches, and ashes by putting water on them first. Before going to bed, check under and around couch cushions for cigarettes that may still be burning.
- Don't allow anyone wearing loose-fitting clothing near a stove, fireplace, or space heater.
- Check the labels on your child's sleepwear to make sure it is not flammable.
- Have your heating system checked and cleaned every year, and have gas appliances checked for leaks or other malfunctions.

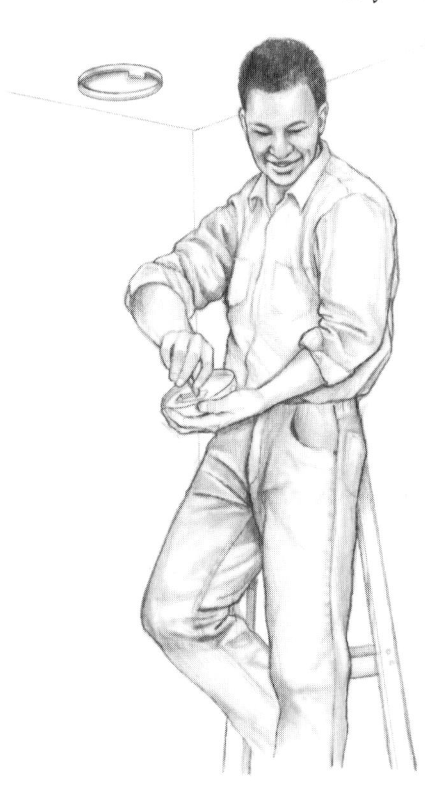

A smoke detector could save your child's life

Smoke detectors are small, battery-powered devices that sound an alarm when they detect fire or smoke. Install smoke detectors on every floor of your home—in the furnace room, at the top of stairways, near the kitchen, and near bedrooms. But your smoke detectors won't warn you if they don't have working batteries. Check the batteries every month but, to be safe, get in the habit of replacing them once a year—on your child's birthday. Never take a battery out of a smoke detector to use in toys, flashlights, or radios. Check the life expectancy of your smoke detector; some need to be replaced every 7 to 10 years.

Fire extinguishers in the home

Fire extinguishers are your first line of defense against small fires. They can save lives by putting out a small fire or containing it until the fire department arrives. Place fire extinguishers on each floor of your home in areas where the risk of fire is greatest, such as the kitchen, furnace room, and any room with a fireplace. Extinguishers should be placed in plain view, above the reach of children, close to an escape route, and away from a stove or heat source.

Fire extinguishers are classified by the types of fires they were designed to put out—those caused by paper and cloth, flammable liquids, or electrical equipment. Some fire extinguishers can fight all three types of fire; look on the package when purchasing a fire extinguisher for your home. Using the wrong kind of extinguisher can make the fire worse. Carefully read the instructions on the extinguisher and try it a few times so you'll know how to use it if you need to. Never use a portable extinguisher to fight a large or spreading fire. Call the fire department immediately.

Class of Extinguisher	Type of Burning Material
A	Ordinary combustibles such as cloth, paper, and wood
B	Flammable liquids such as grease, oil, gasoline, and oil-based paint
C	Electrical equipment such as wiring, appliances, fuse boxes, and circuit breakers

- Check electric appliances and cords regularly for wear or loose connections.
- Install a smoke detector on each floor of your home.
- Supervise children around a campfire or barbecue grill at all times. Never put lighter fluid into a barbecue grill that is already lit.
- Use a fire screen in front of your fireplace. If you have a wood-burning stove, set up a barricade around it to prevent your child from falling against it or touching it.
- If you need a portable heater to provide additional heat in a room, buy an electric one rather than one that runs on kerosene or gas. Make sure it has safety devices, such as an automatic switch that shuts off the heater if it gets knocked over and a thermostat that shuts it off if it gets dangerously hot. Keep the portable heater away from areas where children play and at least 3 feet away from beds and other furniture or from curtains. Teach your children to stay away from the heater.
- Never use flammable fluids, such as paint thinner, in an enclosed space, such as the furnace room.
- At Halloween, teach your children to keep their costumes away from the lit candles in jack-o'-lanterns.

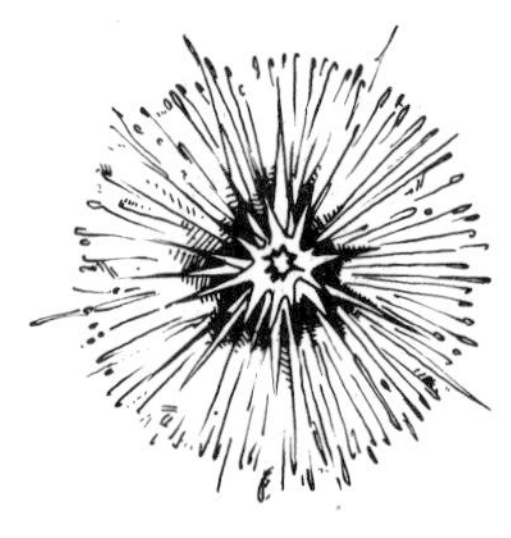

Enjoy fireworks from a distance

Each year, thousands of people are treated in emergency departments for fireworks-related injuries. All fireworks—even sparklers, which burn at very high temperatures—can cause severe injuries, including burns or loss of an arm, leg, or eye. The safest way to enjoy fireworks is to attend a local show given by professionals who are licensed and trained to use them safely.

Home fire drills Every family should have a fire escape plan. When your children are about 3 or 4 years old, get together as a family and work out an escape plan to follow in case of a fire. Be sure to decide who will take charge of each child. Draw a simple picture of your home, showing escape routes, including two ways to get out of each person's bedroom (most home fires occur at night). If you live in a high-rise building, show your children the shortest route to a safe exit and warn them not to use the elevator during a fire. If your house has more than one story or your apartment is on the second or third floor, you may also want to buy a portable ladder that you can store in your closet and hang over the window ledge for escape should the upper floor doors be blocked by fire.

Practice the escape plan often as a family—at night, practice with both the lights on and with them off—and include alternate escape routes. Designate a place outside your home for everyone to meet—pick a neighbor's house or a special place in your yard away from the house. Stress to your children that they should never go back into a burning house—no matter what. Nor should you or any other adult. During your fire drill, activate the smoke alarm so everyone knows what it sounds like. These measures save lives in a real fire.

Many young children die in fires because they try to hide from the fire, often under a bed or in a closet. To avoid the smoke of a fire, teach your children to get low by crawling on their hands and knees. If they are trapped in a smoky room, tell them to get low on the floor, cover their mouths and noses, and shout their name continuously so you can find them. If their clothes catch on fire, they should immediately stop moving, drop to the floor, and roll over and over to smother the flames. Have them practice to "Stop, drop, and roll."

WATER SAFETY

Young children can drown easily, even in shallow water. Drowning is a leading cause of death in children under age 4. Most drownings occur when a child falls into a pool or is left alone in a bathtub. Follow these guidelines to protect your child from drowning:

- Never leave a young child alone or with a sibling in the tub—not even if he or she is in a bathtub seat. The seat is not a safety device and could tip over. If you have to answer the phone, wrap your child in a towel and take him or her with you.
- Empty the bathtub and all buckets completely after use. A child can drown in seconds in a household bucket filled with only 1 or 2 inches of water.
- Watch your child closely at the pool, beach, or lake.
- Keep the bathroom door closed at all times and install a toilet lid lock.
- Sign your children up for swimming lessons at about age 4 or 5. Younger children may forget how to swim and are at a higher risk for ear and respiratory infections from swallowed water. Knowing how to swim does not mean that your child is safe in the water without adult supervision.

Home swimming pool safety

Each year in the United States, hundreds of children under age 5 drown in home swimming pools—usually while being supervised by one or both parents. Toddlers often do unexpected things. It only takes a second for a child to become submerged in a pool—without a splash or screams for help. Some simple measures can reduce the risk of an accident. Put off getting a home swimming pool until your child is at least 5 years old. If you already have a pool, make sure it has a 5-foot-high fence around all four sides, completely separating it from your house and the rest of the yard. Don't use your house as one of the side barriers. The fence should have gates that close and latch automatically and the latches should be higher than your child can reach. Never leave your child alone in or near the pool, even for a second. Keep rescue equipment, such as life preservers, by the pool, as well as a telephone and emergency phone numbers.

- Never allow your children to swim without adult supervision. Make sure the adult who is responsible for watching your child knows how to swim and knows how to perform cardiopulmonary resuscitation (CPR) (see page 668).
- In the winter, caution your children against walking on frozen lakes, rivers, and streams. Make sure they understand the risk of drowning by falling through thin ice.
- When boating, make sure your child wears a regulation life jacket at all times, one that is the right size and worn properly, but remember that a life jacket is no substitute for adult supervision. Never drink alcohol in a boat—whether you're the driver or a passenger.

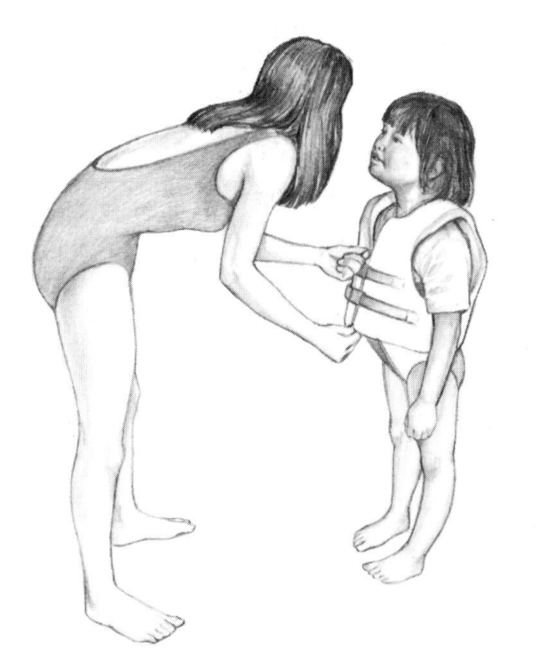

Always put a life preserver on your child near water

A life jacket, or life preserver, can mean the difference between life and death for a child who falls into water. When buying a life jacket for your child, look for one that has been tested by Underwriters Laboratories (UL) and approved by the US Coast Guard (check the label). Make sure the jacket is the right size and type for your child—younger children need a life jacket with a head support so they can float face up. Your child needs to wear the life preserver whenever he or she is in a boat or near any body of water. Put the life preserver on your child yourself so you can make sure he or she is wearing it the right way, but teach your child how to put it on and encourage him or her to wear it in the water to get used to the feel of it. Don't let young children or those who can't swim use inflatable toys, rafts, mattresses, or arm "bubbles" instead of life preservers in water above their waist because these articles are not lifesavers.

Pedestrian safety

One out of four people who dies in a traffic accident is a child under age 16 who is a pedestrian. Half of these deaths occur between 4:00 PM and 8:00 PM, when children are walking home from school and adults are driving home from work. Start teaching your children about street safety as soon as you begin taking walks together–each time you cross the street with your child can be an opportunity for learning. Don't allow your child to cross the street alone until he or she is at least 9 to 10 years old and has developed the judgment to cross safely. Here are some safety rules to teach your young pedestrian:

- When crossing the street, always hold hands with a grownup.
- Never run into the street; drivers can't see a small child over the hood of a car.
- Stop at the curb or edge of the road before crossing a street; cross only at crosswalks or intersections. Obey all traffic signals.
- Listen and look for traffic–look to the left, to the right, and to the left again. (If your child is too young to know left and right, tell him or her to look "this way," "that way," and "this way" again.)
- Wait until the street is clear before starting to cross and keep looking both ways for traffic until you reach the other side.
- Never run in a parking lot because cars may be turning into a lane or parking in a vacant spot. Always look both ways before crossing lanes in a parking lot.

School bus safety

A school bus is generally a safe means of transportation but injuries can occur. Teach your child these rules to make the bus ride a safe everyday experience:

- Wait for the bus away from traffic and at least 3 feet away from the curb.
- Don't run to the curb when the bus comes; wait until the bus comes to a complete stop and the door opens before starting to board.
- Open windows in the bus only if the driver has given permission to do so. Always keep hands, arms, and head inside the bus.
- Don't distract the bus driver; he or she needs to pay attention to driving.
- When exiting the bus, move away from the bus immediately. Don't take things from or hand things to students who are still on the bus.
- Tuck in scarves and keep book bags and purses close to the body so they don't get caught in the school bus door.
- Once you sit down, stay seated for the entire ride. If your bus has seat belts, fasten yours right away. Push your bottom all the way to the back of the seat.

If your child has to cross the street after getting off the bus, teach him or her to follow these additional rules:

- After getting off the bus, walk away from the bus and about 10 steps in front of it on the shoulder or sidewalk.
- Wait until the bus has come to a complete stop.

Playground safety check

Playgrounds are designed to be fun but, during their excited play, children can fall off of monkey bars or slides, be hit by swings, or get cut on loose nails and screws. When you take your child to a park, watch him or her closely at all times. Warn your child never to go near a swinging swing. If your child goes to a friend's house to play, make sure the swing set is safe. If it isn't, don't allow your child to play on it; invite the playmate to your home instead. In backyards and public parks, check playground equipment for basic safety features.

- The surface under play equipment should contain at least 12 inches of wood chips, double-shredded bark mulch, or pea gravel; 10 inches of fine sand; or a rubber outdoor mat that meets safety specifications.
- The shock-absorbing ground surface should cover an area that extends 6 feet from the equipment in all directions.
- All screws and bolts should be capped and nuts and bolts secure; be sure no hardware protrudes.
- All edges should be rounded and smooth to avoid cuts.
- The equipment should sit on a level surface and be anchored firmly to the ground.
- Swing seats should be made of soft material, not wood or metal; swings should be at least 2 feet apart and at least 2½ feet from an adjacent support structure.
- No tree roots, stumps, rocks, or concrete footings should be sticking out of the ground.
- Elevated surfaces that are more than 30 inches above the ground—including platforms, ramps, and bridges—should be surrounded by guardrails.
- Openings in guardrails and spaces between platforms and between ladder rungs should be smaller than 3½ inches or larger than 9 inches.
- Moving pieces of equipment—such as suspension bridges, track rides, merry-go-rounds, or seesaws—should have no accessible parts that could crush or pinch a child's fingers.

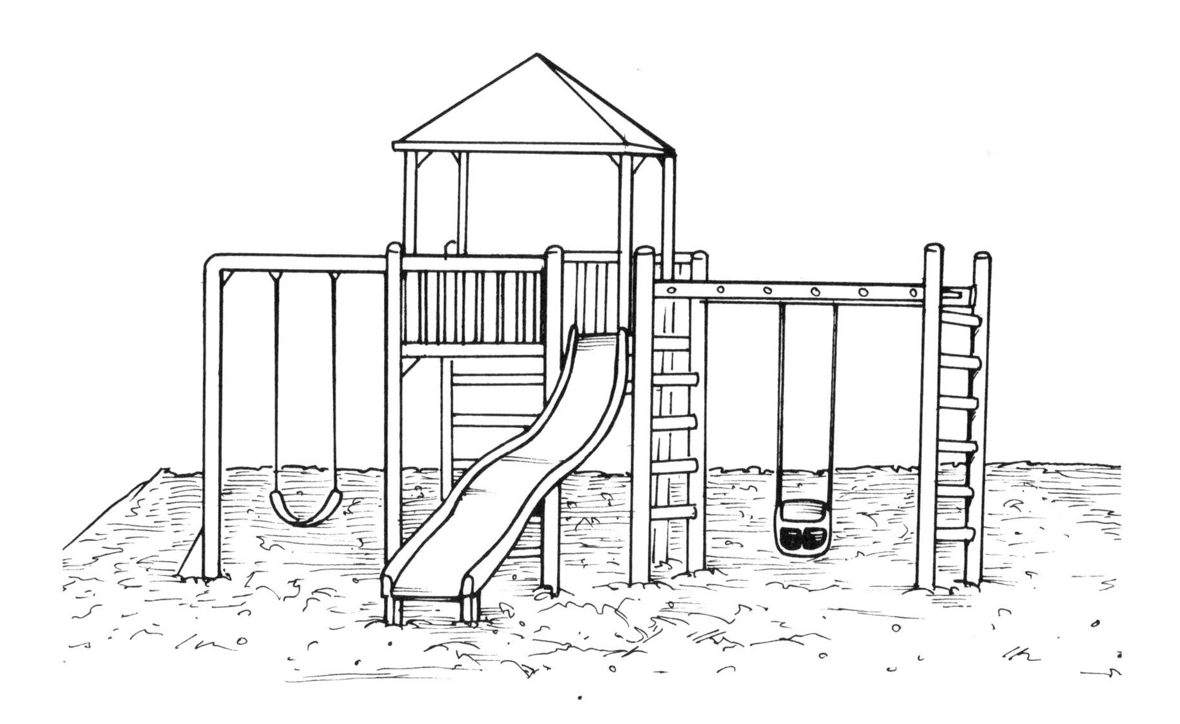

School bus safety

When a school bus stops on the side of the street, it can prevent passing drivers and even the bus driver from seeing around it. Unless they are getting on and off the bus, children should stay at least 10 feet away from it on all four sides (shaded area). The most dangerous areas are those that are out of the view of the bus driver–close to the front of the bus and on the right side, along the back.

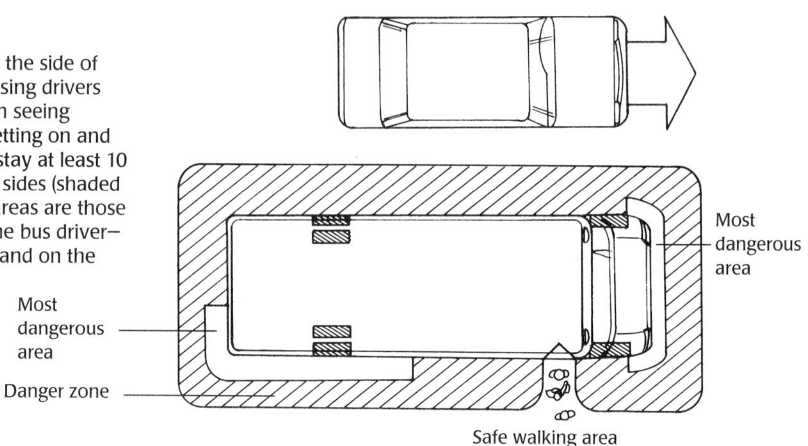

• Check to make sure the red lights at the top of the bus are flashing and the stop arm is extended. Watch for a sign from the driver that it is OK to cross.
• As you reach the edge of the front of the bus, before crossing the street, look for traffic in both directions. Walk across the street slowly–don't run–continuing to look both ways for traffic.

BICYCLE SAFETY

Every child takes a tumble from a bicycle once in a while, especially when just learning how to ride. But your child could sustain a serious head injury (see page 507) resulting in permanent disability after a fall from a bike or from being hit by a car while on a bike. Make sure your young bike rider always wears a helmet to protect his or her head. Buy a bicycle that fits your child properly (see page 317). Take these additional steps to help your child avoid injuries while riding his or her bike:
• Buy a helmet that fits your child's head (see page 318) and check the label to make sure it is marked ANSI, ASTM/SEI, Snell, or CPSC, the accreditations that ensure a high standard of safety. Bring your child with you to pick the helmet out so you can check for proper fit. Then make sure your child always wears the helmet–no matter how short the ride (even up and down the driveway). He or she should wear the helmet low on the forehead, not tilted up. Always wear your own helmet when riding to set a good example for your child.
• Don't push your child to ride a two-wheeler until he or she is ready–usually at about age 5 or 6. Don't switch to a bike with hand brakes until your child is an older and experienced rider.
• Don't allow your children (even older ones) to ride their bike at dusk or at night. Tell them to call home for a ride instead.
• Don't allow your child to wear headphones while bike riding because they reduce the ability to hear the sounds of traffic.

• Don't allow a child under 8 years old to ride in the street. Young children don't have the skills needed to recognize and avoid potentially dangerous traffic situations. Children between 8 and 12 years of age should ride in the street only when accompanied by an older teenager or an adult.
• Teach your child that bicycle riders must obey the same traffic rules that drivers follow.

Rules of the road for safe cycling To make your child's bicycling an enjoyable and safe activity, train him or her to follow these rules of the road:
• Ride near the curb in the same direction as traffic.
• Always ride single file.
• Before turning, always give a hand signal to alert drivers and pedestrians.
• Before entering the street from a driveway, sidewalk, alley, or parking lot, or when crossing an intersection, always stop and look left, right, and left again. Children under age 12 should walk, not ride, a bike through intersections.
• Obey all stop signs and traffic lights.
• Look back and yield to traffic coming from behind before turning left at an intersection.
• Never ride double or attempt stunts on a bicycle.

Buying the right bike
When buying a bicycle for your child, choose one that is the right size for your child at the time—not one that he or she can "grow into." Riding a bike that is too large can be dangerous. Bring your child with you to try it out. He or she should be able to put the balls of both feet on the ground while sitting on the seat. Make sure the bike has reflectors on the front and rear, on the pedals, and on both wheels.

Children as bicycle passengers Doctors and safety experts warn parents never to place their children on the back of a bike or allow their children to be taken for a ride on anyone else's bike. A child on the back of a bike makes the bike unstable and increases the amount of time it takes to stop. Even during a slow ride, an accident can cause severe injury to a child. If you choose to take your child for a ride on your bike, ride at a slower-than-usual speed and only in parks or on bike paths or quiet streets. Never ride in bad weather and don't carry your child in a backpack or frontpack while riding on your bike.

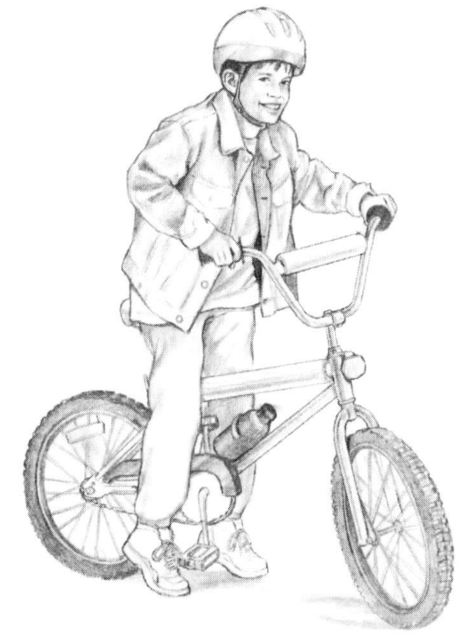

Children younger than 1 year are too small to ride on the back of a bike, and children older than age 4 or 5 are too heavy to ride as passengers. For children between 1 and 4 years, use a rear-mounted seat that is securely installed over the rear wheel. The seat should have spoke guards to prevent the child's feet and hands from being caught in the wheels, a high back, and a sturdy shoulder harness and lap belt. Before you get on the bike, make sure that your child is securely strapped into the seat and is wearing a bike helmet that meets ANSI, ASTM/SEI, Snell, or CPSC standards of safety.

When your child rides in a bicycle buggy that is towed behind your bicycle, strap your child into the buggy securely and put a bicycle helmet on his or her head. Attach a flag to a pole on the back of the buggy to alert other riders and drivers. Ride only on a bike path or quiet street.

Sports safety

As greater numbers of American children participate in organized and recreational sports, they become susceptible to more sports-related injuries. Bicycle riding, in-line skating, and skateboarding are the solo sports that cause the most injuries. In team sports, children are most likely to be injured from falling or being struck by another player or piece of equipment. Wearing protective equipment can greatly reduce the risk of sports injuries, so teach your young athletes the importance of wearing protective gear. If you engage in sports with your child, wear your protective equipment too, to set a good example. Of course, even with protection, children can get injured if they use poor judgment or behave recklessly.

Bicycle helmets save lives

Bicycle helmets protect a child's head and brain by absorbing and distributing the impact of a crash. Buy a bicycle helmet for your child when you buy his or her bike and be sure your child wears it every time he or she rides a bike. Always wear your own helmet when riding a bicycle. When buying a bicycle helmet for your child, look for one with a sticker that has the Snell, CPSC, ASTM, or ANSI label, indicating that the helmet has passed rigorous safety tests.

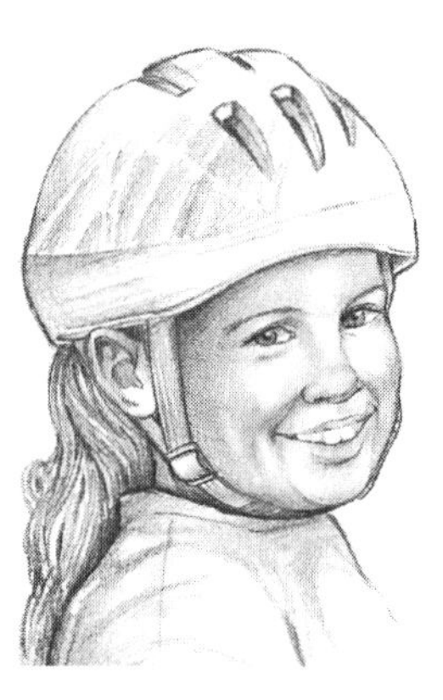

Bicycle helmets: Getting a good fit

A bicycle helmet will protect your child in a fall or crash only if it fits properly. The helmet should sit level on the child's head—not forward or back. It needs to be comfortable and snug but not tight; most helmets come with adjustable pads that can accommodate some growth. Always fasten the strap and make sure it's tight; you shouldn't be able to get the helmet off without unfastening it.

In-line skating

In-line skating has become extremely popular but it is also a major cause of sports-related injuries. The wrist, lower arm, and elbow are most vulnerable to injury, when a skater holds out a hand to break a fall. Before you buy skates for your child, rent a pair and have him or her take a lesson or two to learn how to stop and how to fall. Tell your child to be careful on sidewalks, where uneven surfaces can cause loss of control. Don't allow your young skater to skate in the street. Older children who skate in the street need to follow the same traffic rules bicyclists do.

When choosing a skate, look for one with wheel bearings that have a rating from the American Bearing Manufacturer's Association. (Look for the rating on the bearing itself, on the package, or in package inserts.) The rating indicates that the bearings allow the wheels to spin freely. A good fit is also important. In-line skates should be more snug than shoes—your child's toes should just touch the inside front of the boot (but the child should still be able to wiggle the toes). When your child bends his or her knees, the heels shouldn't lift up.

Gear up for skating safety

Every time your child skates, even if it's just in the driveway, make sure he or she wears the safety equipment shown here. It's best to put the gear on before putting on the skates. Your child can use his or her bicycle helmet for head protection. The child also needs to wear knee and elbow pads and wrist guards in his or her size; buy them with the skates.

Baseball

Millions of children play T-ball, baseball, and softball. But each year, many young players end up in hospital emergency departments with injuries. Using the newer baseballs that have a softer core and newer batting helmets that have face guards can help prevent or reduce many of these injuries and their severity. If your community league doesn't yet have helmets with face guards, ask about getting them. Boys should wear an athletic cup to protect their genitals.

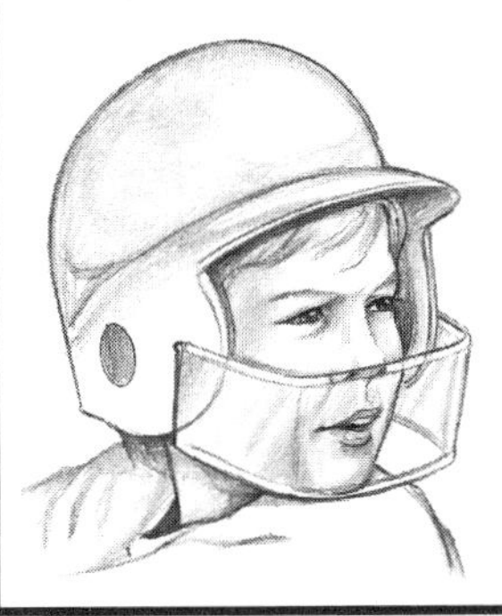

Newer, safer baseball equipment

Most organized community baseball leagues require that all players wear a protective helmet whenever they are up to bat or running bases. The use of helmets—especially those with face guards—has greatly reduced head injuries in young baseball players.

Football

Thanks to improvements in football equipment and coaches who teach their players proper techniques, football has become a safer sport for children. The helmet is the most important piece of safety equipment for football players. Football players should also wear pads on their shoulders, knees, thighs, and hips and tailbone (and girdles over the hip padding to keep it from slipping); vests to protect their ribs; shoes with rubber cleats; and a mouth guard. Boys should wear an athletic cup to protect their genitals. Neck rolls or support shields are also available to prevent the child's neck from bending too far back upon impact with another player.

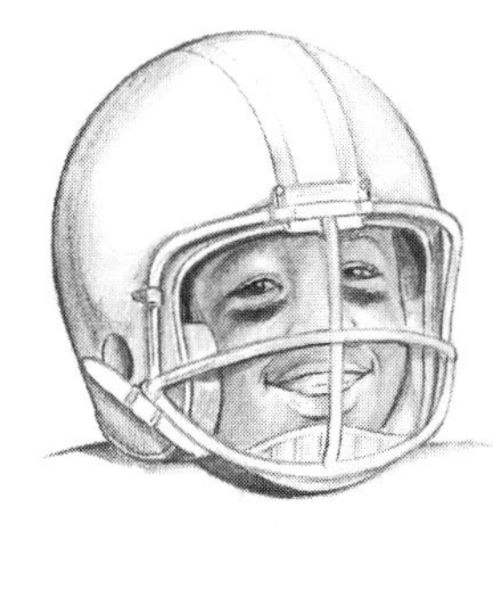

A football helmet that fits

In a properly fitting football helmet, there should be a 1-inch gap between the child's eyebrows and the bottom edge of the helmet. The helmet should fit snugly; inflate the liner on the inside of the helmet to make it snug. If the helmet is hard to put on, have your child remove the jaw pads and reinsert them once the helmet is on. The chin strap must be centered and snug against the chin; if it isn't, your child should ask the coach to tighten it.

Safe skateboarding

Many young skateboarders do not have the balance and body control needed to react quickly enough to prevent injury. Experienced riders can fall while trying difficult stunts. Many sprains, fractures, cuts, and bruises can be avoided by wearing protective equipment, keeping the board in good condition, and avoiding irregular riding surfaces. Instruct your skateboarder never to ride in the street and never to ride holding onto a moving object such as a bike or car.

Check out your child's skateboard to make sure it's safe. Look for loose, broken, or cracked parts; sharp edges; a slippery top surface; or wheels with nicks or cracks. Your child should wear the same protective gear recommended for in-line skaters—a bicycle helmet, knee and elbow pads, and wrist guards. He or she should also wear sturdy, slip-resistant shoes (no sandals), special padded jackets and shorts, and skateboarding gloves to absorb the impact of a fall. Tell your skateboarder to check the riding surface for holes, bumps, rocks, sand, or debris.

Mouth guards

Whenever children participate in activities that put them at risk of falling or bumping their head, they should wear a mouth guard. Mouth guards are made of soft plastic that protects the teeth, lips, cheeks, and tongue. Customized mouth guards provided by a dentist are more expensive than those bought over the counter, but they fit the mouth better—and a proper fit is essential for good protection. Ask your child's dentist which type of mouth guard is best for your child.

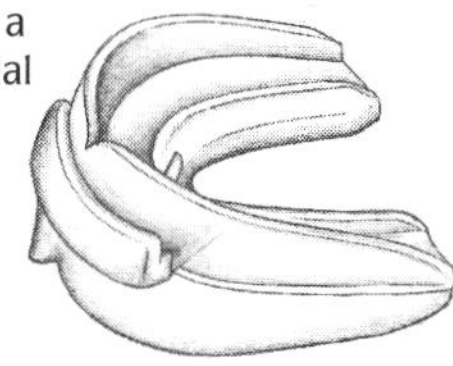

GUN SAFETY IN THE HOME

Half of all homes in the United States contain a gun but statistics show that the personal risk of owning a firearm far outweighs the potential benefits. A person living in a home with a gun is 18 times more likely to be killed with the gun than a stranger. A gun in the home is more likely to injure a child than to protect him or her. Most children who unintentionally kill themselves or others while playing with a gun find the weapon in their home. For these reasons, the best way to protect your child against a gunshot injury is to avoid having guns in your home, especially if any member of your household is depressed, has talked about suicide, is a troubled teenager, is violent toward others, abuses alcohol or other drugs, or has Alzheimer's disease. Explore other ways of protecting your home and family, such as alarms, dead-bolt locks, reinforced bars on windows, additional outdoor lighting, and a guard dog.

If you choose to keep a firearm in your home, reduce the risk of injury and death by keeping it unloaded (with the safety lock on) and stored in a locked cabinet or drawer. Make sure the key is available only to responsible adults because children who know where guns are kept may be tempted to show them off to their friends. Store ammunition in a separate locked cabinet. Teach your children never to touch a gun and tell them what to do if they find one (don't touch it and immediately come and tell you or another adult), even if they aren't sure whether it's real or a toy. Before your child visits the home of a friend or a baby-sitter, ask if there is a gun in the house. If there is, don't allow your child to go there. Instead, invite your child's friend or the baby-sitter to your home.

Handling and storing tools safely

Garden and home repair tools are a common cause of injuries in adults and children. Store all implements out of the reach of your child and be aware of his or her presence while you are using them. When your child is old enough to use these tools, teach him or her how to use them safely and always supervise their use. Certain items—nailers used to install drywall, power tools such as staplers and drills, and work tables with saws—should not be used by children under any circumstances. The following guidelines can help you and your children avoid injuries from common household tools:

- Store all tools out of reach of children. Always put them away after using them.
- Never use a tool without checking to see where your child is first.
- Always wear goggles and gloves to set a good example for your child.
- Use a power lawn mower with a control that can stop the mower if you release the handle. Never leave the mower unattended.
- Don't allow anyone to be in the yard while you are mowing the lawn. A mower can throw sticks, rocks, and other debris, causing serious injury.

Protecting your children from violent crime

Many parents worry that their child may become the victim of a violent crime, such as kidnapping or sexual assault. Unfortunately, increasing numbers of American children are becoming exposed to acts of violence–against themselves, a family member, or a friend. Violent acts can have harmful, long-lasting effects on a child's physical and mental health and quality of life. The best way to protect your child from harm is to teach him or her some basic safety rules and to make sure that he or she understands and follows them.

AVOIDING DANGEROUS CIRCUMSTANCES

You can teach your child how to avoid potentially dangerous situations and what to do if he or she gets into frightening circumstances. As soon as your child is old enough to understand, teach him or her the following safety measures:

- How to give his or her name, address, and phone number (by age 4 or 5).
- Safe routes for walking in the neighborhood and to and from school. He or she should always walk with a friend and walk only in well-lighted, busy areas.
- If your child comes home to an empty house after school, he or she should immediately call you (or another adult).
- If your child gets separated from you in a public place, instead of wandering around looking for you, he or she should go immediately to the checkout counter, security office, or the lost-and-found and tell the person in charge that he or she is lost. On outings, designate a meeting place in case you get separated.
- Never get into a car or go anywhere with anyone unless you have said it is OK to do so.
- If someone follows your child, to stay as far away from that person as possible and to run for help.
- If someone tries to take your child somewhere, to scream or yell and run away.
- To be suspicious of and get away from anyone who asks for directions.
- If someone your child doesn't know well wants to take his or her picture, to refuse and tell you or a trusted adult.
- To tell you, a teacher, other trustworthy adult, or the police about any observed crime or suspicious activity or to call 911 or the emergency number in your area for help.
- To not allow anyone except a doctor, or a baby-sitter helping him or her with a bath, to see him or her unclothed and to not let anyone touch him or her inappropriately.

Here are some things you can do to help keep your child safe:

- Know where your child is at all times. Become familiar with his or her friends and daily activities and routines.
- Don't leave children and young teens alone and unsupervised after school.
- Make sure your child always has enough money to make a phone call in case

he or she needs to call you for a ride home. Teach your child how to make a collect call from a pay phone so he or she can call in the event the money gets lost.

- Be sensitive to changes in your child's behavior; if you notice anything unusual, sit down and talk about it.
- Be alert to a teenager or adult who is paying an unusual amount of attention to your child or giving him or her inappropriate or expensive gifts.
- Teach your child that no one should approach him or her in a way that makes your child feel uncomfortable; if someone does, he or she should tell you immediately. Teach your child that he or she has the right to say "no" to anything that seems wrong.
- If you can't pick your child up from day care, make sure that the day-care attendants know who will be picking him or her up in your place; use a code word that only you, the caregivers, and your child know to identify the designated person.
- Always ask a specific person to be responsible for your child if you leave the area, even for a moment; make sure the child knows who is in charge.
- More children are kidnapped or harmed by people they know than by strangers. While you should teach your children to beware of strangers, you also need to instruct them to be alert to uncomfortable situations with people they know well and to tell you about them immediately.

HARASSMENT AND VIOLENCE AT SCHOOL

For some children, school has become an uncomfortable and even dangerous place. Children may be afraid to go to school because they feel intimidated by their peers. Other students may even carry knives or guns. School violence threatens a child's physical and emotional well-being and undermines the ability to learn. If your child seems reluctant to go to school, he or she may have a good reason. Talk to your child to find out what is going on at school and intervene early to prevent the situation from getting out of control.

Tell the school authorities about any incidences of violence, intimidation, or harassment that your child is aware of and work closely with them to try to resolve the situation. Once you are satisfied that the problem has been solved, insist that your child return to school. The longer your child stays out of school, the more anxious he or she is likely to become and the longer his or her progress will be disrupted. If your child continues to have problems dealing with a given situation, ask for help from a school counselor or a social worker.

TEACHING NONVIOLENT PROBLEM SOLVING

Children can be seriously affected by violence they witness at home, including violence on television. Children who are victims of violence or who have witnessed violent acts are more likely to become violent or aggressive adults. Teach your child how to express his or her emotions without hurting someone else and how to solve problems without resorting to violence.

As a parent, you need to teach your child the difference between assertiveness and aggression. You want your child to be assertive so he or she can stand up for himself or herself without becoming overwhelmed or afraid. But aggressiveness can lead to hurtful or destructive actions. The following guidelines can help you teach your child to distinguish between these two forms of behavior:

- Give your children consistent love and attention. A loving, nurturing relationship with a parent or other adult is essential for healthy development and for making children feel secure and trusting.
- Make sure your children are supervised at all times. Children need adult supervision and guidance so they can learn how to think for themselves. When they get older, such guidance will help them withstand peer pressure to engage in risky or dangerous activities.
- Teach your children positive problem-solving skills. Tell them how to settle arguments through talking instead of through physical violence, and to treat every person with respect.
- Don't use physical punishment. Physical punishment may stop your child from misbehaving today, but it is not effective in the long run. If you hit, slap, or spank your child, he or she may think that hitting other people is a good way to solve problems. Ask your doctor about more positive and effective methods of discipline (see page 126). Try "catching" your child being good and reward him or her for it. Children respond well to positive reinforcement.
- Limit your children's exposure to violence in the media. Seeing a lot of violence on television, in the movies, or in video games can cause a child to behave aggressively toward others. Limit your child's television viewing to nonviolent programming that is appropriate for his or her age. Monitor the type of television shows and movies your child sees and screen the video games he or she plays. Talk with your child about the differences between media violence and violence in real life. Watch television shows and movies with your child and explain that what happens on the screen is not real—for example, that, in reality, guns can kill or seriously injure people.
- Don't allow your child to carry weapons in self-defense. Guns and knives carried for protection can easily be taken and used against your child.

Child abuse

Child abuse—physical abuse, neglect, emotional abuse, and sexual abuse—is a growing problem in the United States. The abuse of children occurs in all socioeconomic, religious, and ethnic groups. Children most at risk are those under age 5 and those who are difficult to care for—premature infants; babies who cry excessively; and children who have a chronic medical condition, a physical or mental disability, or behavior problems. The people who care for the child, including biological or adoptive parents, foster parents, grandparents, boyfriends and girlfriends, baby-sitters, and siblings, are the most common abusers. Factors that increase a person's risk of abusing a child include substance abuse, loneliness, unhappiness, anger, poverty, youth, and being a single parent who did not plan the pregnancy. An adult who was abused as a child is more likely to become an abuser, and exposure to violence increases the likelihood that a person will commit abuse. Child abuse occurs most often in families that are under stress from the loss of a job or home, financial difficulties, marital problems, abuse of alcohol or other drugs, or a physical or mental illness. Families that are socially isolated and lack strong support systems are also vulnerable to child abuse.

PHYSICAL ABUSE, EMOTIONAL ABUSE, AND NEGLECT

Physical abuse is characterized by injury–bruises, burns, and broken bones–that occurs when a person punches, beats, kicks, bites, throws, or burns a child. In many cases, the abuser does not intend to hurt the child, but uses inappropriate physical force to discipline or punish him or her. Physical neglect is the failure to provide a child the basic needs–food, clothing, shelter, and a safe environment–that enable him or her to grow and develop normally.

Emotional abuse is much more difficult to detect than physical abuse, but can be just as damaging. Emotional abuse occurs when a caregiver hurts a child with negative words or behaviors, such as assigning blame to the child or rejecting, isolating, criticizing, or terrorizing the child. Emotional neglect occurs when a caregiver fails to nurture a child with the comforting and encouraging words and acts needed to promote healthy development. Exposing a child to a violent or sexually inappropriate environment is also an example of emotional abuse.

The physical and psychological effects of abuse on a child can be severe and long lasting. Abuse can affect brain development, intellectual capacity, and personality, and can influence a child's behavior and emotions throughout life. Abused children are more likely to experience delayed development of skills such as language and to have low self-esteem. They also display more aggressive behavior, are more unstable emotionally, and have an extremely high risk of depression (see page 467). Child abuse can also cause physical disability, failure to thrive (see page 485), and long-term health problems. Some abused children develop posttraumatic stress disorder (see page 416), producing irritability and sleep problems (including nightmares). Children with posttraumatic stress disorder may have frequent flashbacks (vivid memories) of their experience and may develop physical symptoms when reminded of the traumatic experience.

Recognizing the signs The first step in getting help for an abused child is to recognize the possible signs of abuse. The most common indications include:

- Repeated or unusual injuries that cannot be explained
- Showing fear of a parent or other adults

Never shake a baby

Never shake your baby in anger. You may think that shaking the baby is less harmful than slapping, but shaking can seriously injure your baby. A baby's head is heavy in relation to his or her body and an infant's neck muscles are not yet strong enough to support his or her head. If you shake a baby, you can strain his or her neck muscles and upper spine. Shaking or throwing the baby down in anger can also cause serious brain and eye injuries, which could result in loss of vision, brain damage, or even death.

- Injuries in unusual areas of the body including the stomach, back, buttocks, back of the hands, cheeks, ears, or mouth
- Injuries with characteristic marks left by an object such as a belt, hand, electric cord, cigarette, or iron
- Behavior problems–being passive and withdrawn or hyperactive and aggressive–or changes in behavior
- Persistent sadness or frequent crying
- Showing inappropriate affection, such as sexual advances
- Signs of reticence or fear when asked about life at home
- Self-destructive, delinquent, or reckless behaviors such as substance abuse, crime, multiple sexual encounters, or running away from home
- Low self-esteem
- Learning problems and lack of motivation in school
- Neglected appearance
- Lack of interest in making friends or inviting schoolmates home
- Aggressive or violent acting out
- Depression
- Suicide attempts

Getting help If you suspect that a child you know is a victim of abuse, contact a local agency that provides services for children and families–child protection service agencies, welfare departments, public health authorities–or the police. Do not directly confront the parent or other person you suspect of abuse. The staff at the social service agency will respect the legal and confidentiality rights of the child and family.

If you have abused your own child or think you might be at risk of doing so, get help immediately. Talk to a friend, your doctor, or a member of the clergy. That person may refer you to a social worker or a program in your community designed to help families who are at risk of abuse. More and more communities have programs that provide home visitors who are public health nurses or nurses' aids who visit new parents and teach them how to care for their child in a nurturing way. Joining a self-help group, such as Parents Anonymous, where parents share experiences and learn positive coping skills and parenting techniques, can also be helpful. This kind of support, advice, and increased knowledge can help reduce the pressures within a family that could lead to abuse.

One of the many benefits of taking your child to regular well-child visits to the doctor (see page 237) is learning about each new stage of development as your child grows. Knowing what to expect of your child can help you avoid unnecessary disappointment that can lead to frustration and unwarranted discipline. Your child's doctor can also help you find alternatives to spanking and other physical forms of discipline (see page 126).

One of the most important ways to reduce the risk of abuse in your family is to learn how to prevent your anger from turning into violence in times of severe stress. For example, if you feel as if you are getting out of control, make yourself calm down by leaving the room, taking a walk, taking deep breaths, or counting to 100. Avoid alcohol and other drugs; use of these substances can reduce your ability to control your anger. Fatigue can also make you short-tempered. Take time for yourself; share child-care responsibilities with your partner, rely on relatives to help out, trade baby-sitting with friends who have children, or use day care. Sometimes all a parent needs to reduce the stress in his or her life is a break from the constant demands of small children.

SEXUAL ABUSE

Young children have a natural curiosity about their bodies and those of others. They may want to stare at, touch, and ask you about their bodies and about the differences between girls and boys. As a parent, you need to set limitations on their sexual curiosity and prevent any adult sexual contact and behavior with your child. If your child describes any sexual experience or genital contact with another child or an adult, you should suspect the possibility of sexual abuse.

Child sexual abuse is defined as forcing a child into sexual activity that gives the abuser sexual gratification. In addition to sexual intercourse, the abuse could include undressing, viewing, or fondling the child or photographing the child in the nude. Some abusers pressure the child into agreement with tricks, bribes, or threats. Most, but not all, sexual abusers are male. Incest (sexual activity between family members) is a common form of sexual abuse. Less frequently, a child may be abused by an acquaintance or stranger.

The abuser usually gains the child's trust and the trust of other family members, who are comfortable leaving the child alone with him or her. A growing number of abusers are now under the age of 16–adolescents who are going through puberty and decide to experiment sexually with a younger child who has been temporarily placed under their supervision.

Most children who are victims of sexual abuse feel confused, uncomfortable, and unwilling to talk about the experience to anyone, including their parents and teachers. They may be embarrassed, ashamed, and afraid that no one will believe them or might blame them for the abuse. If the abuser is a relative, they may fear getting the relative into trouble. The child may have been threatened or bribed to keep the abuse a secret. Sometimes children are too young to understand or explain what has happened to them.

Recognizing the signs If you have established an atmosphere of trust and support in your home, your child will be more likely to confide in you. Be alert to the following signs of sexual abuse in your child:

- Bruising, redness, swelling, discharge, or other signs of injury in the genital or rectal area
- Regressive behavior, such as bed-wetting, excessive clinging, or stool incontinence
- Frequent nightmares, fear of going to bed, or other sleep disturbances

- Acting out or an increase in hostile or aggressive behavior
- Fear of certain places, people, activities, or being alone with certain people
- Withdrawal from friends, family, or school activities
- Sexually seductive or promiscuous behavior or having an unusual amount of sexual knowledge or curiosity for his or her age

Long-term consequences Sexual abuse can have long-term effects. The children most severely affected are those who were abused by a parent because the abuse shatters the bond of trust that develops between a parent and a child. Adolescent girls who were sexually abused have a high risk of becoming runaways or prostitutes or of having an unplanned pregnancy. Boys may act out sexually or violently, or become abusive themselves. As adults, these children may have difficulty developing close relationships; many get involved in abusive relationships. Some women who have been victims of sexual abuse have a number of health problems that affect their reproductive and urinary systems. Adults who were sexually abused as children may also need to seek psychiatric help for conditions such as depression (see page 467), anxiety (see page 415), substance abuse (see page 475), or eating disorders (see page 478).

Preventing sexual abuse The most effective way to protect your child from sexual abuse is through education. Talk about ways to avoid sexual abuse in a nonfrightening, matter-of-fact way as early as possible–by about age 3. Teach your child the proper names and function of all of his or her body parts, including the genitals. Make sure your child understands that the parts of the body that are covered by a bathing suit are private and should not be touched by anyone except a doctor during a physical examination or (for very young children) by a parent or caregiver during bathing. Teach them the difference between acceptable and unacceptable behavior by an adult or child, including a close relative or family friend.

Tell your child that, if someone tries to touch his or her body or do anything else that makes him or her uncomfortable, the child should tell the person "no" and come and tell you right away. Your child should also tell you immediately about any secrets he or she has been asked to keep. Teach your child that showing respect for adults does not mean blindly following requests that are unreasonable or confusing.

Maintain an open, honest, and forgiving relationship with your child so he or she will feel comfortable telling you about anything without having to worry about being blamed or punished. Children are never to blame for sexual abuse because a child does not have the emotional maturity to consent willingly to sexual activity and must always be coerced into it by someone older. If your child tells you about a potentially abusive situation, make it clear to the child that you believe him or her. Try to get as much specific information as you can. Respect your child's privacy by not discussing the situation with people who do not need to know about it.

Getting help If you suspect your child may have been sexually abused, get help immediately. Call your child's doctor first. The doctor will evaluate your child's condition and treat any physical problem related to the abuse. He or she can also gather physical evidence and reassure the child that he or she is all right. The doctor may refer you to another doctor who specializes in treating sexually abused children.

Treatment depends on the type of sexual abuse, the age of the victim, the frequency of the abuse, and the identity of the abuser. Children who are abused by a parent usually need the most help because they were harmed by the very person who is supposed to love and protect them. Most abused children can benefit from individual and group therapy with a child psychiatrist, child psychologist, clinical social worker, or rape victim advocate. When choosing a counselor to work with your child, look for someone who has experience treating children who are the same age as yours. Ask the counselor how many sexually abused children he or she has worked with. Other members of the family may also benefit from counseling.

If the abuser is someone outside the family, report the abuse to the police, sheriff's office, district attorney's office, or other law enforcement agency. The agency receiving the report will conduct an investigation and do whatever is necessary to protect the child, including legally prosecuting the abuser.

Remember that, if your child's doctor suspects or becomes aware of any incident of child abuse, he or she is legally bound to report the incident to the proper legal authorities (which may differ depending on the state in which you live). Your child's doctor is interested only in protecting your child, not in pointing a finger of guilt at anyone in particular.

CHAPTER • 12

Your child's emotional health

Your child's emotional health is just as important as his or her physical health. A child who is loved and valued is likely to grow up to be a happy, well-adjusted adult. The family in which a child is raised has a powerful influence on the child's general feeling of well-being. Experiences and relationships within the family determine a child's sense of self, level of self-esteem, and ability to manage stress. But growing economic pressures, divorce, and an increase in the number of single-parent families are sources of stress and anxiety for many families in the United States today.

Boosting your child's self-esteem

Self-esteem is the value people place on themselves based on their beliefs about their abilities and strengths. This self-appraisal defines their character and guides their behavior. People with high self-esteem have confidence in their ability to make decisions, to cope with the challenges of life, and to be successful. The development of a positive self-image begins early in life and is influenced by a child's family, friends, and experiences. As a parent, you can help your child feel good about himself or herself by showing your unconditional love–responding to your infant's cries, kissing your young child's hurt knee, or reassuring your adolescent that you understand and admire him or her. To grow up to be a responsible, caring adult, your child also needs clearly defined rules of behavior that are enforced consistently and fairly.

Your child's early interactions with you and other caregivers–being touched, held, and rocked; being talked to and read to–will determine his or her sense of self-worth. When you respond sensitively to your children's needs, you foster a feeling of trust that will help them confidently explore the world and form positive relationships with other children and adults. You show them that they are important, that their needs and desires matter, and that their actions make a difference.

As children grow and develop, they gain self-assurance from doing things well. You can help your child develop confidence in his or her ability to meet the challenges of life by providing many opportunities to test himself or herself. Give tasks that your child can do on his or her own. Nurture persistence by encouraging your child to work hard to achieve a goal, such as overcoming an obstacle, learning a new skill, or finishing a difficult task.

Some stages of childhood are more difficult than others and can challenge a child's self-esteem. For example, when children start school, many doubt their abilities and fear leaving the security of their homes. During this period, it is especially important to let your child know that you have confidence in his or her ability to succeed in school. Point out specific milestones he or she has already reached. Early adolescence is another vulnerable time as young people undergo the dramatic physical and emotional changes of puberty. Self-esteem tends to fall for both boys and girls at this age because adolescents focus on their physical flaws, which may appear exaggerated and make them feel different.

When your child reaches these vulnerable ages, try to avoid criticizing him or her, even if you think your suggestions are helpful. Your child needs to know that you accept him or her the way he or she is. Help your child understand the things that can be changed, such as a hairstyle, and to accept the things that cannot be changed, such as height. Teach your child to value his or her strengths and not to dwell on weaknesses. You can do a lot to help your children develop a positive self-image:

- Be there. Ready availability of a parent or other caring adult can make a child feel secure and valued.
- Allow children room to explore. From infancy on, give your child as much room as possible to explore and test himself or herself, according to age and ability.

Pick your battles

Children who are constantly criticized by their parents may end up thinking they can't do anything right and may eventually stop trying. Adolescents need acceptance just as much as toddlers do. Set priorities when guiding your child's behavior. For example, enforcing house rules about curfew and homework are more important than disapproving of a current hairstyle or fashion. Don't forget to praise your child when he or she succeeds.

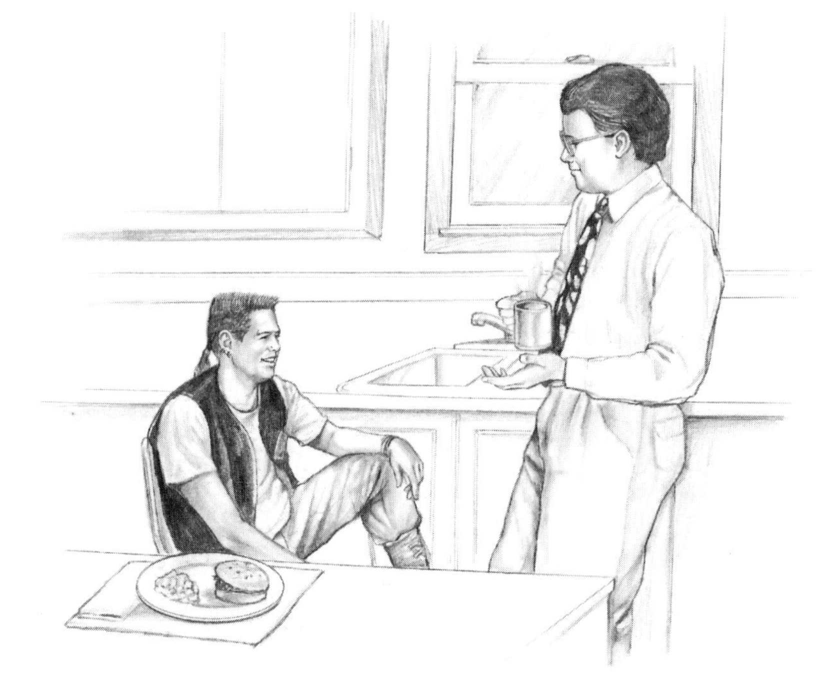

- Give positive feedback. Recognize and praise your child for good behavior, for achieving goals, and for making improvements. But try to avoid giving undeserved praise; it can prevent your child from learning from his or her failures.
- Choose your words carefully. When showing disapproval, say that the child's behavior is unacceptable or "bad"—never the child. Your child may not feel comfortable when he or she makes mistakes, but he or she should never feel defeated. Explain that setbacks are a normal part of life and that your child can learn from them.
- Respect your child's talents. Encourage him or her to develop them.
- Give choices. Let your child make some choices that are suited to his or her age and ability to nurture the capacity to make decisions.
- Have realistic expectations. Understand what your child is able to do so you don't expect either too much or too little from him or her.
- Encourage optimism. Instill optimism in your child by being optimistic yourself. Teach your child that a single defeat does not represent general failure and incompetence. Explain that setbacks are temporary and can be overcome.
- Assign chores. Give your child chores to do around the house so he or she can make a contribution to the household and learn to accept responsibility.
- Encourage self-evaluation. Help your child evaluate his or her work. Ask what he or she likes about it or what could be done to improve it.
- Play games with your children. Playing games helps improve a child's self-esteem, concentration, and planning skills. Set a good example of how to be a gracious loser. Put less emphasis on winning and more on improvement of skills.

Nurturing your child's personality

Children—even those in the same family—may not only look different but also have very different temperaments. Some are easygoing; others are hard to please. Some are curious; others are afraid to explore. Your child's basic temperament determines how he or she responds to circumstances and people and, in turn, how people respond to him or her. Personality and other character traits derive from both a child's environment—inside and outside the family—and his or her genetic makeup. If you have children who are different in temperament, you need to nuture each one's individuality. Don't try to change his or her disposition to conform to your preconceived ideas.

Some children are naturally extroverted. They are dynamic, verbal, become energized from being with other people, and crave interpersonal contact. Other children are inherently introspective, needing time alone to pursue their own interests. As a parent, you need to recognize your own child's temperament and provide the time with others or the time alone that your child needs. But it's important not to label your child. Keep in mind that there is a broad range of normal behavior. If your children are markedly different from one another, their difference isn't good or bad—it's just different.

Children brought up in the same home—even those who are close in age—can have very different experiences. A first child receives plenty of attention until a baby brother or sister comes along, but a second child has to compete for attention from the beginning. That could be why your second child seems so demanding. A second child has an older sibling to look up to; a first child has someone to protect. These roles shape a child's personality, sometimes for life.

You and your partner may respond differently to your child because you have different expectations. Your feelings about your child's behavior are also influenced by your own upbringing, your biases about how girls and boys should behave, your educational background, and your own temperament and personality. There is no correct way to deal with a child—each parent's perspective is valid and usually springs from his or her own experiences with the child. The parent who spends 1 or 2 hours a day playing with a child will observe different behavior than the person who spends 8 hours a day with the child, running errands, preparing dinner, and giving a bath. At the same time, different parenting styles can bring out different responses from a child. Again, these responses help to form your child's distinct personality.

If you sometimes feel that your child is especially difficult to deal with, discuss your feelings with your partner, a close friend or relative, or your child's doctor. Sometimes just acknowledging negative feelings and talking about them can be helpful. Many parents have difficult children. Your child's doctor can help you identify the behaviors that bother you and find ways to cope with them constructively. For example, if your child has difficulty switching from one activity to another, you might prepare him or her with reminders that the activity is going to end at a certain time.

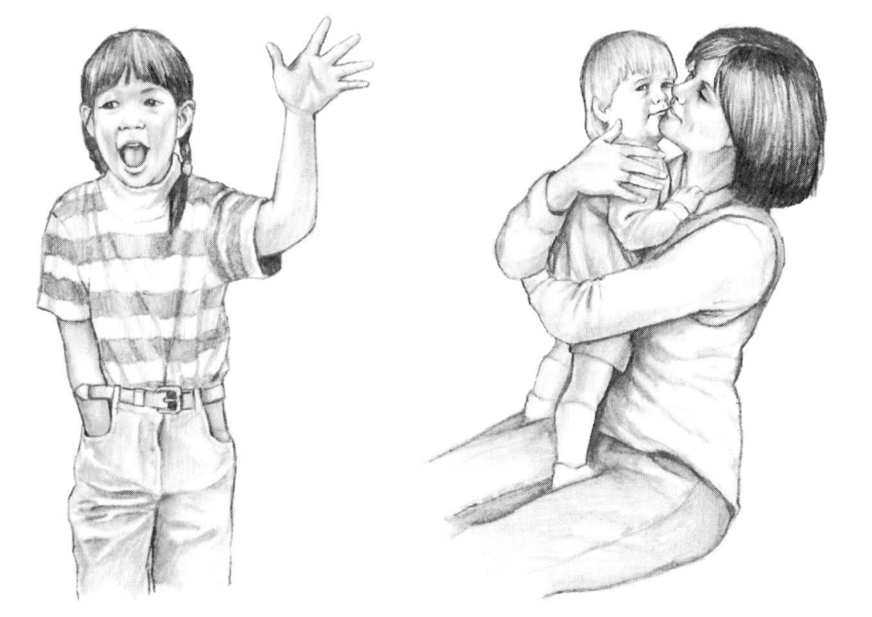

No two children are the same

Some children (near right) adapt easily to new situations and people. They quickly make friends and meet new challenges. Others (far right) are shy, quiet, reserved, and uncomfortable with new people or in new circumstances. Accept your child's individual personality and temperament. Encourage your child to develop his or her talents and pursue his or her particular interests.

The changing family

Families have changed dramatically in the last few decades. Although the two-parent, mom-at-home family is no longer the norm, a family can still be defined as a group of people living together who provide guidance and support for children or other dependent members. The family unit functions with clearly defined roles and rules for interaction that can have a powerful influence on a child's development. Different families have different ways of relating to each other, showing feelings (such as with a hug or kiss, or with just a smile or frown), solving problems, accomplishing daily tasks, and celebrating holidays and birthdays.

Ideally, the family will provide a loving, nurturing, secure environment for a child. Factors such as parents' income, education, employment, marital status, age, or sexual orientation alone do not determine the successful development of a healthy, happy, socially competent child. The most important factor is meeting a child's physical, emotional, social, and educational needs. Successful families tend to be supportive, adaptable, and communicative.

Circumstances such as divorce, the birth of a new child, or the death of a grandparent can disrupt the family. The increasing number of families in which both parents work outside the home, more single-parent families, and less support from the extended family and community put additional stress on families today. The stronger the family relationships, the easier it is to adapt to these changes.

SUPPORTIVE PARENTS

Your child's emotional health is closely linked to yours and your partner's and to the stability of your family. Successful parents are consistently warm, affectionate, sensitive, and responsive to their child's needs. Children who have good early relationships and whose families nurture, love, support, and value them have higher self-esteem, are better able to cope with stress, and have fewer problems such as delinquency, depression, and drug use during adolescence.

Children whose physical and emotional needs are not met or who experience rejection or harsh treatment come to view themselves as unworthy of love. They expect–and often get–further rejection. If you feel overwhelmed and concerned about your ability to care for your children, talk to your child's doctor. He or she can suggest things you can do to get help, such as attending parent support groups or talking to a therapist who can help you understand your feelings and teach you positive ways to cope with your circumstances.

When a parent becomes depressed

When a parent is depressed (see page 467), he or she affects every other member of the family. Depression can interfere with your ability to take care of your child, hindering his or her emotional and intellectual development. The illness can also interfere with your relationship with your partner, disrupting the stability of the family. Children exposed to excessive conflict in the home have a higher risk of developing behavior problems, difficulties in school, and problems getting along with peers. Depression is a serious condition that can almost always be treated. The earlier you seek treatment, the less emotional pain your child will experience.

SIBLING RELATIONSHIPS

Whenever a new child enters the family, he or she changes the dynamics of the family and the day-to-day routine of the household. An older sibling may feel jealous and insecure when a new baby arrives, especially if the older child is under 4 years of age. Toddlers don't want to share their parents with anyone else so they may feel threatened by all the attention paid to the new child. You can limit these feelings by preparing your child for the new sibling while you are pregnant. Tell your child as much as possible about what is going to happen in words that your child will understand. A good way to do this is to read books together about pregnancy and infant care, encouraging your child to ask questions as you read. Ask your child to help you prepare for the new baby–fixing up the baby's room, buying diapers, or picking out a crib.

Make any needed changes, such as moving your older child out of a crib or into a new room, several months before the baby is born. That way, your child will be less likely to connect the change with the baby and feel resentful. This is not the time to toilet train an older child or expect him or her to learn new skills, even if he or she appears ready to do so. Wait until the child has had a chance to adjust to the presence of the new baby; the first few months are the most crucial in helping a child accept a new sibling. Involve your older child in the excitement of the birth by having him or her come to the hospital shortly after the delivery. Make an effort to spend time alone with the older child each day–and encourage grandparents and other relatives and friends to do so. On initial visits, encourage friends and relatives to fuss over the older sibling's new big brother or big sister status and to pay less attention to the baby (who won't miss it anyway). This consideration will help minimize jealousy. Let your older child help out with the new baby and talk to the older child as you are caring for the infant. In response to the arrival of a new sibling, a young child may regress to behaviors such as thumb sucking during the adjustment period; accept this as a temporary need for comfort and give him or her a little extra attention. Encourage the child to talk about his or her feelings–both positive and negative–about the baby.

Adjusting to a new sibling

The arrival of a new baby can be difficult for an older sibling who now has to share his or her parents with another child. You can minimize your child's insecurity by encouraging him or her to help you care for the baby. A child who is 5 or 6 years old can learn to hold, feed, comfort, and play with an infant. As the baby grows and develops, he or she will look to the older child as a model.

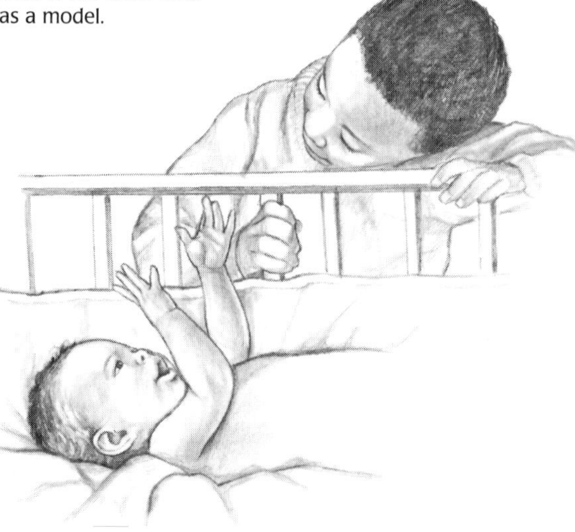

As siblings grow up together, they usually become close friends and companions. But they also bicker and fight–usually over possessions or privileges such as who gets to sit where in the family car. For the most part, these battles are normal and healthy and help children learn to share, to compromise, and to stand up for their rights. Make it clear to a younger child that some privileges given to an older child are based on his or her age only and that the younger child will eventually be given the same privileges. The following guidelines can help reduce sibling jealousy:

- Treat your children as unique individuals; avoid comparing them with each other or anyone else. Show each child that he or she is loved and valued. Listen to each child and spend some special time alone with each one whenever possible.
- Acknowledge your children's feelings and encourage them to talk about them. Explain that it is normal to get angry at a sibling but that it is not OK to be hurtful–physically or emotionally.
- Offer constructive alternatives to fighting, such as taking turns.
- Never show favoritism or take sides.
- Praise your children when they cooperate with each other.
- Divide household chores evenly among your children based on their ability. Make sure they all take turns doing tasks everyone dislikes.
- Allow your children to settle their own arguments. By staying out of their fights, you give them the chance to learn how to negotiate, solve problems, and compromise. Step in if a fight gets too loud, or if it degenerates into physical violence, breaking things, or name-calling. Set a good example for your children by settling your own disputes calmly and rationally.
- If you need to punish a child, do it privately.
- Discourage tattling. Encourage your child to tell you about safety concerns ("He keeps banging his truck against the glass door") but not about squabbles ("He called me names").

SINGLE-PARENT FAMILIES

More and more children in the United States live in single-parent homes for at least part of their lives. One out of four children is born to a single mother and many single mothers are still in their teens. More single women are choosing to adopt children or become pregnant, and many men gain custody of their children after a divorce. The idealized version of the family, in which children live with both parents, makes some children in single-parent homes feel as if their own family is second-rate. But the most important characteristics of a well-adjusted family are the relationships within the family and the children's sense of security and happiness.

Most single parents enjoy a rewarding family life. They often develop closer relationships with their children than do parents in traditional two-parent families. Other relationships may become more important too–those with aunts, uncles, grandparents, teachers, and coaches. But being a single parent is always demanding. Many single parents have no one with whom to share the endless responsibilities waiting for them after work. If you are a single parent, it's important for you to take steps to prevent yourself from becoming physically and emotionally exhausted. If you are overwhelmed by the pressures at home and work, you won't be there for your children, who need you. It is in both your interest and your child's that you maintain some balance in your life.

Here are some guidelines for helping to prevent burnout:

- Set aside some time each day to unwind and rest—even though you feel you don't have any extra time. It's all right to let the housework go until later.
- Encourage your children to talk about their feelings to relieve concerns.
- Maintain consistent, fair discipline. Learn effective ways to guide your child's behavior by reading books about parenting or taking parenting classes.
- Get help and support from other people. Single parents and their children do better when they have a strong support system. Enlist grandparents, aunts, uncles, brothers, sisters, good friends, coaches, or members of the clergy. Choose people who can develop a supportive, trusting relationship with your child and who are willing to step in when you cannot. Join support groups such as Parents Without Partners. Web sites on the Internet can also help single parents to exchange experiences, parenting tips, and encouragement.
- Take care of your own needs. To be a good parent to your child, you need to feel good about yourself. Take time out from parenting to socialize with other adults and maintain and nurture friendships.
- Give your child household chores to take some of the burden off of yourself. But avoid asking him or her to take on adult responsibilities.
- Don't try to be a superparent. Don't feel guilty about what you can't do or give to your children.

CHILDREN AND DIVORCE

Although divorce is always difficult for children, it doesn't have to be debilitating. When parents place a priority on nurturing their children and helping them adjust, the children do just as well as those in two-parent families. In fact, the most important predictor of a child's long-term adjustment to divorce is the way in which his or her parents adapt to the situation. Children whose parents are divorcing have many different emotions. Most feel frightened, confused, angry, and insecure during the difficult transition or worried that their parents might abandon them. No matter how bad their parents' relationship was, all children view a breakup as a loss.

Depending on their age and stage of development at the time of a divorce, children will show their feelings in different ways. For example, preschoolers may seem afraid of being separated from a parent or of being with other people. They may also have temper tantrums, or develop sleeping, eating, or toilet-training problems. Some blame themselves for the divorce. School-age children may be moody, whiny, angry, distracted, aggressive, afraid to go to school, or have tantrums. They may talk about their sadness and how much they want their parents to get back together, and worry about dividing their loyalty between their parents. Intense anger is the predominant emotion in older children and adolescents, who usually take sides and place the blame on one of the parents. They may also withdraw from family and friends, become aggressive, worry about the financial effects of divorce, experience depression, and feel pessimistic about their own future intimate relationships. Many teenagers act out by engaging in harmful behaviors, such as using alcohol and other drugs.

After a divorce, you need to handle the new family dynamics with your child's best interests in mind. The following guidelines can help your child adjust to life after your divorce:

- Set aside old conflicts and focus on the well-being of your child. A child does best when both parents work together to establish firm guidelines, a consistent routine, and similar rules and discipline practices in both homes.
- Encourage your child to talk about his or her feelings. Avoid the temptation to tell your child how he or she should feel. Your child may withdraw and be less likely to share his or her feelings with you.
- Don't say negative things about the other parent. When you denigrate your ex-partner to your child, you will make your child feel caught in the middle. Your child will feel much better about himself or herself if he or she has a positive view of both parents.
- Encourage your child to have a good relationship with the other parent and allow as much contact as possible. Don't ask your child to choose one parent over the other.
- Don't use your child as an intermediary between you and your former partner. Communicate directly and privately with the other parent about matters such as scheduling visits, or school or discipline problems.
- Try to avoid custody battles. Custody disputes can make a child feel insecure about his or her future. Don't split up siblings unless an adolescent states a clear preference to live in a different home from his or her sibling.
- Don't expect your child to adjust quickly and easily to your dating. After a divorce, parents' dating relationships cause adjustment problems for children under the best of circumstances. During this transition, give your child lots of extra time and patience.
- Take care of your own needs. Your child will cope more easily if you are adjusting well yourself. If you have an especially hard time getting on with your life after a difficult divorce or separation, get help. Seek out community programs designed for single parents. If you feel hopeless, helpless, or worthless and find little enjoyment in anything, talk to your doctor. You may have depression (see page 467), which can be treated.

BLENDED FAMILIES

A blended family, or stepfamily, is one that includes an adult couple with one or more children from a previous relationship. The couple may be married or unmarried, or gay or straight. Half of all people in the United States will experience a stepfamily relationship at some time in their lives–as a stepparent, remarried parent, or stepchild.

A child in a blended family has strong emotional connections to a parent who lives in another household or to a parent who has died. In many cases, a child moves back and forth between two households that often have very different rules and expectations. This adjustment period can be even more stressful than a divorce or living in a single-parent home. Children may feel angry, anxious, or depressed because a parent's remarriage eliminates the hope that their mother and father will reunite. They worry that they won't be able to have as much contact with either parent.

Stepfamilies in which both adults have children from a previous relationship have the biggest problems to overcome. Children in such families may worry that their own parent will have less time to spend with them, that they will have to share their bedroom or possessions with a stepsibling they hardly know, or that their place in the family hierarchy will change (for example, from being the oldest or youngest in the original family to being a middle child in the stepfamily). Rules and daily routines may be different. All these new experiences can put stress on a child. Many remarried parents, who are caught up in their own romantic relationship, may not notice how disturbing the changes can be for their children.

During this period, your child may display his or her feelings through disruptive behavior. For example, your child may become withdrawn; angry or defiant; disruptive or destructive; have frequent temper tantrums or fight with siblings, stepsiblings, or friends. He or she may also perform poorly in school. Give your child time to adjust to the current situation, to become familiar with the new family members, and to get used to the working structure of the household. Stepfamilies who work together to solve problems eventually find a living arrangement they can all be happy with. Once you make it through the difficult early years, you will probably find that being part of a stepfamily is a rewarding, enriching, fulfilling experience.

The following tips can help make living in a stepfamily easier for everyone involved:

- Put a priority on the couple relationship; a secure relationship between the two adults is essential for a successful blended family. In many stepfamilies, couples spend so much time dealing with child issues that they don't nurture their own relationship.
- Agree with your partner on a few important rules and spell them out to the children. Always support each other in front of the children.
- Be patient in establishing a relationship with a stepchild–it takes time. And be cautious when taking on a parenting role, especially with a teenager, who may never accept you as a parent. Instruct your stepchildren to always treat you with respect and courtesy and treat them the same way.
- Supervision of children is especially important in a blended family. It can be very tempting for an unsupervised older child to stretch the rules with a younger or smaller stepsibling when the two are left alone.
- Have regular family meetings to discuss the week's activities or any problems that come up. Open communication helps establish healthy relationships among all family members.
- Take most of the responsibility for disciplining your own child. Give the step-

parent time to establish a trusting relationship with your child before beginning to set rules for him or her. Make sure that all children in the household are disciplined equally and fairly.

• If your partner will be alone with the children for a time, make your rules and expectations clear. Delegate authority to your partner in your absence.

• Resolve any personal differences between a stepparent and stepchild or between stepsiblings promptly and directly; unresolved problems get worse over time.

• Set aside time for one-on-one activities between family members. Stepchildren need to spend time alone with their parent; stepparents should do things alone with stepchildren; and the two adults should spend time alone with each other.

• Participate in a support group for stepfamilies. You'll see that you are not alone and can learn a lot from the experiences of other stepfamilies.

• If your children are part of their other parent's stepfamily, support that family and cooperate with both of the adults involved. Competition and tension between two households can cause the children to suffer emotionally.

YOUR ADOPTED CHILD

An adopted child has the same emotional and physical needs as any other child. As a parent of an adopted child, you have the same responsibilities and concerns as any other parent. But adoption adds another dimension to parenting. The fact that adopted children are not living with either of their biological parents can be a source of insecurity and apprehension for both children and parents. It's important for parents to come to terms with this difference openly and honestly and make sure that they treat their adopted child the same way they would treat a biological child. If your child was adopted, he or she may also experience many conflicting emotions–grief, fear, anger, identity confusion–about the adoption. The best way to help your child deal with such emotions is by communicating about the adoption openly. In the end, most adopted children are secure, happy, and well adjusted and have a deep, loving, long-lasting relationship with their adoptive parents.

Some children are adopted when they are older, after spending some time in one or more foster homes or in an orphanage. The environment in which a child was previously raised can have a significant impact on his or her physical and emotional health. Some children may not have received affection, stimulation, adequate medical care, or even basic needs, such as adequate nutrition, in their previous home. Some may have been physically abused and incurred severe emotional problems. The long-term consequences of these early experiences on a child are often difficult to predict. Learn as much as you can about the child's early experience, so you will be able to give the child the necessary support and understanding. Many families can get their adopted children on the right track simply by providing a warm, secure, and loving home in which they can reach their full potential.

If you have adopted a child from another country, teach your child about the country in which he or she was born to instill an appreciation of its culture and history. Form a play group with other parents who have adopted children from the same country so your child has playmates with a similar life experience. If your child is of a different race from you, he or she will like having friends who resemble him or her. Your adoption agency can help you find resources, such as an ethnic cultural center or summer camp, devoted to preserving the culture of your child's birth country. You may even want to give your child language lessons in his or her native tongue. Above all, always show that you accept and love your child just as he or she is.

Experts agree that adopted children raised in a family that feels comfortable talking about adoption are more likely to be emotionally well adjusted. As parents, your level of comfort in talking about adoption with your child will disclose how you feel about adoption and will influence your child's own feelings about it. He or she may think there is something bad about being adopted if it is kept a secret. The worst way for your child to find out that he or she is adopted is from someone other than you. Hearing about the adoption from you lets your child know that adoption is good and that you can be trusted.

Begin telling your child that he or she was adopted during infancy to make being adopted part of the child's identity from a young age. Don't just talk about the adoption once; repeat the story, adding more and more information

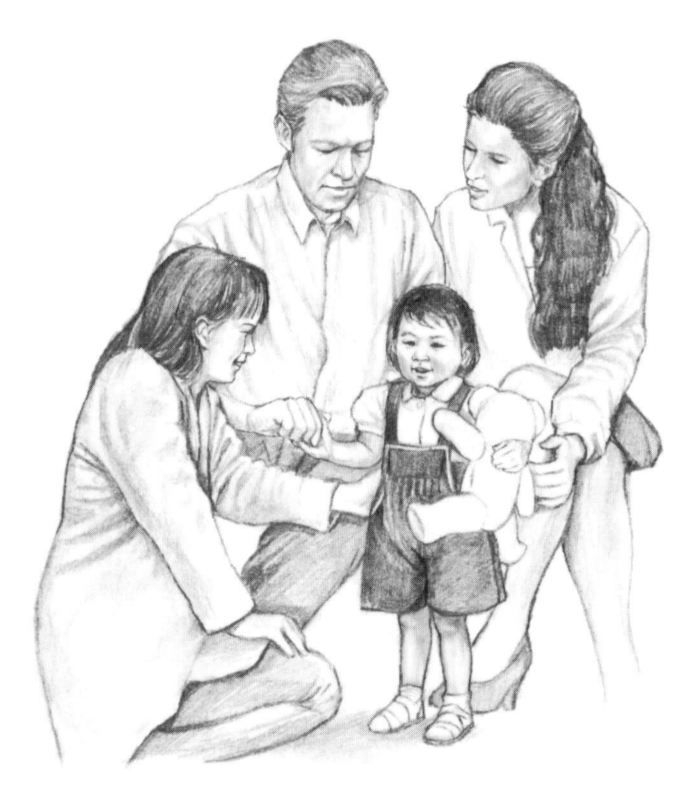

Adopting a child from another country

If you have adopted a child internationally, bring him or her to the doctor right away for a thorough medical examination. In some countries, children who are waiting to be adopted may live in orphanages without adequate nutrition, mental or emotional stimulation, or health care—all of which are necessary for proper development. The doctor can assess your child's level of development, administer all the necessary immunizations, and diagnose any medical condition or special need he or she may have.

Open adoption

In an open adoption, the adoptive parents meet the birth mother or parents before the child is placed in the adoptive parents' home—sometimes even before the child's birth. The birth parents remain in contact with the child to a varying extent as he or she gets older. Open adoption can have the following advantages for the child's emotional well-being:

- Knowing his or her own family background and social identity
- Availability of the child's medical history and genetic predisposition for disease
- Greater understanding of the birth parents' life circumstances and motives for adoption placement.

On the other hand, open adoption also raises the following potentially troublesome issues that could affect the child's emotional health:

- Interruption of the bonding process between the adoptive parents and the child
- Increased insecurity of the adoptive parents about how long they can keep the child
- Confusion in the child ("If my parents didn't want me, why do they keep coming over?")

If you are considering an open adoption, or if your child was placed with you in an open adoption, take full advantage of the counseling services offered by your adoption agency, or talk to a counselor on your own. Such services will help you work together with the birth parents to provide a loving and nurturing long-term arrangement that fosters the best interests of your child.

as your child gets older and begins to understand more. Answer your child's questions about the adoption whenever they arise. Using positive language—such as "Your birth mother planned the adoption" rather than "Your real mother gave you up"—will help develop your child's feelings of self-worth.

If your adopted child is determined to find his or her biological parents, try to stay neutral, neither encouraging or discouraging the search. You should, however, explain any special circumstances—such as state guidelines or specific requests by birth parents not to be identified—that may make the search difficult. In most cases, contact between birth parents and children is done with the help of support groups.

The initial contact between an adopted child and a birth parent churns up emotions in everyone involved—the child, the birth parents, and the adoptive parents. Although every situation is different, keep in mind that your child does not belong to his or her birth parents. They are not his "real" family—you are—and your child needs to understand this. He or she is probably apprehensive about making contact with a birth parent even if he or she wants to, so your support and love are essential at this time.

An adoption support group can be a helpful source of information and encouragement for parents. The national organization known as Adoptive Families of America sponsors local support group meetings and produces a newsletter and other information. Books explaining adoption are available for both parents and children; some are designed for children adopted internationally. Ask the staff at your adoption agency for a list of suggested books.

If you are having difficulty bonding with your child, or if you feel your child is having trouble accepting you and his or her new home, talk to friends who have adopted or join an adoption support group to talk about your concerns and reduce your anxiety. If the situation seems serious, talk to your child's doctor. He or she may be able to help you or refer you to a therapist. Depending on the situation, the therapist may recommend therapy sessions for the whole family or for the child alone.

Children and stress

Most demands on a child's life are normal and healthy and can challenge a child to do well in school or learn a new skill. But demands that become overwhelming can cause both physical and emotional harm. Events that can be highly stressful for a child include moving to a new home, changing schools, frequent parental arguing, overly high expectations of achievement, and of course parental separation or divorce. A constant source of stress for many children in the United States is the regular exposure to violence in their home, neighborhood, or school.

Children show that they are under stress in different ways. Some regress to behavior they have outgrown, such as thumb sucking. Others experience sleep disturbances or nightmares, become hyperactive, complain of stomachaches, cry,

Recognizing signs of stress

Children often have a hard time recognizing that they are under stress. If you are concerned that your child may be experiencing an unusual amount of stress, especially if it lasts for more than a month, talk to your child's doctor. He or she may be able to help you, or refer you to a counselor, such as a child psychiatrist or psychologist. Here are some common signs of stress in children:

- Irritability
- Worsening performance in school
- Recurring problems with friends or siblings
- Moodiness
- Withdrawal from friends and family
- Lack of interest in formerly enjoyable activities
- Abuse of alcohol or other drugs
- Poor hygiene
- Acting out with unacceptable behavior such as lying or stealing
- Worsening of a chronic condition such as asthma (see page 420) or diabetes (see page 471)
- Frequent complaints of vague physical problems such as headaches or stomachaches
- Change in sleep patterns or appetite

or withdraw from activities. These forms of behavior can vary depending on the child's temperament, stage of development, and past experience. A child who is under severe stress may have more frequent colds and digestive problems and is at higher risk of being injured in an accident than one who experiences little tension or anxiety. Children under stress for long periods may be at increased risk for such conditions as high blood pressure and heart disease as adults.

Your child will be better able to handle stress if he or she has your support. You may not realize that your child is undergoing a stressful time so try setting aside time alone with him or her every day—even if it's only for 10 or 15 minutes—to explore your child's feelings about the things that are going on in his or her life. Share your own experiences in difficult or stressful situations and explain how you dealt with them to show your child that he or she is not the only one struggling to overcome problems. Here are some other things you can do to help your child manage stress:

- Teach your child how to handle stress positively by your example.
- Encourage your child to work out problems—either on his or her own or with your guidance. Finding solutions to problems can give your child a sense of accomplishment.
- Encourage your child to get into the habit of regular exercise from a young age. Exercise relieves stress in both children and adults.
- Encourage your child to engage in imaginative games and playacting, so he or she can express his or her feelings in indirect, nonthreatening ways.
- Don't overload your child with too many household responsibilities. Children need to have chores, but too many demands, such as frequent requests to watch a younger sibling, can be overwhelming and may discourage a child from taking on any responsibility at all.
- Don't overstructure your child's day. Although it's beneficial to challenge your child and encourage him or her to learn new skills, it's also good to allow for some unstructured activities so your child can pursue his or her own interests.
- Place less emphasis on grades and more on the sheer joy of learning.
- Never compare one child to his or her siblings or to other children. A child who feels he or she can never measure up to a parent's expectations lives under constant stress.

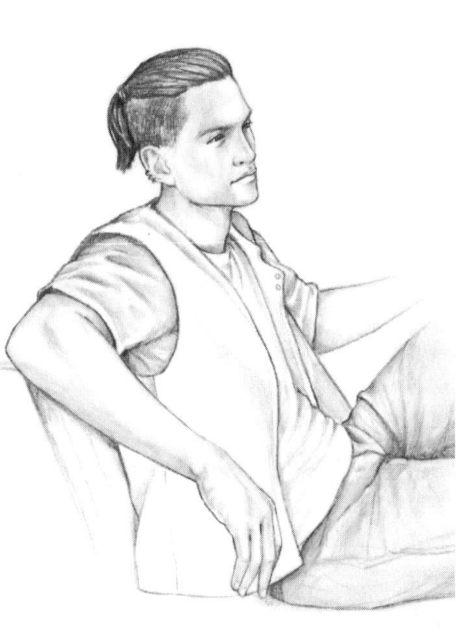

When your child is under stress

Like adults, children deal with stress in different ways. Many children, especially adolescents, cannot discuss their feelings with parents or anyone else and may withdraw into themselves. They may also act out their feelings through unacceptable behaviors, such as lying or stealing. If you think your adolescent is having problems, try to get him or her to open up to you by asking nonjudgmental questions. Often just talking about feelings and frustrations can make your child feel better.

Helping your child understand death

Grief is an inevitable part of life. How much you tell your child about the death of a loved one depends on his or her level of maturity. Let your child ask questions, and give direct answers in words he or she can understand.

Preschool children tend to see death as temporary and reversible—like the cartoon characters they see on TV. Children this age also tend to confuse reality with fantasy and have trouble understanding cause and effect. For example, if a child has been angry at a parent for disciplining him or her and then the parent dies, the child may feel responsible for the death. Make sure you tell your child that he or she is not to blame in any way for the death of a family member or close friend. By ages 5 to 9, children begin to understand more about death and, after a death in the family, they may become concerned that they or their parents will get sick or die. During this time, they need plenty of reassurance to help deal with their fears.

Sometimes adults are so upset about a death that they can't talk about it at all, or their grief may make them emotionally unavailable at a time the child needs comforting the most. By exhibiting grief openly, you show your child that crying and anger are natural responses to death and you give the child permission to show his or her own feelings.

Let your child express feelings in his or her own way. Children may grieve intermittently—over a long period of time and at unexpected times. Or they may not appear to grieve at all. Because young children have a hard time describing their feelings, they often show their confusion and fear by becoming clingy or by reverting to earlier behaviors such as bed-wetting (see page 429). They may act out their anger about the death by becoming irritable or aggressive. Older children who aren't comfortable talking about their feelings may describe them in a story, private journal, or poem.

After the death of a loved one, try to maintain a familiar routine in your home to reassure your child that many parts of his or her life are the same. Explain that the loss will hurt less as time passes. Allow your child to participate in ceremonies, such as a funeral, but don't force it if he or she is afraid or resistant.

Some children just can't cope with loss and develop long-term emotional problems. If your child has any of these symptoms, talk to the doctor:

- A prolonged period of sadness and loss of interest in daily activities
- Prolonged fear of being alone
- Inability to sleep
- Loss of appetite
- Acting younger than his or her age for a prolonged period
- Constant imitation of the dead person or wanting to join the dead person
- Withdrawal from friends and family
- A sharp drop in school performance or refusal to attend school

Your child's doctor may recommend counseling by a therapist who can help your child accept the death and go through the grieving process.

CHAPTER • 13

Children with special health needs

Children with special needs can have a variety of problems–chronic illness or a mental or physical disability–but they and their families face similar challenges. If your child has a special health need, you must act as his or her advocate to ensure that the child receives the care and services required. No matter what condition your child has, the most important goal should be to make his or her quality of life as high as possible.

Children with special needs include those who have chronic illnesses such as asthma or diabetes, developmental delays, physical handicaps, mental retardation, learning disabilities, and emotional or behavioral problems such as autism or an attention disorder. Some children may have more than one of these conditions. But special needs are most usefully defined by a child's limitations in development or functioning, not by a particular illness or disability.

Many of these disorders require ongoing care from a number of health care providers, programs, and agencies. The professionals who collaborate to care for a child with special needs can be thought of as a health care team, directed by the child's doctor. You will need to work closely with this team of professionals to make sure that your child achieves his or her potential and can live as independently as possible.

Above all, remember that your child is much more than his or her illness or disability. He or she is a sensitive, perceptive person who responds to your care and attention, just like any other child. Think of your child as differently abled rather than disabled. That way you can value, encourage, and celebrate the many abilities your child does have.

Your family

Having a child with special health needs alters the dynamics of any family. Each family member needs to make adjustments–in daily routines, priorities, values, and beliefs. Many families are made stronger by the experience of having a child with a special need in the home, acquiring new skills and insights and broader attitudes that make them better able to meet the challenges of life. The family's response to the condition affects the child's ability to understand and come to terms with it.

EFFECTS ON YOU AS PARENTS

It's normal to react to the diagnosis of your child's disability or chronic illness with grief, shock, anger, fear, denial, guilt, or anxiety. Your response will depend on your personality, support system, the condition your child has and its severity, the treatment it requires, and the demands and limitations the condition places on your family. You may grieve over losing your dream of a healthy child. You may worry about whether you will be able to afford all the treatments–therapy sessions, special equipment, and special schooling–your child needs. You may feel angry about having to give up your own dreams of buying a home or taking a vacation. The requirements of your special-needs child may prevent you from providing opportunities to your other children.

Eventually you will come to terms with your child's diagnosis and acknowledge the implications of his or her condition, even though it may always be difficult to accept. From time to time, you will probably feel sad that your child can't do all the things that other children can. Again, these feelings are normal.

It's essential to try and balance your child's needs with the needs of each family member. The following suggestions can help minimize the stresses and strains involved in coping with a chronic illness or disability:

- Take care of your own needs. When you feel you need a break, find a babysitter and go to a movie or out to dinner.
- Nurture your relationship with your partner.
- Don't focus attention solely on the child with special needs. Enjoying activities with your other children will draw all of you together as a family.
- Try to fit your child's treatment regimen into family routines.
- Work closely with the professionals who care for your child.
- Talk about your feelings and encourage other family members to do the same.
- Be flexible in setting rules and defining expectations within the family.
- Find a few good people you can count on to share the day-to-day care of your child; involve extended family members and close friends.
- Be realistic about your child's situation and capabilities but encourage him or her to achieve goals to the best of his or her ability.
- Make realistic plans for your child's future.
- Share experiences with other parents who have children with similar conditions.
- Get counseling when you need it. It's normal to feel sad and frustrated once in a while, but if you are persistently feeling despondent and helpless, you need to get help. Ask your child's doctor, a social service agency, or a local medical center for the name of a professional who can help you.

EFFECTS ON YOUR OTHER CHILDREN

Siblings of a child with special needs often experience the same feelings that parents do–grief, guilt, anger, and resentment. They may feel guilty that they somehow caused the disability or feel jealous and resentful of the attention given to the child. Many siblings who love and care for their brother or sister within the family may be embarrassed when their friends laugh at or make fun of him or her. On the other hand, having a sibling with a chronic illness or disability can have a positive effect. It can enable the sibling to learn to be responsible, unselfish, patient, caring, and more sensitive to other people.

When explaining your child's condition to your other children, speak simply and clearly. Allow them to ask questions and explain only as much as you think they can understand. As they get older and their understanding increases, tell them more. Don't keep information from them or they may think the disability is too frightening to talk about or that you don't trust them with the knowledge. When a sibling's friends come to visit, tell them briefly about your child's condition to make them feel more at ease. Make sure that all of your children's teachers know about the child's condition and the family situation; this information can give them insight into any problems that may arise.

Involve siblings in the day-to-day care of your special-needs child–but give them only as much responsibility as they can handle. Find or start a support group for your other children so they can meet other siblings of children with disabilities or chronic diseases. In a relaxed setting, they can talk about common concerns, learn from each other, and understand more about the implications of their sibling's special needs. Go to these sessions occasionally to learn about some of their shared concerns.

Managing your child's care

At home, you will have the primary responsibility for managing your child's overall care. You will have to coordinate your child's medical appointments, meet with teachers or home tutors to plan lessons tailored to your child's needs, find specialized equipment such as a wheelchair, fill out insurance forms, and

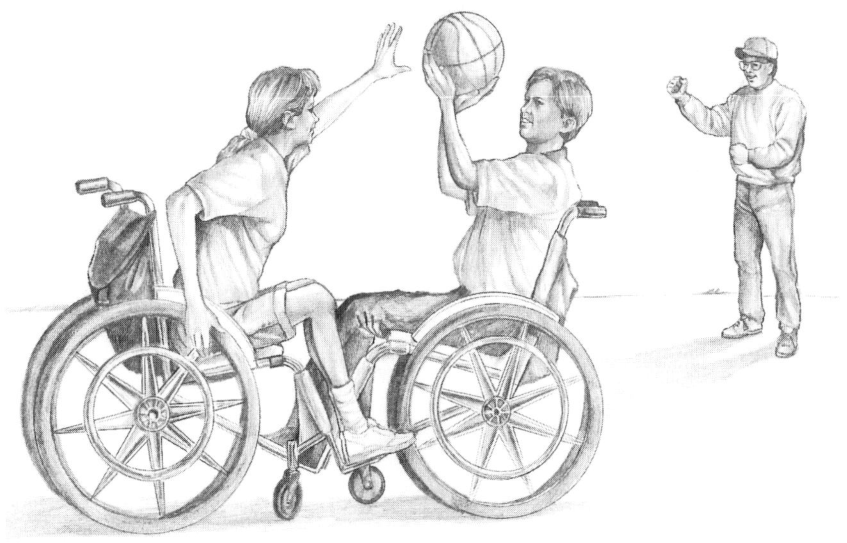

Being a part of the fun

Children with a disability or chronic medical condition need to feel that they can do some of the same things as other children. Give your special-needs child the chance to take part in the kinds of activities that all children enjoy, even if the activity has to be modified a bit.

arrange transportation to and from school and doctor's appointments.

You may also have to learn how to perform certain medical procedures to care for your special-needs child at home. For example, if your child is a diabetic, you might have to learn how to measure his or her blood sugar level. You might need to be trained to give fluids or medication intravenously or to dispense oxygen. You may also need to learn certain procedures that are not medical but are essential to the care of your child. For example, if your child has a spinal cord injury, you will probably have to learn how to insert a catheter into his or her bladder to drain urine. You will have to learn how to recognize signs of distress in your child that could signal a medical emergency. Your child's doctor will probably encourage you to take a course in cardiopulmonary resuscitation (see page 668). If you don't understand a certain aspect of your child's care, ask your doctor or visiting nurse, or call the nurse who coordinated your child's care the last time he or she was in the hospital for an explanation or equipment demonstration. In some communities, local agencies sponsor workshops that train parents how to manage their child's complex care. Check with the social service department of a nearby hospital about programs in your community.

Children with special needs often require individualized learning techniques that compensate for their disability. A child with hearing loss may need to have material presented visually or through touch. One who has a learning disability may only be able to learn if the lesson is kept short or is repeated and reinforced. Children with a physical handicap may require special aids or equipment. Lengthy hospitalizations may demand special schooling arrangements, such as allowing the child to do schoolwork in his or her hospital room. Ask your child's doctor about your child's individual learning needs. Then, meet with your child's teachers to talk about ways to meet these needs in the classroom. As your child gets older, involve him or her in educational planning.

Allow your child to be independent, within his or her limitations. An older child or adolescent may be able to handle certain aspects of his or her care, such as giving himself or herself insulin injections. Mastering some self-care can help your child achieve a certain amount of control over the circumstances. Encourage and praise your child for learning tasks that are especially difficult because of his or her condition.

Respite care—getting help when you need it

All parents need relief from the day-to-day care of a child with special health needs. You will be a better parent if you can take a break from your responsibility once in a while. To do this, you need to find people you can trust to take over the care of your child from time to time. Try the following suggestions when looking for potential caregivers:

- Ask your child's therapists, teachers, other parents in your support group, and people in your church or synagogue for recommendations of caregivers they have used.
- Find out about available community and government programs, such as temporary placement services, day care, respite care, and in-home family support services.
- Check preschools; they often have extended day care.
- Ask a social worker at your local hospital about "relief families" who offer to care for children with special needs from a few hours to a week or more.
- Send your child to a specialty camp, where he or she can spend time with other children in similar circumstances and feel independent from your family.
- Ask grandparents to help out as much as they can.
- Hire a reliable babysitter for a day or evening.

Your child's health care team

You and your special-needs child will work with a team of health professionals who specialize in a variety of disciplines–nursing, physical or occupational therapy, social work, and nutrition–to minimize the effects of the disease or disability. Your child's doctor will coordinate the treatment and monitor your child's progress over time.

YOUR CHILD'S DOCTOR

Ideally, the doctor who coordinates the care of your special-needs child should be experienced in caring for children with your child's specific condition. If you live in a small town or a rural area, your child may be the only child with that condition under his or her doctor's care. When choosing a doctor for your special-needs child, ask if the doctor is comfortable working with children who have special health needs, and if he or she can spend the time needed to manage your child's problems. If the doctor does not seem to have the time or desire to care for your child, ask him or her to refer you to another doctor. You could also ask for recommendations from other parents of disabled children, a local chapter of the national organization that represents your child's condition such as the United Cerebral Palsy Association, the state chapter of the American Academy of Pediatrics (ask for a list of pediatricians who have a subspecialty in disabilities), or a children's hospital. You and your child will benefit most from working with a doctor who:

- Respects the impact your child's condition has on your family.
- Listens to your concerns and values your opinions.
- Encourages your child to communicate his or her needs and feelings.
- Includes you and the child in decisions about treatments.
- Shares new information about the condition with you and your child.
- Speaks in easy-to-understand language.
- Answers all of your questions.
- Is willing to work with schools, therapists, community health nurses, and neighborhood agencies to help you gain access to services, support, and education.
- Gives information and guidance appropriate for your child's development.

OTHER HEALTH CARE TEAM MEMBERS

Other health care professionals–nurses, physical or occupational therapists, speech-language pathologists, social workers, or child psychologists–may work with your child from time to time. Your child's doctor may also refer your child to one or more physician specialists. Each professional will set goals for your child and will decide the type and length of therapy your child needs to accomplish them. Your child's doctor will probably recommend a therapist but you might also get names from your local school district, other parents in your support groups, or community agencies that help children with special needs. The team of health care professionals assigned to your child's care may include:

• **Nurses** Visiting nurses make home visits to perform a variety of medical procedures and to teach parents how to care for their child at home. In the hospital, nurses are responsible for a child's day-to-day care, prepare children for medical procedures, and plan for discharge from the hospital.

• **Physical therapists** Physical therapists work with children who have disorders affecting movements of the large muscles, such as those in the arms and legs. They use techniques, such as range-of-motion exercise, and adaptive equipment, such as braces and wheelchairs, to help children make the most of their physical potential.

• **Occupational therapists** These specialists teach the skills a child needs to carry out the activities of daily living–such as eating, dressing, or using the toilet–so the child can live as independently as possible. Occupational therapists help children learn to perform the tasks needed for school and, eventually, a job.

• **Speech-language pathologists** If your child has difficulty communicating, feeding, or swallowing, he or she will be evaluated by a speech-language pathologist. The pathologist will design a program for your child that might include individual or group sessions from one to five times a week.

• **Child psychologists** These experts work with children who have emotional or behavioral problems, or trouble socializing with their peers. They see children in individual therapy sessions and in group therapy with other children.

• **Social workers** Social workers work in the community and in the hospital to help children and their parents find sources of financial aid and gain access to services within the community, such as respite care and school re-entry after a hospitalization.

Communicating competently

Like other children, a child with special needs must be able to communicate to be successful in school and life. The health care team can make the most of a child's ability to convey his or her needs. For example, hearing-impaired children can learn to communicate with their family, teachers, and peers by using sign language.

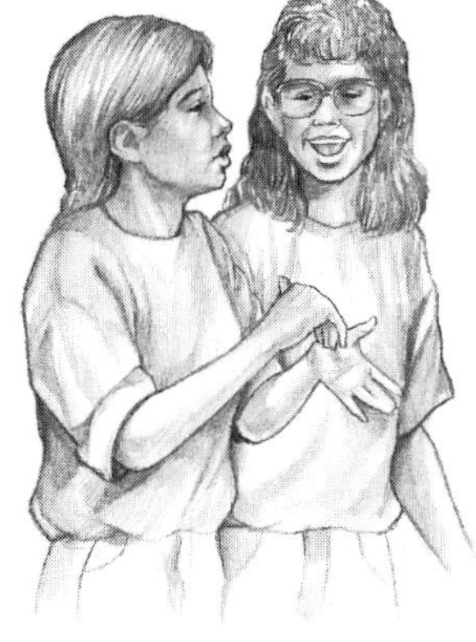

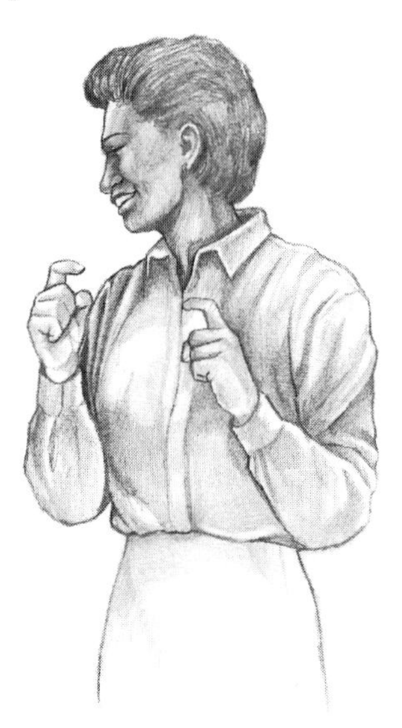

• **Child life specialists** A child life specialist plans play activities that help hospitalized children deal with their fears (therapeutic play) or learn material they missed while absent from school.

• **Registered dietitians** If the doctor has placed your child on a special diet because of a medical condition such as diabetes or galactosemia, a registered dietitian will meet with you and your child to explain the dietary restrictions. The dietitian will also make sure your child is getting enough nutrition to grow and develop.

• **Chaplain** When your child is in the hospital, you may find it comforting to talk to the hospital chaplain for spiritual guidance.

Insurance and financial issues

Millions of Americans lack private or public health insurance for at least part of each year, and the number of uninsured continues to grow. Children under the age of 18 make up a large percentage of the uninsured, even though their parents work. Many families who do have health insurance face high out-of-pocket expenses for deductions and copayments or for medical services that are not covered. Families with children who have special needs often experience financial hardship from inadequate insurance, limitations on benefits, lack of coverage for certain types of services or equipment, and limits on maximum lifetime benefits in addition to the burden of day-to-day care for their child.

Some health insurance plans do not cover pre-existing conditions, or require you to wait a certain length of time before the condition will be covered. If you are switching to a new health care plan, make sure your child's condition will be covered. Read the insurance policy carefully or ask your employee benefits representative or insurance agent exactly what types of services will be covered.

Most services provided in a hospital are covered by insurance and managed care plans, but many community-based services–nursing services, social work, nutrition services, physical and occupational therapy, respite care, and family counseling–are not covered or are only partially covered. You may have to pay for such services yourself. If you feel that your child has been wrongly denied coverage for a service, contact your employee benefits department, insurance agent, or the state department of insurance.

If you do not have private health insurance or have a modest policy that leaves many medical bills inadequately covered, ask your child's doctor, a social worker, or a local advocacy group for information about public and private sources of financial help. Civic, social welfare, and religious groups sometimes have funds available for at least emergency or short-term medical needs. Local charitable foundations can also be a source of assistance. Ask your chamber of commerce about local businesses that donate money to causes that help children. Be creative, resourceful, and patient in your search for help.

Children with extreme medical needs often qualify for the federal Medicaid health insurance program, but eligibility requirements vary from state to state. Many other government programs have been established to help families through a crisis or to meet their basic needs, such as for food. These programs include emergency and temporary cash assistance programs, the food stamp program, the Supplemental Security Income program, Aid to Families with Dependent Children, and food distribution programs. See if your child is eligible for any of these programs. To find out what benefits may be available to you, contact your state public assistance agency, your local Social Security office, and local chapters of national advocacy organizations.

Reductions in federal and state income taxes are available to all taxpayers who incur excessive expenses from caring for a child with a chronic illness or disability. For information about federal income tax rules, contact the nearest Internal Revenue Service district office. To find out about rules governing state income taxes, contact your state department of revenue. Because laws dictating income tax deductions, exemptions, and credits can change, check with these agencies each year before you file your return.

Your child's rights

Since the 1970s, numerous federal and state laws have been passed to ensure that children with chronic illnesses or disabilities have the same educational and developmental opportunities as other children. Many states have initiated programs to identify children with disabilities at a young age to help minimize developmental delays and reduce the long-term dependency that could otherwise afflict a special-needs child.

BEING AN ADVOCATE FOR YOUR CHILD

Children with a chronic illness or disability deserve to live with their family and to share in the everyday experiences most of us take for granted. In many states, programs for children with special health needs are inadequate and new laws are often implemented slowly. That's why you need to be an advocate for your child. Try to work within the system to obtain the services and programs that your child is entitled to.

Make your child's interests and needs known to the professionals you work with. Ask your child's doctor to help you gain access to local resources. Work with community, state, and national programs to address your child's needs, to improve access to services, and to enhance the quality of those services. Parent activism has often been the force behind increases in local and federal support for children with disabilities. Do your part by participating on boards, councils, and committees and being active in local, state, and federal legislatures.

A number of state and national groups can help parents who want to be effective advocates for their children. Protection and advocacy agencies, staffed mainly by lawyers and social workers, can help you understand specific federal laws and court rulings relating to the rights of children with special needs. Parent training and information centers are part of a national network of parent-run projects to help parents work more effectively with professionals to meet the educational needs of their children.

Support groups exist for almost every disorder, many sponsored by hospitals and social service agencies. In a support group, parents can share experiences, concerns, and practical solutions to everyday problems, and give each other emotional support. They often find that, as a group, they have more power to bring about the changes needed to increase special services for their children.

EARLY INTERVENTION

Every state is legally required to establish a Child Find Program to identify and refer children with disabilities from birth through age 21. (To locate a Child Find office near you, contact your state director of special education.) States are also encouraged, at their discretion, to develop early intervention services for children from birth to 3 years of age who have mental, physical, social, or emotional delay or a condition that could result in developmental delay. These early intervention programs are designed to both stimulate the child's development and provide training and support for the family.

As part of the program, each child receives an evaluation called an Individual Family Service Plan, provided at no cost to families. The evaluation includes a statement about the specific early intervention services the child and family need. These services may be provided through a public or private agency either in the child's home or in a clinic, day-care center, hospital, or the local health department. Examples of available services include prescribing glasses for a 2-year-old and developing a physical therapy program for an infant with cerebral palsy.

If your child is eligible for services under this program, a case manager (called a service coordinator) will be assigned to your family to make sure your child gets the care he or she needs. Your service coordinator can tell you about the policies for early intervention programs in your state and help you find needed services in your community, such as recreation, child care, or family support groups. Keep in mind that the earlier your child receives the care he or she needs, the more he or she will benefit.

YOUR CHILD'S EDUCATION

With the passage of the Individuals with Disabilities Education Act, all children with chronic illnesses or disabilities were given the right to benefit as fully as possible from public school programs. The goal of this law is to increase the child's independence. In addition to mandating free public education for all children from ages 6 through 21, the law requires the following conditions:

- Schools must provide the services children need to participate in integrated educational programs that place special-needs children in regular classrooms with peers who are not disabled, at least for some classes. Such services may include transportation to and from school, physical therapy, and medical care.
- Each child with a developmental delay must receive an individualized education program (IEP). The program must include statements about the child's present level of educational performance, long- and short-term goals, the type of special services the child needs, the amount of time he or she will spend in regular classrooms, and criteria for evaluating success in meeting the goals.
- The IEP must be updated each year by a team of medical and educational professionals, with input from the parents. Periodic monitoring is also required to determine the need for a change in placement or in the program.

- Parents must be included in team meetings and in decision-making about their child's education. The child and family must have a way to challenge any decision made about the child's education program.

Some parents object to the special education process because they fear it stigmatizes their child, creating self-image problems. They may be concerned that, once placed in special education, their child will remain there forever. All IEPs are reviewed every year to avoid such permanent placement. If you don't agree with your child's placement in special education classes, you can appeal.

Planning ahead for your child's future

The time will come when your child will want to live independently from your family or when you will no longer be able to meet your child's needs. For many families, this change occurs around the time their child turns 18. Although it may be difficult to imagine anyone else taking care of your child or your child leaving home and living on his or her own, it's important to plan for your child's future. Include your child in the planning as much as you can.

As your child grows up, prepare him or her for the eventual separation from your family by involving him or her in recreational activities outside the family, such as team sports or summer camp. Help your child make friends and develop skills in decision-making to ease the transition to community living. Show your child how to use public transportation and manage money.

The ultimate goal is for your child to live, work, and play within the community, and to have meaningful personal relationships. Look for an environment that provides protection and support as well as independence. If you are unsure about the types of living situations available in your community, talk with a social worker at your local hospital to find out what options your child has.

A child with a physical disability that requires periodic care or one who is mentally disabled may benefit from a semi-independent living or working arrangement. Group homes are residences in which four to six disabled people live together with one or two support staff. Group homes offer many of the comforts of home while helping the child become self-sufficient.

Children who need ongoing care may need to be placed in a long-term care facility or specialized rehabilitation center that offers care for an extended period. If your child needs long-term care, carefully consider all of the emotional and financial implications of placing your child in such a facility. Ask your child's doctor or a social worker at the hospital where the doctor has staff privileges to recommend a qualified long-term care center. Visit the facility before placement so you can feel comfortable with the staff and surroundings. Don't feel guilty that you have abandoned your child after placement. Your child's doctor will recommend long-term care only if your child needs it. If you have difficulty coming to terms with your child's placement in long-term care, ask the doctor to recommend a therapist you can talk to.

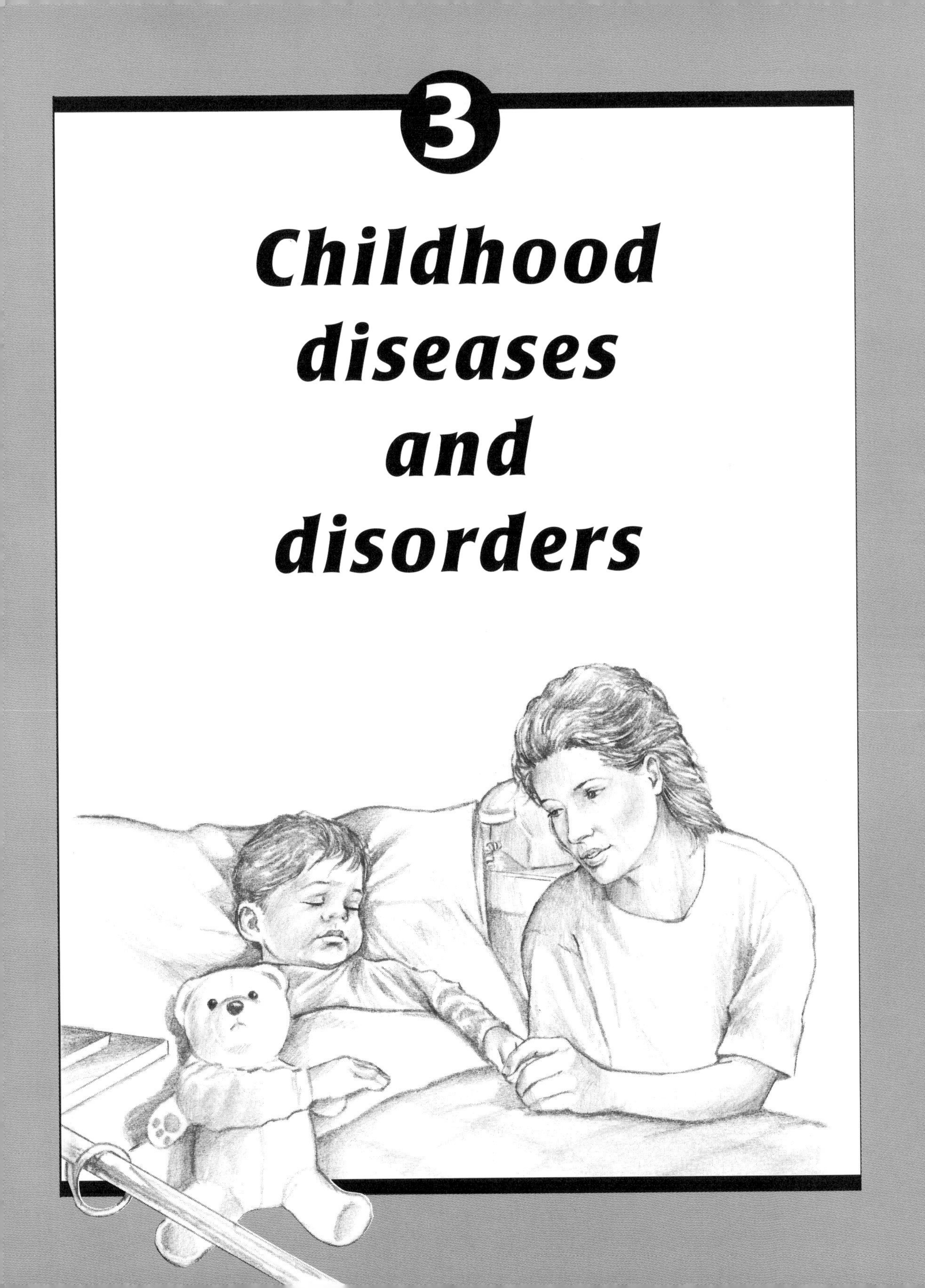
3
Childhood
diseases
and
disorders

QUICK REFERENCE GUIDE
SYMPTOM CHARTS

The charts on pages 358 to 400 lead you through a question-and-answer format to help you find the possible causes and significance of many common symptoms. The alphabetical listing below refers you to the chart you need.

Infants

Children

INFANTS

CRYING

Persistent sobbing, whimpering, or screaming that tells you your baby does not feel well.

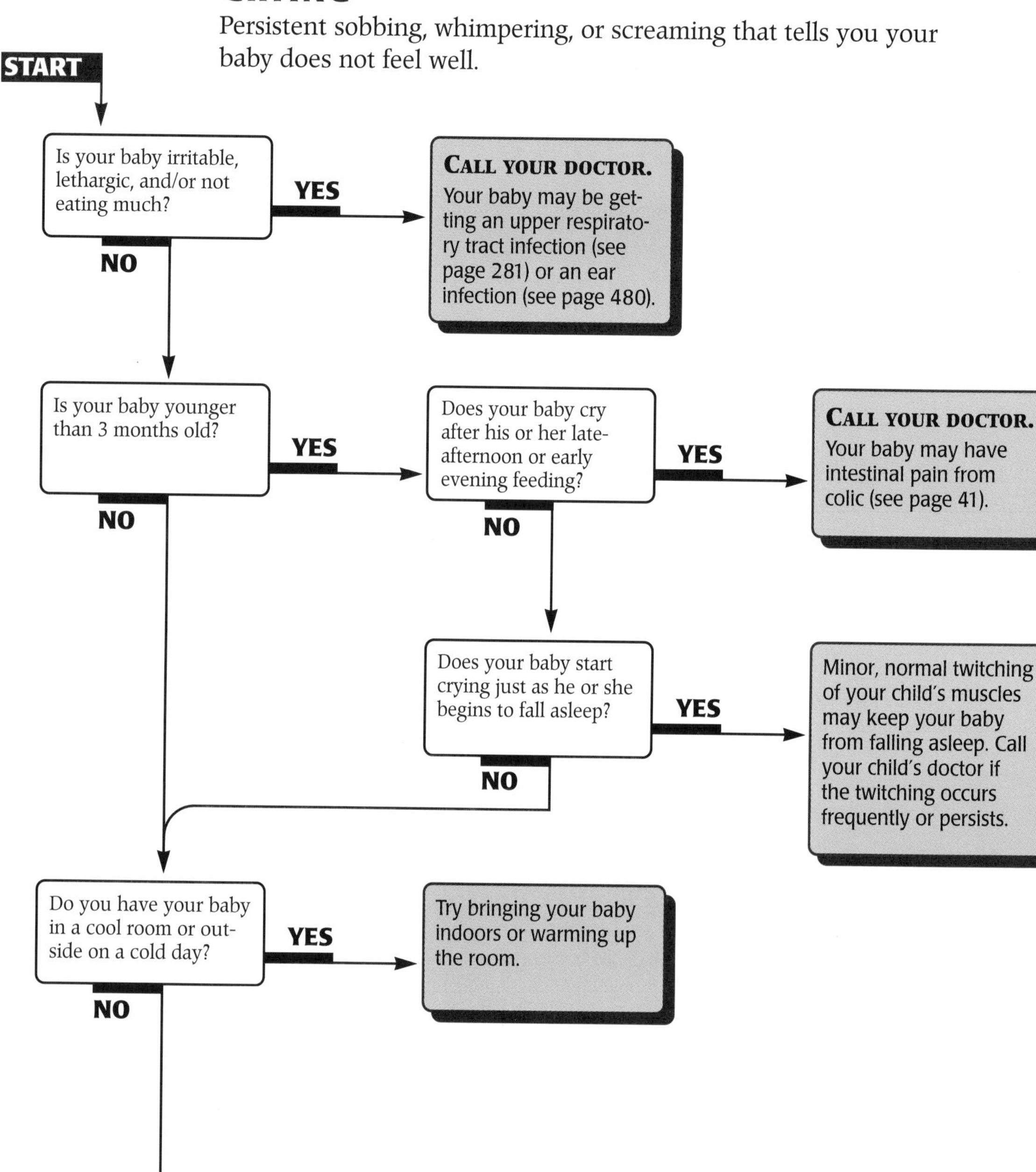

Continued on next page.

Continued from previous page.

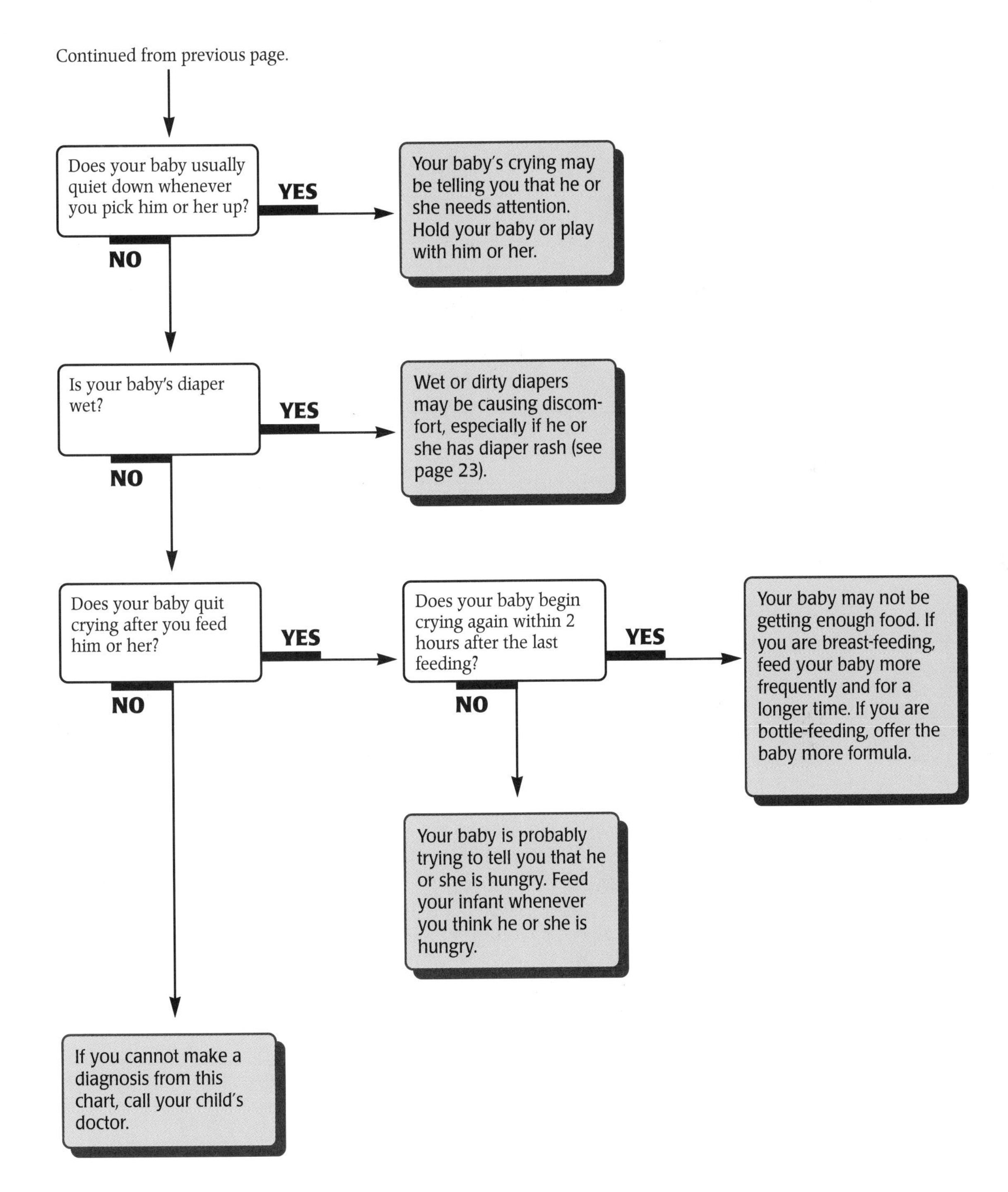

INFANTS

FEVER IN CHILDREN UNDER 1 YEAR

Temperature of 101°F or higher in a child 12 months of age or younger.

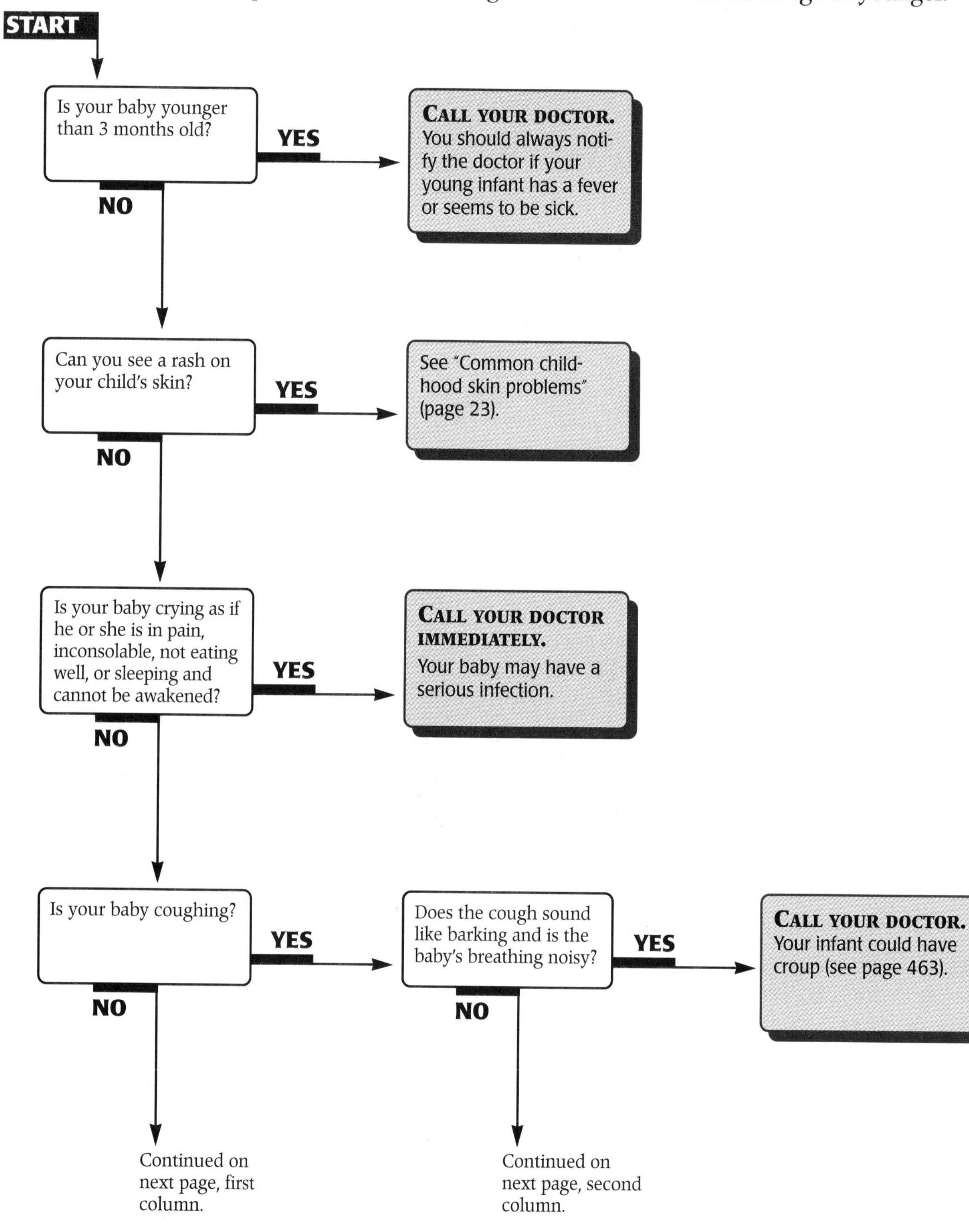

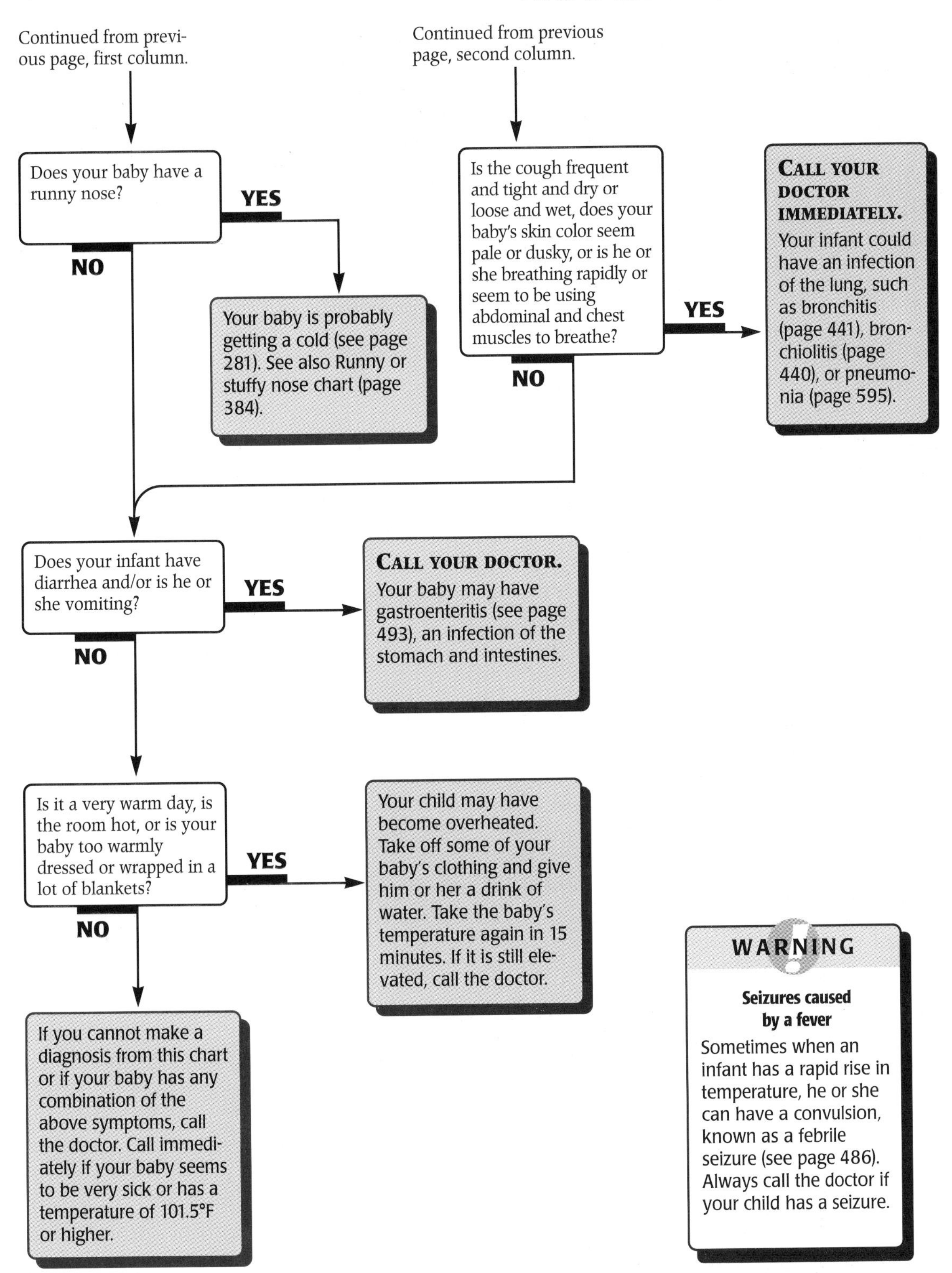
Continued from previous page, first column.
Does your baby have a runny nose?
YES
Your baby is probably getting a cold (see page 281). See also Runny or stuffy nose chart (page 384).
NO
Continued from previous page, second column.
Is the cough frequent and tight and dry or loose and wet, does your baby's skin color seem pale or dusky, or is he or she breathing rapidly or seem to be using abdominal and chest muscles to breathe?
YES
CALL YOUR DOCTOR IMMEDIATELY.
Your infant could have an infection of the lung, such as bronchitis (page 441), bronchiolitis (page 440), or pneumonia (page 595).
NO
Does your infant have diarrhea and/or is he or she vomiting?
YES
CALL YOUR DOCTOR.
Your baby may have gastroenteritis (see page 493), an infection of the stomach and intestines.
NO
Is it a very warm day, is the room hot, or is your baby too warmly dressed or wrapped in a lot of blankets?
YES
Your child may have become overheated. Take off some of your baby's clothing and give him or her a drink of water. Take the baby's temperature again in 15 minutes. If it is still elevated, call the doctor.
NO
If you cannot make a diagnosis from this chart or if your baby has any combination of the above symptoms, call the doctor. Call immediately if your baby seems to be very sick or has a temperature of 101.5°F or higher.
WARNING
Seizures caused by a fever
Sometimes when an infant has a rapid rise in temperature, he or she can have a convulsion, known as a febrile seizure (see page 486). Always call the doctor if your child has a seizure.

INFANTS

FEEDING PROBLEMS

Reluctance to feed; constant hunger or crying; swallowing of air, causing spitting up or abdominal discomfort; difficulty swallowing food; or vomiting after feedings.

START

Does your baby seem uninterested in feeding?

YES → Has your infant had a good appetite in the past?

NO → Do you breast-feed your baby?

Has your infant had a good appetite in the past?

YES → You should call your child's doctor immediately if your infant is younger than 6 months old and has not eaten within 4 to 6 hours of his or her normal feeding time, or if he or she seems uncharacteristically sleepy or irritable or shows any signs of being ill.

NO → Is he or she gaining weight normally (see page 238)?

Is he or she gaining weight normally (see page 238)?

YES → Many babies become uninterested in eating from time to time. Don't worry, as long as your baby seems alert and is gaining weight normally. Call the doctor if your baby seems to be sick in any way.

NO → **CALL YOUR DOCTOR.** Your baby could have some underlying disorder that is causing an abnormally slow weight gain.

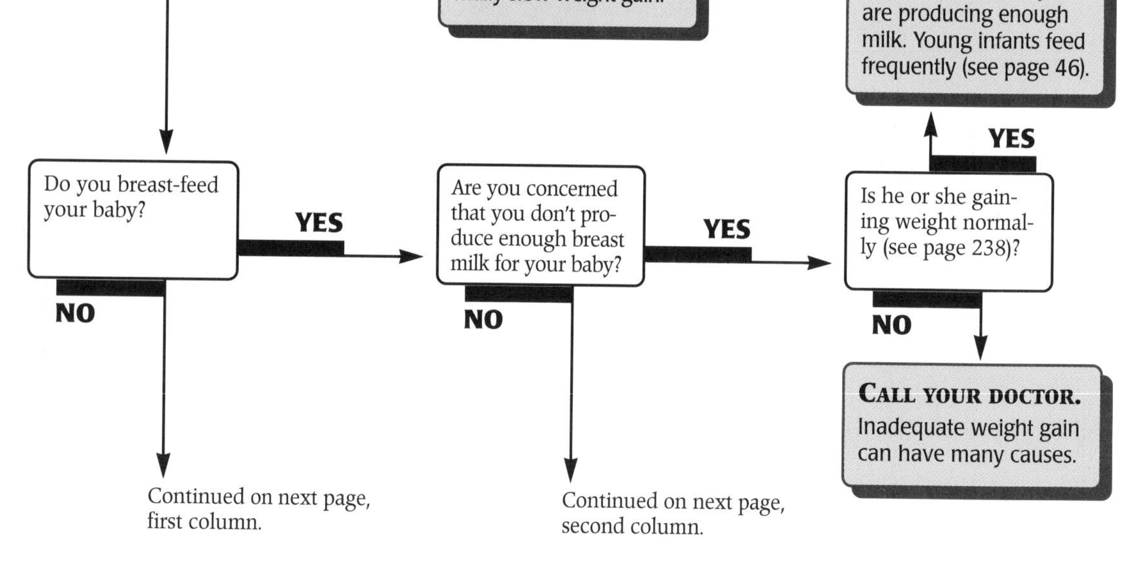

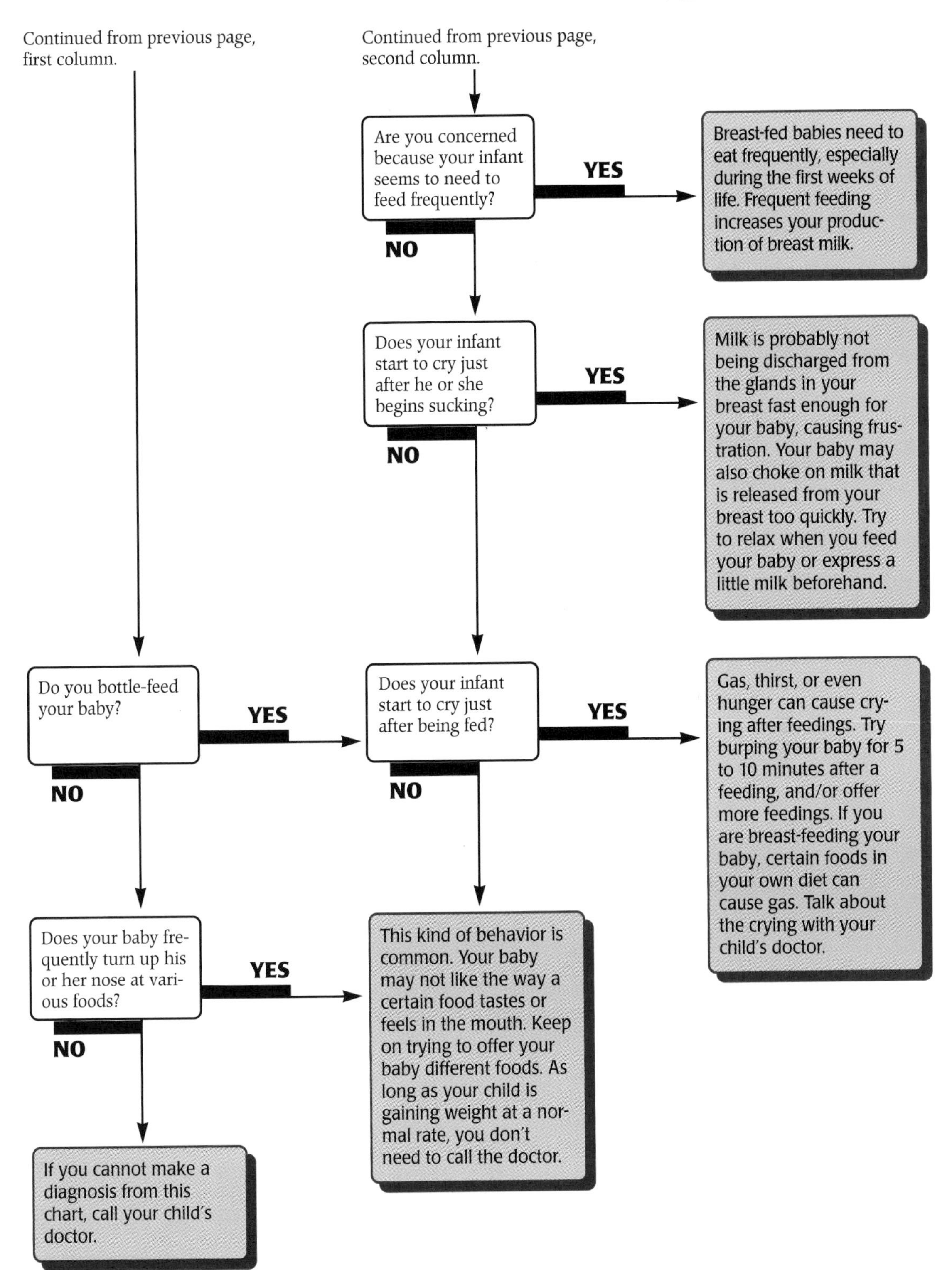
Continued from previous page, first column.
Continued from previous page, second column.
Are you concerned because your infant seems to need to feed frequently?
YES
Breast-fed babies need to eat frequently, especially during the first weeks of life. Frequent feeding increases your production of breast milk.
NO
Does your infant start to cry just after he or she begins sucking?
YES
Milk is probably not being discharged from the glands in your breast fast enough for your baby, causing frustration. Your baby may also choke on milk that is released from your breast too quickly. Try to relax when you feed your baby or express a little milk beforehand.
NO
Do you bottle-feed your baby?
YES
Does your infant start to cry just after being fed?
YES
Gas, thirst, or even hunger can cause crying after feedings. Try burping your baby for 5 to 10 minutes after a feeding, and/or offer more feedings. If you are breast-feeding your baby, certain foods in your own diet can cause gas. Talk about the crying with your child's doctor.
NO
NO
Does your baby frequently turn up his or her nose at various foods?
YES
This kind of behavior is common. Your baby may not like the way a certain food tastes or feels in the mouth. Keep on trying to offer your baby different foods. As long as your child is gaining weight at a normal rate, you don't need to call the doctor.
NO
If you cannot make a diagnosis from this chart, call your child's doctor.

INFANTS

VOMITING IN CHILDREN UNDER 1 YEAR

Forceful expulsion of the stomach contents from sudden contraction of the muscles in and around the stomach.

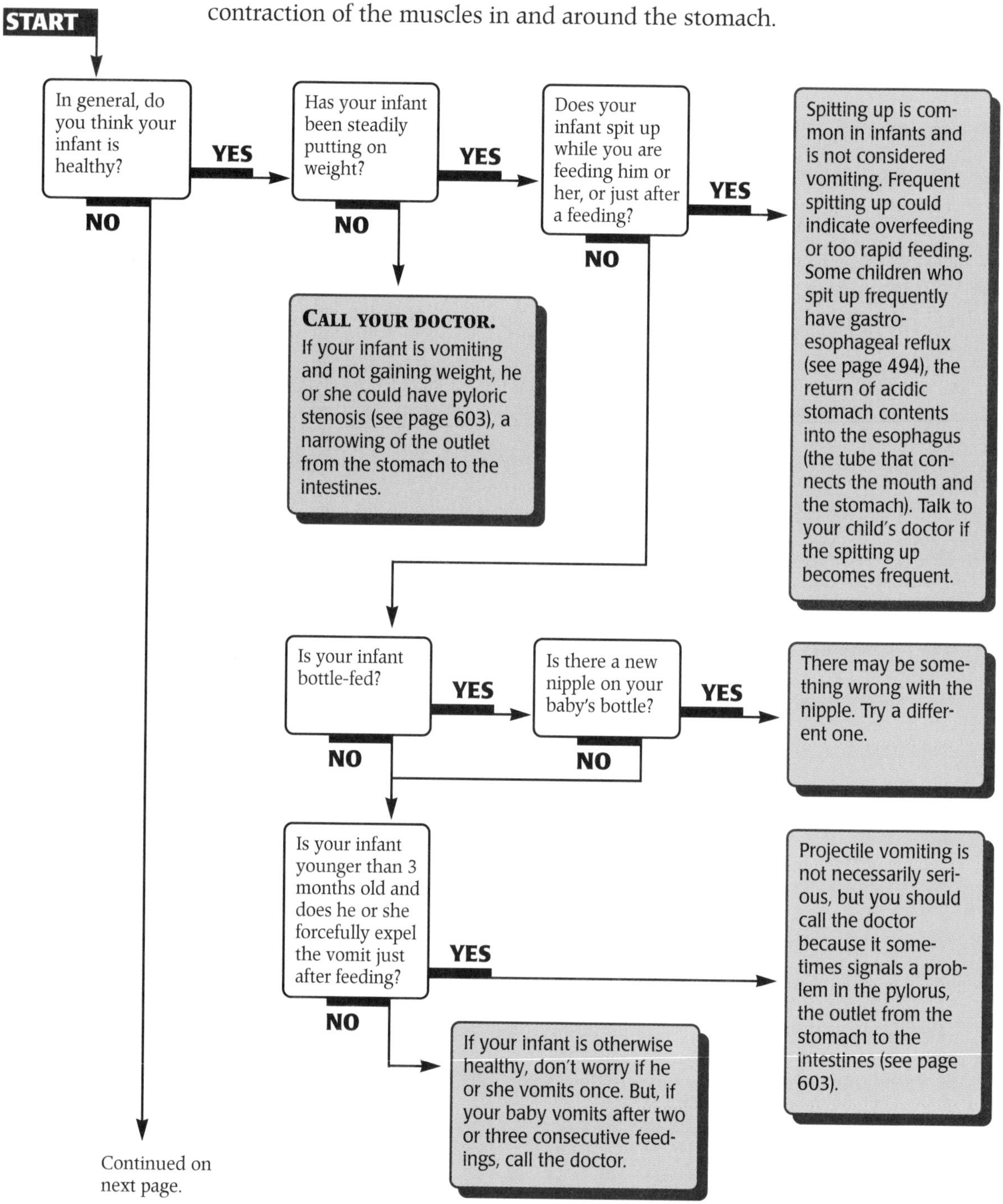

START

In general, do you think your infant is healthy?

YES →

Has your infant been steadily putting on weight?

YES →

Does your infant spit up while you are feeding him or her, or just after a feeding?

YES →

Spitting up is common in infants and is not considered vomiting. Frequent spitting up could indicate overfeeding or too rapid feeding. Some children who spit up frequently have gastroesophageal reflux (see page 494), the return of acidic stomach contents into the esophagus (the tube that connects the mouth and the stomach). Talk to your child's doctor if the spitting up becomes frequent.

NO (weight) →

CALL YOUR DOCTOR.
If your infant is vomiting and not gaining weight, he or she could have pyloric stenosis (see page 603), a narrowing of the outlet from the stomach to the intestines.

NO (spit up) →

Is your infant bottle-fed?

YES →

Is there a new nipple on your baby's bottle?

YES →

There may be something wrong with the nipple. Try a different one.

NO →

Is your infant younger than 3 months old and does he or she forcefully expel the vomit just after feeding?

YES →

Projectile vomiting is not necessarily serious, but you should call the doctor because it sometimes signals a problem in the pylorus, the outlet from the stomach to the intestines (see page 603).

NO →

If your infant is otherwise healthy, don't worry if he or she vomits once. But, if your baby vomits after two or three consecutive feedings, call the doctor.

NO (healthy) →

Continued on next page.

Continued from previous page.

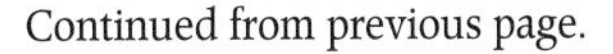

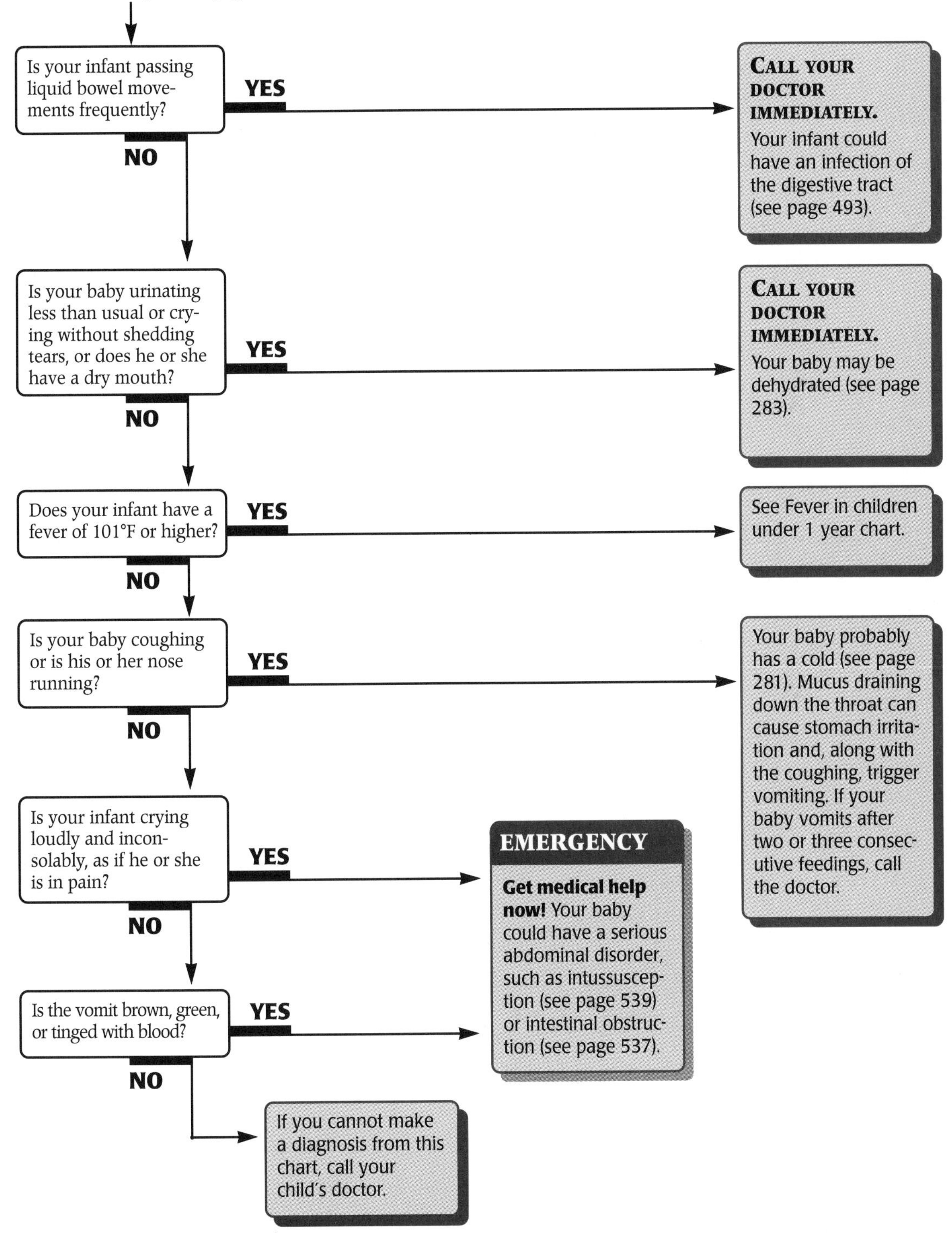

INFANTS

Diarrhea in Children Under 1 Year

Passing watery stools more frequently than usual.

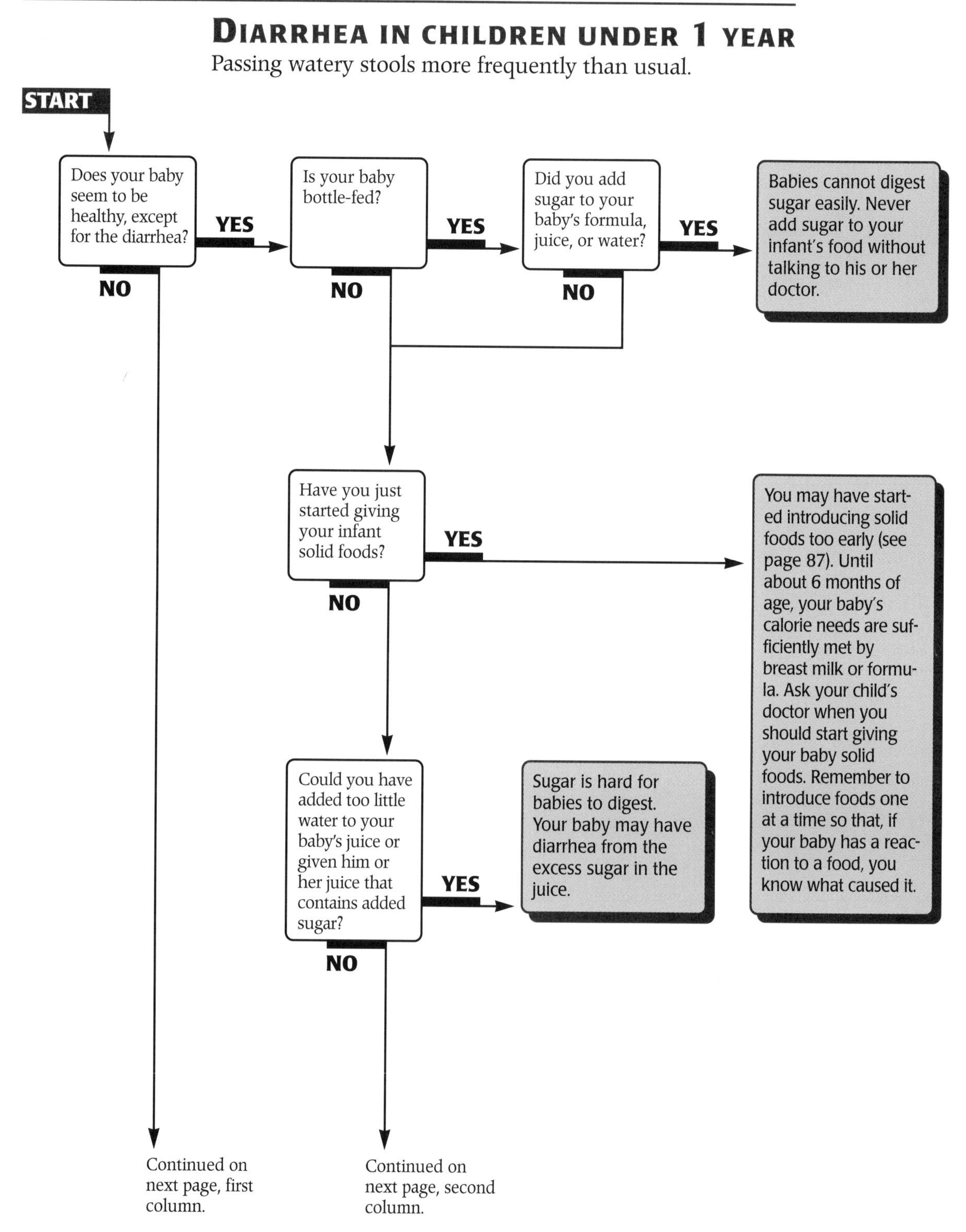

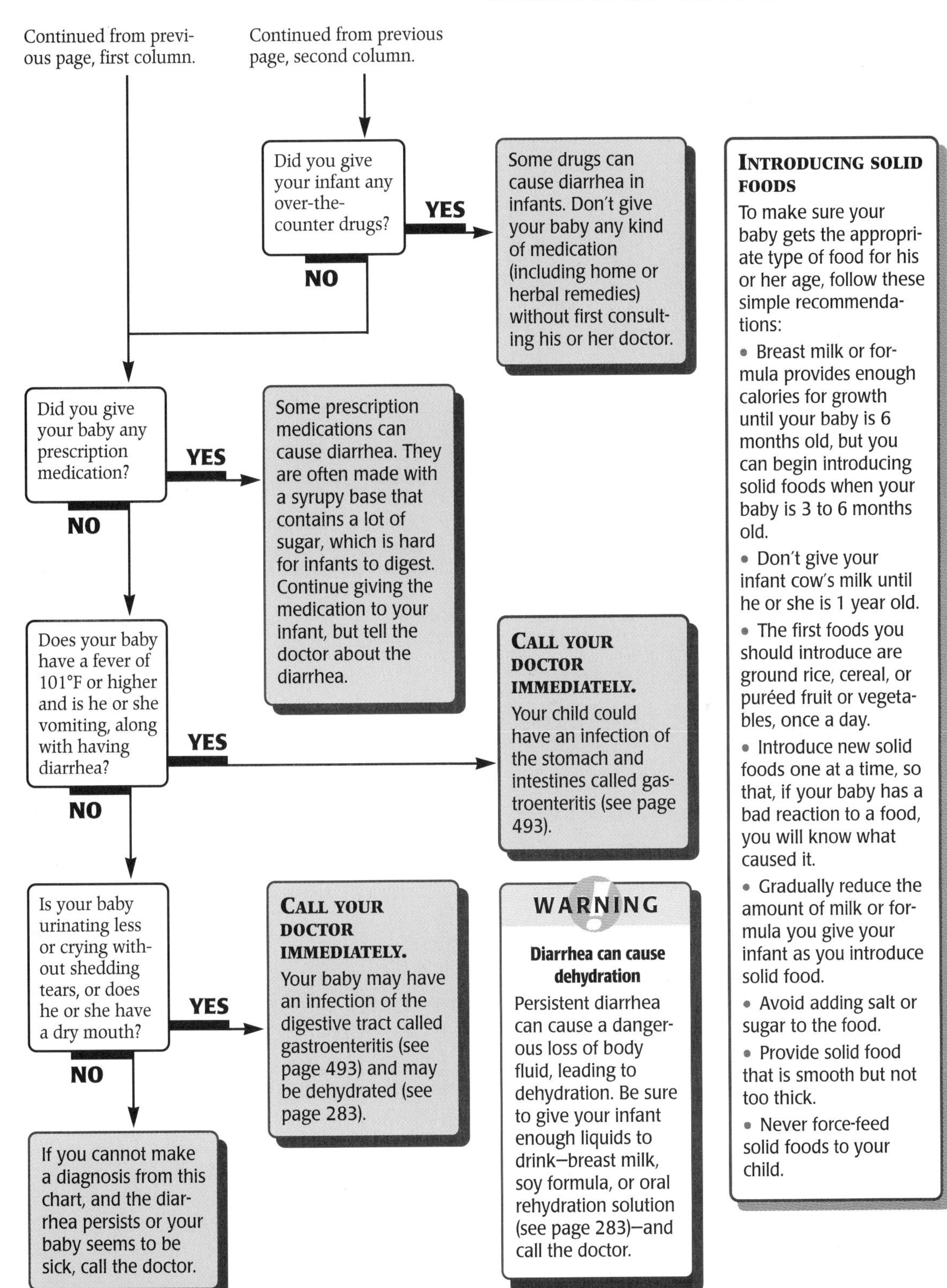

WARNING

Diarrhea can cause dehydration

Persistent diarrhea can cause a dangerous loss of body fluid, leading to dehydration. Be sure to give your infant enough liquids to drink—breast milk, soy formula, or oral rehydration solution (see page 283)—and call the doctor.

INTRODUCING SOLID FOODS

To make sure your baby gets the appropriate type of food for his or her age, follow these simple recommendations:

- Breast milk or formula provides enough calories for growth until your baby is 6 months old, but you can begin introducing solid foods when your baby is 3 to 6 months old.
- Don't give your infant cow's milk until he or she is 1 year old.
- The first foods you should introduce are ground rice, cereal, or puréed fruit or vegetables, once a day.
- Introduce new solid foods one at a time, so that, if your baby has a bad reaction to a food, you will know what caused it.
- Gradually reduce the amount of milk or formula you give your infant as you introduce solid food.
- Avoid adding salt or sugar to the food.
- Provide solid food that is smooth but not too thick.
- Never force-feed solid foods to your child.

INFANTS

SLOW WEIGHT GAIN

Failure to put on weight at a normal rate (see growth charts, pages 239–243).

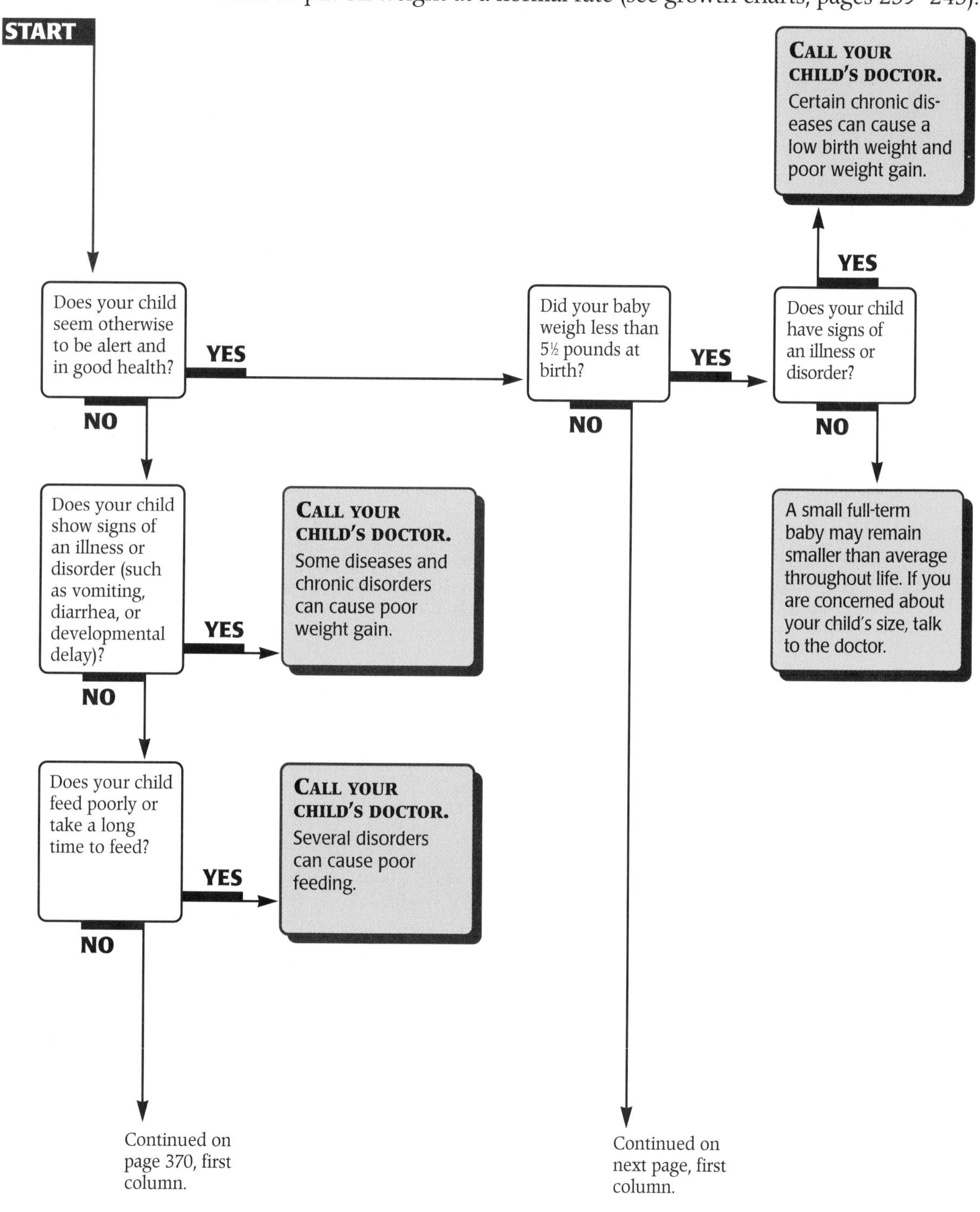

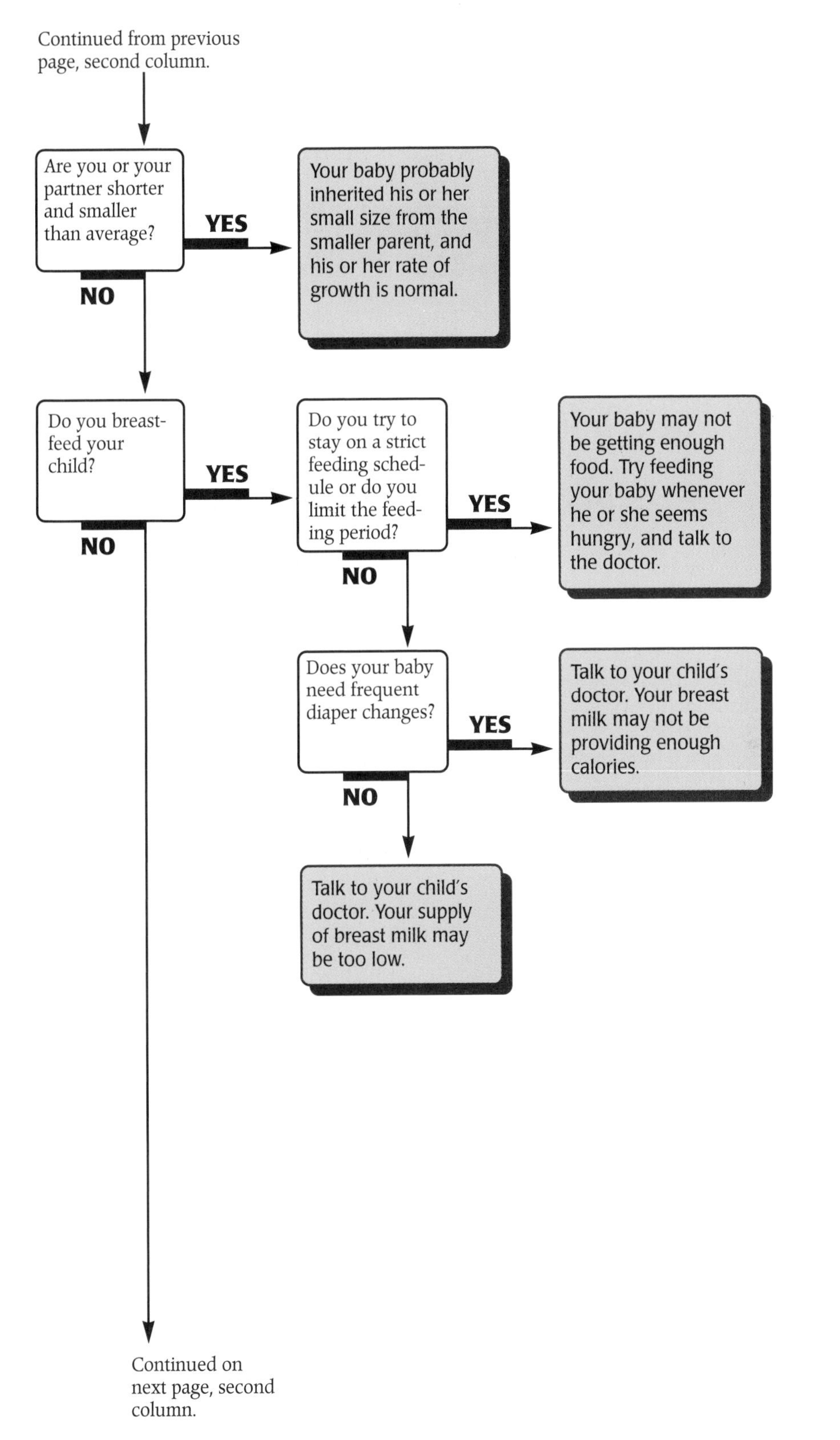
Continued from previous page, second column.
Are you or your partner shorter and smaller than average?
YES
Your baby probably inherited his or her small size from the smaller parent, and his or her rate of growth is normal.
NO
Do you breast-feed your child?
YES
Do you try to stay on a strict feeding schedule or do you limit the feeding period?
YES
Your baby may not be getting enough food. Try feeding your baby whenever he or she seems hungry, and talk to the doctor.
NO
Does your baby need frequent diaper changes?
YES
Talk to your child's doctor. Your breast milk may not be providing enough calories.
NO
Talk to your child's doctor. Your supply of breast milk may be too low.
NO
Continued on next page, second column.

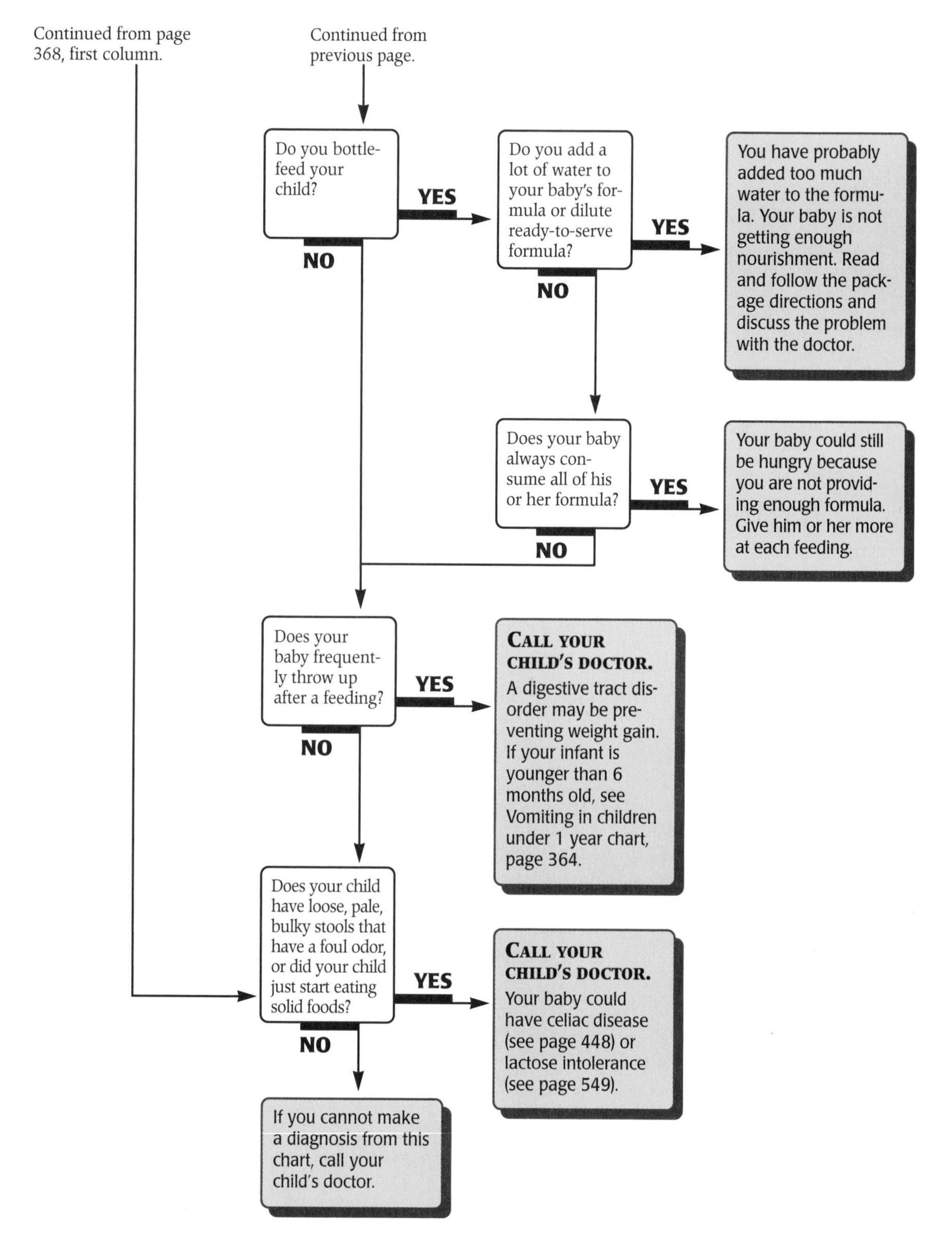
Continued from page 368, first column.
Continued from previous page.
Do you bottle-feed your child?
YES
NO
Do you add a lot of water to your baby's formula or dilute ready-to-serve formula?
YES
NO
You have probably added too much water to the formula. Your baby is not getting enough nourishment. Read and follow the package directions and discuss the problem with the doctor.
Does your baby always consume all of his or her formula?
YES
NO
Your baby could still be hungry because you are not providing enough formula. Give him or her more at each feeding.
Does your baby frequently throw up after a feeding?
YES
NO
CALL YOUR CHILD'S DOCTOR.
A digestive tract disorder may be preventing weight gain. If your infant is younger than 6 months old, see Vomiting in children under 1 year chart, page 364.
Does your child have loose, pale, bulky stools that have a foul odor, or did your child just start eating solid foods?
YES
NO
CALL YOUR CHILD'S DOCTOR.
Your baby could have celiac disease (see page 448) or lactose intolerance (see page 549).
If you cannot make a diagnosis from this chart, call your child's doctor.

CHILDREN

HEAD INJURY

Any headache, unusual drowsiness, blurred vision, problems with coordination or concentration, or loss of consciousness after a head injury.

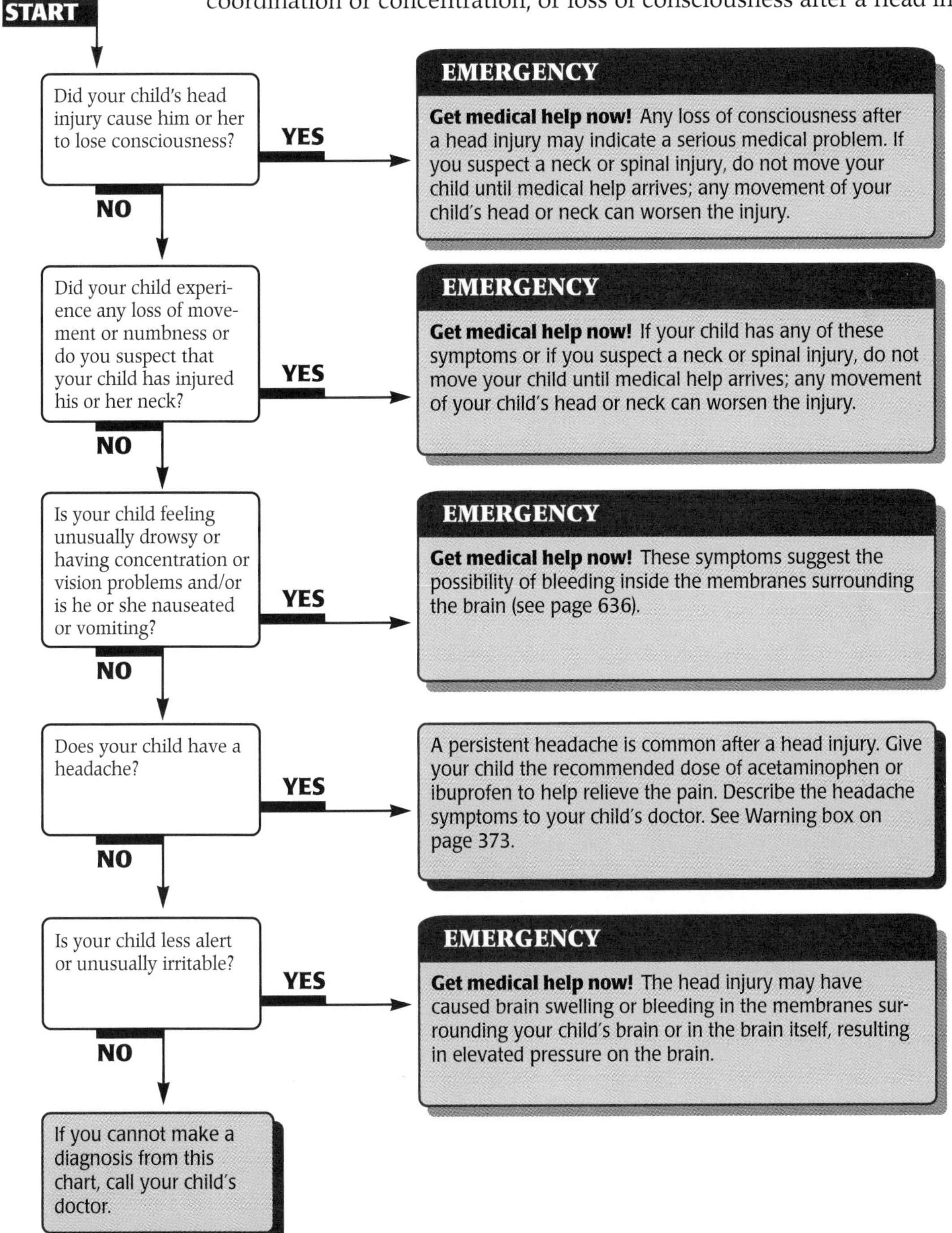

CHILDREN

FAINTING, DIZZY SPELLS, AND SEIZURES

Faintness and unsteadiness, dizzy spells, loss of consciousness, periods of "blankness," and attacks during which your child has uncontrolled body movements.

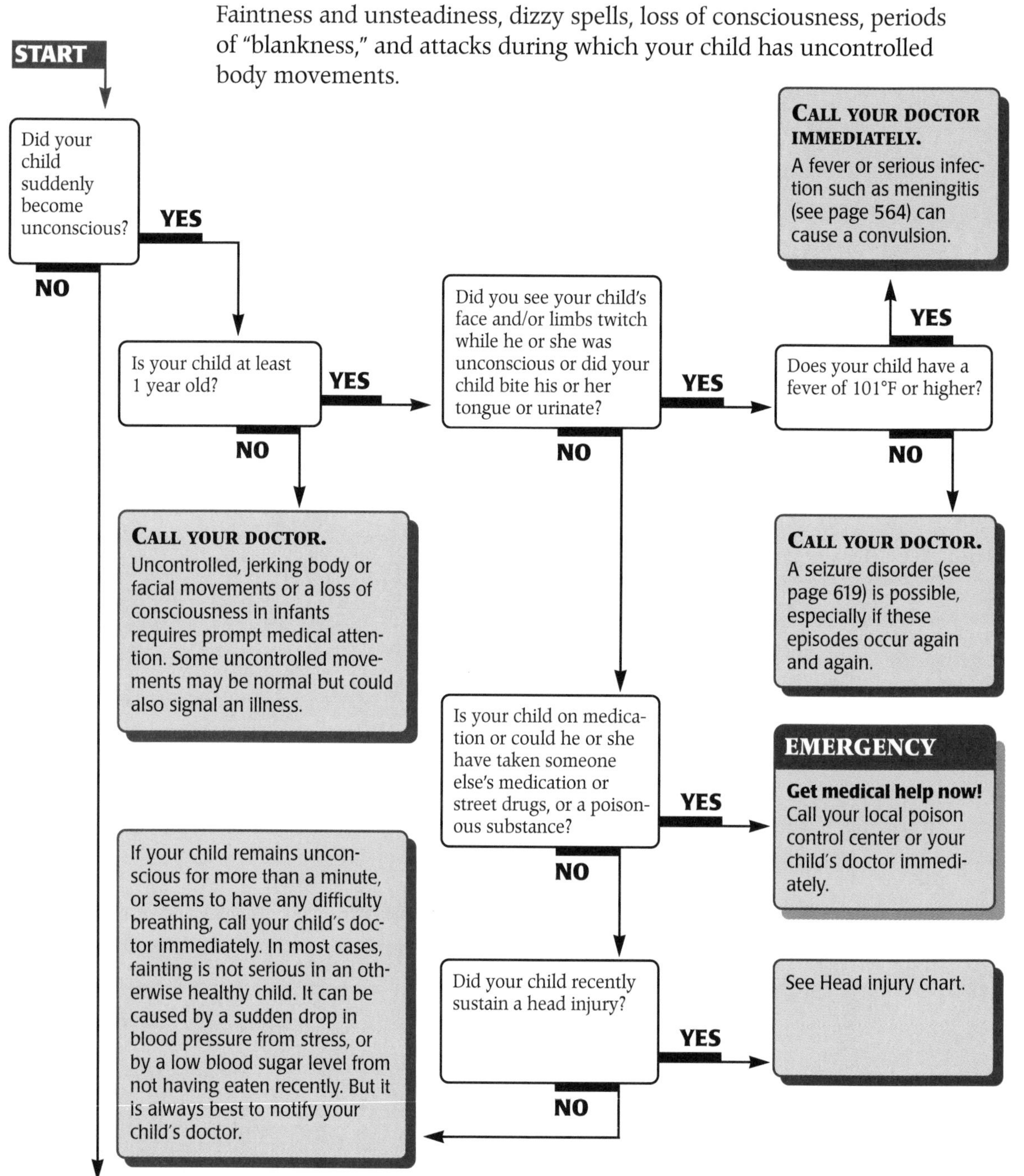

Continued on next page.

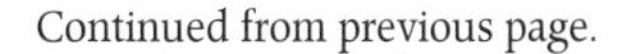
Continued from previous page.

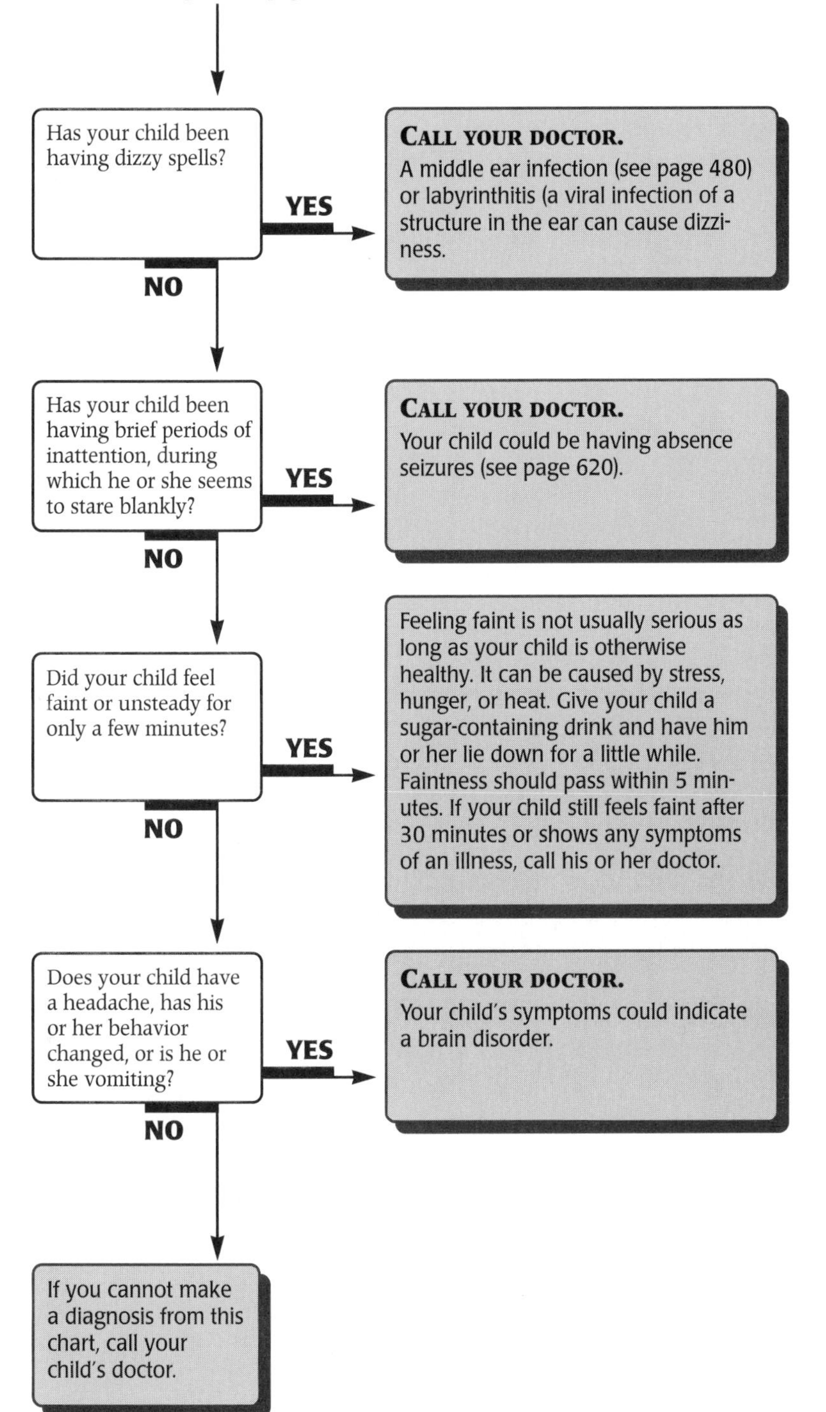

WARNING

Head injuries can be serious

If your child has had a head injury (even if he or she did not lose consciousness), you need to observe him or her closely for 24 hours (see Head injury chart). Be sure to wake your child every 4 hours and see how he or she is feeling. If your child develops any of the following signs, call your child's doctor immediately:

- Change in behavior (such as drowsiness or unusual irritability)
- Vomiting two or more times
- Change in coordination or concentration
- Problems with vision

CHILDREN

Waking during the Night

Night waking that causes your child to cry or call out for you.

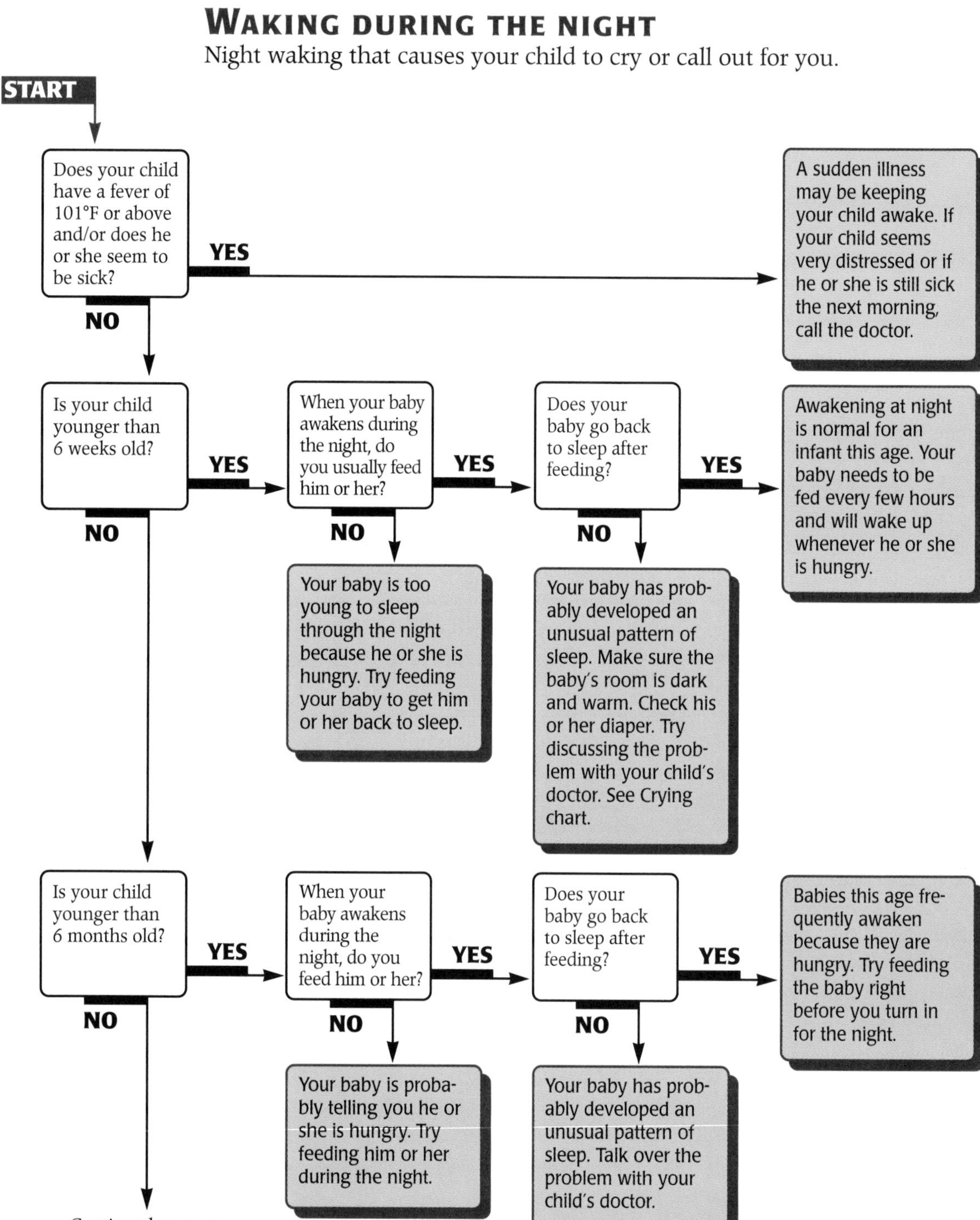

Continued on next page.

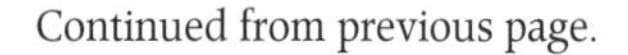
Continued from previous page.

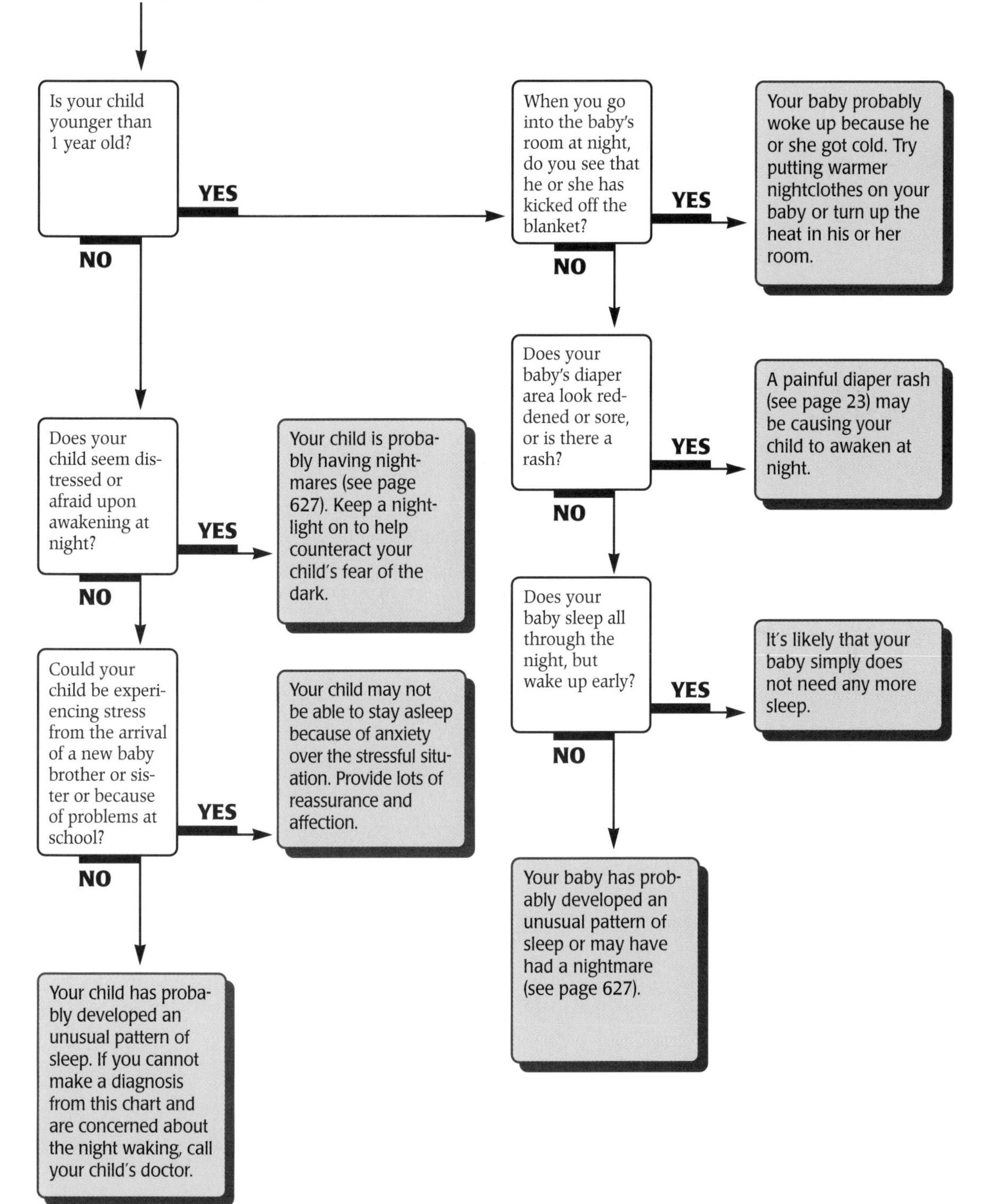
Is your child younger than 1 year old?
YES
NO
When you go into the baby's room at night, do you see that he or she has kicked off the blanket?
YES
Your baby probably woke up because he or she got cold. Try putting warmer nightclothes on your baby or turn up the heat in his or her room.
NO
Does your baby's diaper area look reddened or sore, or is there a rash?
YES
A painful diaper rash (see page 23) may be causing your child to awaken at night.
NO
Does your baby sleep all through the night, but wake up early?
YES
It's likely that your baby simply does not need any more sleep.
NO
Your baby has probably developed an unusual pattern of sleep or may have had a nightmare (see page 627).
Does your child seem distressed or afraid upon awakening at night?
YES
Your child is probably having nightmares (see page 627). Keep a nightlight on to help counteract your child's fear of the dark.
NO
Could your child be experiencing stress from the arrival of a new baby brother or sister or because of problems at school?
YES
Your child may not be able to stay asleep because of anxiety over the stressful situation. Provide lots of reassurance and affection.
NO
Your child has probably developed an unusual pattern of sleep. If you cannot make a diagnosis from this chart and are concerned about the night waking, call your child's doctor.

CHILDREN

SCHOOL PROBLEMS

Learning problems or behavior problems, including reluctance to go to school.

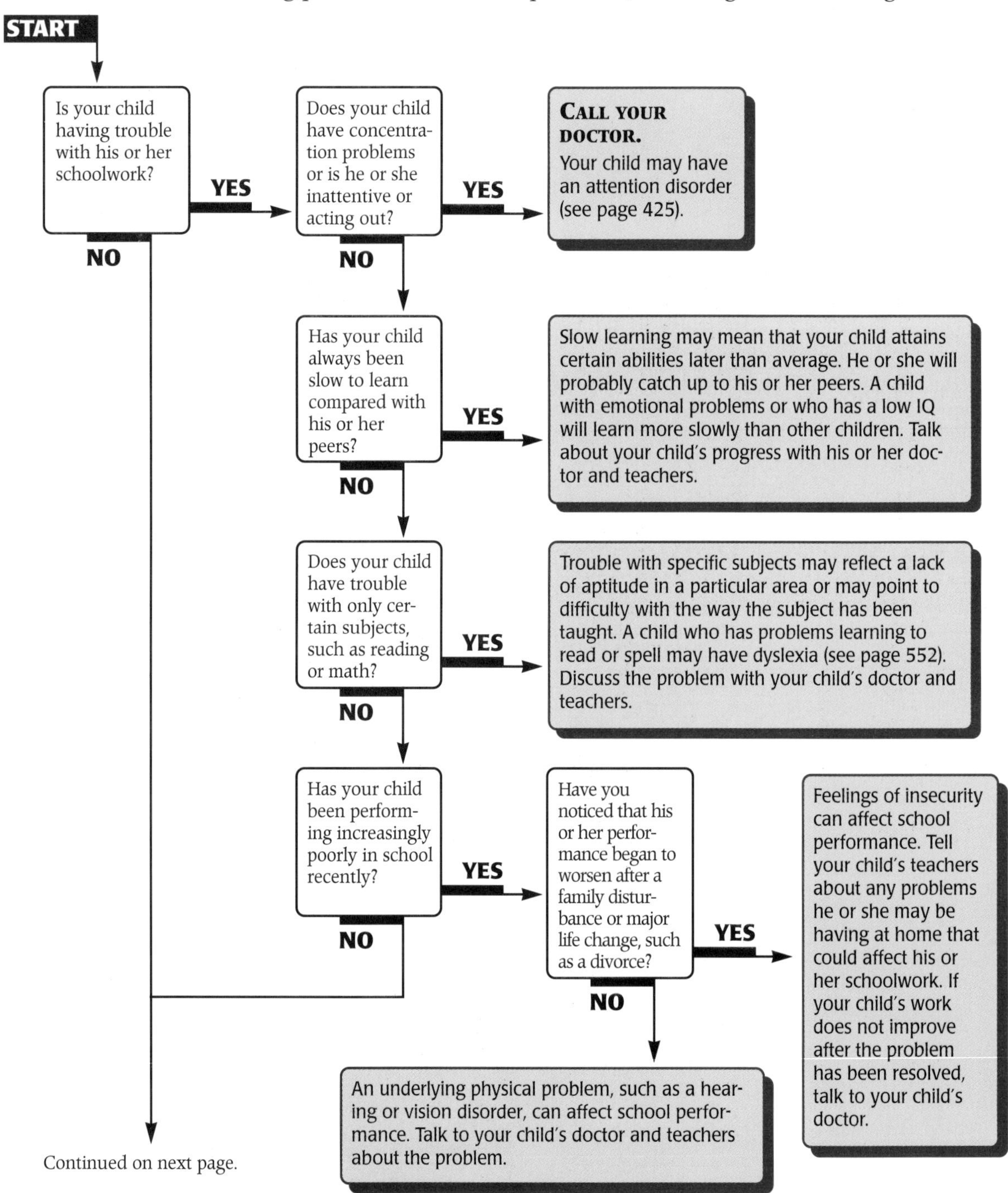

Continued from previous page.

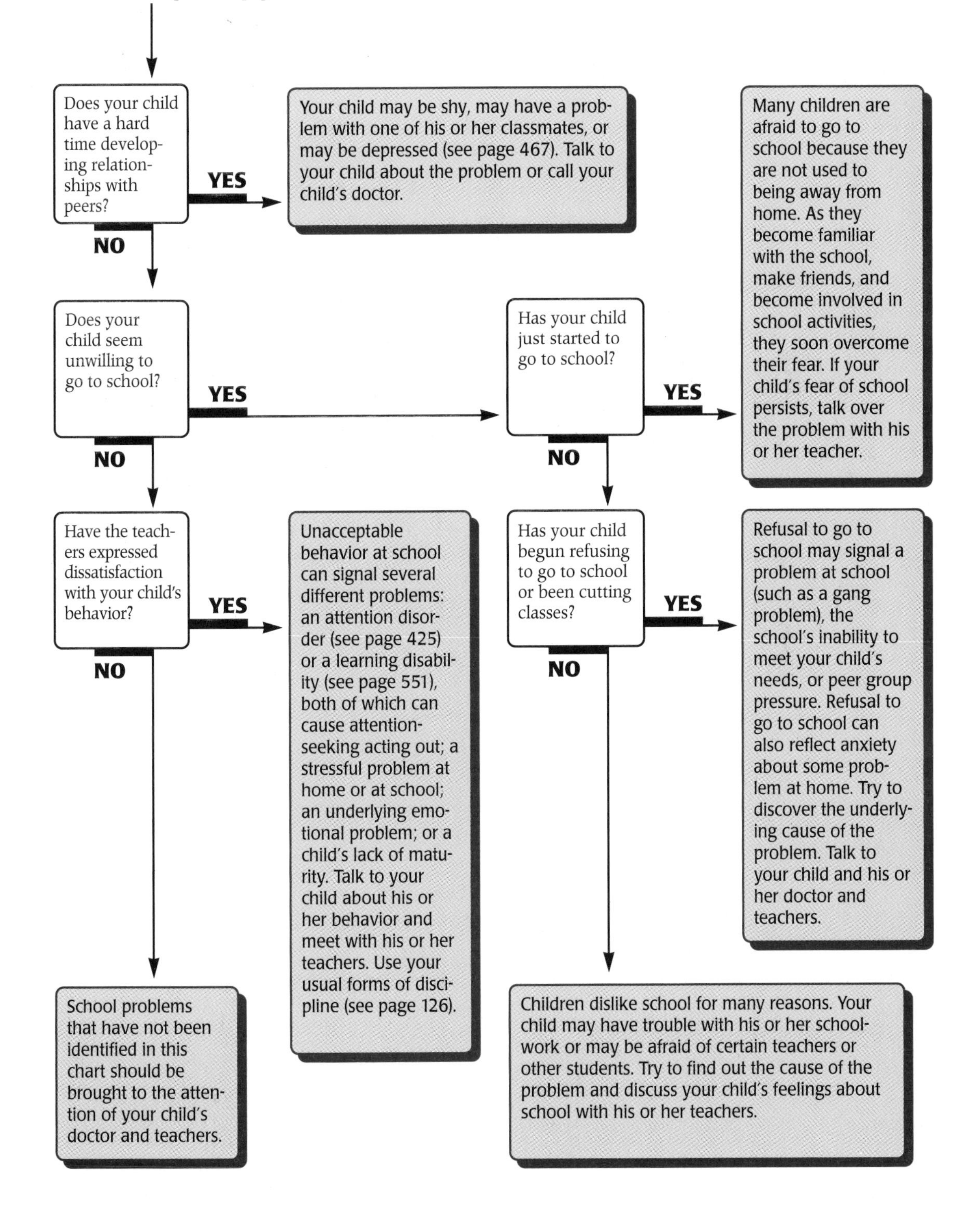

CHILDREN

ADOLESCENT BEHAVIOR PROBLEMS

Difficult or unacceptable behavior and conflict with authority figures.

START

Have you seen a sudden change in your child's behavior?

YES → Could he or she be worried about something at school or does the behavior problem occur mainly while he or she is at school?

YES → See School problems chart.

NO → Has your child been uncharacteristically drowsy or irritable, alternatively experiencing periods of unexplained elation or jitteriness?

YES → Your child may be using drugs, drinking alcohol, or inhaling solvents. Be alert for a sudden switching of friends or change in school performance, a neglect of hygiene, secretiveness, and theft of money from your home. A child who is using drugs or alcohol also often drops out of activities he or she used to enjoy. If a child is depressed or anxious, he or she could have an emotional problem. Talk to your child to find out what the problem is. If your child denies having a substance abuse problem, discuss the matter with his or her doctor.

NO → Has your child seemed unusually "down" for a while, not eating very much, neglecting to wash, sleeping badly, and withdrawing from family and friends?

YES → Many adolescents periodically become depressed (see page 467) for a short time, but long bouts of depression could be dangerous. Talk to your child to try to help resolve any emotional problems. If your child experiences a prolonged period of depression, call his or her doctor.

NO → Could your child be worried about something, such as parental fighting or problems with a boyfriend or girlfriend?

YES → Talk to your child about the problem. If you cannot help your child or if you have trouble uncovering the cause of his or her anxiety, talk to his or her doctor.

NO ↓ (and NO from "Have you seen a sudden change in your child's behavior?")

Continued on next page.

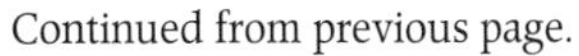
Continued from previous page.

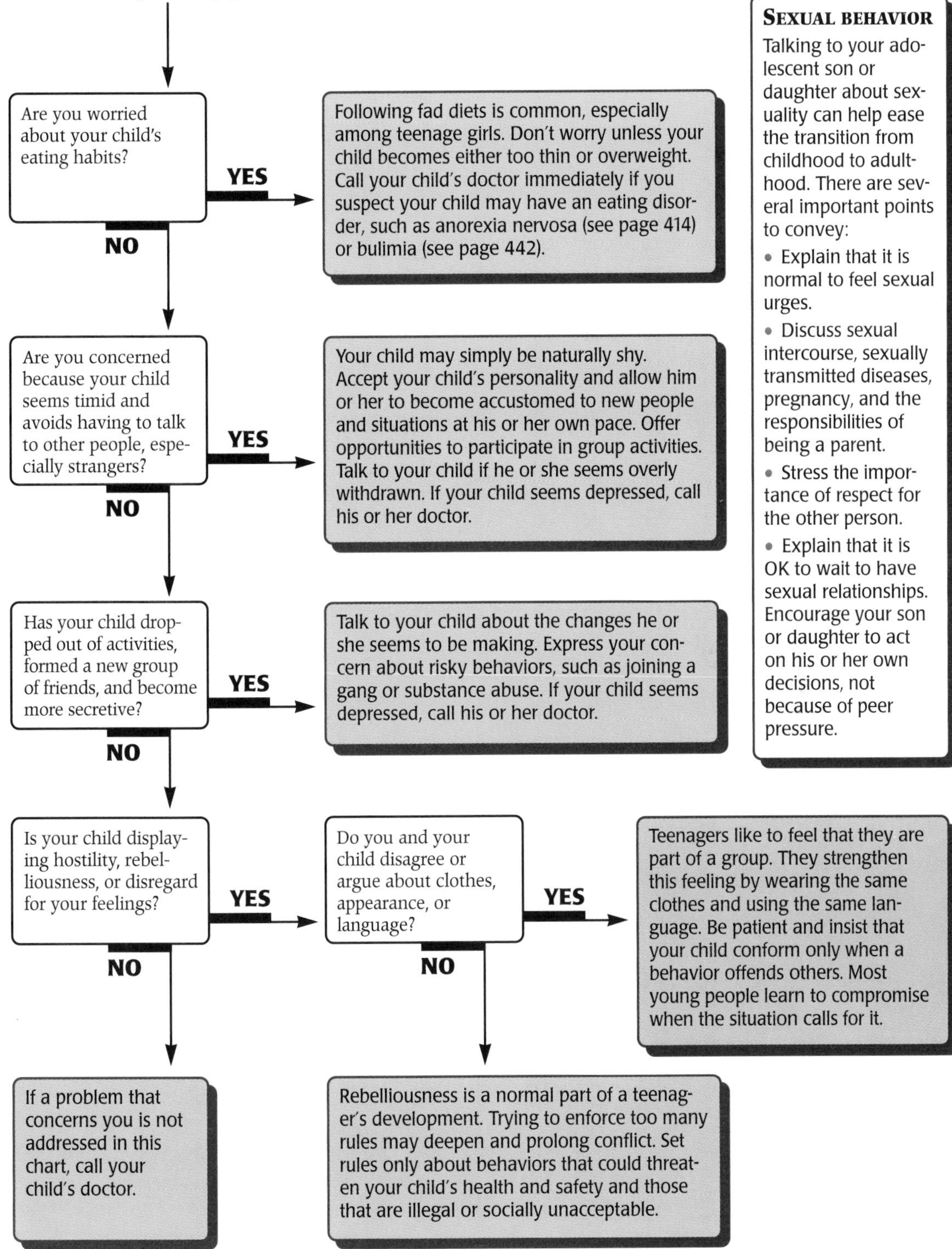

SEXUAL BEHAVIOR

Talking to your adolescent son or daughter about sexuality can help ease the transition from childhood to adulthood. There are several important points to convey:

- Explain that it is normal to feel sexual urges.
- Discuss sexual intercourse, sexually transmitted diseases, pregnancy, and the responsibilities of being a parent.
- Stress the importance of respect for the other person.
- Explain that it is OK to wait to have sexual relationships. Encourage your son or daughter to act on his or her own decisions, not because of peer pressure.

CHILDREN

FEVER IN CHILDREN OVER 1 YEAR

Temperature of 101°F or higher.

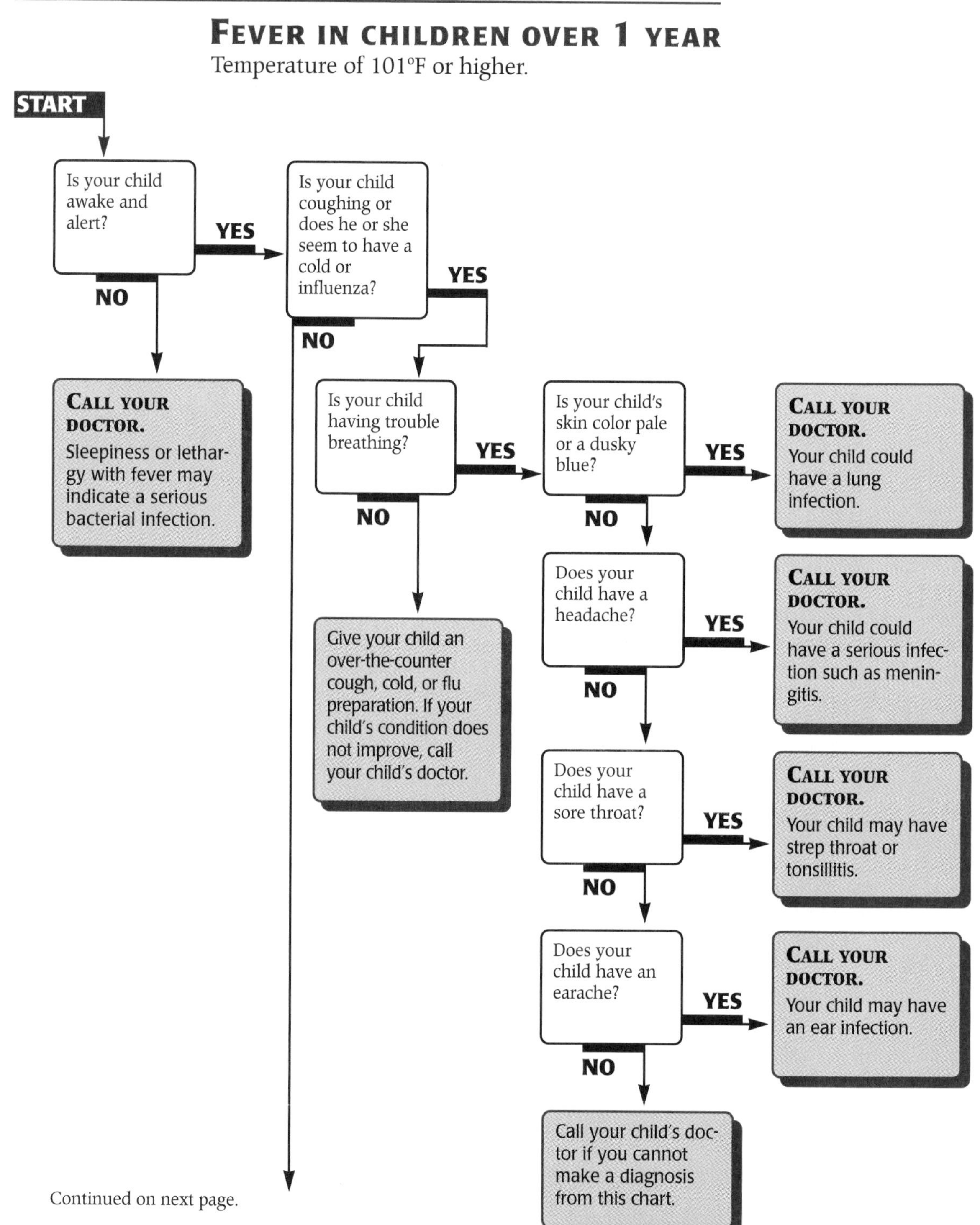

Continued on next page.

Continued from previous page.

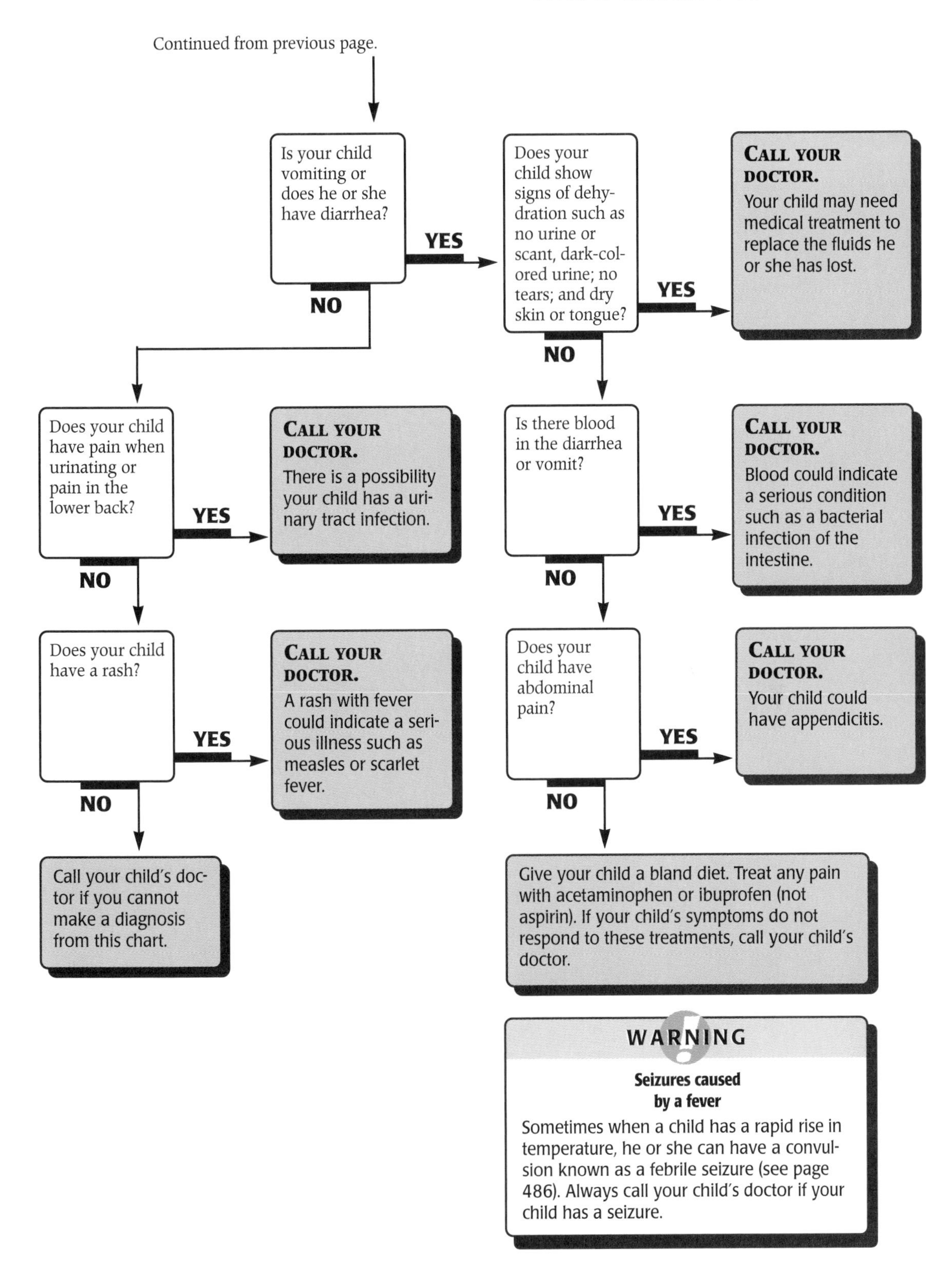

WARNING

Seizures caused by a fever

Sometimes when a child has a rapid rise in temperature, he or she can have a convulsion known as a febrile seizure (see page 486). Always call your child's doctor if your child has a seizure.

CHILDREN

BREATHING PROBLEMS

Noisy breathing, coughing, or wheezing.

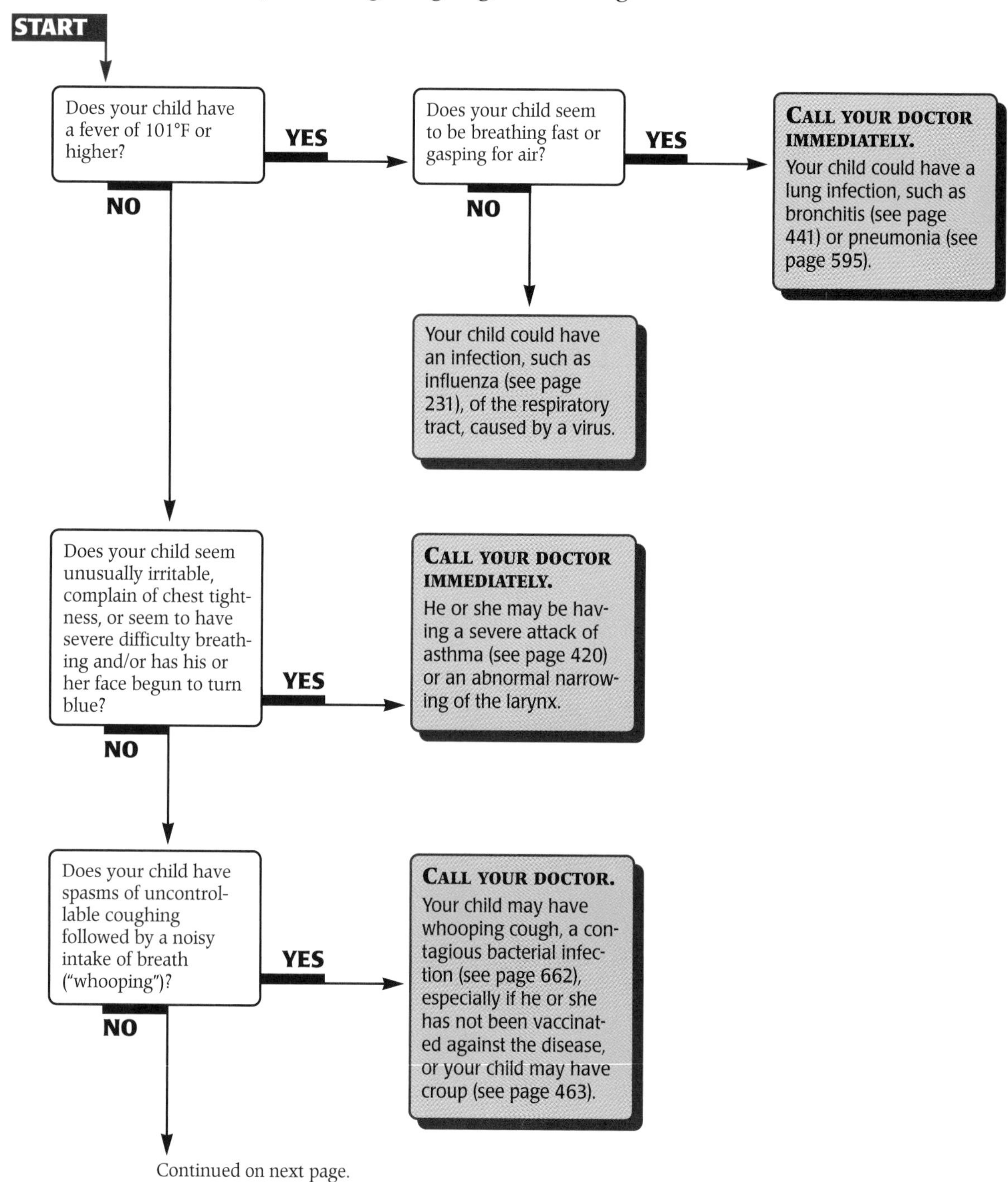

Continued on next page.

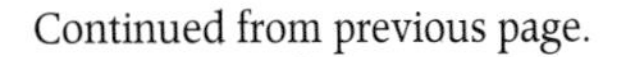
Continued from previous page.

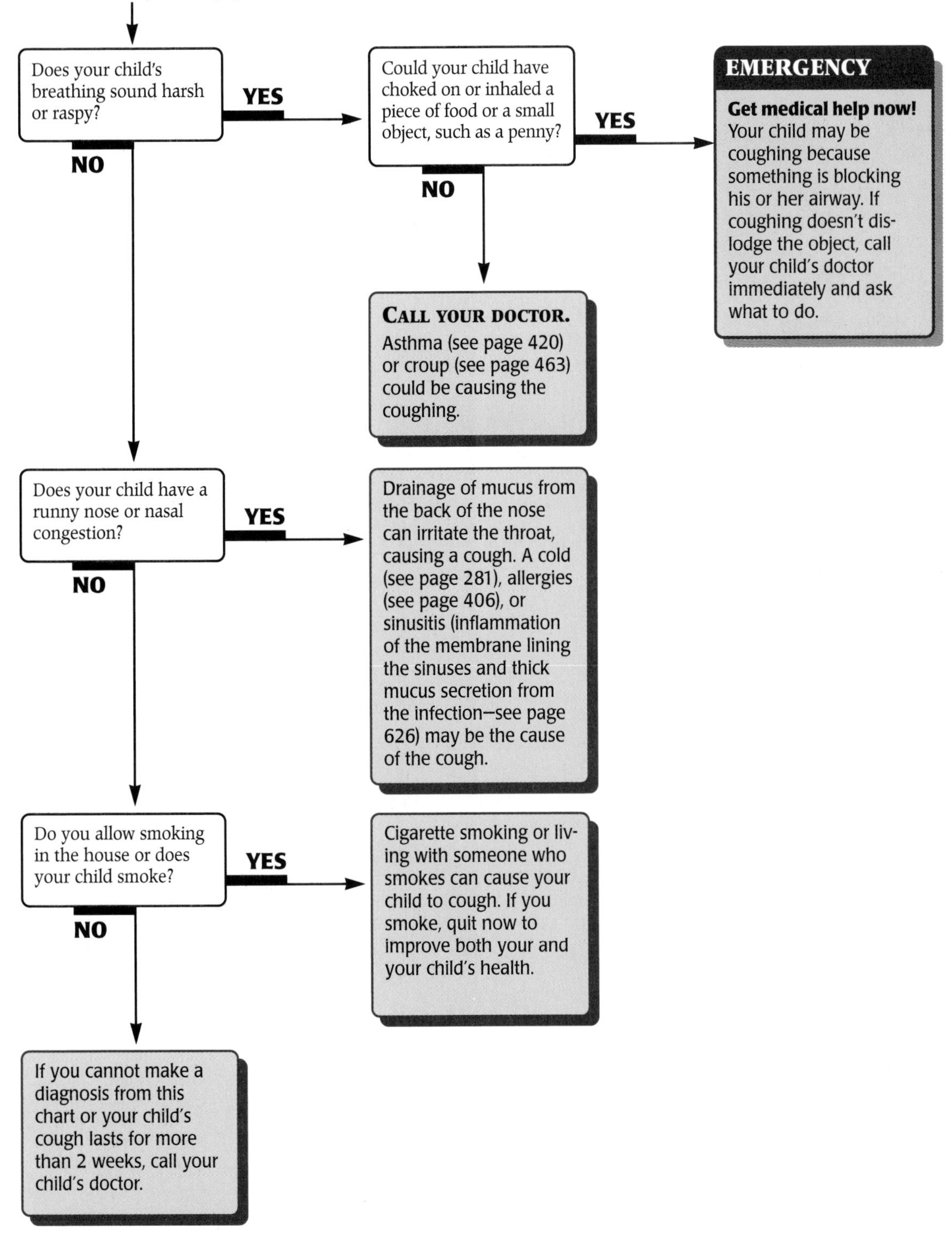
Does your child's breathing sound harsh or raspy?
YES
NO
Could your child have choked on or inhaled a piece of food or a small object, such as a penny?
YES
NO
EMERGENCY
Get medical help now!
Your child may be coughing because something is blocking his or her airway. If coughing doesn't dislodge the object, call your child's doctor immediately and ask what to do.
CALL YOUR DOCTOR.
Asthma (see page 420) or croup (see page 463) could be causing the coughing.
Does your child have a runny nose or nasal congestion?
YES
NO
Drainage of mucus from the back of the nose can irritate the throat, causing a cough. A cold (see page 281), allergies (see page 406), or sinusitis (inflammation of the membrane lining the sinuses and thick mucus secretion from the infection—see page 626) may be the cause of the cough.
Do you allow smoking in the house or does your child smoke?
YES
NO
Cigarette smoking or living with someone who smokes can cause your child to cough. If you smoke, quit now to improve both your and your child's health.
If you cannot make a diagnosis from this chart or your child's cough lasts for more than 2 weeks, call your child's doctor.

CHILDREN

RUNNY OR STUFFY NOSE

Discharge from the nose (usually accompanied by sneezing) or a stuffy nose.

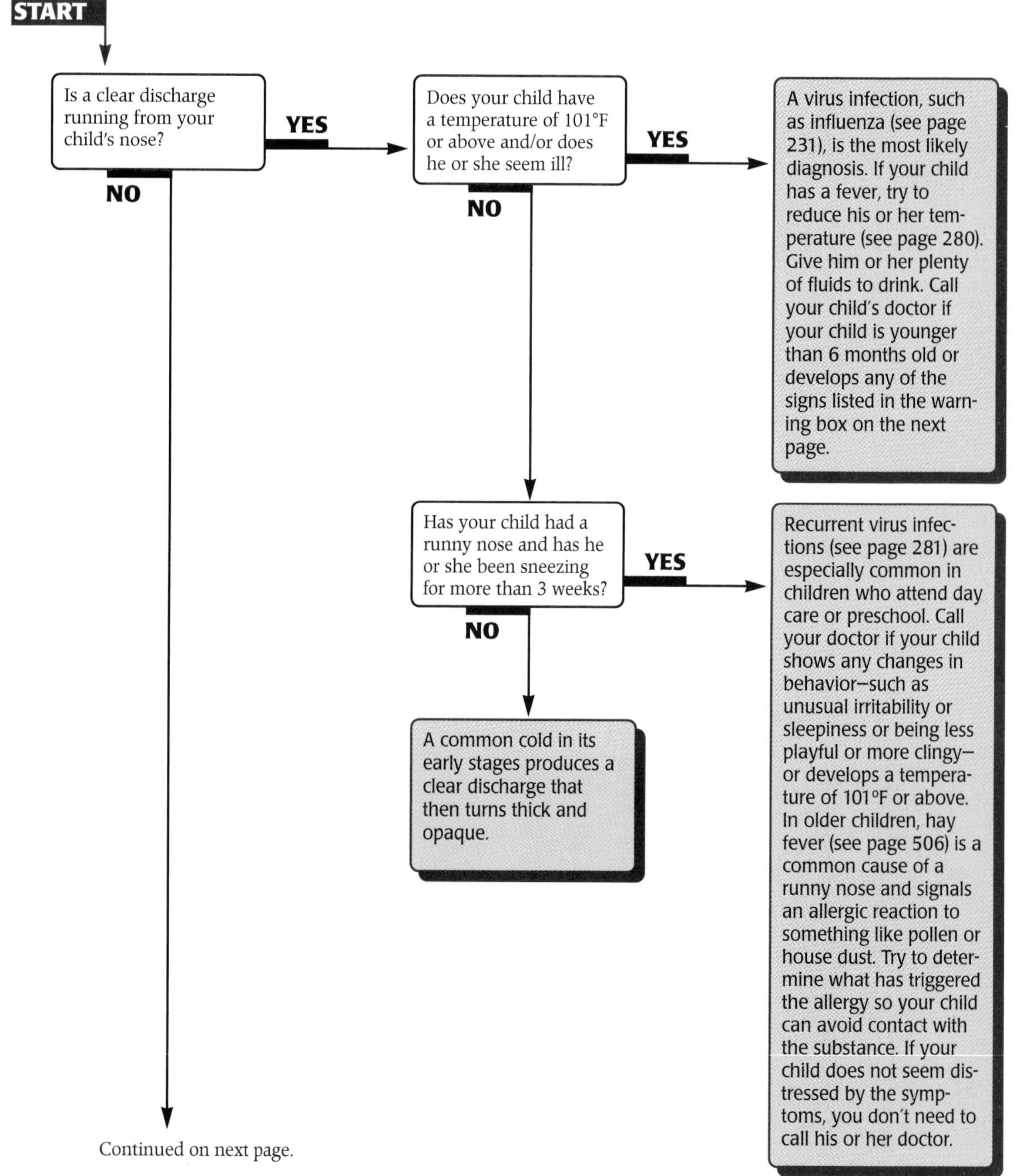

Continued on next page.

Continued from previous page.

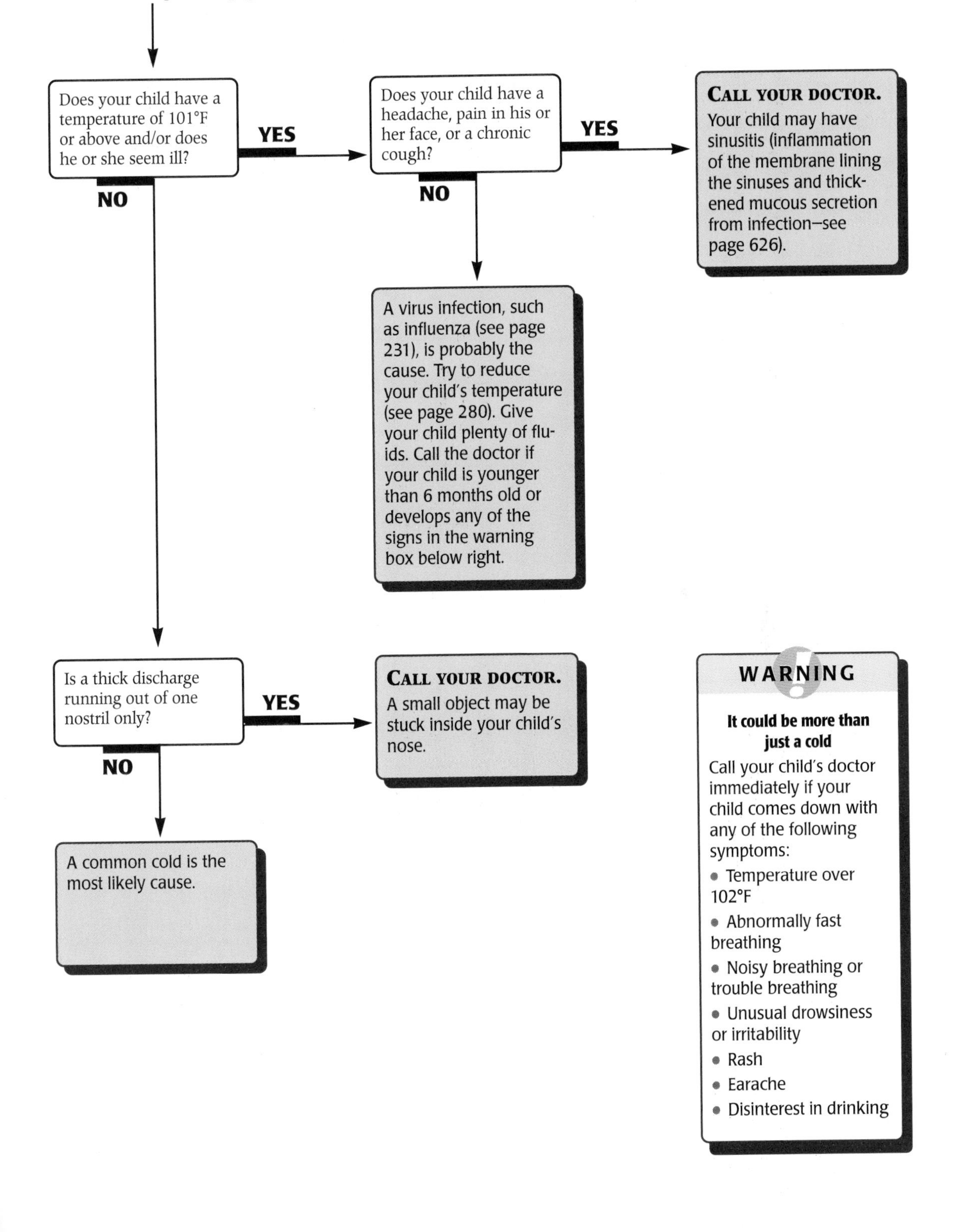

CHILDREN

SWOLLEN GLANDS OR SORE THROAT

Swelling, sometimes with tenderness, of one or more of the glands (lymph nodes) in the neck, or throat pain.

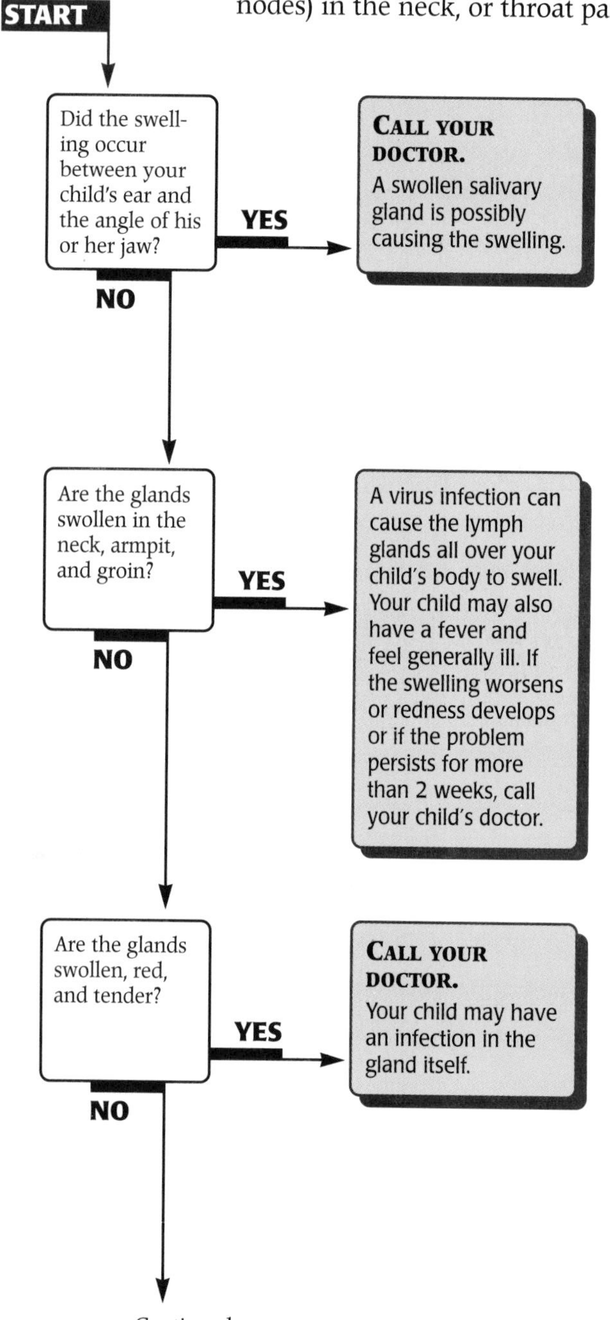

Continued on next page.

Continued from previous page.

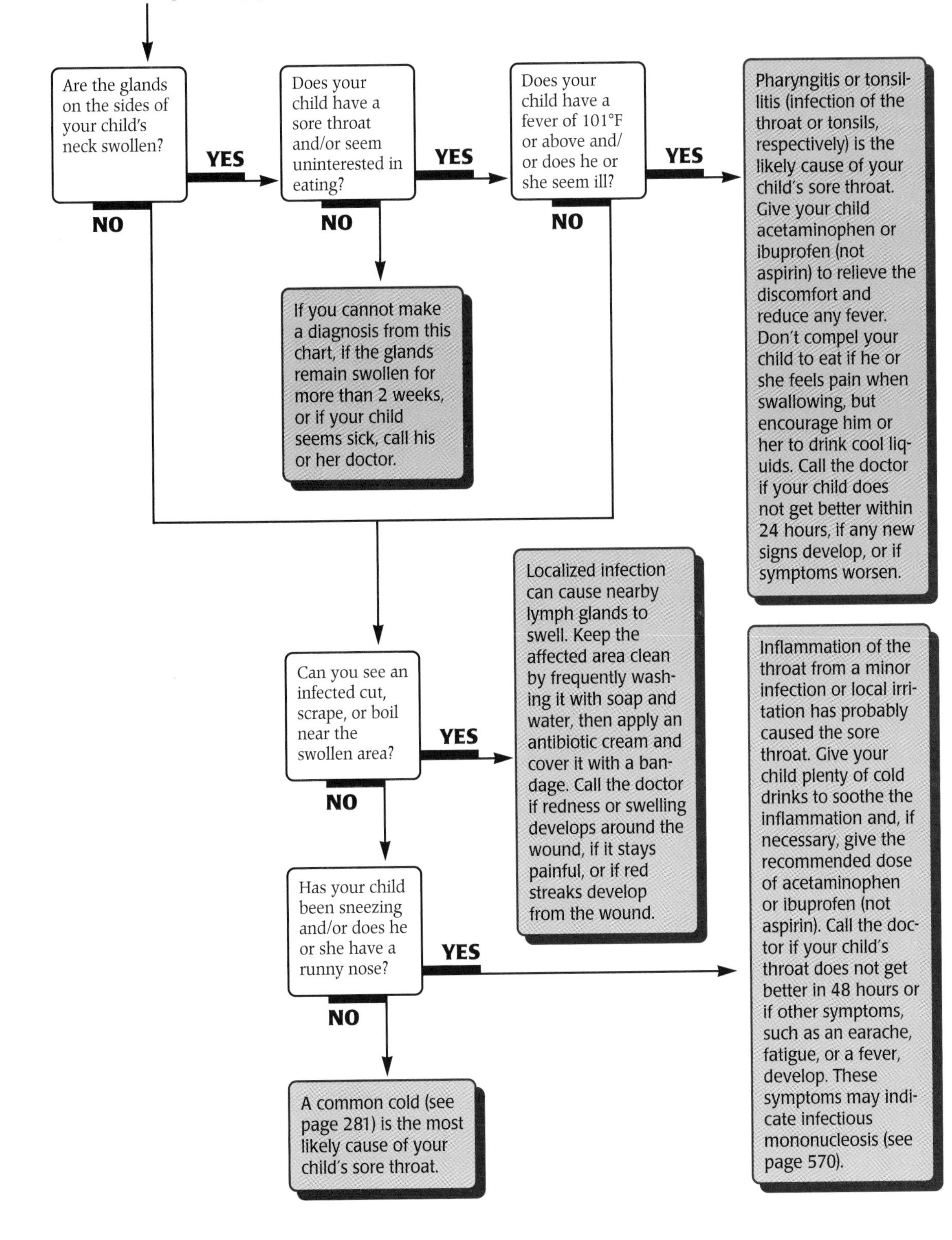

CHILDREN

EARACHE

Ear pain, often causing prolonged crying, shrieking, pulling at the affected ear, or waking at night.

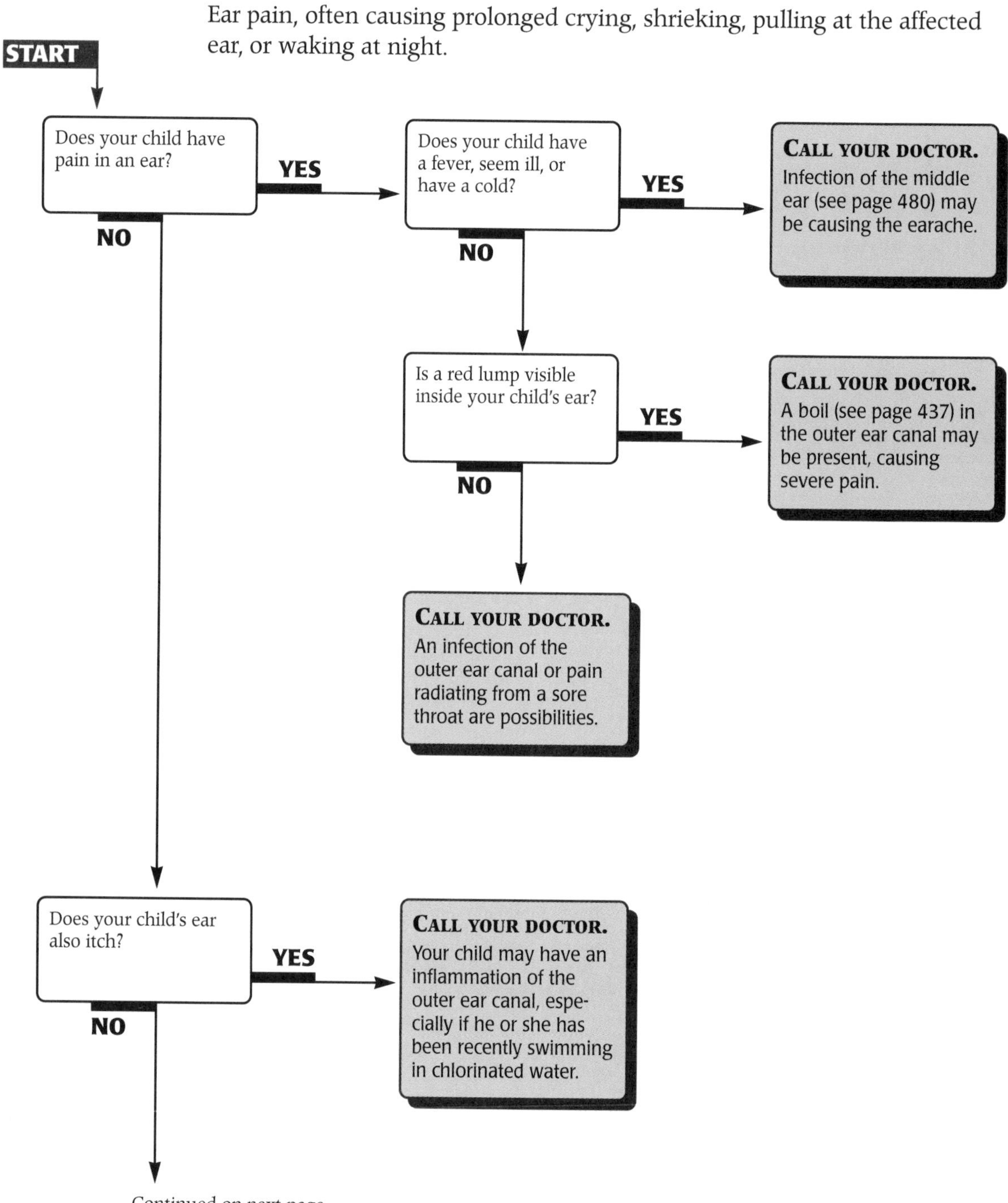

Continued on next page.

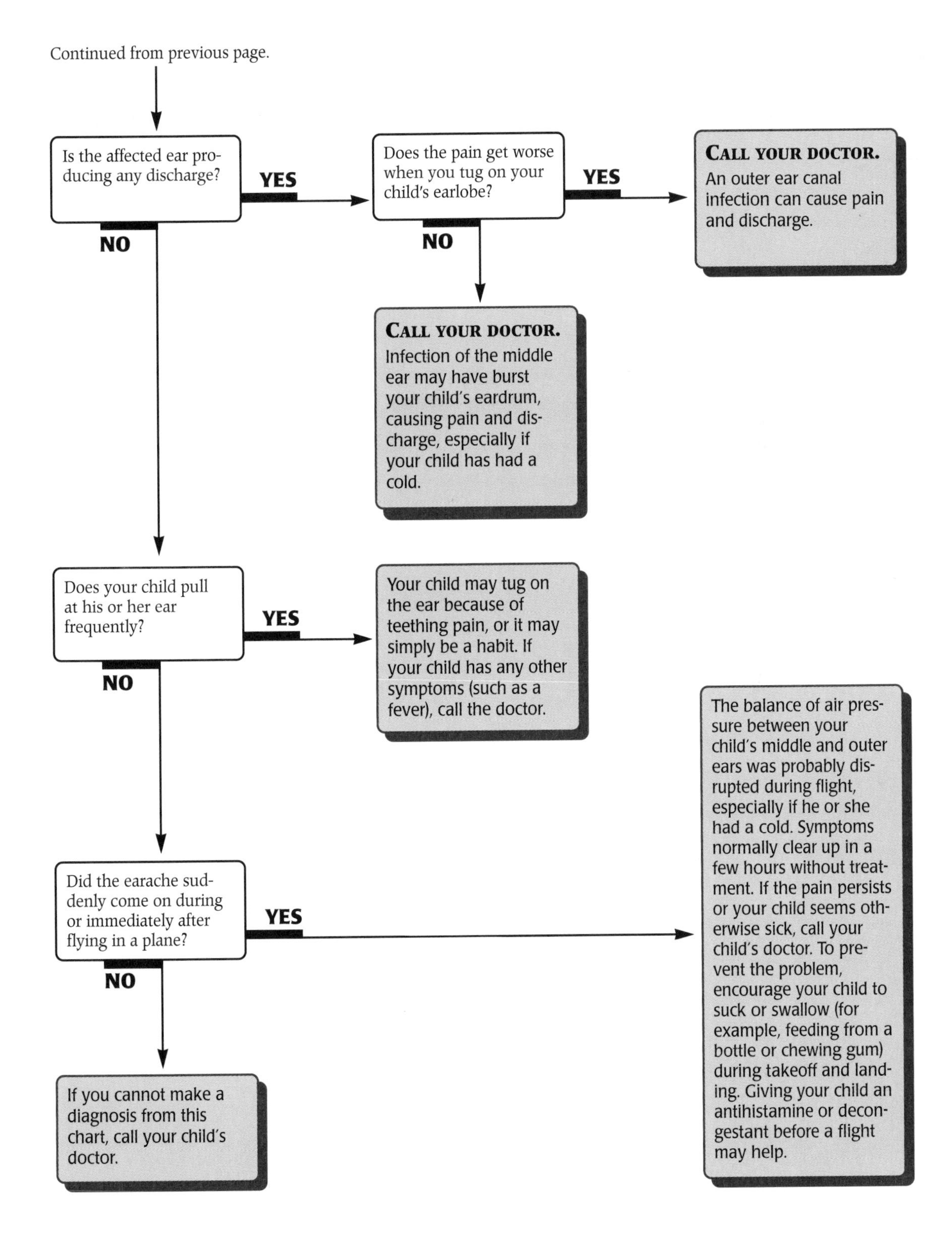
Continued from previous page.
Is the affected ear producing any discharge?
YES
NO
Does the pain get worse when you tug on your child's earlobe?
YES
NO
CALL YOUR DOCTOR.
An outer ear canal infection can cause pain and discharge.
CALL YOUR DOCTOR.
Infection of the middle ear may have burst your child's eardrum, causing pain and discharge, especially if your child has had a cold.
Does your child pull at his or her ear frequently?
YES
NO
Your child may tug on the ear because of teething pain, or it may simply be a habit. If your child has any other symptoms (such as a fever), call the doctor.
Did the earache suddenly come on during or immediately after flying in a plane?
YES
NO
The balance of air pressure between your child's middle and outer ears was probably disrupted during flight, especially if he or she had a cold. Symptoms normally clear up in a few hours without treatment. If the pain persists or your child seems otherwise sick, call your child's doctor. To prevent the problem, encourage your child to suck or swallow (for example, feeding from a bottle or chewing gum) during takeoff and landing. Giving your child an antihistamine or decongestant before a flight may help.
If you cannot make a diagnosis from this chart, call your child's doctor.

CHILDREN

VOMITING IN CHILDREN OVER 1 YEAR

Ejection of the stomach contents from a sudden contraction of the muscles in and around the stomach.

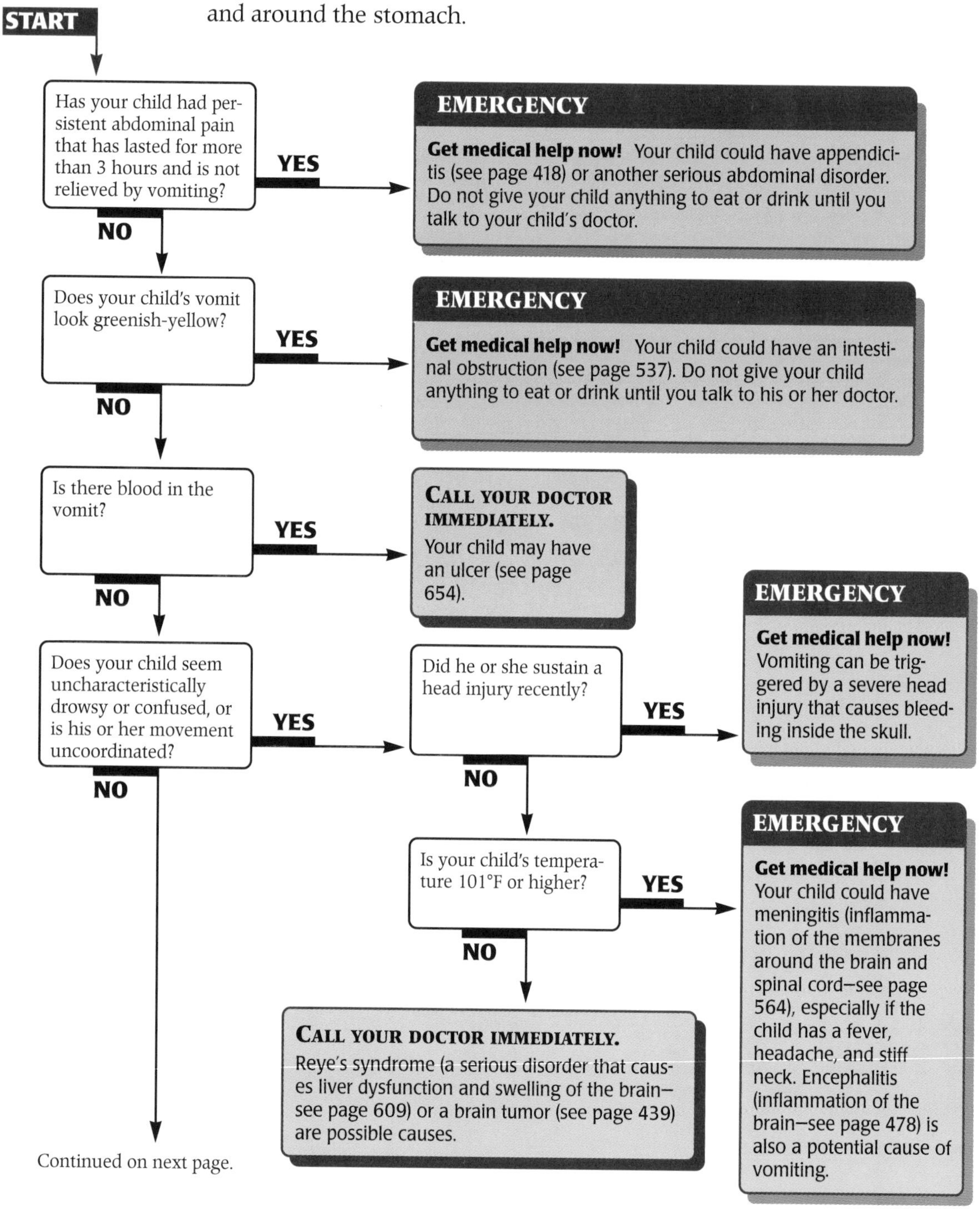

START

Has your child had persistent abdominal pain that has lasted for more than 3 hours and is not relieved by vomiting?

YES →

EMERGENCY

Get medical help now! Your child could have appendicitis (see page 418) or another serious abdominal disorder. Do not give your child anything to eat or drink until you talk to your child's doctor.

NO ↓

Does your child's vomit look greenish-yellow?

YES →

EMERGENCY

Get medical help now! Your child could have an intestinal obstruction (see page 537). Do not give your child anything to eat or drink until you talk to his or her doctor.

NO ↓

Is there blood in the vomit?

YES →

CALL YOUR DOCTOR IMMEDIATELY.

Your child may have an ulcer (see page 654).

NO ↓

Does your child seem uncharacteristically drowsy or confused, or is his or her movement uncoordinated?

YES →

Did he or she sustain a head injury recently?

YES →

EMERGENCY

Get medical help now! Vomiting can be triggered by a severe head injury that causes bleeding inside the skull.

NO ↓

Is your child's temperature 101°F or higher?

YES →

EMERGENCY

Get medical help now! Your child could have meningitis (inflammation of the membranes around the brain and spinal cord—see page 564), especially if the child has a fever, headache, and stiff neck. Encephalitis (inflammation of the brain—see page 478) is also a potential cause of vomiting.

NO ↓

CALL YOUR DOCTOR IMMEDIATELY.

Reye's syndrome (a serious disorder that causes liver dysfunction and swelling of the brain—see page 609) or a brain tumor (see page 439) are possible causes.

NO ↓

Continued on next page.

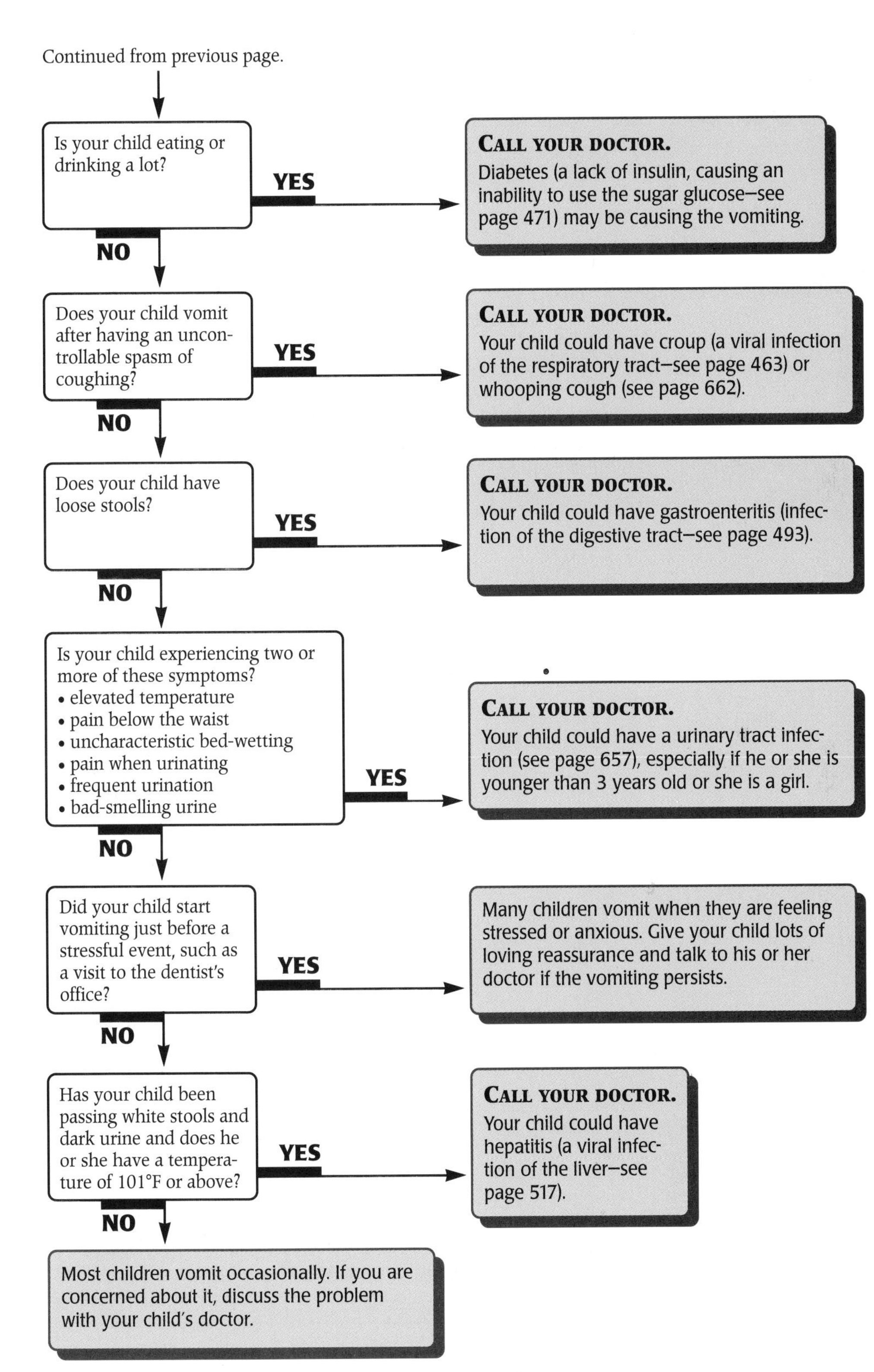
Continued from previous page.
Is your child eating or drinking a lot?
YES
CALL YOUR DOCTOR.
Diabetes (a lack of insulin, causing an inability to use the sugar glucose—see page 471) may be causing the vomiting.
NO
Does your child vomit after having an uncontrollable spasm of coughing?
YES
CALL YOUR DOCTOR.
Your child could have croup (a viral infection of the respiratory tract—see page 463) or whooping cough (see page 662).
NO
Does your child have loose stools?
YES
CALL YOUR DOCTOR.
Your child could have gastroenteritis (infection of the digestive tract—see page 493).
NO
Is your child experiencing two or more of these symptoms?
• elevated temperature
• pain below the waist
• uncharacteristic bed-wetting
• pain when urinating
• frequent urination
• bad-smelling urine
YES
CALL YOUR DOCTOR.
Your child could have a urinary tract infection (see page 657), especially if he or she is younger than 3 years old or she is a girl.
NO
Did your child start vomiting just before a stressful event, such as a visit to the dentist's office?
YES
Many children vomit when they are feeling stressed or anxious. Give your child lots of loving reassurance and talk to his or her doctor if the vomiting persists.
NO
Has your child been passing white stools and dark urine and does he or she have a temperature of 101°F or above?
YES
CALL YOUR DOCTOR.
Your child could have hepatitis (a viral infection of the liver—see page 517).
NO
Most children vomit occasionally. If you are concerned about it, discuss the problem with your child's doctor.

CHILDREN

DIARRHEA IN CHILDREN OVER 1 YEAR

Passing unusually runny stools more often than usual.

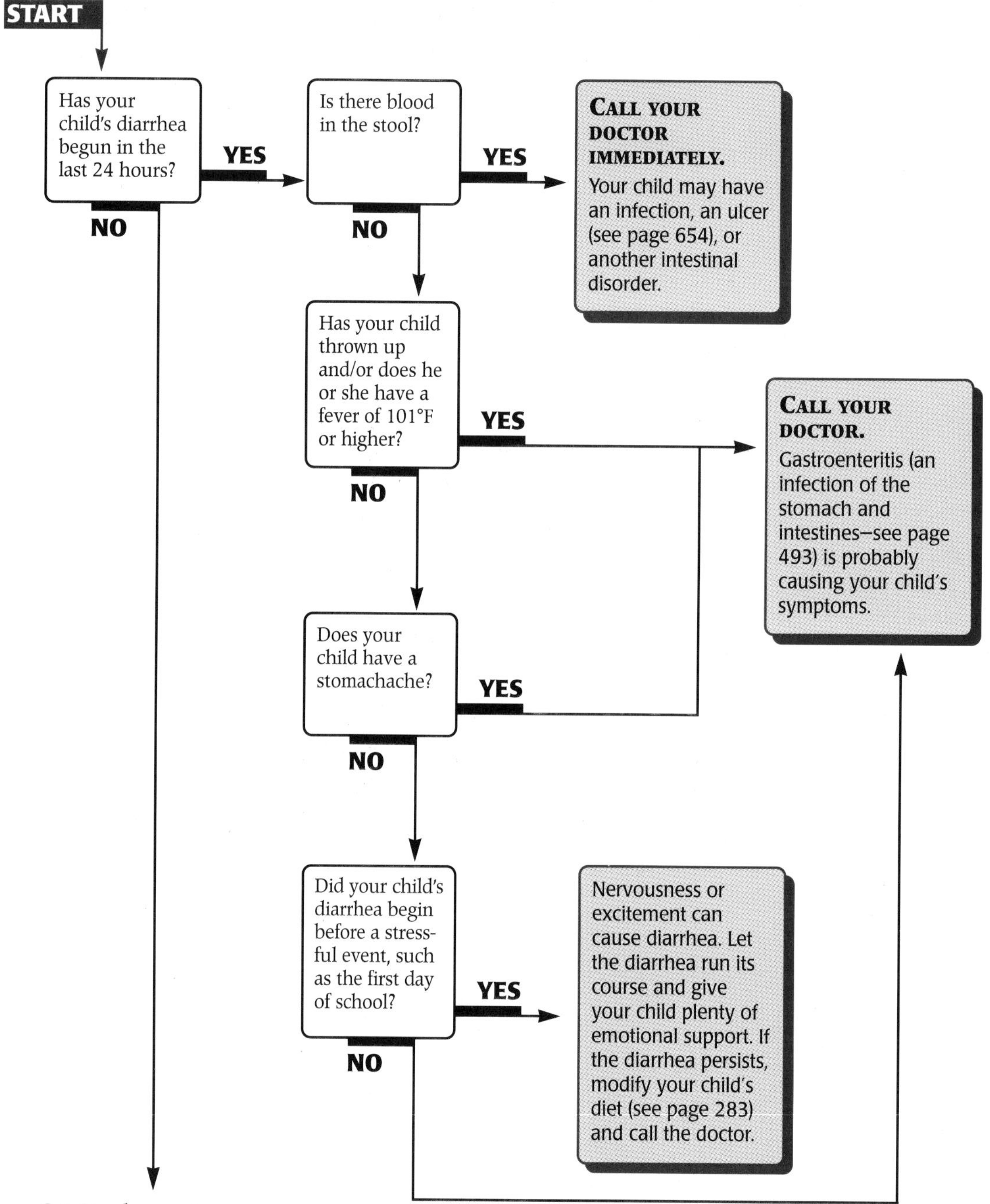

Continued on next page.

Continued from previous page.

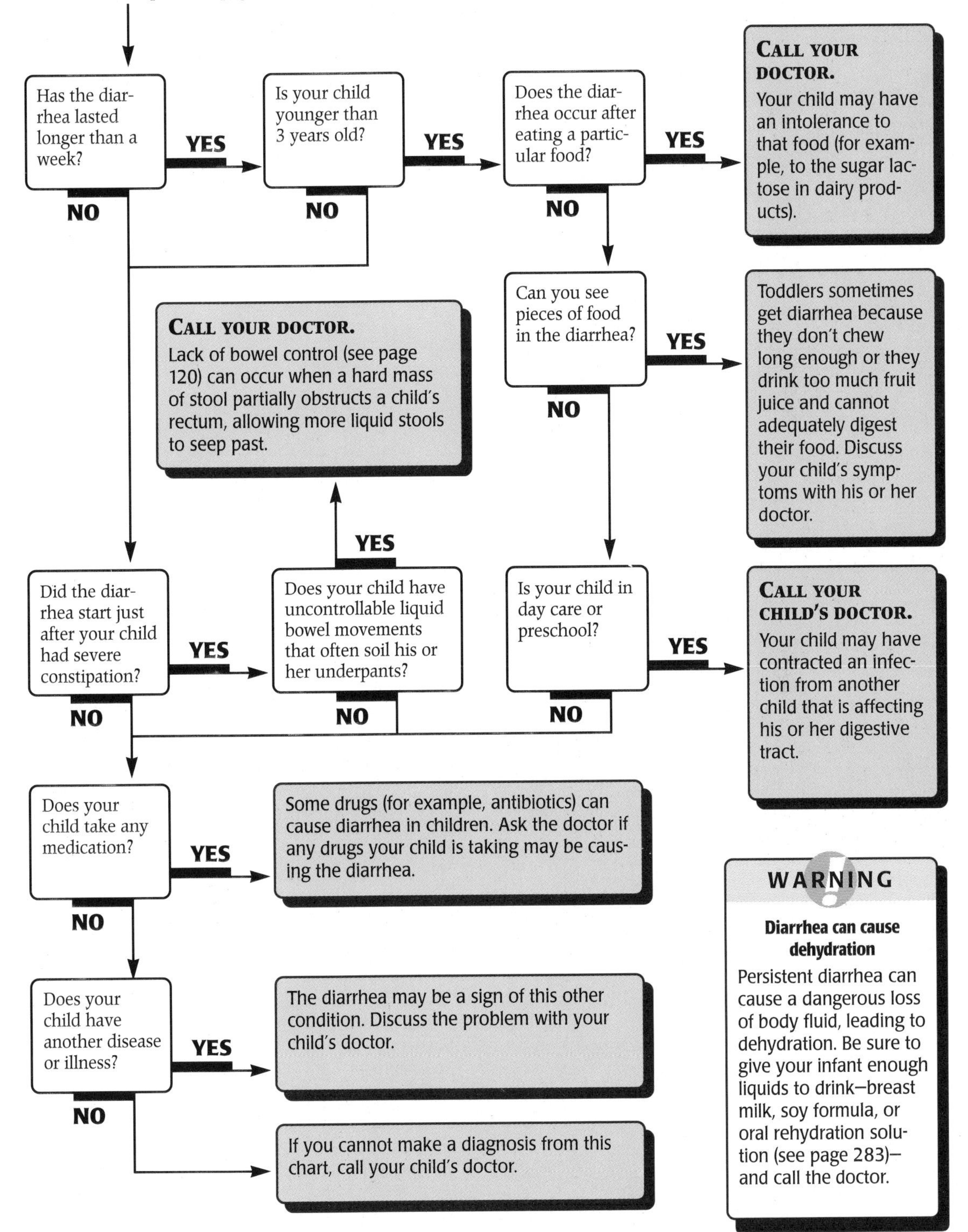

WARNING

Diarrhea can cause dehydration

Persistent diarrhea can cause a dangerous loss of body fluid, leading to dehydration. Be sure to give your infant enough liquids to drink—breast milk, soy formula, or oral rehydration solution (see page 283)—and call the doctor.

CHILDREN

TOILET PROBLEMS

Lack of or changes in the ability to control urination or bowel movements.

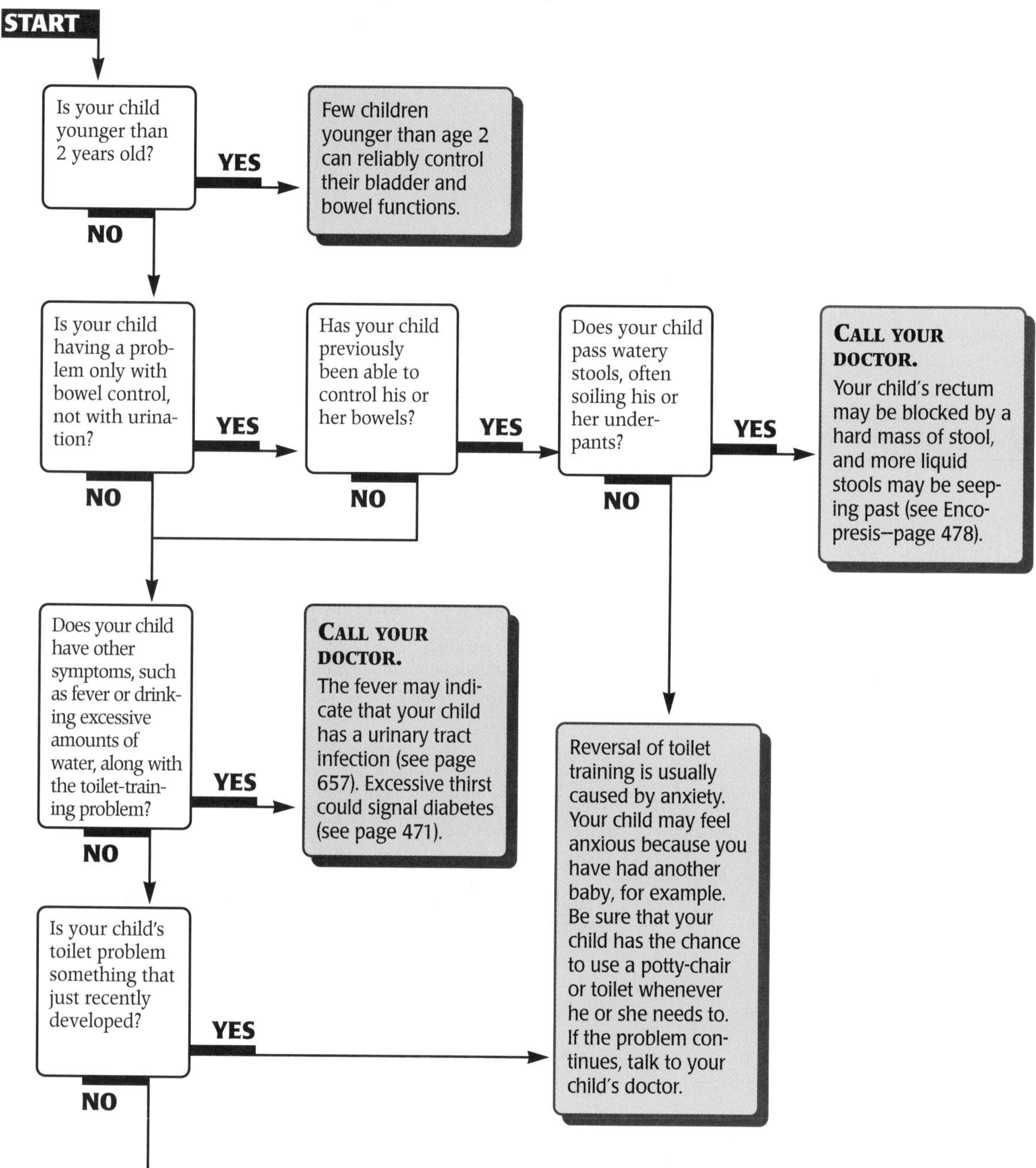

Continued on next page.

Continued from previous page.

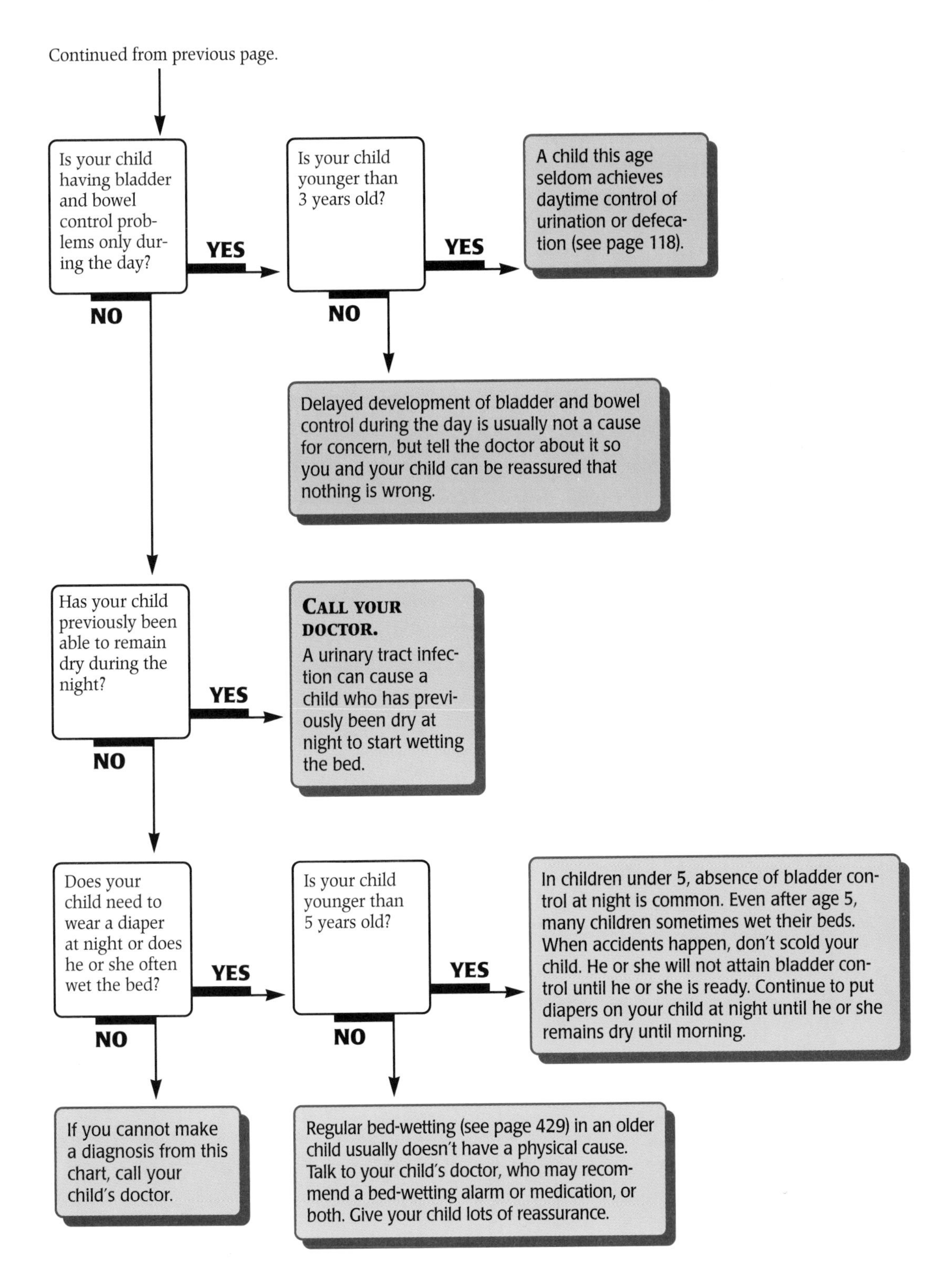

CHILDREN

URINARY PROBLEMS

Pain when passing urine, urinating more frequently than usual without a noticeable increase in fluid intake, passing urine more than once an hour, passing small amounts of urine frequently, waking several times during the night to pass urine, or discoloration of urine.

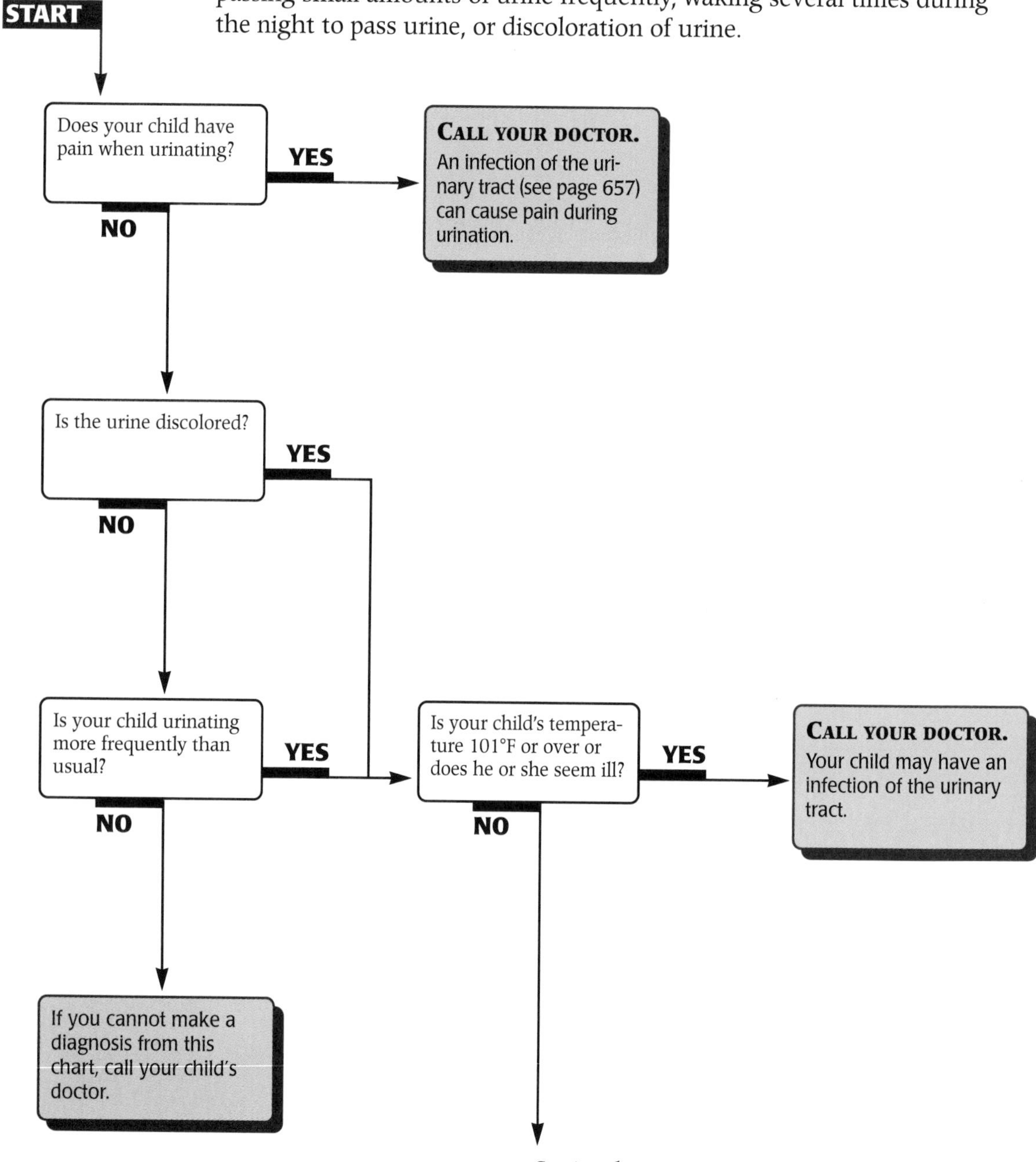

Continued on next page.

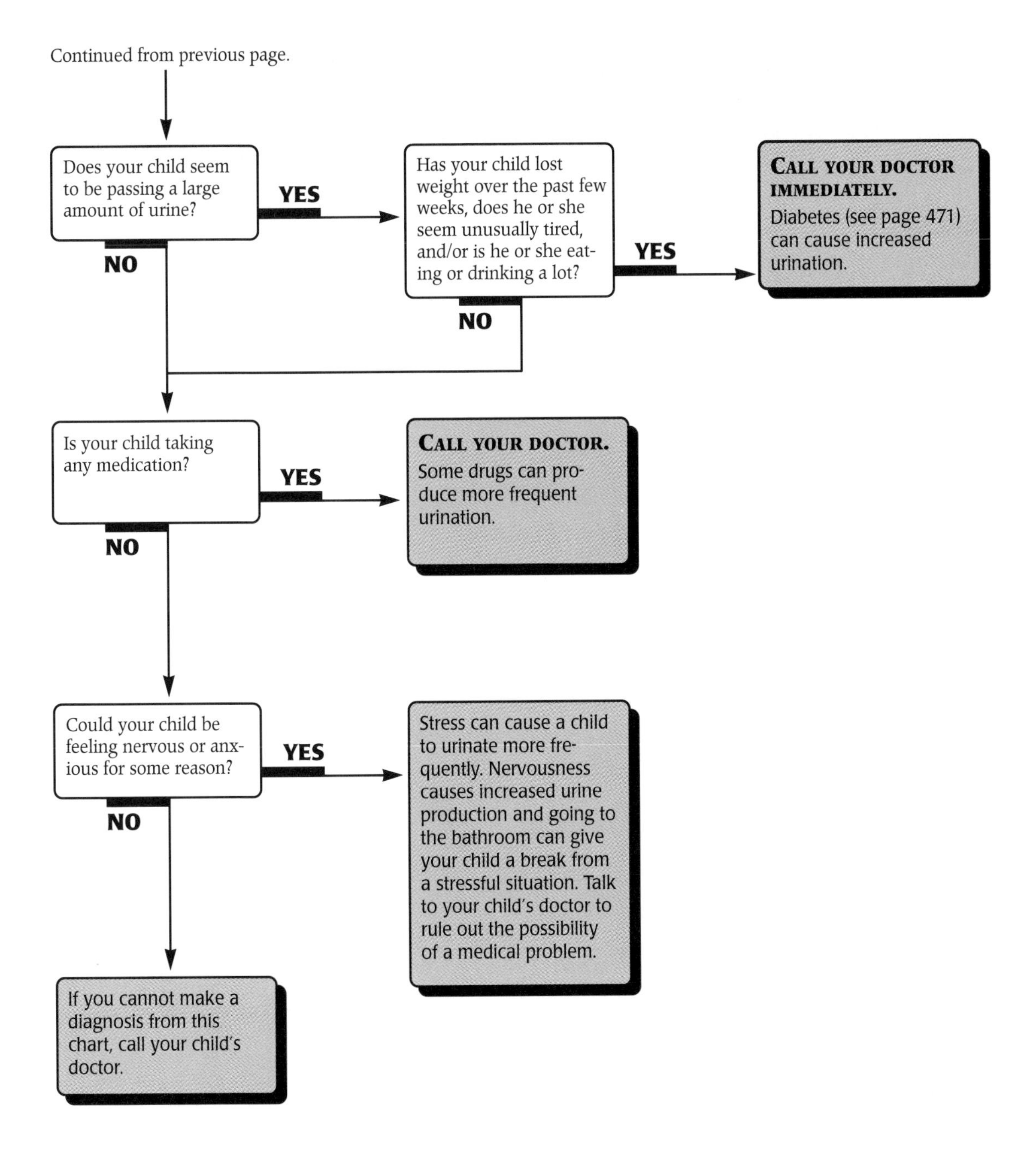
Continued from previous page.
Does your child seem to be passing a large amount of urine?
YES
NO
Has your child lost weight over the past few weeks, does he or she seem unusually tired, and/or is he or she eating or drinking a lot?
YES
NO
CALL YOUR DOCTOR IMMEDIATELY.
Diabetes (see page 471) can cause increased urination.
Is your child taking any medication?
YES
NO
CALL YOUR DOCTOR.
Some drugs can produce more frequent urination.
Could your child be feeling nervous or anxious for some reason?
YES
NO
Stress can cause a child to urinate more frequently. Nervousness causes increased urine production and going to the bathroom can give your child a break from a stressful situation. Talk to your child's doctor to rule out the possibility of a medical problem.
If you cannot make a diagnosis from this chart, call your child's doctor.

CHILDREN

GENITAL OR ANAL PROBLEMS IN BOYS

Pain or swelling inside the scrotum (the sac that encloses the testicles) or in the penis or itching or irritation around the anus.

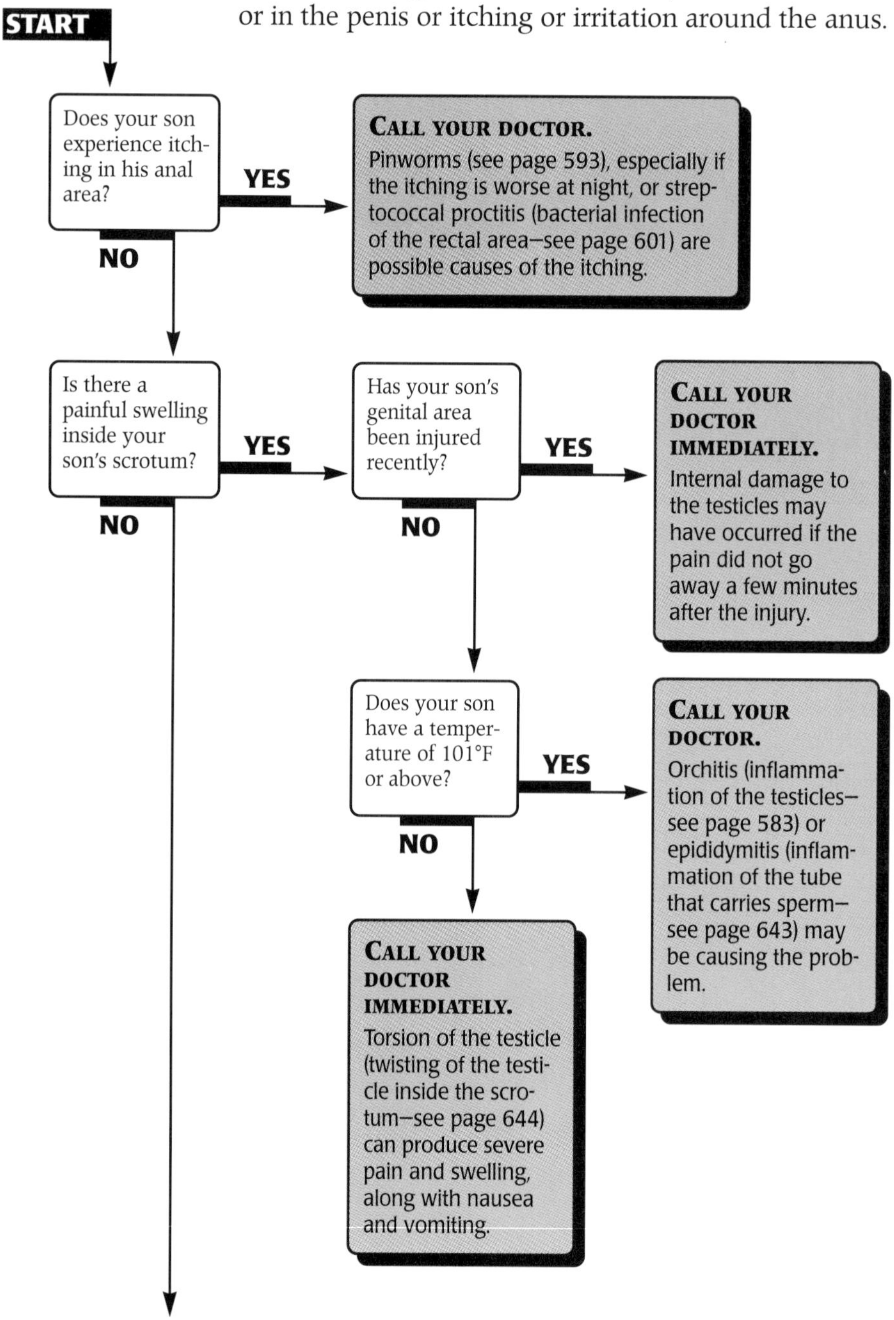

START

Does your son experience itching in his anal area?

- YES → **CALL YOUR DOCTOR.** Pinworms (see page 593), especially if the itching is worse at night, or streptococcal proctitis (bacterial infection of the rectal area—see page 601) are possible causes of the itching.
- NO ↓

Is there a painful swelling inside your son's scrotum?

- YES → **Has your son's genital area been injured recently?**
  - YES → **CALL YOUR DOCTOR IMMEDIATELY.** Internal damage to the testicles may have occurred if the pain did not go away a few minutes after the injury.
  - NO → **Does your son have a temperature of 101°F or above?**
    - YES → **CALL YOUR DOCTOR.** Orchitis (inflammation of the testicles—see page 583) or epididymitis (inflammation of the tube that carries sperm—see page 643) may be causing the problem.
    - NO → **CALL YOUR DOCTOR IMMEDIATELY.** Torsion of the testicle (twisting of the testicle inside the scrotum—see page 644) can produce severe pain and swelling, along with nausea and vomiting.
- NO ↓

Continued on next page.

Continued from previous page.

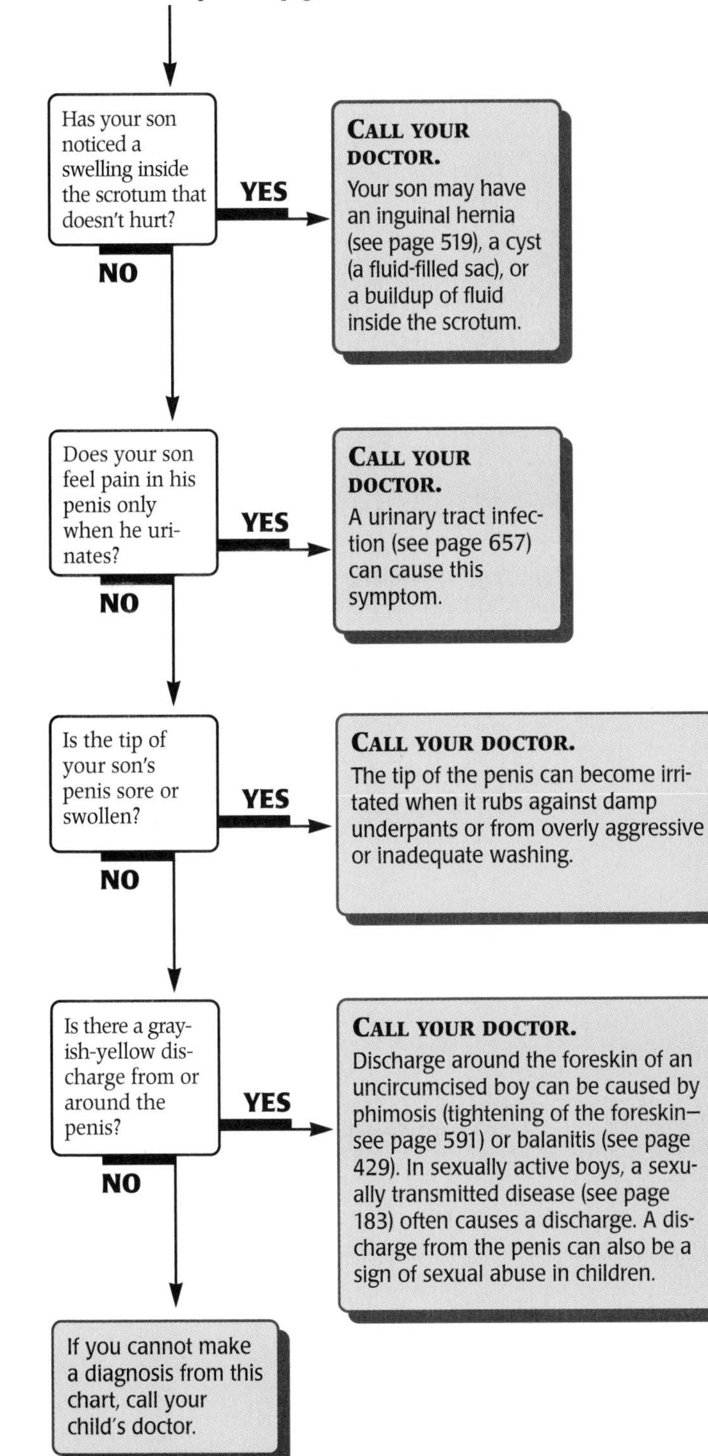

CHILDREN

GENITAL OR ANAL PROBLEMS IN GIRLS

Itching and inflammation of the vulva (the outer genital area), pain during urination, an unusual vaginal discharge, or itching or irritation around the anus.

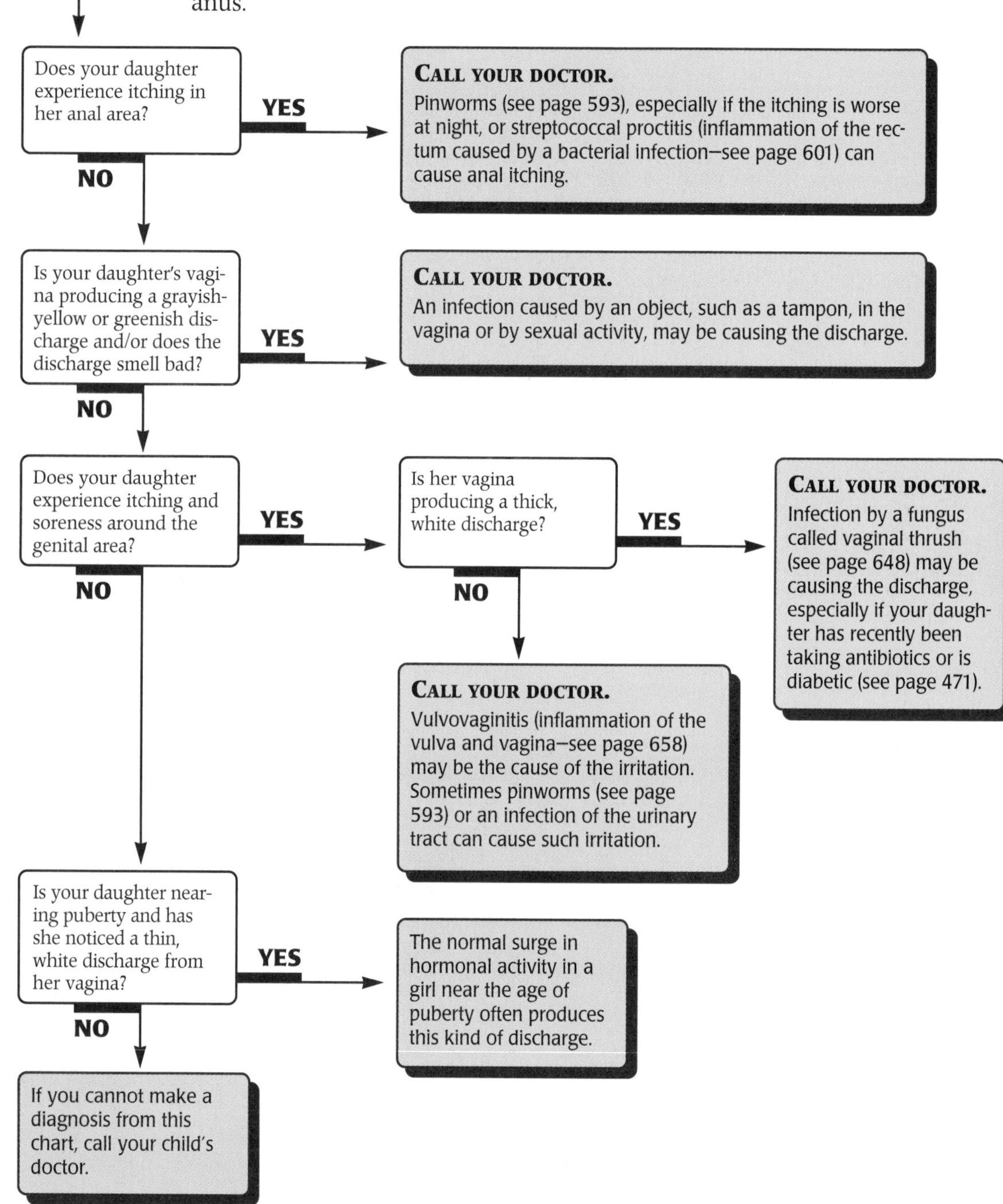

If you see a word that appears in italics (*chromosome*) while reading the description of a disorder, look up its definition in the glossary on page 681. If you see a word that appears in small capital letters (LICE), you can read a full explanation of the condition in the alphabetized entry for that disorder.

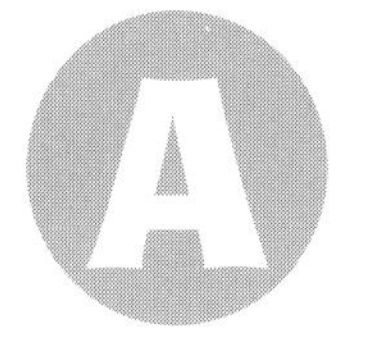

Abuse, drug and alcohol

See Drug and alcohol abuse

Abuse, physical, sexual, and emotional

See page 323

Acne

Acne is a skin disorder that occurs when hair follicles (the cavities in which hairs grow) and oil ducts in the skin become blocked with excess oil. It is the most common skin disorder in adolescents, with about 85 percent of all teenagers affected. In adolescence, acne is usually caused by the normal increases in hormone levels during puberty. Higher hormone levels increase the size of the oil ducts, especially those in the face, neck, chest, shoulders, and back. Your child may be more likely to develop acne if other people in your family had acne as teenagers.

Signs and symptoms Acne produces characteristic pimples, blackheads, and whiteheads. The blocked oil ducts and hair follicles become infected easily, producing red, inflamed pimples or cysts. Some cysts can leave permanent scars.

Diagnosis Your child's doctor will examine your child to determine the extent and distribution of the acne. He or she will also note whether the acne mainly takes the form of pimples, blackheads, or whiteheads. During the examination, the doctor will talk to your child about the cause of acne and will explain how he or she intends to treat it.

Treatment Acne may persist for years, but several treatments are available to keep it under control. Your teenager can use over-the-counter medications that contain benzoyl peroxide to help clear the plugged oil ducts and kill the bacteria that can cause skin infections. He or she can start with a mild 2.5 or 5 percent benzoyl peroxide lotion or gel, rubbing a small amount over the eruptions and the surrounding area. If the acne does not start to clear up after 4 to 6

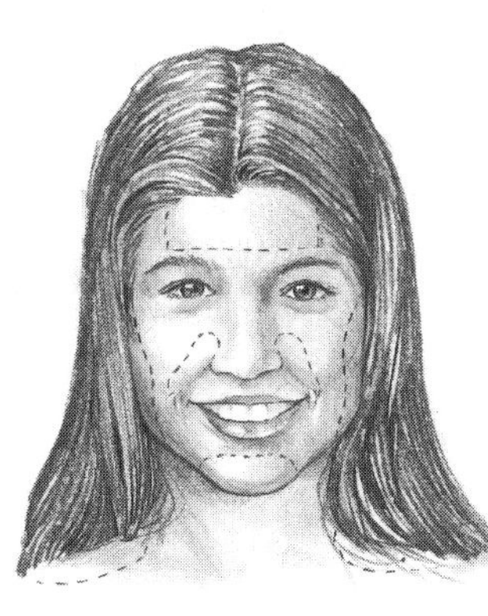

Common sites of acne
Oil ducts in an adolescent's skin overproduce an oily substance that clogs pores, causing pimples, blackheads, and whiteheads. The most likely places for acne to occur are on the cheeks, chin, and forehead and around the nose.

weeks, he or she could progress to using a 10 percent solution. At each strength, your teen should use the medication once a day for a week, then twice a day, unless the medication irritates the skin. Make sure your teen avoids exposure to the sun while using benzoyl peroxide because the medication can make the skin more sensitive to burning.

Acne that does not improve with treatment at home can be treated with the prescription medication tretinoin in cream or gel form. While using tretinoin, your teen should try to avoid excessive sun exposure and tanning parlors because this drug also increases the skin's sensitivity to sunlight. Your teenager should continue using the medication as long as his or her skin remains prone to acne. His or her doctor might also prescribe antibiotics to be taken by mouth or applied to the skin. The antibiotics help kill the bacteria in the skin that promote acne.

For severe forms of acne that do not respond to other treatments, the doctor may refer your child to a dermatologist, a doctor who specializes in skin disorders. Dermatologists sometimes prescribe a medication called isotretinoin for severe cases of acne. This drug can have serious side effects—bone and muscle pain, NOSEBLEEDS, nausea, vomiting—and can affect your child's liver. It can also increase the fat content of the blood (a risk factor for heart disease) and cause brain inflammation. If the dermatologist prescribes isotretinoin, he or she will test your child's blood regularly to see if the drug is causing any changes in his or her blood chemistry. Isotretinoin must not be taken 1 month before or during pregnancy because it can cause serious birth defects.

Encourage your teenager to wash his or her skin frequently to help keep dirt and oil out of the pores and minimize the formation of acne, although hard scrubbing of the skin can irritate it. Squeezing or popping the pimples can cause them to become infected. Hats, headbands, and chin straps can also irritate skin with acne. Some cosmetics can block the oil ducts and increase skin eruptions. Sweating, heat, and humidity can all make acne worse. Menstrual periods and birth-control pills can also aggravate acne, as can emotional stress. Acne usually clears up on its own as your adolescent gets older, but serious cases can lead to permanent scarring if left untreated.

Above all, be sensitive to your child's embarrassment about acne. Appearance and peer approval are enormously important to a child during adolescence.

ACQUIRED IMMUNODEFICIENCY SYNDROME

See AIDS

ADDISON'S DISEASE

Addison's disease is a rare disorder of the adrenal glands that causes a deficiency of *corticosteroid* hormones, which the adrenal glands secrete. The disease is also called adrenal insufficiency. The adrenal glands of a child with Addison's disease fail to produce enough of two corticosteroids—cortisol, also known as hydrocortisone, and aldosterone—because something has damaged the cortex (the outer part) of the adrenal glands. This damage is most often caused by an AUTOIMMUNE DISORDER, but it may also be caused by infection, bleeding, and other disorders.

SIGNS AND SYMPTOMS Children with Addison's disease have a poor appetite and gradually lose weight over several months or years. They feel extremely weak and tired. They can also experience abdominal pain, nausea, vomiting, HEADACHE, and diarrhea. The skin around the mouth and in the creases of the palms may look abnormally dark. Low blood pressure is common. Addison's disease can also cause a life-threatening crisis during times of extreme physical stress, such as surgery, injury, or infection. A person going through such a crisis experiences extreme muscle weakness and seizures, and can go into a coma.

An addisonian crisis is a medical emergency, so, if your child has symptoms of such a crisis, take him or her to a hospital emergency department immediately.

DIAGNOSIS To diagnose Addison's disease, the doctor will order blood, urine, and hormone level tests. The doctor may also order X-rays and *computed tomography.*

TREATMENT Replacing the deficient hormones is the usual treatment for Addison's disease. Before corticosteroid therapy became available in the 1950s, the disease was always fatal. Today a child with Addison's disease is given hydrocortisone by mouth, *intravenously,* or by injections to replace the deficiency of corticosteroids in his or her body. The child also receives replacement doses of aldosterone, another hormone secreted by the adrenal glands that is needed to maintain the balance of salt in the blood. The hormone-replacement drugs effectively control the symptoms of this disease, allowing the child to grow and develop normally. Your child will need to take these drugs for life. To avoid an addisonian crisis, the doctor will instruct your child to take larger and more frequent doses of the corticosteroids when he or she is under extreme physical stress, such as after an injury, an infection, or surgery. The doctor may also recommend injections of the drug during these times.

What do the adrenal glands do?

The two tiny adrenal glands (see page 531), located on top of each kidney, are made up of an outer part, known as the cortex, and an inner part, called the medulla. The cortex releases corticosteroid hormones, including cortisol (also known as hydrocortisone) and aldosterone, into the bloodstream. These corticosteroids play a role in the body's use of nutrients and in the balance of salt in the blood. The medulla secretes two so-called stress hormones known as epinephrine (also called adrenaline) and norepinephrine in response to stress, fear, or physical exercise. The release of these two hormones into the bloodstream increases the heart rate and widens the airways, preparing the body for action in times of stress.

ADENITIS

Adenitis is the inflammation of lymph nodes or glands (organs in the lymphatic system, one of the body's defenses against infection). Lymph nodes are located throughout the body, but most commonly become infected in the neck, armpits, or groin. The condition is usually caused by a bacterium or virus or by an allergy.

Your child may get adenitis after having strep throat (see STREP INFECTION), mononucleosis (see MONONUCLEOSIS, INFECTIOUS), TONSILLITIS, or a tooth abscess. Infections from a skin wound can spread to the lymph glands and cause adenitis in the armpits or groin. Less common causes include TUBERCULOSIS, toxoplasmosis, and CAT-SCRATCH FEVER.

SIGNS AND SYMPTOMS The glands in the child's neck, armpits, or groin become swollen and tender and the skin may become reddened. The child may also have a fever, but otherwise has no symptoms.

DIAGNOSIS If your child's symptoms persist for more than a day, take the child to your doctor. The doctor will perform a physical examination to determine the cause of the adenitis. If no obvious cause exists, the doctor may do a blood *culture,* a *complete blood cell count,* a mononucleosis test, and a tuberculosis skin test (see page 234). The doctor will receive the results of the skin test within 48 hours.

TREATMENT Treatment varies depending on the cause, but most children with adenitis need to take oral antibiotics. The doctor will want to see your child again in 3 to 4 days to see if the glands are shrinking and the infection is improving.

AIDS

AIDS (acquired immunodeficiency syndrome) is a contagious, life-threatening disease that weakens the immune system, the body's natural defense against infection. It is caused by the human immunodeficiency virus (HIV). AIDS is one of the leading causes of death among children 1 to 14 years of age in the United States. Most children with AIDS become infected with HIV before or during birth. HIV is probably transmitted when the mother's blood enters the fetus's bloodstream through the placenta or when the baby passes through the mother's birth canal at delivery. The virus can also be transmitted through breast-feeding.

Adolescents and sexually abused children (see page 326) can become infected with HIV by sexual contact with an HIV-infected person. HIV is spread during heterosexual or homosexual intercourse through blood, semen, and secretions from the vagina or rectum. HIV infected many young adults who now have AIDS as teenagers (see page 180). Sharing needles contaminated with HIV can also infect adolescents and children who inject drugs. In the past, HIV was transmitted to children and teens who needed blood transfusions (see HEMOPHILIA) through HIV-infected blood and blood products but, since 1985, the nation's blood supply has been tested for HIV. Transmission through blood transfusions is now unlikely.

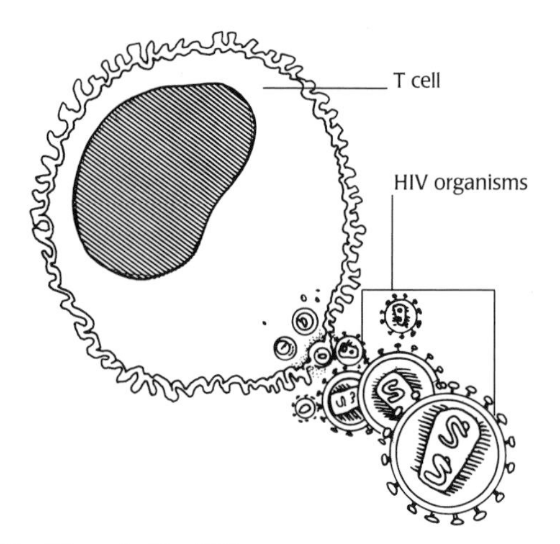

T cell invaded by HIV

T cells (also known as T lymphocytes) normally control the way other lymphocytes attack and destroy organisms that cause infection. The destruction of a T cell by HIV leaves the body vulnerable to infection. Above, the virus enters and weakens a T cell.

SIGNS AND SYMPTOMS Because HIV weakens the body's immune system (see illustration), infected children are vulnerable to cancer and infections, especially serious bacterial infections (so-called opportunistic infections) that the immune system would normally fight off. It usually takes time before HIV weakens the immune system enough to allow these infections to take hold. About one in five children infected with HIV becomes seriously ill in the first year of life. In the remaining affected children, the disease takes longer to develop; these children may not become seriously ill until they are at least school age or in early adolescence.

Some of the first signs of infection with HIV are loss of appetite, poor weight gain or weight loss, persistent fever, persistent swelling of the lymph nodes, diarrhea, and fatigue or constant lack of energy. AIDS develops with the onset of unusual and recurrent infections, cancer, or brain disease. If the child's brain is affected, his or her intellectual and nervous system functioning is also affected. Infected children are often slow to develop motor (movement) skills, such as crawling, and intellectual skills, such as speaking (see DEVELOPMENTAL DELAY). Growth is also slowed. Affected children have frequent bacterial infections that can cause PNEUMONIA, high fevers, severe diarrhea, dehydration (see page 283), and seizures. They may develop YEAST INFECTIONS known as thrush or candidiasis, which cause white spots in the mouth and throat and a persistent diaper RASH. Rapid weight loss may develop. Infected children also frequently develop a lung disease called lymphocytic interstitial pneumonitis, which makes breathing difficult. The leading cause of death among children with AIDS is a specific type of pneumonia known as *Pneumocystis carinii.*

DIAGNOSIS If your infant or child has any symptoms of AIDS or has been exposed to HIV, see the doctor immediately. He or she will order a blood test that can identify the presence of HIV in your child's blood. Your child may need to have this blood test done again or have other blood tests if he or she has been exposed to HIV but does not yet have symptoms. If your infant is born with HIV, you and your partner must also be tested for HIV. A negative test result does not always mean the person is not infected with HIV. It may take several months after infection before HIV can be detected in the blood. Also, being infected with HIV does not mean the child has AIDS; AIDS occurs as the HIV infection progresses. Early on, HIV-infected individuals may not have any signs or symptoms of AIDS. The average time it takes to develop symptoms is 10 years. It is 2 years for infants born HIV infected.

TREATMENT There is no cure for AIDS. Researchers have developed a number of drugs that are successful in slowing or stopping the progression of the disease in some children. Doctors begin treatment before AIDS develops. Combining drugs has been successful in fighting AIDS and in delaying its onset in HIV-infected individuals. HIV-infected infants and children who become seriously ill are usually hospitalized for the treatment of the specific infection they have.

ALLERGIC RHINITIS

See Hay fever

Living with a child who has AIDS

Parents or guardians of children with AIDS need to keep them healthy so they can avoid infections that could overwhelm their immune system. Children with AIDS also need an environment in which they can lead as normal a life as possible. Here are some guidelines if your child has AIDS:

- Know the facts. Because HIV is not spread through casual contact, show your child your love and support by hugging, kissing, and playing with him or her. Assure your child that he or she is not a danger to playmates or schoolmates. Explain how to handle any situations, such as a nosebleed, that need special safety precautions.
- Provide a healthy diet. Talk to your child's doctor about the best foods to feed your child. Your child needs the best nutrition so he or she can not only grow and develop, but also fight the disease.
- Encourage your child to be active. Regular exercise will strengthen your child's muscles. Also, interaction with friends is an important part of any child's life—especially a child with AIDS.
- Make sure your child gets plenty of sleep. Rest and sleep help your child gather strength to fight the disease.
- Get regular medical and dental care. Your child needs frequent medical and dental examinations and checkups to monitor the progress of the disease and to keep him or her in good physical condition.
- Keep everything clean. Teach your child to wash his or her hands often and stay away from anything that could harbor infection-causing organisms. Keep your child's toys and surroundings clean to reduce the risk of picking up an infection.
- Give your child the recommended medication. Make sure your child takes all the medication that has been prescribed.
- Encourage your child to share his or her feelings. Be ready to answer tough questions straightforwardly with plenty of love and reassurance.
- Talk to your child's teachers. Make sure they know the facts about your child's illness so they can prepare other children and their families with sound information.

ALLERGIES

An allergy is an oversensitive physical reaction to a specific substance, called an allergen. Common allergens include pollen, mold, household dust, cigar or cigarette smoke, animal dander (microscopic particles of skin and hair), feathers in pillows or comforters, foods (see ALLERGIES TO FOOD), drugs (see ALLERGIES TO MEDICINE and SERUM SICKNESS), and venom from a bee or wasp sting (see page 289). Some common allergies in children include ASTHMA, HAY FEVER, food allergies, eczema (see ATOPIC DERMATITIS), and CONTACT DERMATITIS. HIVES is a common reaction to some allergens. Some children outgrow allergies by the time they become adolescents or adults.

Allergens are substances that are harmless to most people. Children with allergies have an extreme sensitivity to these substances. Their immune system (the body's natural defense mechanism against infection) identifies an allergen as foreign, which causes a reaction. The immune system forms *antibodies* to fight the invading allergens by binding to them. Then the antibodies attach themselves to specialized cells in human tissue known as mast cells, which release a strong chemical known as histamine along with other chemicals into the child's tissues and blood. These chemicals irritate tissue throughout the body, causing itching, swelling, and other allergic symptoms.

SIGNS AND SYMPTOMS Different allergens cause different allergic symptoms. Allergens that children inhale—such as pollen, mold, and dust—usually cause itchy, red, swollen, and watery eyes and nose. The child's throat may feel sore and he or she could develop asthma symptoms. Allergens that affect the skin generally cause an itchy RASH, HIVES, and sometimes BLISTERS on different parts of the body. Food allergies can cause rashes, abdominal pain, vomiting, diarrhea, and breathing and circulation problems.

DIAGNOSIS If your child seems to have hay fever or allergies that affect the nasal passages, the doctor will look for two telltale signs. One sign is an upward-turned nose that results from the child constantly wiping an itchy or runny nose with his or her hand by pushing the nose upward. The other sign is known as an "allergic shiner." The child has what look like black bags under his or her eyes because nasal congestion interferes with the flow of blood in the veins beneath the eyes. The lower eyelids look swollen and dark and may have creases in them. Children

Allergy tests

The doctor needs to find out what specific substance, or allergen, is causing your child's allergic reaction. Here are the most common testing methods doctors use:

- **Skin tests** Skin tests are most often used to test for allergies to pollens, other inhaled allergens, or food. A small amount of the suspected substance is injected under the skin (your child will experience little more than a pinprick sensation) or applied on top of the skin with a patch. Your child may experience itching at the site of application if he or she is allergic to the substance. The child's doctor or an allergist will then look for any redness and swelling that would indicate a positive reaction.
- **Elimination tests** These tests are used most often for food allergies. Under strict supervision, your child will receive samples of various foods, such as milk or eggs, one by one, to see how he or she reacts to them. If your child has no reaction, then that food is eliminated from the list of possible allergens.
- **RAST tests** Using a radioallergosorbent test (RAST), the doctor can find out what is causing your child's allergy by determining if *antibodies* to any allergens are present in a sample of the child's blood.

with hay fever or allergies that affect the nasal passages commonly breathe through their mouths. Your child's doctor may use skin tests or blood tests to determine if your child has allergies to any common allergens.

TREATMENT The best treatment for allergies is to avoid the allergen that causes a physical reaction. To combat air-borne allergens, such as pollen and dust, which are hard to avoid, the doctor may prescribe antihistamines with or without decongestants to combat the itching, sneezing, and stuffy or runny nose. He or she may also prescribe bronchodilators to open the child's airways, especially if your child has asthma, or *corticosteroids* to reduce swelling and irritation in the airways. If prescription medications fail to control symptoms or cause unwanted side effects, your child's doctor or an allergist may administer allergy shots. The shots consist of injections of small amounts of the pollen, dust, or other allergens causing your child's allergy. Eventually, the immune system reacts less strongly to the allergen, causing fewer symptoms.

Preventing allergic reactions at home

You can do a number of things at home to minimize your child's exposure to substances that bring on allergic reactions. Try the following suggestions:

- Damp-mop or wipe down all horizontal surfaces once or twice a week to remove dust.
- Consider replacing wall-to-wall carpeting, which traps dust, with smaller area rugs.
- Vacuum upholstered furniture regularly or replace it with wood, plastic, or leather-covered furniture.
- If a family pet seems to be causing your child's allergy, find a good home for your pet. Washing a cat weekly dramatically reduces the presence of dander.
- Wash pillows and bed clothes every week to minimize dust and don't use pillows or quilts that contain feathers.
- Keep your home's humidity low by using a dehumidifier on humid days to reduce mold. Keep your child out of damp basements. Thoroughly clean humidifiers weekly with bleach.
- Avoid buying foods that contain sulfites if your child is sensitive to them (see page 419).
- Never smoke around your child.

ALLERGIES TO FOOD

A food allergy is an adverse reaction of the body's immune system (the body's natural defense against infection) to certain foods. Your child could have a significant allergic reaction up to 3 hours after eating the food. About 5 percent of young children are diagnosed with food allergies, often within the first year of life, but many children outgrow them. The most common foods that cause childhood allergies are cow's milk, eggs, fish and shellfish, nuts, corn, and wheat. Allergies to milk and eggs sometimes disappear by the time the child is 3 to 5 years old. Other food allergies may last longer, even a lifetime.

Food allergies run in families. A child with one affected parent is twice as likely as other children to develop a food allergy. If both parents have a food allergy, the child is four times as likely to develop the allergy. Children with food allergies commonly have other types of ALLERGIES as well.

SIGNS AND SYMPTOMS Within a few minutes or a few hours after eating some food that causes an allergic reaction, the child's lips, mouth, or throat begin to swell or itch. The child's skin may break out in HIVES (a raised, red RASH), itch, and look red. A scaly rash known as eczema (see ATOPIC DERMATITIS) may occur if the child is repeatedly exposed to the food allergen. The child can also sneeze and have a stuffy or runny nose, or develop ASTHMA and shortness of breath. When the food reaches the child's stomach, it can cause abdominal pain, nausea, vomiting, cramps, and diarrhea. In rare cases, a child may have a severe allergic reaction known as anaphylaxis. The symptoms of anaphylaxis include excessive sweating; quick and shallow breathing; wheezing; a weak pulse; cold, clammy skin; hives; dizziness; and fainting. The child's pulse may be weak. If anaphylaxis is not treated right away, it can be fatal.

DIAGNOSIS AND TREATMENT If your child has a severe reaction to a food, take him or her to a hospital emergency department immediately. A child with a history of asthma and food allergies should be taken to the doctor immediately if he or she eats a known food allergen, whether a reaction occurs or not. The doctor will teach you how to give your child a drug known as epinephrine to prevent anaphylaxis. He or she will order blood tests to rule out possible causes.

To identify a specific food allergy, your child's doctor may ask you to keep a diary of the foods your child eats and how he or she reacts to them. Identifying a food allergy may be done through a process of elimination or by a skin test in which an extract of food is placed on or injected underneath the skin (see page 406). Once the food that caused the allergic reaction is identified, the best treatment is to avoid it altogether. You and your child will need to read labels carefully and ask about the ingredients in dishes prepared in restaurants (for example, peanuts can be used to thicken chili) to make sure they contain no food allergen. Some children are able to eat small amounts of the food without getting an allergic reaction. You and your child should always carry a premeasured dose of epinephrine with you in case he or she accidentally eats a known food allergen.

ALLERGIES TO MEDICINE

An allergy to medicine is an adverse, sometimes life-threatening, physical reaction to a specific drug or medication. Your child can have a reaction to a medicine even if he or she has taken it many times before.

SIGNS AND SYMPTOMS Signs and symptoms can develop either immediately or after having taken the medicine for several weeks. Allergic reactions can occur whether your child is taking a drug orally, inhaling it, applying it directly to the skin, or injecting it either into the muscle or *intravenously*. Skin rashes are the most common reactions. The RASH consists of tiny, itchy, raised bumps and flat, red patches that initially develop on the arms and legs and then spread onto the trunk. The child can develop HIVES that may look like red, thick, swollen patches of skin or BLISTERS. The child's eyelids, lips, tongue, and mouth can swell and the child may have difficulty breathing. Another type of skin reaction known as ERYTHEMA MULTIFORME can appear. This type of rash tends to spread and join together and the skin may peel. The child can develop round or oval patches of darkened skin that vary in size. Painful, peeling mouth sores and bloody diarrhea can also occur. In rare cases, a child can have a severe allergic reaction known as anaphylaxis. The symptoms include excessive sweating, quick and shallow breathing, a weak pulse, cold and clammy skin, dizziness, and fainting. If not treated right away, anaphylaxis can be fatal.

DIAGNOSIS AND TREATMENT If your child has a severe reaction to a drug, get him or her to a hospital emergency department immediately. For milder reactions, have your child stop taking the medication and see his or her doctor. The doctor will probably order blood tests to rule out other possible causes of your child's reaction. Skin tests (see page 406) are available for a few medications. The doctor will tell you to stop giving your child the medication and will recommend an alternative if one is available. Your child will be allergic to the medication for the rest of his or her life. If your child has erythema multiforme or anaphylaxis, he or she may need to be hospitalized. Your child should wear a medical identification tag to identify his or her drug allergy. Be sure to note the allergy on all medical forms in the doctor's office and on school records.

ALOPECIA

Alopecia is the medical term for the loss or absence of hair, which can affect children as well as men and women. There are three types of alopecia. In alopecia areata, hair falls out in patches in different places on the scalp. A second type, alopecia totalis, occurs when most or all of the hair on the scalp falls out. The third type is alopecia universalis, in which hair falls out all over the body.

The cause of alopecia is unknown, but some experts think that heredity, stress, anxiety, and diseases that attack the immune system (the body's major defense against disease) are linked to the hair loss. Some children exhibit a behavior disorder known as trichotillomania, or compulsive hair pulling, which can also cause hair loss. Hair pulling may indicate that the child is under stress. Infection by a fungus, disorders of the thyroid gland, and pregnancy can also cause hair loss.

SIGNS AND SYMPTOMS Children with alopecia have sudden and rapid hair loss. There are no other physical signs. Hair loss can cause children to be teased by playmates or schoolmates and lead to DEPRESSION and low self-esteem. Children who lose hair because of compulsive hair pulling may show signs of this behavior in early childhood, before age 5. Casual hair pulling probably calms the child and may be a phase he or she outgrows.

DIAGNOSIS Your child's doctor will diagnose alopecia from a physical examination. He or she may ask you if your child has been under a lot of stress lately or may ask about signs of disorders, such as a thyroid disorder, that can cause alopecia.

TREATMENT Balding caused by alopecia usually stops after several months. Most cases of alopecia require no treatment, except for calm reassurance. Many children with mild alopecia see their hair grow back on its own. Your child's doctor may prescribe *corticosteroids* that your child can rub into his or her scalp or onto other affected parts of his or her body. The doctor may also give injections of corticosteroids and have your child take cortisone (a corticosteroid) in pill form. Some children with alopecia can achieve hair regrowth using a lotion that contains the drug minoxidil, which is now sold over the counter. If hair loss results from infection by a fungus, it will be treated with antifungal medication. Hair loss caused by a thyroid disorder will be treated with thyroid medication.

Children who lose hair because of compulsive hair pulling may need counseling and behavior-modification therapy (therapy that attempts to treat an emotional disorder by changing behavior rather than through psychoanalysis). If your child pulls his or her hair because of a movement disorder, such as a tic (a repeated, uncontrolled muscle contraction), or obsessive-compulsive disorder, he or she can be treated with medication.

ANEMIA, APLASTIC

Aplastic anemia is a blood disorder that affects bone marrow, the tissue in the core of your child's bone that forms red blood cells, white blood cells, and platelets (cells needed for blood clotting). The bone marrow fails to produce the blood cells in a child with aplastic anemia. The condition may be temporary or permanent.

The disease can be inherited or caused by certain medications (antibiotics and drugs used to treat cancer), infections with certain viruses such as the hepatitis B virus, excessive exposure to poisonous chemicals such as benzene (found in insecticides and model-airplane glue), or exposure to *radiation* (from radioactive materials or radiation therapy for cancer). Many cases of aplastic anemia arise from unknown causes.

SIGNS AND SYMPTOMS A child with aplastic anemia has fewer red blood cells than normal, producing fatigue, pale skin, and weakness. In severe cases, anemia can cause your child to be short of breath, have an unusually rapid heartbeat, or faint.

With fewer white blood cells than normal in his or her bloodstream, your child will be more likely to get infections. Aplastic anemia causes fewer platelets to form, so your child's blood will not clot properly. Your child might get frequent nosebleeds, bruises that appear suddenly, purple spots on his or her skin, and bleeding from the mouth or injured areas. The low number of platelets can cause bleeding into or around the brain after an injury or even spontaneously. Adolescent girls can get frequent, heavy, and prolonged menstrual bleeding.

DIAGNOSIS If your child's doctor suspects aplastic anemia, he or she will order a *complete blood cell count* to look for evidence of the disease. A doctor who specializes in blood disorders (hematologist) will need to remove a small amount of your child's bone marrow through a needle and look at it under a microscope to make a definite diagnosis of aplastic anemia.

TREATMENT For aplastic anemia caused by a certain medication or therapy, your child's doctor will stop the drug or therapy and try to find a substitute. If your child is somehow being exposed to poisonous chemicals or radioactive materials, you need to immediately remove the chemicals from your home and keep your child away from the harmful materials.

Your child's doctor will treat any infections that occur as a result of the disease with antibiotics. To combat your child's fatigue, pale skin, weakness, and blood-clotting problems, the doctor will order blood and platelet transfusions. If your child's condition does not improve in a few weeks, he or she may need medication called granulocyte-stimulating factor, which stimulates the bone marrow to produce the white blood cells needed to fight infection. Your doctor may also give your child *corticosteroids* or other medications to stimulate his or her bone marrow to resume normal function and to overcome any natural suppression of the bone marrow by your child's own immune system.

In severe cases, your child may need a bone marrow transplant. This procedure requires a compatible bone marrow donor, such as a sister or brother. The donor's bone marrow is injected into your child's vein, and the donor marrow travels through the bloodstream to your child's own bone marrow where it begins to produce the needed blood cells. It takes from 10 to 20 days for the new blood cells from the donated marrow to mature enough to function. During this time, your child will be placed in isolation in a special unit of the hospital to minimize the risk of infection. There is a chance that your child's body may reject the new cells from the donated marrow, but rejection is less likely with marrow from a compatible donor. With bone marrow transplantation from a compatible donor, your child's chances of a complete recovery are about 80 percent.

ANEMIA, BLOOD-LOSS

Blood-loss anemia occurs when your child bleeds so much that he or she no longer has enough red blood cells to carry adequate amounts of oxygen throughout his or her body. Your child can lose blood for a number of reasons, such as a bleeding ulcer, or other intestinal disorders that cause bleeding. Adolescent girls sometimes experience heavy menstrual bleeding that could lead to blood-loss anemia. Any large wound that causes a loss of blood can produce anemia. Even small amounts of blood lost over long periods of time can produce anemia.

SIGNS AND SYMPTOMS The most common symptoms of anemia are fatigue, weakness, pale skin, a general lack of energy, shortness of breath during play or other activities, and changes in behavior. If your child has a bleeding ulcer, he or she may vomit blood; produce black, tarlike stool; and have abdominal pain. Heavy bleeding from any site—the nose, rectum, vagina, or a wound—can produce significant blood loss and anemia.

DIAGNOSIS Take your child to your doctor immediately if he or she has lost a lot of blood or seems to have signs of anemia. Your doctor will take a *complete blood cell count* to assess the severity of the anemia and may conduct a number of other tests, depending on the suspected cause of the anemia. For example, if your child's doctor thinks intestinal bleeding may be the cause, he or she will perform a rectal examination and check your child's stool for blood.

TREATMENT Your doctor will probably give your child iron and folic acid (a B vitamin) supplements. In severe cases, your child might need a blood transfusion. The doctor will also treat the specific cause of the blood loss. If your child has a serious case of blood-loss anemia, he or she may need to be hospitalized.

What is blood made of?

Blood is made up of a fluid, called plasma, that contains water, minerals, sugar, fats, and proteins. Inside this plasma soup swim three different types of cells: red blood cells, white blood cells, and platelets. All three types of blood cells are created inside bone marrow, the tissue inside bone, and have very distinct functions:

- Red blood cells are the most abundant type of cells in blood. Their main purpose is to carry oxygen from the lungs to all the other cells in the body. They also transport carbon dioxide, a waste product of cells, back to the lungs for disposal. Hemoglobin, a protein containing iron that resides in red blood cells, is essential for oxygen transport. Any condition, such as anemia, that reduces the amount of iron in the blood lowers the amount of oxygen carried throughout the body. The bone marrow immediately boosts the rate of red blood cell production.
- White blood cells are part of the immune system, the body's main defense against infection. There are six different types of white blood cells, all with specific infection-fighting jobs. Some specialize in destroying foreign organisms. Others fight inflammation. Still others are active in allergic reactions.
- Platelets are cells that clump together at sites of injury to stop bleeding by plugging the holes in injured blood vessels. They also help the blood to coagulate (clot).

ANEMIA, HEMOLYTIC

Hemolytic anemia is a blood disorder in which an excessive number of red blood cells are destroyed at an abnormally high rate. Red blood cells form in your child's bone marrow (the tissue inside bone) and are released into his or her bloodstream. The cells normally live in the bloodstream for about 3 months and are constantly replaced by new red blood cells. Anemia occurs when the bone marrow cannot replace the destroyed red blood cells fast enough to transport a steady supply of oxygen throughout the body.

This high rate of red blood cell destruction can be caused by abnormalities in the red blood cells themselves. Such abnormalities include inherited defects in the cell membrane (the covering of the cell), such as hereditary spherocytosis (see SPHEROCYTOSIS, HEREDITARY) or in the hemoglobin (the protein in red blood cells that carries oxygen), such as SICKLE CELL ANEMIA. Abnormalities can also stem from inherited defects in an enzyme (a protein that speeds up a chemical reaction in the body) within the red blood cells. For example, lack of the enzyme known as glucose-6-phosphate dehydrogenase causes inadequate red blood cell nutrition, leading to early cell destruction and hemolytic anemia.

Red blood cells can also be destroyed by obstructions in the bloodstream, such as blood clots or artificial heart valves, which "tear" the red blood cells, and by some medications. Some diseases—such as LUPUS, other autoimmune diseases (diseases caused by a reaction of a person's immune system against his or her own body), and certain types of infections—damage red blood cells, causing anemia.

Signs and symptoms A child with hemolytic anemia experiences all of the common symptoms of anemia—fatigue, weakness, pale skin, a general lack of energy, and shortness of breath during vigorous activities. He or she may also have a pale yellow color to his or her skin and eyes from JAUNDICE, caused by a buildup of bilirubin, a byproduct of red blood cell destruction, in the bloodstream. A swollen spleen (an organ in the upper left abdomen that fights infection) is also a common sign of hemolytic anemia. The child's urine may be darker than usual and he or she may eventually develop gallstones (tiny stones in the gallbladder).

Diagnosis Your doctor will diagnose hemolytic anemia on the basis of your child's medical history, a physical examination, and laboratory tests of his or her blood, including the number of red blood cells present in the blood. A microscopic examination of your child's blood will show any unusually shaped red blood cells, an abnormal number of newly formed red cells, or evidence of red blood cell damage. Other tests may be needed to find out what is causing the red blood cell damage and to see how it is affecting the organs of your child's body.

Treatment There are many different causes of hemolytic anemia and, in many children, treating the underlying cause will eradicate the anemia. If your child's doctor diagnoses an inherited blood disorder that causes hemolytic anemia, he or she may decide to remove your child's spleen, the organ that collects and destroys worn-out red blood cells, to minimize red blood cell destruction. Removing the spleen can relieve many of your child's symptoms but, after removal of the spleen, your child's body will be less able to fight certain bacterial infections. Hemolytic anemia that is caused by an autoimmune disease requires drugs that treat the autoimmune disorder so that your child's immune system will stop destroying his or her red blood cells. Your child's doctor will find a substitute for any medication that may be causing the hemolytic anemia. If your child's hemolytic anemia is caused by an infection, it will be treated with drugs designed to fight the specific infection. If your child's symptoms are serious or life threatening, the doctor will order transfusions of red blood cells or whole blood to stabilize his or her condition.

Anemia, iron-deficiency

Iron-deficiency anemia is characterized by insufficient amounts of hemoglobin (a protein in red blood cells that carries oxygen throughout the body), from a deficiency of iron in a child's body. Iron is needed for the production of hemoglobin by bone marrow, the tissue inside bone that creates red blood cells. Iron deficiency is the most common cause of anemia in children.

Your child's blood can become deficient in iron for a number of reasons. In children and teenagers, especially girls, the most common cause is a diet lacking in the essential mineral iron (see box on facing page for dietary sources of iron). Children under age 3 who drink excessive amounts of milk or juice do not consume a well-balanced diet and may become deficient in iron. Young people on fad diets often have an iron deficiency. Babies under 1 year old who are taken off breast milk or iron-enriched formula and given solid foods lacking in iron can become iron deficient. Children under 1 year of age who drink cow's milk can become iron-deficient because the milk can cause intestinal bleeding and because the iron in cow's milk is not readily absorbed. Don't give your child cow's milk until he or she is 1 year old. Premature babies can develop an iron deficiency because they do not get the large amounts of iron available during the last weeks of pregnancy.

A pregnant teenage girl or one who is breast-feeding can easily become deficient in iron because the baby obtains nutrients such as iron from the mother. Intestinal bleeding from ulcers, diseases that cause MALABSORPTION, and inflammatory bowel disease can also produce iron-deficiency anemia.

SIGNS AND SYMPTOMS At first, iron-deficiency anemia can be present with no symptoms at all. Once they develop, symptoms include pale skin (especially on the hands), fatigue, and weakness. Other, less common symptoms include shortness of breath during play or exercise, an unusually fast heartbeat, fainting, loss of appetite, a mild stomachache, and a sore mouth or tongue. You may also notice changes in your child's behavior, such as moodiness, hostility, and a shorter attention span.

DIAGNOSIS If your child's doctor suspects iron-deficiency anemia, he or she will test your child's red blood cell count and iron level to evaluate the blood's ability to bind with iron. Your doctor may also check your child's stool for blood. If blood is present in your child's stool, the doctor will order other tests, such as an X-ray or examination of his or her intestines through a scope, to determine whether there is internal bleeding and what might be causing it.

TREATMENT Your doctor will give your child iron medication in tablet or syrup form to be taken daily. If your child needs to take the medication by mouth, he or she should take it immediately after a meal to avoid an upset stomach. Don't give your child over-the-counter iron pills without talking to your doctor first because the extra iron might make it harder for the doctor to diagnose the problem and could cover up the cause of your child's anemia.

Your child's condition should improve in 2 to 4 weeks with treatment. To replace the iron stores in your child's body, your doctor will want you to continue giving your child the iron medication for 2 months. If your child consumes a diet that is deficient in iron, he or she will need to start eating more iron-rich foods. Iron-deficiency anemia caused by internal bleeding will require further treatment, depending on the site of the bleeding. The prospects for full recovery are excellent once your child's doctor has identified the cause of the anemia and has treated it.

Boosting your child's intake of iron-rich foods

Red blood cells need iron to transport oxygen throughout the body. Full-term infants are born with a store of iron that lasts up to 6 months. Breast milk contains only small amounts of readily absorbable iron so, by 6 months of age, your child's nutritional needs exceed the amount of iron available in breast milk or iron-fortified formula. You need to start giving your baby iron-fortified cereals and other foods by the sixth month of life. As your child gets older, he or she needs to continue eating iron-rich foods. Teenagers need extra iron because they build a lot of muscle during adolescence, another function that needs iron. Adolescent girls need even more iron than boys because of their monthly blood loss during menstruation. The best dietary sources of iron include:

- Beef, pork, lamb, dark-meat poultry, and organ meats
- Dried beans and peas
- Iron-fortified cereals and breads
- Leafy green vegetables, such as spinach

Iron is most abundant in animal protein, such as red meat. The iron in animal protein is also the most easily absorbed by the body. If your child is a vegetarian or prefers not to eat red meat, he or she can obtain sufficient amounts of iron by eating other foods that are good sources of the mineral. Foods high in vitamin C—citrus fruits; green, leafy vegetables; green and red bell peppers; and tomatoes—and vitamin C supplements can help your child's body better absorb iron.

ANEMIA, SICKLE CELL

See Sickle cell anemia

ANENCEPHALY

Anencephaly is a rare but serious BIRTH DEFECT marked by incomplete development or absence of a brain and skull in a fetus or newborn. About 65 percent of fetuses with anencephaly die before birth and are stillborn. Infants who survive birth die within a few days. The risk of having a baby with anencephaly increases if the mother has had a previous baby with the same defect. Anencephaly occurs more frequently in certain geographic areas of the world, especially in Ireland.

The suspected causes of this birth defect include CHROMOSOMAL ABNORMALITIES, hyperthermia (a very high body temperature) in the mother, and a lack of certain nutrients, such as zinc and copper, in the mother.

SIGNS AND SYMPTOMS An affected fetus or infant has no brain or only part of a brain. Infants with anencephaly often have malformed skulls, faces, and bodies at birth.

DIAGNOSIS A blood test that looks for certain proteins called alpha-fetoprotein and acetylcholinesterase can be done to screen for anencephaly in the fetus. If the levels of these proteins are elevated, the doctor will do an *ultrasound* of the fetus to look for abnormal brain or skull development and may recommend *amniocentesis.*

TREATMENT There is no treatment for anencephaly. Without a brain, the infant cannot function. Depending on when the defect was diagnosed, you can talk to your doctor about your options, including terminating the pregnancy. Because of their increased risk of having another child with anencephaly, parents should seek genetic counseling (see page 497) before having more children.

ANOREXIA NERVOSA

Anorexia nervosa is an eating disorder marked by an intense fear of gaining weight that leads to self-starvation. The vast majority of children who have this disorder are girls between the ages of 14 and 18 years, although it can affect children of all ages and both sexes. Anorexia often coincides with the onset of puberty. In many cases, the disorder begins when the adolescent feels social pressure to be thin and starts dieting. The adolescent with anorexia goes beyond normal weight loss and eventually refuses to eat sufficient amounts of food to maintain normal body weight for his or her age and height.

Anorectics see themselves as overweight even if they are extraordinarily thin. They may think or talk about food all the time and are obsessed with their own body image. They become conscious of every bite of food they eat. They may also exercise compulsively to keep their weight down. Affected children may feel insecure, have low self-esteem, and be motivated by a strong desire to be in control of their bodies. They are frequently perfectionists; many excel in sports. Other family members may have a history of eating disorders or depression and communication

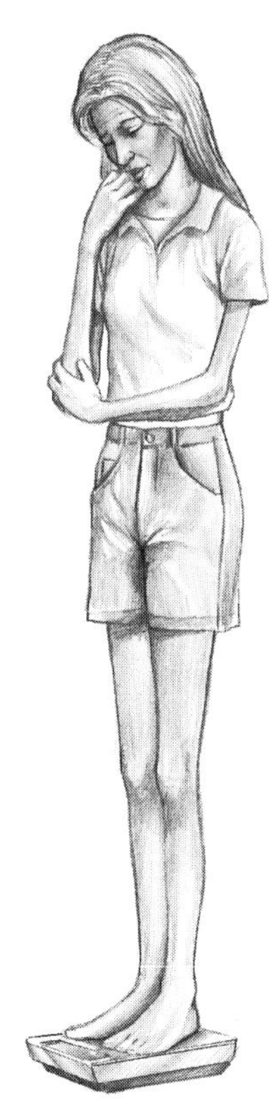

Obsessed with weight
A teenage anorectic is obsessed with weight. The child has a distorted body image, seeing herself or himself as overweight no matter what the scale or mirror shows. The limbs of a teenager with anorexia are so thin the bones may stick out at the joints. The child's eyes become hollow and, in a girl, the chest may be boyishly flat.

problems may exist within the family. Anorectics can become isolated and may be secretive about their weight control. They may also take diet pills excessively and use laxatives, enemas, and diuretics to prevent weight gain. Some anorectics also have BULIMIA—a condition in which the person engages in binge eating and then self-induces vomiting to purge the body of the excess food. Although not always dangerously thin, bulimics can have life-threatening body chemical imbalances. If the self-starvation process is not reversed, it can be fatal.

SIGNS AND SYMPTOMS The physical symptoms of anorexia are brought on by starvation and every part of the body is affected. The most obvious initial symptom is weight loss so extreme that the child becomes dangerously thin. Anorectics weigh less than 85 percent of the normal body weight for their age and height. The child's bones become visible beneath the skin and, in extreme cases, his or her abdomen may protrude from a lack of protein. (The child usually perceives the bloated look of the abdomen as weight gain.) His or her eyes become hollow and vacant looking. A deficiency of vitamins and protein make the skin dry and yellow and the hair and fingernails brittle. Fine, downy hair appears on the child's arms, legs, back, and face, but the hair on his or her head tends to fall out.

The child may also have abdominal pain and constipation. Menstrual periods stop or, if the anorectic girl has not yet had her first period, may never begin. Many anorectics become anemic (see ANEMIA, IRON-DEFICIENCY), look tired and pale, and lack energy. Because of the loss of fat and muscle, they may feel cold all the time. Some continue to be very physically active. Eventually, the long-term lack of nourishment can cause kidney and liver damage and heart problems, such as low blood pressure, an abnormal heartbeat (see ARRHYTHMIAS), and heart failure (see HEART FAILURE, CONGESTIVE). The anorectic may ultimately die of a heart attack or the starvation itself. Some commit suicide.

DIAGNOSIS AND TREATMENT Other diseases can mimic anorexia, so it is important for your child to see his or her doctor for an examination. If your child shows signs of the disorder, the doctor will do a thorough physical examination and will order blood, urine, and stool tests, along with a thyroid function test. The doctor may also refer your child for a psychological evaluation. If your child's weight loss is severe, he or she may need to be hospitalized and nourished through a feeding tube.

Most anorectics deny their illness and resist therapy. Treatment requires a team of health care professionals, including a pediatrician, psychiatrist or psychologist, and nutritionist, who work together to counteract the disorder. Nutritional counseling is essential to help the child plan meals and establish weight goals. Mental health counseling can help change the child's unhealthy behavior, helping him or her to improve his or her self-image. Counseling might include the entire family and may need to be continued consistently for a long period. The doctor will monitor your child's progress and weight gain. With successful treatment, your child should gain weight gradually over 1 to 2 months. But the disorder is difficult to treat and the child may have further episodes of anorexia. Recovery can take many years. It is important to maintain your child's routine health care over the years.

ANXIETY

Anxiety is an emotional state characterized by uneasiness, worry, or fear, which can be mild or extreme. A certain amount of anxiety is normal as your child passes through the different stages of childhood. For example, anxiety over separation from parents or close relatives is common in children from about 7 months of age until the time they start school. Young children often also fear the dark, lightening, strangers, and many other things they can't understand or see as threatening. You need to be concerned when your child's anxiety does not seem to be related to any particular thing or event or when it interferes with your child's ability to function normally (for example, when your child is afraid to go to school). Extreme anxiety can develop into an anxiety disorder.

TYPES OF ANXIETY DISORDERS The most common types of anxiety disorders include generalized anxiety disorder, panic disorder, phobias, post-traumatic stress disorder, and OBSESSIVE-COMPULSIVE DISORDER.

Generalized anxiety disorder A child with generalized anxiety disorder is constantly afraid or worried and the emotions are unrelated to or out of proportion to a specific cause. The child's feelings can hinder normal activity. The child may be short of breath, is unable to concentrate, loses sleep, feels dizzy, is irritable, trembles, and has a rapid heartbeat (see ARRHYTHMIAS) and dry mouth.

Panic disorder A child who has panic disorder experiences brief periods of intense fear, commonly known as panic attacks, for no apparent reason. The child may suddenly feel chest pain or pressure, his or her heart may pound and beat rapidly, and dizziness, light-headedness, and a choking feeling may occur. Other symptoms include sweating, shortness of breath, chills, hot flashes, tingling in the feet or hands, fear of losing control or even dying, and a sense of being out of touch with reality.

Phobias Irrational fears of specific things or circumstances, such as crowds, snakes, or heights, are known as phobias. Usually experienced by older children and adolescents, phobias can trigger panic attacks. One common phobia, known as agoraphobia (a fear of being out in public or in open places) causes a child to fear leaving the house without feeling intense anxiety. When in public places, the child with agoraphobia suffers panic attacks.

Post-traumatic stress disorder This anxiety disorder is a response to a frightening, violent event—such as surviving an automobile collision or tornado, witnessing someone being shot, or experiencing severe child abuse or rape—that causes physical or emotional trauma. The child relives the event over and over in memories or dreams and may become withdrawn and feel emotionally numb. He or she may also fear involvement in anything that triggers memories of the event. Other symptoms include DEPRESSION and panic attacks. The child may also develop a pessimistic view of the future.

Obsessive-compulsive disorder This anxiety disorder produces persistent, obtrusive thoughts (obsessions), such as "Germs are everywhere," that cause the child to repeat ritualized acts (compulsions), such as hand washing.

DIAGNOSIS AND TREATMENT If your child displays symptoms of an anxiety disorder, the doctor will refer him or her to a psychiatrist or psychologist for an evaluation. Once diagnosed with an anxiety disorder, your child may need prescription medication to reduce the anxiety, along with psychotherapy to deal with its underlying causes. Other members of your family may need to attend the therapy sessions. With treatment, your child can overcome his or her anxiety and learn how to better deal with day-to-day stresses. Talking with your child about his or her worries or problems may help alleviate day-to-day anxieties and fears.

APNEA

Apnea is a temporary cessation of breathing that occurs because of an interruption in the nerve signals sent from the brain to the muscles in the chest and diaphragm or from an obstruction in the airway, or both. The child's breathing can stop for 20 seconds or more or be so inadequate that the child's skin becomes blue and his or her heart rate decreases. The problem usually occurs during sleep. Frequent or prolonged episodes of apnea can cause brain damage because of inadequate oxygen levels in the brain. It can also cause heart disease later in life from long-term low oxygen levels. Apnea can even be fatal.

Preterm (premature) babies may develop apnea of prematurity because their brain, nervous system, and muscles used for breathing are not yet fully developed. Enlarged adenoids (two clusters of tissue at the back of the roof of the mouth that are part of the body's immune system) can cause apnea in an older child when they obstruct the upper airway during sleep. The child typically wakes up momentarily to change position and open the blocked airway many times during the night. Other causes of apnea include seizures, malformation of the airway, feeding abnormalities, gastroesophageal reflux (see GASTROESOPHAGEAL REFLUX AND HIATAL HERNIA), OBESITY, infection, a swallowed or inhaled object, or a spinal cord injury. SIDS is a type of sleep apnea.

SIGNS AND SYMPTOMS If your child has apnea, you will notice that your child stops breathing for at least 20 seconds or that his or her airflow is inadequate. Your child may become frightened, lethargic, or irritable. Prolonged periods of apnea may cause a bluish discoloration of the lips and loss of consciousness. Snoring may be a sign of obstructive sleep apnea from enlarged adenoids. A seizure can cause an episode of apnea. In a premature baby, apnea may be present from the first few days of life until the infant reaches his or her term due date. If your child is choking on an inhaled object, he or she will take gasping breaths and will not be able to make a sound.

DIAGNOSIS Your child's doctor will diagnose apnea based on your description of your child's symptoms. The doctor will try to find out the cause of your child's apnea and treat the underlying condition.

TREATMENT The treatment of apnea can vary depending on the cause and the age of the child. A premature infant may need a medication known as theophylline, which stimulates breathing. Corrective surgery is the recommended treatment for enlarged adenoids or airway malformation. A child with spinal cord damage may need to be placed on a machine called a ventilator that

Home monitors to treat apnea

It can be a frightening experience to see your baby stop breathing. To help you monitor your infant's breathing, the doctor may prescribe a home apnea monitor that you can use while your baby is at home or in a car. Use the monitor until your baby outgrows apnea or the underlying cause is treated.

The electric monitor connects to conductors placed on your child's chest that record your baby's breathing and heart rate. The doctor analyzes these recordings to assess your baby's breathing over time. If your baby's breathing stops or his or her heart rate drops, an alarm goes off. When the monitor sounds, check your baby right away. The monitor sometimes sounds false alarms because of loose connections. If your baby is breathing normally, turn off the alarm, check the connections, and reset the alarm. If your baby has stopped breathing, nudge him or her gently to try to stimulate breathing. After your baby has started breathing again, record the baby's skin color, how long the apnea lasted, and whether or not the baby started breathing again on his or her own in the chart that comes with the monitor. Look at the heart rate monitor and record the baby's heart rate on the chart. Talk to your child's doctor about the apnea episode. If you cannot rouse your baby with nudging, call your local emergency number and begin cardiopulmonary resuscitation right away.

Your child's doctor will want you to wait until your baby has been successfully treated before you take him or her off the home monitor. Expect to use the home monitor until no more true apnea alarms occur for 2 or 3 months.

helps with breathing. If your child has apnea because he or she is choking, you will need to remove the inhaled object (see page 668).

The doctor may prescribe a continuous positive airway pressure device for apnea, to be used at home. During sleep, your child would wear a mask connected to an air compressor that uses pressure to keep his or her airways open. Home oxygen therapy may also be prescribed. If you have a child with apnea, you should take a class in cardiopulmonary resuscitation (CPR) (see page 668) so you can perform CPR during a severe or prolonged episode. In serious cases, your child will have to go to a hospital emergency department. Your child's doctor may prescribe a home monitor to alert you to pauses in your baby's breathing or decreases in his or her blood oxygen levels. Some children need home nursing care so their breathing can be carefully monitored overnight.

APPENDICITIS

Appendicitis is an acute inflammation of the appendix, a small pouchlike appendage branching off the first part of the large intestine in the lower right part of a child's abdomen. Inflammation occurs when the appendix becomes blocked by feces, causing infection, or when tissue in or around the appendix swells. Appendicitis occurs most often in children and young adults between the ages of 10 and 20.

SIGNS AND SYMPTOMS Early symptoms include indigestion and intermittent pain around the child's navel. The pain becomes more constant and intensifies within a few hours. Fever, vomiting, and loss of appetite follow. The intense pain and tenderness then move to the lower right portion of the child's abdomen.

If appendicitis is not treated right away, the child's appendix can rupture, spilling bacteria and intestinal contents into the child's abdomen. A ruptured appendix can cause peritonitis (a serious infection of the abdominal lining) or an abscess (a collection of pus) in the abdomen. Untreated, peritonitis can be fatal.

DIAGNOSIS Appendicitis can be life threatening, so take your child to the doctor or a hospital emergency department right away if he or she develops intense pain and tenderness in the lower right part of his or her abdomen.

Appendicitis can be difficult for a doctor to differentiate from other abdominal disorders. The doctor will perform blood and urine tests, and may order an abdominal X-ray or an *ultrasound.* Surgery may be needed to confirm the diagnosis.

TREATMENT The only cure for appendicitis is surgery to remove the appendix. If your child has appendicitis, he or she will be hospitalized and given general anesthesia. A surgeon will make a small incision on the lower right part of the child's abdomen and remove the appendix. Your child may be able to go home in a day or two if the appendix did not rupture, but he or she will probably need to stay in the hospital for 4 to 7 days after a ruptured appendix, receiving nourishment and antibiotics *intravenously.* Once

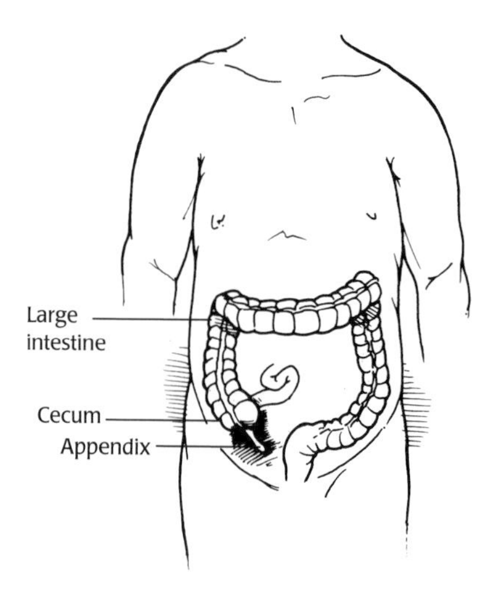

The appendix: No known function
The appendix is a small pouch that extends down from the cecum, the first segment of a child's large intestine.

your child's digestive system starts working fully, he or she will be able to take food by mouth. After discharging your child from the hospital, the doctor will tell you when your child can gradually begin to resume regular activities.

ARRHYTHMIAS

An arrhythmia is an abnormal heartbeat. There are two major types of arrhythmias: bradycardia, which is a slower-than-normal heartbeat, and tachycardia, which is a faster-than-normal heartbeat. Sometimes, the heartbeat alternates between beating too fast and beating too slowly. Infants and children up until their midteen years normally have a faster heartbeat than do adults. Children who exercise a lot or train for sports may have a slower-than-normal heartbeat because their heart is working more efficiently.

Serious problems occur when the child's heartbeat is extremely slow (under 40 beats per minute) or extremely rapid (over 200 beats per minute). These heartbeat rates can lead to heart failure (see HEART FAILURE, CONGESTIVE). Variations in a child's heartbeat can also indicate an underlying heart condition, such as RHEUMATIC FEVER, CARDIOMYOPATHY, or congenital heart disease (see HEART DISEASE, CONGENITAL). Other causes of arrhythmias include drugs, poisons, infection, and disorders of the endocrine (hormonal), nervous, and respiratory systems.

SIGNS AND SYMPTOMS Often the child has no symptoms at all, especially in mild cases. Infants with severe arrhythmia may look pale, feed poorly, and become less active. Children who have an arrhythmia become aware of their own slow, rapid, or irregular heartbeat. They may also experience shortness of breath, dizziness, or weakness, and may look pale and faint suddenly. An underlying heart condition can cause chest pain.

DIAGNOSIS Your child's doctor may be the first to notice abnormalities in your child's heartbeat during a routine physical examination. To confirm a diagnosis of arrhythmia, the doctor may order an *electrocardiogram* (ECG) test, which uses an external monitor to measure electrical activity in the heart. The test is painless. In some cases, your child may need to be monitored with a portable ECG device called a Holter monitor over a 24-hour period. The doctor may also order blood tests and an *echocardiogram* (an *ultrasound* of the heart) to find out what is causing the arrhythmia.

TREATMENT If your child has only a mild arrhythmia, he or she will probably receive no treatment. In severe cases, the doctor may prescribe antiarrhythmia drugs, which usually control symptoms. Extreme cases sometimes require an electric shock given to the heart through paddles applied to the chest. An artificial pacemaker is an option for long-term arrhythmia problems.

ARTHRITIS, JUVENILE RHEUMATOID

See Juvenile rheumatoid arthritis

ARTHRITIS, SEPTIC

Septic arthritis is inflammation of a joint caused by a bacterial infection. The bacteria usually spread to the joint through the bloodstream from a wound or another site of infection or after surgery on the joint. This uncommon but serious condition rarely affects more than one joint. If the infection is not treated quickly, the child's joint can be permanently damaged or destroyed.

This type of arthritis can occur in children of all ages, but appears most commonly in children under age 3. The hip and knee joints are the most common sites of infection, but the shoulders, ankles, and elbows can also be affected. In children under age 2, infections in the nose and throat cause about half of the cases of the disorder. Infected skin wounds most commonly bring about septic arthritis in children over age 2. Most cases of the disease in adolescents are linked to GONORRHEA.

SIGNS AND SYMPTOMS Infants or toddlers with septic arthritis may not be able to move the arm or leg near the infected joint because it is too painful. When you move the infected joint, the child may cry. For example, a child with an infected hip will cry when you change his or her diaper. The child may also have a fever and be irritable. A young child or adolescent may experience swelling, redness, warmth, and pain in the joint along with a slight fever and may find it too painful to move the joint. Chills can also occur in rare cases.

DIAGNOSIS To confirm a diagnosis of septic arthritis, your doctor may order a *complete blood cell count*, blood *cultures*, an X-ray of the infected joint, and a culture of the fluid in the joint for evidence of infection.

TREATMENT Prompt treatment with antibiotics is essential for recovery. Your child will receive antibiotics injected into a *catheter* in the vein. The doctor may give antibiotics even before he or she has gotten back any test results because of the danger of damage to the untreated joint.

If fluid builds up rapidly in the joint, the doctor may remove the fluid with a needle inserted into the joint. Otherwise, surgical drainage may be needed to extract excess fluid and prevent joint damage.

To ease the pain, keep your child's joint immobile and elevated. Apply warm, wet cloths over the joint. Your child should get plenty of rest. Once the antibiotics have begun to take effect, the child will need to do certain exercises to regain mobility and strengthen the joint. The outlook for complete recovery is good if treatment is prompt.

ASTHMA

Asthma is a chronic disease that affects the breathing passages connecting the lungs to the windpipe. These airways are very sensitive to irritation from a variety of triggers (see box). When irritated, the airways swell, become clogged with mucus, and constrict, making breathing difficult. The sudden breathing difficulty is commonly known as an asthma attack. Asthma is the most common chronic disease among children; nearly 5 million children and adolescents in the United States have the disorder. It tends to run in families and affects boys more often than girls. Although children can develop asthma at any age, most get it before they enter school. Asthma

What triggers an asthma attack?

A number of common substances in your child's environment can trigger an asthma attack or make the condition worse. Here are some common asthma triggers:

- **Infection** Ear, nose, and throat infections are frequent triggers of asthma in children. Other respiratory infections, such as SINUSITIS or PNEUMONIA, can also trigger asthma.
- **Environmental irritants** Tobacco smoke, perfume or hair spray, house dust mites, cockroaches, pollen, air pollution, mold, animal fur, paint or other fumes, and cold air or sudden changes in temperature can trigger asthma.
- **Exercise** Exercise-induced asthma is fairly common. Sometimes a child coughs, wheezes, and feels short of breath about 10 minutes after he or she stops exercising. Exercise in cold weather or when the humidity is low is more likely to bring on an asthma attack than activity done in a warm, humid environment.
- **Stress** Emotional stress can trigger an asthma attack or make it worse.
- **Drugs and food** Aspirin and ibuprofen can both trigger an asthma attack, but you should never give aspirin or aspirin-containing medications to children anyway because of the risk of REYE'S SYNDROME. Certain foods—such as dehydrated soups—that contain a preservative known as sulfite or the flavor enhancer monosodium glutamate can also bring on an attack. Other foods, such as nuts, milk, eggs, and cola drinks, that cause allergic reactions may also trigger an asthma attack.

can flare up once in a child's life, appear periodically, or produce frequent attacks. It sometimes disappears in adulthood.

SIGNS AND SYMPTOMS Symptoms of an asthma attack can range from mild to life threatening. Persistent coughing may be the first and, in mild cases, the only sign of asthma. In more serious cases, the child's chest hurts or feels tight and breathing becomes rapid and labored. The child will commonly wheeze (see REACTIVE AIRWAY DISEASE). While the child is struggling for breath, muscles in the child's neck, chest, and stomach sometimes noticeably strain. It can take the child twice as long to breathe out as to breathe in. Other symptoms are shortness of breath, coughing or spitting up mucus, excessive sweating, and paleness. The symptoms often get worse at night and can wake the child up. In severe cases, an affected child could panic and become confused and anxious (see ANXIETY). The child may also be drowsy. Because the child is not getting enough oxygen, he or she may turn blue or gray, especially around the lips. If untreated, an asthma attack can be fatal.

DIAGNOSIS If your child develops any of the symptoms of asthma, take him or her to the doctor. If the attack is severe, take your child to a hospital emergency department right away. The doctor will order blood tests, a chest X-ray, and additional tests to rule out other possible causes of your child's breathing problems. The doctor may also ask your child to perform a breathing test using a device known as a peak flow meter that measures the flow of air during periods of normal breathing, during an asthma attack, and immediately after inhaling asthma medication. Skin tests (see page 406) are available to determine some of the triggers of asthma.

TREATMENT Doctors prescribe several types of medication to treat asthma. Your child may need only one type or a combination of drugs. The three major types of drugs used to treat asthma are:

- **Bronchodilators** These medications relax the muscles in the airways and open up the bronchial tubes. They can be taken by mouth or inhaled. Some bronchodilators are given *intravenously* in the hospital.
- **Corticosteroids** *Corticosteroids* fight the inflammation that causes swelling and irritation in the airways. They are usually inhaled so they can act directly on the airways. In severe cases, your

Foods that contain sulfites

Some children are allergic to a preservative known as sulfite found in many common foods. Sulfites can be either sprayed onto foods, such as french fries, before cooking or added to preserve freshness. Sulfites can trigger life-threatening asthma attacks in sensitive children. Always check food labels to see whether a packaged food contains sulfites. When buying food, such as shrimp, in bulk, look for a sign at the counter that lists the food's ingredients or ask a store clerk. Always carry your child's asthma inhaler with you to restaurants. In 1986, the Food and Drug Administration banned the use of sulfites on foods—such as fruits and vegetables in salad bars—meant to be eaten raw. Foods that can contain sulfites include:

- Processed meats, such as bologna, hot dogs, and sausages
- Baked goods, such as breads and rolls
- Condiments, such as ketchup and mustard
- Dried fruits
- Canned vegetables
- Bottled jams, gravies, maraschino cherries, and molasses
- Dehydrated or precut potatoes and french fries served at restaurants
- Shrimp and lobster
- Dried soup mixes
- Guacamole
- Beer, wine, hard cider, fruit and vegetable juices, and tea

child may need to take corticosteroids by mouth or intravenously.

- **Cromolyn sodium** Cromolyn sodium is an inhaled drug that prevents the release of chemicals in the airways that trigger an attack. It is usually taken to prevent an attack before exercise or exposure to other asthma triggers. It does not work when taken during an asthma attack.

If specific ALLERGIES trigger your child's asthma, the doctor may give your child allergy shots to decrease his or her sensitivity to allergens such as pollen or dust. Your child should avoid whatever triggers his or her asthma as much as possible. In severe cases, your child may need to

Taking drugs for asthma

The doctor will teach you and your child the proper way to use an inhaler (center). Your child will need to shake the metal canister, exhale, and hold the mouthpiece up to his or her mouth. The lips must stay open so the medicine can swirl into a fine mist before it is inhaled. He or she should press down the top of the canister while taking a deep breath at the same time. The doctor will probably recommend taking two puffs from the inhaler.

Some inhalers have a small, tubelike attachment called a spacer that fits between the child's mouth and the mouthpiece on the inhaler (left). An inhaler with a spacer works better if the child closes his or her lips around the mouthpiece so he or she will get the correct dose.

Young children often find it difficult to use an inhaler properly so doctors frequently prescribe a machine called a nebulizer (right) to deliver bronchodilator drugs during or after an asthma attack. The nebulizer turns the drug into a fine mist that flows through a tube into a face mask. The child inhales the drug through the mask while breathing normally.

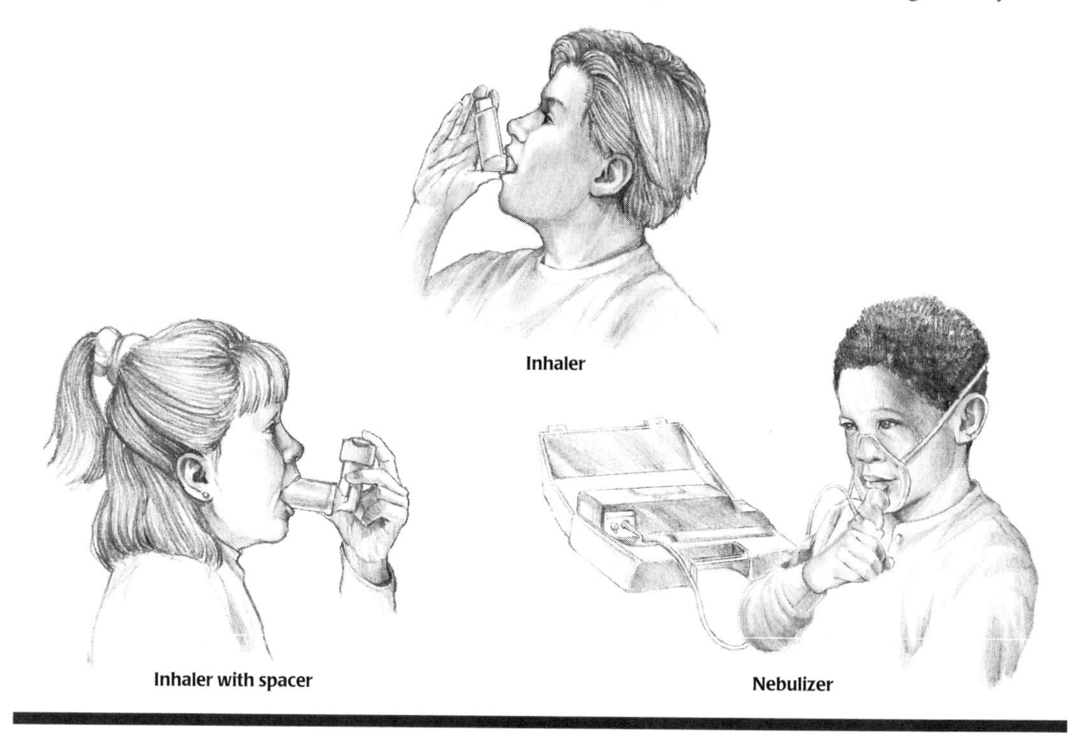

Inhaler

Inhaler with spacer

Nebulizer

Common questions about asthma

Q Does my child's asthma have a psychological cause?

A Some people think that asthma only occurs in people who have an underlying psychological problem. Emotional stress or anxiety can trigger attacks or make them worse, but asthma is a physical disease, not a mental or psychological condition.

Q Will my daughter outgrow asthma?

A About two thirds of children do outgrow asthma; others never will, especially if the disorder appeared before age 3. But even for children whose asthma persists, the outlook is positive because asthma can be controlled well with treatment. It's important for your child's asthma to be correctly diagnosed to avoid potentially life-threatening attacks.

Q Will my son's asthma inhibit his participation in sports?

A There's no reason why it should. Asthma attacks can be triggered by strenuous exercise, but, if your son warms up gradually and takes his medication properly, he can continue to participate in sports. Don't try to limit your son's athletic activities; instead encourage his participation, as long as he follows his doctor's instructions to prevent an asthma attack.

be hospitalized or treated in a hospital emergency department. Your child may be given oxygen in addition to bronchodilators and corticosteroids.

ATHLETE'S FOOT

Athlete's foot is a common infection, caused by a fungus, affecting the skin of the feet, especially the soles and the area between the toes. It can affect people of all ages but is most common among teenagers. The fungus grows especially well on damp feet and can be passed from person to person in locker rooms or showers.

SIGNS AND SYMPTOMS Your child will experience itching or burning and a red, scaly rash will appear on the skin. The skin will crack and peel between the toes, especially the fourth and fifth toes. The foot smells musty and sometimes has small blisters on it.

DIAGNOSIS You will probably be able to recognize athlete's foot and treat it on your own with an over-the-counter medication. But your child should see the doctor if the infection spreads over the whole foot or if a fever develops. The doctor may take a sample of affected skin and examine it under a microscope.

TREATMENT Treat athlete's foot at home with an over-the-counter athlete's foot powder, cream, or ointment, according to package directions. Your child will need to bathe his or her feet daily, remove the scaly skin between the toes with a clean cloth or tissue, and dry the feet carefully—especially between the toes.

How to avoid athlete's foot

You and your child can do a great deal to prevent athlete's foot:

- Bathe the feet every day and dry them thoroughly.
- Change socks daily.
- Wear cotton socks because they absorb sweat better than socks made of synthetic fibers.
- Wear shoes made of natural materials, such as leather or canvas. Synthetic materials can cause the feet to sweat.
- Go barefoot as much as possible. During warm weather, wear sandals or other open shoes that allow your feet to breathe.
- If a family member develops athlete's foot, make sure that person wears shower sandals or thongs in the bathroom to avoid spreading the infection.
- Wear sandals or shower thongs in public showers and dressing rooms.

For a severe case of athlete's foot that spreads to the toenail, your child's doctor may prescribe a stronger medication that is either applied directly to the skin or taken by mouth. With proper treatment, athlete's foot should clear up in 2 or 3 weeks.

If your child uses a public shower or locker room at school or at a health club, he or she should wear shower sandals or thongs to avoid becoming reinfected or spreading the infection to others.

Atopic dermatitis

Atopic dermatitis, also known as eczema (see page 23), is a common childhood skin RASH marked by red, itchy, scaly, dry areas of skin or weepy small BLISTERS. The rash can occur on any part of the body, but appears most frequently on the face, neck, inside of the elbows, and backs of the knees and affects only the outer layers of the skin. Atopic dermatitis most commonly affects infants, who usually get it on their face and scalp and in the skin folds of their elbows and knees. About half of all cases among infants clear up by the time the baby reaches 18 months. Most children outgrow the condition by their early teens, although some continue to have flare-ups into adulthood. The condition tends to run in families and it often affects children who also have ALLERGIES, ASTHMA, HAY FEVER, or PSORIASIS (the word "atopic" refers to the inherited tendency to develop allergies). Eczema is not contagious and the skin eruptions will not leave a scar, but eczema is a chronic condition, meaning that it keeps coming back, even after treatment.

Signs and symptoms If your infant has atopic dermatitis, he or she will have itchy red spots on his or her skin that can ooze with fluid and crust over. Because the spots itch, your infant will rub them with his or her hand or with a pillow or toy. Some children scratch the sores so badly, especially at night, that the skin starts to bleed and can easily become infected. The affected areas become dry, brown-gray, and covered by thick, scaly skin if the eczema continues beyond 18 months of age.

Adolescents with atopic dermatitis usually have scaly spots on the backs of their knees and the insides of their elbows, but the spots can also occur on the face, neck, chest, wrists, and ankles.

Diagnosis Your child's doctor will make a diagnosis based on whether there is a family history of atopic dermatitis or allergies and a careful examination of the rash on your child's skin.

Treatment Keep the affected areas moist by applying moisturizing lotions several times a day. When flare-ups occur, give your child very brief baths or showers in lukewarm (not hot) water daily or every other day. Bathing helps prevent the skin eruptions from becoming infected. It's best to use only small amounts of a moisturizing soap because harsh soaps can irritate the skin. Immediately after a bath or shower, apply lotion to your child's damp skin to seal in the moisture.

Your doctor may recommend an over-the-counter *corticosteroid* ointment or cream, such as hydrocortisone cream, to reduce the inflammation. Apply the cream to your child's skin lightly to avoid irritating the skin further.

Eczema is aggravated by dry skin, wool clothing, harsh soaps, excessive perspiration, stress, some cosmetics, and the perfume in lotions and soaps. Scratching makes the condition worse and can cause infection, so keep your child's fingernails short and put long-sleeved clothing on him or her if the rash extends to the arms. Ask your child's doctor if he or she recommends using an over-the-counter antihistamine, such as diphenhydramine, to reduce the itching, but remember that antihistamines can cause drowsiness.

Attention-deficit disorder

See Attention disorders

ATTENTION-DEFICIT HYPERACTIVITY DISORDER

See Attention disorders

ATTENTION DISORDERS

An attention disorder is a behavior problem in which a child is easily distracted, has difficulty paying attention, and acts impulsively. There are two major types of attention disorders. One is attention-deficit disorder (ADD); the other is attention-deficit hyperactivity disorder (ADHD), which includes hyperactivity as a symptom.

Three to 5 percent of all school-age children have an attention disorder. ADHD is more common in boys. Both types seem to run in families. Although doctors don't know for sure what causes attention disorders, possible causes include a genetic disorder, a brain injury, slower-than-normal brain development, or a nervous system abnormality that affects the way chemical messages are sent to the child's brain. Babies born to mothers who used alcohol or street drugs—such as cocaine, heroin, and amphetamines—during pregnancy have a greater risk of developing attention disorders. Premature infants are also at greater risk of attention disorders.

SIGNS AND SYMPTOMS All children have trouble paying attention and act impulsively from time to time, but children with attention disorders have these problems consistently for at least 6 months. Many children have symptoms throughout childhood and adolescence, and the disorder can continue into adulthood. Attention disorders often cause difficulties in school and can lead to low self-esteem.

A child cannot be diagnosed until about age 3, when he or she has reached a certain level of development. Common symptoms include:

Inattention Affected children from age 3 to 5 years are easily distracted, may play with toys for only brief periods, quickly go from one activity to another, and have trouble following simple instructions. Children over 6 may not finish school assignments or chores. They do not pay close attention to instructions or details, often make careless mistakes, and perform poorly in school. They may be disorganized and lose things frequently.

Impulsive activity From 3 to 5 years of age, an affected child may seem noisier than other children, misbehave a lot, have trouble waiting to take turns or sharing, and take things away from others. Children over 6 may disrupt class, interrupt others, yell out answers in school before being called on, and have difficulty waiting in line. They may also engage in dangerous activities without thinking.

Hyperactivity Young children with an attention disorder are in constant motion, cannot sit still for meals, and may talk constantly. Children over 6 fidget and squirm in their seat, wander around the classroom, cannot sit quietly and read, run and climb at inappropriate times, and talk a lot.

Other symptoms include trouble sleeping (see SLEEP DISTURBANCES), acting or playing aggressively, insisting on instant gratification, an inability to keep friends, LEARNING DISABILITIES, intellectual DEVELOPMENTAL DELAY, withdrawal, a lack of motivation, and depression. Adolescents with ADHD or ADD may have difficulty in social situations and can have trouble keeping a job.

DIAGNOSIS An attention disorder may become apparent when your child starts going to school, where the order and discipline of the classroom may reveal it to your child's teacher. The disorder might be more difficult to see in children who are not hyperactive and are quiet and withdrawn. The doctor will determine whether your child's symptoms indicate an attention disorder by asking questions about his or her behavior patterns. The doctor will also do a thorough physical examination and order laboratory studies to rule out other diseases or disorders that may mimic an attention disorder. He or she may refer your child to a psychiatrist or psychologist for an evaluation. While most affected children have all of the characteristic symptoms from time to time, doctors diagnose ADD or ADHD based on the persistence of the symptoms and the degree of distress and dysfunction they cause.

Attention disorder: Managing your child at home

If your child has an attention disorder, you can do a number of constructive things at home to help change your child's behavior and manage his or her disruptive activities:

- Don't get angry. Children with attention disorders can be difficult to deal with, but try not to lose your temper. Never hit, spank, or slap your child when he or she misbehaves or seems out of control. Instead, be patient. ADD is not your child's fault. Try using time-outs (see page 126) to calm your child down. Sit your child down away from other people in a quiet, nondistracting environment for several minutes—about 1 minute for every year of life. For example, a 7-year-old would get a 7-minute time-out.
- Reward your child for good behavior. Show your child love and respect every day and praise him or her for behaving well. Be consistent. Correct the bad behavior with time-outs rather than scolding so your child does not think he or she can get attention by behaving badly.
- Develop routines. Put your child on a regular schedule. Set times for waking, eating, going to school, playing, doing homework and housework, and going to bed. A strict schedule will help establish order and discipline in your child's life.
- Tune in to your child's environment. Try to appreciate how he or she experiences the world. Minor distractions, such as rustling papers or hissing radiators, may be difficult to tune out. Try to create a soothing, calm environment and be aware of overstimulating situations that could put him or her on edge.

TREATMENT Treatment options include drugs, behavior modification techniques, and individual or family therapy. Sometimes all three treatments are used in combination. Most children with attention disorders respond well to drug therapy combined with behavior modification techniques. Your child's doctor or psychiatrist may prescribe one of several stimulant drugs that appear to work by balancing the brain chemicals responsible for behavior. Stimulants can have certain side effects, such as HEADACHES, DEPRESSION, sleep loss, appetite loss, and growth delay. In some cases, your child's doctor may prescribe antidepressant medications instead.

Behavior modification attempts to change the child's behavior by teaching him or her desirable behavior responses instead of undesirable ones. It takes cooperation between parents and teachers. Your child may need special education or a tutor. His or her teachers may need to take extra time explaining assignments and expectations to your child. You may need to be a vocal advocate for your child to ensure that he or she gets all the help he or she needs and you will probably need to monitor your child's school assignments, homework, test dates, and project deadlines to make sure your child complies. Therapy can address self-esteem issues to boost your child's self-confidence. Finding activities that your child does well, along with improving social skills and compliance with school assignments will help create a sound self-image.

AUTISM

Autism is a nervous system disorder that affects the way a child's brain functions, causing impaired social, emotional, and language development. The disorder affects boys four times more often than girls. Children with mild autism may seem almost normal, while severely autistic children may seem profoundly mentally retarded (see MENTAL RETARDATION) or have seizures. Some autistic children have a high intelligence quotient (IQ) masked by an inability to communicate. All children with autism have developmental impairments that in some way affect their social interaction, communication abilities, and overall behavior. The cause of autism is unknown. The child's developmental problems may be apparent in early infancy or may not become obvious until age 2 or 3.

SIGNS AND SYMPTOMS An autistic infant may stiffen or become limp to avoid physical contact when parents or nurses try to pick him or her up. These reactions arise from sensory impairment and an inability to withstand normal stimulation. Some autistic infants are quiet and passive, while others cry a lot and seem agitated most of the time. Some fail to bond with their mothers and avoid eye contact. Head banging and rocking are common manifestations of autism.

In early childhood, some autistic toddlers learn to crawl, walk, and talk early; others are considerably delayed for their age. About a third develop normally until about age 2 or 3. Autistic children may withdraw from normal social relationships with other children and often become isolated. Children with severe autism may not even seem to be aware that other people are around them. Their communication skills fall behind others their age and they may not be able to express themselves or appear to understand simple sentences, commands, or questions. They may repeat words or phrases over and over again mechanically.

Some autistic children manifest repetitive behavior, such as hand flapping or teeth grinding. They may hurt themselves by biting their hands or banging their heads repeatedly and may seem insensitive to pain. Autistic children often have trouble sleeping and eating and exhibit hyperactivity. They rarely make eye contact.

Autistic children like routine and may throw a tantrum if you change their schedule or move objects or furniture in the house. They like to go the same way to school every day and may want to eat the same foods at every meal.

DIAGNOSIS There are no medical tests available to diagnose autism. Psychological testing is the usual means by which children are tested for the disorder.

TREATMENT Autism affects a child for life. The mainstays of treatment are special education and a supportive family. Some children may need medication to reduce agitation or seizures. The symptoms of some autistic children with food allergies may be improved by changes in diet. Other autistic children who have problems processing visual information may be helped with special eyeglasses. Some autistic children can live at home with their parents; others need to move into residential facilities or group homes. Some autistic adults can eventually learn to live independent lives. Usually only those with very severe autism are placed in institutions.

Raising an autistic child can be extremely difficult and stressful for parents. If your child is autistic, ask your doctor or a social worker at a local hospital for the names of organizations in your community that provide respite care. You may also find it helpful to join a support group made up of other parents with autistic children.

AUTOIMMUNE DISORDERS

Autoimmune disorders are a group of diseases in which the immune system, the body's natural defense against infection, reacts against a child's own organs or tissues. This reaction occurs when the immune system activates abnormally or when cells change and the immune system mistakes them for dangerous foreign substances and attacks them. The immune system normally recognizes the body's own cells and tissues and does not harm them. In a child with autoimmune disorders, the immune system releases antibodies to attack some of the child's body's cells, tissues, and organs. Bacteria, viruses, and some drugs are thought to trigger an autoimmune response in children who have inherited a predisposition to these disorders.

Autoimmune disorders can destroy cells and tissues, cause an organ to grow abnormally, or change the normal function of an organ. They can affect only one organ or type of cell or tissue, or many. Such disorders frequently attack blood cells, blood vessels, organs, joints, muscles, and skin.

Common autoimmune disorders occurring in children include ADDISION'S DISEASE, DERMATOMYOSITIS, diabetes (see DIABETES MELLITUS, TYPE I), HYPERTHYROIDISM, HYPOTHYROIDISM, JUVENILE RHEUMATOID ARTHRITIS, LUPUS, and THYROIDITIS.

SIGNS AND SYMPTOMS The signs and symptoms of autoimmune disorders will vary according to the specific disorder, but common symptoms include an overall feeling of ill health, fatigue, lack of energy, dizziness, and chronic fever. Autoimmune disorders can cause an organ to become larger than normal—for example, when the thyroid gland becomes enlarged from thyroiditis. They can also destroy an organ, such as the pancreas, causing diabetes, or cause tissue to fail to function normally.

TREATMENT Treatment of a childhood autoimmune disorder will vary depending on the specific type, but in general, treatment seeks to either replace hormone deficiencies when present or suppress the overproduction of hormones with medication. Blood transfusions may be needed to correct anemia or dialysis may be needed to treat kidney failure. Treatment also attempts to bring the immune system under control with drugs, such as *corticosteroids* or immunosuppressant drugs that suppress the child's immune system. Immunosuppressant drugs can have serious side effects, such as susceptibility to infection, anemia, nausea, diarrhea, and hair loss, so they must be used with extreme caution.

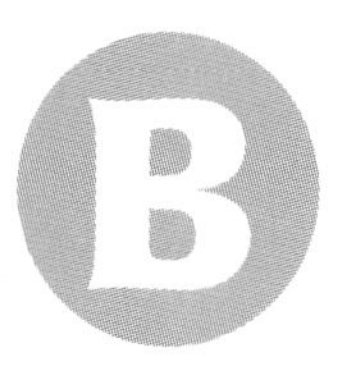

BACTEREMIA

Bacteremia (also called blood poisoning) is an infection caused by bacteria in the bloodstream. Bacteria can enter a child's bloodstream through a cut or wound; from infections such as TONSILLITIS, PNEUMONIA, or APPENDICITIS; and from minor surgery, including routine dental procedures like tooth extractions.

Left untreated, bacteremia can lead to more serious and life-threatening diseases as the bacteria spread through the bloodstream to other parts of the body. Some bacteria also produce *toxins* in the blood.

SIGNS AND SYMPTOMS A high fever (102°F or higher) is the main symptom of bacteremia. If the bacteria spread throughout the bloodstream, your child will also have chills, loss of appetite, irritability, exhaustion, and an overall feeling of ill health. The illness can progress to SEPTICEMIA, which can cause shock (see page 678).

DIAGNOSIS Call the doctor immediately if your child displays the symptoms of bacteremia so the doctor can treat the infection before it spreads throughout the child's body. During the examination, the doctor will check for low blood pressure and a quick pulse rate. He or she will test a sample of the child's blood and may also analyze a sample of urine and spinal fluid to identify the source of infection.

TREATMENT The doctor will give your child antibiotic drugs to kill the bacteria that caused the infection. If the child looks well enough, aside from a high fever, the doctor may give the child antibiotics by mouth or through injection into a muscle. The doctor may admit a sicker child to a hospital so that the antibiotics can be given *intravenously* and to monitor the child's condition.

BALANITIS

Balanitis is the inflammation of the head of a boy's penis. It can be caused by infection from a bacterium or fungus, a tight or unretractable foreskin, or irritation from chemicals in clothing, diapers, latex condoms, or contraceptive creams. Bacterial or fungal infections usually develop from poor hygiene or sexual contact. Boys with an uncircumcised foreskin are more likely to get balanitis than those who have been circumcised.

SIGNS AND SYMPTOMS The head of the penis, and sometimes the foreskin, becomes red, swollen, and painful. The penis may have ulcers (open sores) on it, and the glands in the groin may be swollen. In rare cases, the boy may feel a burning sensation while urinating, and may see a discharge of clear, thick fluid from his penis.

DIAGNOSIS The doctor will diagnose balanitis by examining your son's penis and by ordering a *culture* of any discharge from the penis.

TREATMENT If your son has balanitis, his doctor will probably prescribe a *corticosteroid* cream to bring down the swelling, antibiotics or antifungal medication to fight infection, and a pain and fever reliever (acetaminophen or ibuprofen). Make sure your son washes the affected area every day. If your son has not been circumcised and the balanitis recurs, the doctor may recommend circumcision (see page 32).

BED-WETTING

Bed-wetting is involuntary urination during sleep. The problem is more common in boys than in girls and occurs in children who have no physical malformation, such as a spinal cord abnormality, that could cause a child to lose control of his or her bladder. Most children achieve bladder control at night at about 5 years of age. Because children develop nerve and muscle control at different rates, bed-wetting is a common problem. Research shows that from 10 to 20 percent of all 5-year-olds wet their beds at night. But the numbers drop as children get older.

Most often, bed-wetting is caused by the inability of the child during deep sleep to sense the need to urinate. The child could also have an underlying illness, such as a URINARY TRACT INFECTION or diabetes (see DIABETES MELLITUS, TYPE I). A small bladder can also predispose a child to bed-wetting. Urine builds up in the bladder overnight and, if the child's bladder is not large enough to hold it, he or she wets the bed. Emotional stress may also be a factor. Bed-wetting is known to run in families and may be related to a child's diet; caffeine, chocolate, carbonated drinks, and citrus juice have all been implicated.

DIAGNOSIS Your child's doctor will do a thorough physical examination and ask you and your child questions about the bed-wetting problem. To check for evidence of diabetes or a urinary tract infection, the doctor will take a sample of your child's urine and send it to a laboratory for analysis. If the interview or examination reveals the possibility of another disorder, the doctor will also order other tests, such as X-rays of the lower spine or an *ultrasound* of your child's kidneys and bladder.

TREATMENT The doctor will treat any underlying disorder and recommend steps you can take to help your child gain bladder control. If your child has a small bladder, your doctor may recommend medications to help relax the bladder so it will stretch. For special occasions, the doctor can prescribe hormonal treatment, taken through the nose, that will keep your child dry overnight by causing the body to retain water. This treatment will not cure the bed-wetting, but can help your child avoid the embarrassment of bed-wetting at camp or a sleepover.

Your child's doctor will probably recommend some type of alarm system to help your child stop wetting the bed. The system uses a moisture-sensitive pad, attached to your child's underpants, that senses when he or she begins to urinate and sounds an alarm or buzzer that wakes up your child so he or she can urinate in the toilet. The alarm helps your child become sensitive to the need to urinate and awaken on his or her own to use the bathroom. You won't have to withhold liquids or wake your child during the night to use the bathroom if you are using a program that includes an alarm, medication, and/or dietary changes. It's important to encourage your child to stick with the plan to be successful. It usually takes about 2 or 3 months for a child's bed-wetting problems to resolve.

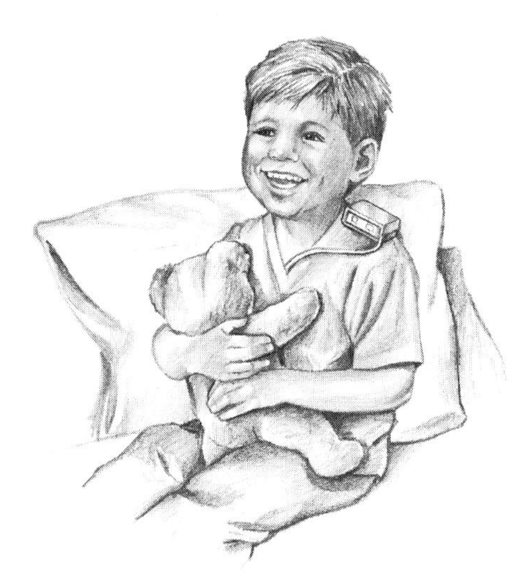

A bed-wetting alarm system

A bed-wetting alarm system can help your child become aware of the need to awaken during the night in time to go to the bathroom. The alarm system uses a moisture-sensitive pad attached to your child's underwear. A wet pad triggers a buzzer attached to the child's pajama top. When your child hears the buzzer, he or she can wake up and go to the bathroom to urinate. Within 2 to 3 months, your child will learn to get up and use the bathroom on his or her own, without the alarm.

What you can do to help stop bed-wetting

Bed-wetting is a common problem that most children outgrow. But you can try some simple techniques at home to help your child gain bladder control. These methods work best when used with an alarm system or medication:

- Never scold, criticize, punish, or blame your child for wetting the bed because you will only make the situation worse. Be supportive and encouraging.
- Don't give your child foods or drinks—carbonated drinks, chocolate, caffeine, or citrus fruit—that might cause bed-wetting.
- At dinnertime, avoid dishes, such as pizza, that contain cheese and dairy foods. About 10 percent of children have a sensitivity to these foods, which can irritate the bladder.
- Encourage your child to urinate right before bedtime.
- Put a plastic cover on your child's mattress.
- Dress your child in pajamas or thick underwear instead of diapers or plastic pants for bed. Diapers are humiliating for an older child and will lower his or her motivation.
- Keep a dry set of pajamas or underwear near the bed so your child can change if he or she needs to. Provide clean sheets so he or she can replace wet ones.
- Praise and encourage your child when he or she stays dry.
- If other family members have had experiences with bed-wetting, encourage them to talk about them.

BILIARY ATRESIA

Biliary atresia is a rare disorder in which a child is born with abnormally developed bile ducts, the tiny tubes that carry the digestive fluid bile through the liver and into the small intestine. The bile becomes trapped in and damages the child's liver. The condition can be fatal by 2 years of age.

Signs and symptoms Up to a month after birth, an affected baby's skin and eyes turn yellow (see JAUNDICE). Then his or her liver enlarges, causing the baby's abdomen to swell and become tender. The infant produces dark-colored urine and pale stool. During the first year of life, the infant's growth and overall health are affected because the baby does not get enough nourishment. The child appears weak and becomes irritable. Unless treated, children with biliary atresia do not survive.

Diagnosis If your newborn has jaundice, the doctor will test his or her blood for bilirubin, a bile pigment that, in excess, causes jaundice. If the test results suggest biliary atresia, the doctor may order more blood tests, *ultrasound,* or a *radionuclide scan* of your baby's liver to confirm the diagnosis. The doctor may also want to do a liver *biopsy* to rule out other possible causes of your baby's jaundice.

Treatment If your baby has biliary atresia, he or she will need surgery to join the small intestine directly to the liver. The operation usually minimizes the baby's symptoms, but your infant may need a liver transplant (replacement of a diseased liver with a healthy, donated one) to cure the disease.

Bipolar disorder

Bipolar disorder, also known as manic-depressive illness, is a mood disorder marked by extreme emotional swings from mania (highs) to DEPRESSION (lows). Among children, this disorder most often begins in adolescence, usually in teenagers between the ages of 15 and 19, but it can also occur in children as young as 6 or 7 years old. No one knows for sure what causes bipolar disorder, but possible causes include a brain disorder, the use of certain drugs, and stressful life events. The child's mood swings may alternate between depression and mania or he or she may experience mania alone. Bipolar disorder seems to run in families.

Signs and symptoms The symptoms of depression include hopelessness, extreme guilt, withdrawal from family and friends, and thoughts of death and suicide. The child may also be very tired for long periods, sleep during the day and have trouble sleeping at night, have difficulty concentrating, lack energy, and become disinterested in his or her normal activities and in personal hygiene. The child's appetite may either diminish or become excessive.

The symptoms of mania include an exaggerated sense of self-importance and well-being, extreme restlessness and hyperactivity, constant talking, racing of thoughts, trouble sleeping, and excessive levels of social activity or sexual promiscuity. The child may also gain weight, be unable to control his or her temper, become paranoid, and spend too much money.

Some children, known as rapid cyclers, may have mania or depression several times a week, while others may experience highs and lows that last weeks, months, or years. In the first few years of the disorder, children may have more manic episodes than depressive episodes.

Diagnosis and treatment If your child has symptoms of bipolar disorder, the doctor will refer him or her to a psychiatrist or psychologist for a complete psychological evaluation. The doctor will also examine your child for any physical problems that could be causing his or her symptoms and will order tests that can rule out other disorders, such as hyperthyroidism, that can mimic the symptoms of bipolar disorder. Hospitalization is sometimes necessary to treat extreme mood swings. Your child may be given antidepressant drugs for depression or antipsychotic drugs for the manic episodes. He or she will also need a course of psychotherapy, which may include other family members.

Once your child's symptoms are under control, the doctor will prescribe a drug called lithium to prevent the symptoms from returning. Lithium therapy is usually very effective but the dosage must be very carefully monitored because the dose needed to stabilize mood is very close to the level that can produce toxic symptoms. The doctor will measure the levels of lithium in your child's blood regularly to avoid any adverse effects from the drug. Your child may need to continue taking lithium for the rest of his or her life to keep bipolar disorder under control. Some children need to take other drugs, known as neuroleptic medications, to control manic symptoms.

BIRTH DEFECTS

Birth defects are abnormal physical or mental conditions that appear in newborns or are detected in infants in the first few months of life. They are also called congenital defects because they are conditions that are present at birth.

Birth defects include a wide range of conditions that may be minor, such as a birthmark, or very serious and even life threatening, such as congenital heart disease (see HEART DISEASE, CONGENITAL). They can be inherited as GENETIC DISORDERS; be caused by environmental factors affecting the developing fetus, such as smoking or alcohol use by the baby's mother during pregnancy; arise from a combination of genetic and environmental factors; or be caused by spontaneous mutation of a gene or defective formation of a fertilized egg. Medical science does not know the cause of some birth defects.

MALFORMATIONS Parts of a newborn's body can become deformed during the time the fetus was developing in its mother's womb. Almost any part of the baby's body can become malformed. Some examples of common malformations are SPINA BIFIDA, HYDROCEPHALUS, CLEFT LIP AND CLEFT PALATE, CLUBFOOT, a deformed hand or fingers, and a deformed heart or other organ.

Some malformations, such as abnormally small lungs, occur because the fetus has small kidneys that produce too little fluid to surround it in the uterus. Others, such as malformed hearts, can develop because of CHROMOSOMAL ABNORMALITIES or diseases in the mother. Certain malformations are caused by harmful substances in the fetus's environment, such as the mother's consumption of alcohol or use of street drugs during pregnancy.

GENETIC DEFECTS A newborn may inherit certain birth defects, such as chromosomal abnormalities or INBORN ERRORS OF METABOLISM in the genes received from his or her parents.

Chromosomal abnormalities occur in a child when the father's sperm or the mother's egg con-

Extra toes

A birth defect that produces extra fingers or toes is called polydactyly. The extra digit may not be fully formed, resembling a fleshy outgrowth. It is usually surgically removed shortly after birth.

Testing for birth defects

Early in your pregnancy, your doctor will order tests to screen for birth defects. For example, a blood test for a blood protein called alpha-fetoprotein (AFP) helps determine the risk for spinal cord and brain defects. Farther along in the pregnancy, your doctor may do *ultrasound, amniocentesis* (taking a sample of fluid from the amniotic sac that surrounds the fetus), or *chorionic villus sampling* (taking a sample from the placenta). Based on these test results, you and your partner may wish to get genetic counseling (see page 497).

tains an abnormal number of *chromosomes,* when the chromosomes do not separate properly during development of the embryo, or when the chromosomes carry extra pieces or are missing pieces. Some examples of chromosomal abnormalities include DOWN SYNDROME and KLINEFELTER'S SYNDROME.

Inborn errors of metabolism include GALACTOSEMIA, GAUCHER'S DISEASE, UREA-CYCLE DISORDERS, and PKU. They are caused by defects in a single gene the baby inherits from one or both of his or her parents.

Genetic defects can produce blood disorders, such as SICKLE CELL ANEMIA and THALASSEMIA, bone deformities and other physical malformations, BLINDNESS, organ damage, and MENTAL RETARDATION. Some genetic defects, such as Gaucher's disease and TAY-SACHS DISEASE, can cause the death of a newborn or the early death of a child.

DEFECTS CAUSED BY MATERNAL INFECTIONS Certain infections, such as GERMAN MEASLES (rubella), in a pregnant woman can cause birth defects and even death of the newborn. The virus that causes German measles in a pregnant woman can also produce blindness, deafness (see HEARING LOSS), heart defects, and mental retardation in her baby. Sexually transmitted diseases in the mother can cause a newborn to have bone malformations, eye infections, blindness, infections in other organs, and brain damage. They could even cause the newborn to die.

DEFECTS CAUSED BY THE MOTHER'S LIFESTYLE Lifestyle choices that the mother makes during pregnancy, such as smoking, drinking alcohol, and taking drugs, can affect the developing fetus and cause birth defects. Women who smoke during pregnancy are more likely to have a stillborn baby, a miscarriage, or a low-birthweight baby. Babies born underweight for their age have a greater risk of birth defects, learning disabilities, and death than normal-weight babies. Women who drink alcohol during pregnancy put their babies at risk of FETAL ALCOHOL SYNDROME, which can cause heart defects, cleft palate, a small brain, deformed joints, and mental retardation. Street drugs (such as cocaine, heroin, or amphetamines) taken during pregnancy increase the risk of miscarriage, premature, low-birthweight babies,

Reducing the risk of birth defects

As prospective parents, you can do several things to help reduce the risk of your baby having a birth defect. The most important step a pregnant woman can take is to get regular checkups and prenatal care during pregnancy to make sure she and her fetus are in good health. Take these additional preventive measures:

- If you have a family history of chromosomal abnormalities, inborn errors of metabolism, or other genetic disorders, seek genetic counseling (see page 497) before conceiving a child.
- Have a medical examination before trying to conceive to rule out or treat any infections or other illnesses in yourself or your partner.
- Eat a well-balanced diet before and during pregnancy and take prenatal vitamins daily during pregnancy.
- If you have a chronic disease, such as diabetes, get regular treatment for it so the disease will be controlled and you can be in the best of health.
- If you are taking any medications, or if your doctor prescribes any medications while you are pregnant, make sure he or she knows that you are pregnant and ask if the drug will affect your fetus.
- Don't smoke cigarettes or use other tobacco products during pregnancy.
- Don't drink alcoholic beverages during pregnancy.
- Avoid exposure to high doses of X-rays, toxic chemicals, or environmental pollutants during pregnancy.
- Never use street drugs, such as cocaine, heroin, or so-called "designer drugs," during pregnancy.

birth defects, and brain damage. Some prescription drugs, such as seizure medications, can also cause birth defects.

Women who do not get adequate nutrition during pregnancy can also have babies with birth defects because the developing fetus does not get the nutrients it needs to grow properly. Older women have an increased risk of having a child with a chromosomal disorder.

DEFECTS CAUSED BY MATERNAL DISEASE Certain chronic diseases present in the mother can cause birth defects in the newborn. For example, diabetes mellitus can increase the risk of heart malformations and newborn lung disease.

DEFECTS PRODUCED BY THE ENVIRONMENT The developing fetus can be damaged if the mother receives high doses of X-rays or *radiation* for cancer early in her pregnancy. Exposure to excessive amounts of toxic chemicals, lead, and other pollutants in the environment during pregnancy may also cause birth defects, but more studies are needed to prove a direct link.

BITES

See page 672

BLEEDING DISORDERS

Bleeding disorders are caused by a deficiency or abnormality in the blood components known as platelets and clotting factors, which are needed for blood clotting. Platelets control bleeding by plugging small breaks in injured blood-vessel walls. When the platelets are abnormal or their number is reduced, they cannot begin the clotting process and stop bleeding. Clotting factors are proteins that complete the clotting process. Bleeding disorders can be inherited or acquired.

TYPES OF BLEEDING DISORDERS The most common bleeding disorders are HEMOPHILIA, von Willebrand's disease, and thrombocytopenia.

Hemophilia Hemophilia is a group of inherited bleeding disorders caused by deficiencies in different blood-clotting proteins (factors) needed to clot blood (see page 516).

Von Willebrand's disease Von Willebrand's disease is an inherited bleeding disorder caused by an abnormality or a deficiency in von Willebrand's factor and factor VIII clotting factor. When these factors are abnormal or deficient, they cannot cause the platelets to stick together and adhere to the walls of blood vessels to form a clot and stop bleeding. Most cases of the disease are mild.

Thrombocytopenia Children with thrombocytopenia have a lower-than-normal number of platelet cells in their blood so they tend to bleed from small blood vessels into their skin and other parts of their bodies. Thrombocytopenia can be caused by infections or medications or it can be inherited. Certain other diseases, such as CANCER and AUTOIMMUNE DISORDERS, can also cause thrombocytopenia.

SIGNS AND SYMPTOMS All bleeding disorders produce prolonged or excessive bleeding or bleeding that occurs in unexpected ways. Such commonplace events as a tooth extraction, an injury, a fall, surgery, or even a minor bump can become a high-risk incident that causes a child to bleed or bruise excessively.

The specific symptoms of von Willebrand's disease include prolonged bleeding after injury or surgery, extensive bleeding of the gums after a tooth extraction, prolonged NOSEBLEEDS, and excessive menstrual bleeding in adolescent girls. Children with this disease also get BRUISES easily after an injury.

The symptoms of thrombocytopenia include flat, purplish-red spots on the skin; nosebleeds; and bleeding in the mouth. Children with thrombocytopenia also have a tendency to bruise easily. Adolescent girls may experience heavy or prolonged menstrual bleeding.

Giving your child non-steroidal anti-inflammatory drugs may make the bleeding worse. A number of other prescription and over-the-counter drugs—sulfa drugs (used to fight bacteria), tranquilizers, diabetes medications, antihistamines, and some of the ingredients in cough medicines—can also make the symptoms of bleeding disorders worse.

DIAGNOSIS To diagnose a bleeding disorder, your child's doctor will do a thorough physical examination. The doctor will also question you and your child about bruising, nosebleeds, bleeding from other parts of the body, his or her general symptoms, and the drugs your child is taking to determine if the bleeding disorders are caused by a reaction to medication. Because these disorders are sometimes inherited, your doctor will also ask about a family history of bleeding problems. He or she will draw some blood from your child and have it analyzed for the number of platelets and clotting factors. Tests for specific clotting factors may be needed. The doctor may also need to obtain a sample of your child's bone marrow if he or she has diagnosed the condition called thrombocytopenia and is uncertain about the cause.

TREATMENT Your child may not require any treatment for either von Willebrand's disease or thrombocytopenia because the diseases tend to be mild. Your doctor will recommend that your child avoid taking drugs that could affect the condition. Specific treatment of thrombocytopenia depends on the underlying cause, but could include *corticosteroid* medication, immunoglobulins (proteins that help suppress the destruction of platelets), or a platelet transfusion.

For severe symptoms of von Willebrand's disease, your child may receive injections of factor VIII and other clotting factors *intravenously* to help restore his or her blood-clotting ability. Some types of von Willebrand's disease can be treated with a medication known as desmopressin acetate, which increases the amount of von Willebrand's factor in your child's blood.

Mild bleeding symptoms of thrombocytopenia and von Willebrand's disease should improve within a few hours to a few weeks. Severe bleeding episodes may require hospitalization.

What you can do if your child has a bleeding disorder

If your child has a bleeding disorder, he or she needs to take extra precautions in all activities of daily life. Here's what you can do to help ease your child's fears and control extensive bleeding:

- Stop nosebleeds by applying a cool, wet cloth and gentle pressure over the bridge of your child's nose (see page 677).
- To stop bleeding in other parts of the body, place a cool, wet cloth over the wound and apply gentle pressure. Elevate the affected part of the body.
- Encourage your child to avoid rough contact sports like football, hockey, rugby, or boxing. Use knee pads, elbow pads, wrist guards, shin guards, and helmets to protect vulnerable areas during other sports or physical activities such as skating or bicycling.
- Be sure to tell your dentist or surgeon about your child's bleeding disorder. Avoid surgery, including dental surgery and tooth extractions, for your child unless it is absolutely necessary.
- Never give your child aspirin. In addition to the dangers of Reye's syndrome, it could make the bleeding disorder worse.
- If you know that your child needs to have a shot, tell the nurse or doctor about the bleeding disorder so he or she can apply gentle pressure to the site for 5 minutes after the injection to prevent bleeding.
- Make sure that your child wears a medical identification tag as a necklace or bracelet that will forewarn medical personnel of the bleeding disorder in an emergency.

BLINDNESS

Blindness is a total or partial loss of vision that cannot be corrected with eyeglasses. Some children are born blind, others become blind from injury, disease, or a physical disorder that affects the child's eyes. In the United States, the legal definition of blindness is vision of 20/200 or less in the less-affected eye (corrected with eyeglasses) or peripheral (side) vision no greater than 20 degrees. This definition means that a child with 20/200 vision sees at 20 feet away what a child with normal vision sees at 200 feet (normal vision is 20/20). A child with peripheral vision no greater than 20 degrees cannot see to his or her side beyond a limited angle (20 degrees).

Some babies are born with cataracts (cloudy lenses in the eyes) or GLAUCOMA that can leave them legally blind. Babies born prematurely can become blind from a disease known as RETINOPATHY OF PREMATURITY that affects the retina (the light-sensitive membrane at the back of the eye). Other causes of blindness in children include BRAIN TUMORS and eye or head injuries.

SIGNS AND SYMPTOMS A newborn or young child who is blind may not be able to focus on an object such as your finger and may not be able to follow it if you move it from side to side. The child's eyes might move in a random or jerky way and he or she may not blink when you move toward the child suddenly. Because so much of a child's development depends on vision, a blind infant may show signs of DEVELOPMENTAL DELAY.

If the child is totally blind, he or she will not be able to perceive light at all and will not close his or her eyes when a strong light is shined into them. Partially blind children may be able to perceive hand movement but may not be able to count fingers placed close to their faces. Children who become blind after they enter school may fall behind in their classes.

DIAGNOSIS A child who has any of the symptoms of blindness should be examined by an ophthalmologist (a doctor who specializes in disorders of the eye). The child will undergo a variety of vision tests—including one called visual evoked responses that measures brain activity stimulated by vision—so the doctor can confirm the diagnosis.

TREATMENT A blind child's treatment will depend on the cause of the blindness. For example, if a brain tumor or cataracts are causing blindness, surgery may be recommended to remove the tumor or the cataracts and improve vision. If a child's blindness cannot be treated, he or she will need special education to learn the skills needed for everyday life.

BLISTERS

A blister is a round, raised area on the skin that is filled with fluid and covered by a thin layer of skin. Blisters form as a protective reaction when blood vessels under the skin are damaged—for example, when a tight shoe rubs against the skin, or from a burn, including SUNBURN. Blisters can also be caused by such conditions as ATOPIC DERMATITIS, or by infections such as IMPETIGO, CHICKENPOX, and COLD SORES. Allergic reactions to plants (POISON IVY) or mites (SCABIES) can also produce small, red blisters. Infants sometimes get sucking blisters on their lips from nursing (see illustration on facing page). Blisters can occur anywhere on your child's body.

SIGNS AND SYMPTOMS Blisters are round or oval fluid-filled areas that develop under the outer layer of skin.

DIAGNOSIS You or your child can usually detect a blister easily and you can treat it yourself. But if your child has many blisters, if they are unusually large or painful, or if your child has a fever or may have developed a blister from using some medication, take your child to see the doctor to determine the cause.

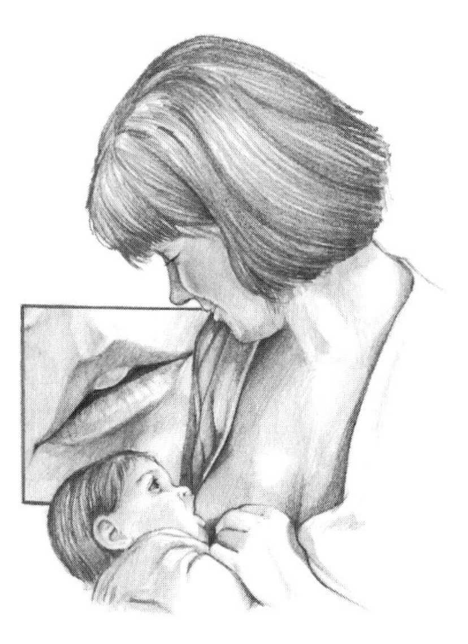

Sucking blisters
When your baby sucks on a bottle or nipple, he or she can get a small, harmless blister on his or her lips. Sucking blisters rarely interfere with feeding. Do not try to pop the blister. If it spreads to other parts of your baby's face or body, call your child's doctor.

TREATMENT Blisters usually heal on their own once the skin underneath the blister heals. It's all right to pop the blister with a sterilized needle, but leave the loose skin to cover the skin below; otherwise, the underlying skin could become infected.

Wash the skin gently (without removing the loose skin) and apply an antiseptic cream or ointment, then cover the area with a bandage to protect it against infection. At night, remove the bandage so the wound can dry and heal. To avoid getting blisters on his or her feet, your child should always wear socks and properly fitting shoes.

Your child's doctor will treat blisters caused by an infection by prescribing medication for the underlying infection.

BLOOD POISONING

See Bacteremia; Septicemia

BOILS

Boils are common, painful bacterial infections of the hair follicle (the small cavity in which hair grows) that are usually caused by staphylococcus bacteria that enter the hair follicle and spread to deeper layers of skin. Boils tend to cluster when the bacteria spread underneath the skin. Clusters of boils are known as carbuncles. Boils and carbuncles can occur in both children and adults and are commonly found on the skin of the face, neck, armpits, breasts, thighs, and buttocks.

SIGNS AND SYMPTOMS Boils appear suddenly as tender, red, solid bumps that enlarge over a 24-hour period by filling with pus. They sometimes itch and cause mild pain. Occasionally the lymph glands near the infection swell up. In rare cases, your child may have a fever. The boils can open up on their own and drain pus onto the surrounding skin. The infection can spread through the bloodstream to other parts of the body. Boils can be extremely painful in the ear canal, nose, or around the rectum.

DIAGNOSIS You will probably be able to recognize a boil on your own. Your child's doctor can diagnose it during a physical examination.

TREATMENT Small boils usually open up, drain, and heal spontaneously on their own in 10 to 20 days. Don't squeeze or lance a boil to drain it because the infection can spread. Instead, cover the boil and the surrounding area with a clean, warm, moist cloth several times a day for 20 minutes to draw the infection to the surface so the boil will open and drain on its own.

Keep the boil and the surrounding skin clean at all times and be especially careful to clean the boil when it is draining. You and your child should wash your hands after touching a boil. Use clean washcloths and towels each time you wash the infected skin and your hands. Over-the-counter antibiotic ointments or creams and antibacterial soaps may help heal the boil.

Call your child's doctor if the boil does not heal within 2 weeks; is painful; looks like it's growing larger; is located in or near your child's nose, ear, or rectum; or is accompanied by a fever. In these cases, it probably requires treatment with oral antibiotics to prevent the infection from spreading to other parts of your child's body. The doctor will open the boil with a needle or scalpel (surgical knife) to drain the pus and alleviate the pain.

BONE CANCER

See Ewing's sarcoma; Osteogenic sarcoma

BOTULISM

Botulism is a rare but potentially life-threatening form of poisoning that is usually caused by eating food contaminated with botulism bacteria. The bacteria, found in incompletely cooked or contaminated foods, produce a *toxin* that can cause paralysis.

The most common form of botulism, infant botulism, affects children less than 1 year old (most frequently infants younger than 6 months old), primarily those who have eaten raw honey. The second most common form is food-borne botulism, found in improperly home-canned vegetables, fruits, or fish, or undercooked sausage and smoked meats. An extremely rare type, known as wound botulism, can occur after an outdoor injury becomes infected by botulism bacteria found in soil.

SIGNS AND SYMPTOMS An infant with botulism initially shows weakness, constipation, dry mouth, and dilated (widened) pupils. Signs of paralysis start in the head and move down the body. The infant has a weak cry, loss of head control, drooping eyelids, drooling, slow eye movement, a slow gag reflex, facial paralysis, and, finally, difficulty moving the arms and legs.

Children with food-borne botulism are nauseated and vomit. They experience blurred vision, difficulty swallowing, weakness in the neck muscles, slurred speech, dry mouth, and sensitivity to light. Eventually, the toxin causes complete paralysis of the arms and legs and the muscles that control breathing. It can be fatal. Symptoms of food-borne botulism usually appear 12 to 36 hours after the child eats contaminated food.

Wound botulism is marked by progressive paralysis beginning in the head, followed by double vision, slurred speech, and dry mouth. Symptoms of wound botulism develop within 4 to 14 days after infection.

DIAGNOSIS If you see any signs of botulism in your infant or child, call your doctor and get the child to a hospital immediately. Do not give the child food or liquids. If possible, take some of the suspected contaminated food with you for testing. The doctor will examine your child and test the child's stool and the suspected food for botulism toxins.

Preventing botulism food poisoning

To prevent your child from getting botulism, take these precautions:

- Never feed your infant honey or put medicines in honey to hide the taste.
- Never feed your infant uncooked or undercooked foods.
- Don't feed your family preserved foods if the can bulges, the lid leaks, or the food smells bad.
- If you preserve food at home, sterilize it by cooking the food in a pressure cooker at 250°F (120°C) for 30 minutes to kill the bacteria. Boiling food for 10 minutes also destroys the toxin.
- Call the health department if you suspect your child has gotten botulism food poisoning from a restaurant or food store. Be alert for warnings in the news about poisonings in certain foods.
- For information about safe food canning, call your local cooperative extension service, or the Consumer Nutrition Hotline of the American Dietetic Association (800-366-1655).

B

TREATMENT In the hospital, an infant with botulism may require intensive care and be put on a ventilator to help him or her breathe. A child with botulism is usually hospitalized and may also require intensive care. The child may receive antibiotics and an *antitoxin*. Botulism antitoxins prevent the condition from getting worse but can cause serious side effects, such as shock (see page 678). They are not useful in treating infants with botulism.

Recovery can take weeks because the body needs time to rid itself of and heal the damage from the toxin. With prompt treatment, the outlook for survival is good, but the child may have long-term muscle or heart damage.

BRAIN TUMOR

A brain tumor is an abnormal growth in the brain. Brain tumors that do not spread are known as benign tumors. Doctors define a brain tumor that is cancerous as being malignant (able to invade and destroy surrounding tissue and spread to other parts of the body). Brain cancer is the second most common cancer of childhood, after LEUKEMIA.

Both malignant and benign brain tumors occur most frequently in children between the ages of 3 and 12. Childhood brain tumors can occur anywhere in the brain. As a tumor grows, it puts pressure on the brain inside the confined space of the skull and interferes with the child's normal physical and mental functions. The cause of brain tumors remains unknown.

Tumors that first appear in the brain are known as primary brain tumors. Tumors that spread to the brain from other parts of the body are called secondary brain tumors.

SIGNS AND SYMPTOMS The symptoms of brain tumor can vary according to the location and size of the tumor, but the most frequent symptoms are HEADACHES that are most severe in the morning or when your child is lying down, nausea, sudden or persistent vomiting, loss of feeling or weakness in your child's arms or legs on either or both sides of the body, or dizziness. Changes in coordination, personality, or development and seizures can also occur. Abnormal eye movements, changes in speech and vision, loss of the sense of smell, and excessive drowsiness are additional signs of a brain tumor.

DIAGNOSIS Take your child to the doctor immediately if he or she shows any of the symptoms described above because the outlook is better if the tumor is diagnosed and treated early, before it grows very large.

Your child's doctor will do a thorough physical examination, checking your child's mental alertness, physical reflexes, coordination, muscle strength, and response to pain. The doctor will use an ophthalmoscope (an instrument with a lighted end) to look for swollen blood vessels in your child's retina (the light-sensitive lining at the back of the eye) that could be caused by pressure from a tumor. Your doctor may also request *computed tomography* or *magnetic resonance imaging* of your child's brain.

Other tests that your doctor may request include an X-ray of the skull to look for any changes; an electroencephalogram, a painless procedure that records electrical impulses in the brain to detect any seizure activity; or a *lumbar puncture*, in which a needle is inserted into the spine to sample your child's spinal fluid for tumor cells. Your doctor may also take X-rays of other parts of your child's body, such as the chest, to check for cancers that might have originated there and then spread to the brain.

TREATMENT Initially, your child may be given *corticosteroids* to reduce swelling of the brain tissue caused by the tumor. He or she may also receive anticonvulsant drugs to control seizures and pain relievers to treat severe headaches. Both benign and malignant brain tumors need to be removed surgically to relieve pressure on the brain. Your child's brain tumor may be treated with *radiation* or *chemotherapy*, either alone or in combination. Your child may be given chemotherapy in pill form or injected into a vein or muscle.

Both radiation and chemotherapy produce unpleasant side effects. Radiation causes fatigue, nausea, vomiting, and hair loss. Because chemotherapy attacks all rapidly dividing cells in the body, not just cancerous ones, it can affect the bone marrow, lining of the intestines, and hair follicles, causing hair loss.

BRONCHIOLITIS

Bronchiolitis is a common infection of the bronchioles, tiny breathing passages inside the lungs. It is usually caused by a virus, most commonly one known as respiratory syncytial virus. Bronchiolitis most often occurs in infants and children under 2 years of age, with a peak occurrence at about 6 months. The virus that causes bronchiolitis infects children most frequently in winter and early spring. It can be spread when an infected person coughs or sneezes the virus into the air or onto a child's toys. The child touches the toy and then transfers the virus to his or her eyes or nose.

SIGNS AND SYMPTOMS Bronchiolitis usually begins with cold symptoms, such as sneezing, a stuffy or runny nose, and a mild cough, for a day or two. The child may also have a fever up to 103°F. The infection causes the bronchioles to swell and fill with mucus, making breathing difficult. The child wheezes (see REACTIVE AIRWAY DISEASE) and breathes rapidly, taking shallow breaths 60 to 80 times a minute and drawing in the neck and chest with each breath. A rapid heartbeat may also occur. Most children have mild symptoms that last only a few days. With a more severe infection, the child may get worse quickly and not be able to get enough air into the lungs despite labored breathing. The skin around the mouth or nails can turn blue from lack of oxygen and the child can become dehydrated (see page 283) because he or she cannot eat or drink.

DIAGNOSIS AND TREATMENT If your infant or child has symptoms of bronchiolitis, he or she should see the doctor, who may take a sample of your child's nasal secretions and check for the presence of respiratory syncytial virus. He or she may also order blood tests and X-rays of your child's lungs.

Antibiotics do not work against this disease (unless your child also develops a bacterial infection) because it is caused by a virus, against which antibiotics are ineffective. Your child's doctor may prescribe a bronchodilator to control wheezing and will advise you to put a cool-mist vaporizer or humidifier in your child's room to keep his or her air passages moist and clear. To avoid accumulation of bacteria in the appliance, clean it daily. Your child needs to drink plenty of fluids. Give your child acetaminophen (not aspirin) to relieve fever and pain. If the symptoms become severe, your child may need to be hospitalized for more aggressive care and oxygen treatment.

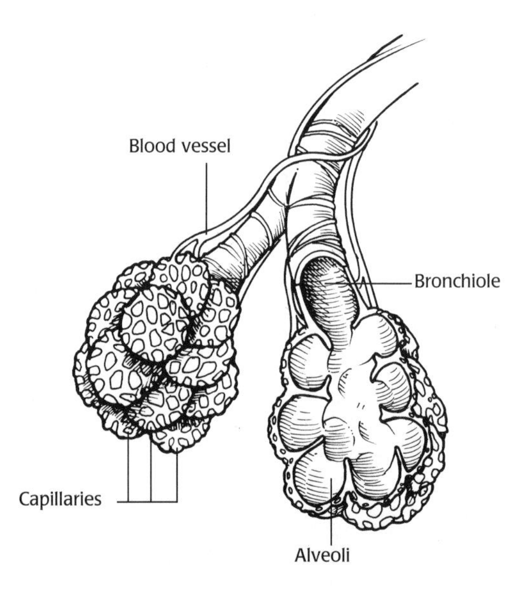

Bronchiolitis

Bronchiolitis affects the tiny airways, called bronchioles, in the lungs that end in microscopic air sacs known as alveoli. The air that your child inhales enters the alveoli and the carbon dioxide in his or her blood is exchanged for inhaled oxygen. Minute blood vessels known as capillaries carry the blood to the walls of the alveoli.

B

BRONCHITIS

Bronchitis is an inflammation of the bronchi, the air passages that connect the lungs to the trachea (windpipe). In children, acute bronchitis, which begins suddenly and lasts a short time, may begin as a runny nose and develop into a dry persistent cough over 3 to 4 days. It usually clears up in 10 to 14 days. Chronic bronchitis, which lasts at least 3 months and recurs over a 3-year period or more, is a disorder seen mostly in adults. The inflammation can be triggered by a viral infection–such as a cold or influenza that spreads to the child's air passages–or by air pollution, especially cigarette smoke. Children with bronchitis commonly get a bacterial infection along with it.

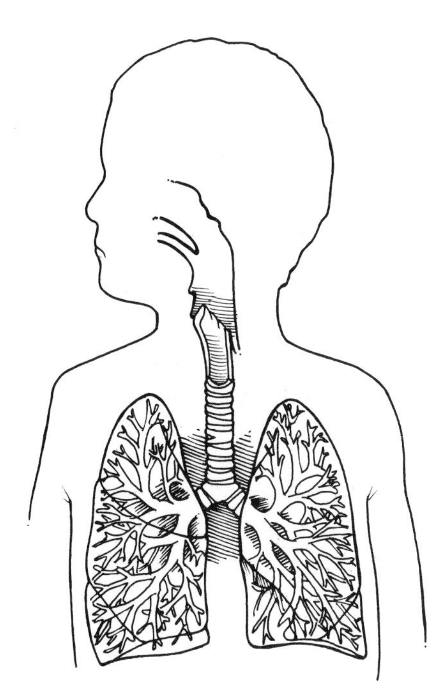

Normal bronchial tree

A child's bronchial tree is a branching network of airways that get successively smaller until they reach microscopic air sacs, known as alveoli, in the lungs. In a child with bronchitis, the airways become inflamed and congested with mucus.

SIGNS AND SYMPTOMS The bronchi become swollen, congested, and filled with mucus. Children with acute bronchitis wheeze (see REACTIVE AIRWAY DISEASE), have difficulty breathing, and have a cough that initially is dry but later may produce yellow or green sputum (phlegm). The child may also have a fever of less than 101°F and chest pain. The symptoms usually clear up in a few days. Children with chronic bronchitis have similar symptoms that persist for a long time but they usually do not have a fever. Acute and chronic bronchitis can lead to complications, such as PNEUMONIA and pleurisy (inflammation of the lining of the child's lungs).

DIAGNOSIS AND TREATMENT The doctor will do a thorough physical examination and will ask how your child's symptoms progressed. He or she may order blood tests, chest X-rays, sputum *cultures*, and lung-function tests to confirm the diagnosis of bronchitis. Your child's doctor may prescribe bronchodilators (drugs that open up the bronchi) to be taken by mouth or in inhaler form. He or she may also prescribe antibiotics for bacterial infections, expectorants to thin out your child's phlegm, and cough suppressants. At home, you can put a cool-mist vaporizer or humidifier in your child's room to keep your child's breathing passages moist and clear. Clean the appliance daily to avoid a buildup of bacteria. Don't expose your child to cigarette smoke, and minimize exposure to other air pollutants, such as dust or chemical fumes, as much as possible.

BRONCHOPULMONARY DYSPLASIA

Bronchopulmonary dysplasia is a chronic lung disorder caused by prolonged oxygen therapy and long-term breathing assistance with a ventilator in infants who are being treated for such conditions as RESPIRATORY DISTRESS SYNDROME or congenital heart disease (see HEART DISEASE, CONGENITAL).

Both the long exposure to high concentrations of oxygen and the high pressure of the ventilator damage the child's airways and lungs. Premature infants are more prone to develop the disorder.

Signs and symptoms The affected infant's breathing is rapid and labored and he or she may wheeze or make other noises when breathing. The child has frequent lung infections and his or her skin may turn blue. The infant may also experience a delay in growth and have difficulty feeding. He or she usually needs extra oxygen to breathe.

Diagnosis and treatment The doctor can diagnose bronchopulmonary dysplasia with a chest X-ray and by asking you questions about your child's condition. Your infant will require oxygen therapy with a ventilator to keep his or her damaged lungs inflated, although the level of oxygen and the amount of pressure the child receives will be slowly reduced as he or she gets better. Once removed from the ventilator, your child may be given oxygen through a removable mask or small tube placed in the nose for several weeks or months. Your infant can be fed by mouth or through tubes placed into the stomach through the nose or directly into the stomach through the abdominal wall. The child may also receive medication to open his or her airways and prevent fluid from building up in his or her lungs. Your infant's condition should improve gradually over time, although he or she may wheeze or have difficulty breathing during a respiratory infection or physical activity for many years.

Bruises

Bruises are discolored spots under a child's skin caused by injured blood vessels that leak blood into the surrounding tissue. The child's blood vessels may be damaged from an injury or a disease. Bruises are common among children, who often bump into things during play and sports. Most bruises are harmless. However, if bruises appear spontaneously on a child's skin for no apparent reason, if they fail to disappear within 2 weeks, or if they become large following a minor injury, they can signal an infection or underlying disease, such as HEMOPHILIA or other BLEEDING DISORDERS, aplastic anemia (see ANEMIA, APLASTIC), or LEUKEMIA.

Signs and symptoms Bruises change color as they heal. When they first appear, they are purple-red. In 1 to 4 days, they turn dark blue to brown. In 5 to 7 days, they become greenish-yellow. After 7 days, they turn yellow and begin to fade. A bruise can be either flat or slightly raised and may or may not be tender or painful. Sometimes bruises do not fade away in a week or two. They may even get bigger if the body's natural defenses seal off the blood to form a hematoma (a pool of blood or blood clot).

Diagnosis and treatment In most cases, bruises disappear on their own. If your child has a painful bruise, place an ice pack or a towel filled with ice directly on the bruise for about 30 minutes to ease the pain and minimize the bruising. Have your child raise his or her bruised limb above the level of the heart so that less blood will flow to the area.

If the bruise lasts more than a couple of weeks, seems unusually large, or has no apparent cause, take your child to the doctor. The doctor may order blood tests and any additional examinations needed to diagnose the problem. If your child has bruises that are severe or an unusual shape, or if they are in an unusual location such as the genital area, the doctor will probably ask about the possibility of physical abuse.

Bulimia

Bulimia is an eating disorder marked by episodes of secret binge eating followed by either self-induced vomiting or the ingestion of large amounts of laxatives or diuretics (drugs that cause the body to lose water) to lose weight.

Some children with bulimia also exercise excessively. Bulimia is more common than ANOREXIA NERVOSA, another eating disorder, but the two often overlap; an anorectic can have bulimic episodes. Bulimia typically begins in adolescents who have tried dieting. They discover that vomiting, laxatives, diuretics, or inordinate amounts of exercise help them control their weight. The bingeing and purging episodes can occur twice a week or more. Episodes of binge eating may be triggered by DEPRESSION, boredom, ANXIETY, or loneliness, or by an upsetting event. Bulimics are usually so preoccupied with food that the disorder interferes with their social and academic life. They may act impulsively and even shoplift, abuse alcohol or other drugs, or become sexually promiscuous.

Ninety percent of bulimics are female adolescents or college-age women; the balance are teenage boys. Adolescents at greatest risk are those with a family history of eating disorders or DRUG AND ALCOHOL ABUSE or sexually abused teens (see page 326). Those who think that they have to be exceptionally underweight to be a model, dancer, or actor are also at risk.

SIGNS AND SYMPTOMS Many bulimics appear to be healthy and are able to hide their illness for years. Their weight may vary, but they do not usually experience extreme weight loss. When physical symptoms occur, they generally stem from the vomiting. The first physical sign may be a scrape mark or scar on the back of the adolescent's hand, from sticking the hand in the mouth to induce vomiting. Repeated vomiting can weaken the enamel on the teeth and cause frequent cavities, tooth discoloration, and sensitivity to hot and cold liquids or food.

A bulimic adolescent may also have frequent HEADACHES, weakness, muscle cramps, or irregular or absent menstrual periods (see MENSTRUAL DISORDERS); urinate often; and be extremely thirsty. Overuse of laxatives can cause severe diarrhea or blood in the stool. Vomiting can cause the salivary glands in the adolescent's cheeks to become sore and swollen. Vomiting can also produce open sores in the back of the throat. Vomiting, excessive exercise, and overuse of diuretics and laxatives can cause life-threatening dehydration (see page 283) marked by rapid breathing, a fast heartbeat, confusion, dizziness, and eventually unconsciousness. Overuse of syrup of ipecac, an over-the-counter drug used to induce vomiting, can damage the heart and potentially even cause sudden death.

DIAGNOSIS Your child's doctor will do a thorough physical examination and will ask your child about his or her eating habits to try and detect any unreasonable concern with body image or weight. The doctor will also examine your adolescent's teeth and mouth to look for physical signs of the disorder. He or she will order blood tests to rule out other diseases that can cause similar signs and symptoms.

TREATMENT The aim of treatment is to change your child's binge-purge cycle of behavior and underlying psychological issues. Your adolescent may need to be hospitalized for several weeks if his or her behavior is out of control and the medical complications are severe. While hospitalized, he or she might have to receive food and liquid through a feeding tube. Whether or not your child is hospitalized, he or she will need psychological counseling to improve his or her self-image and identify the underlying feelings that are causing the bulimia. Nutritional counseling teaches your child healthy ways to manage his or her weight. Group therapy, family therapy, and support groups can also help. Your child's doctor may prescribe antidepressant drugs. Recovery can be slow and your child may relapse weeks or months after initial treatment, but the outlook is good. With treatment, the majority of people with bulimia recover from their disorder.

BUNIONS

See Calluses, corns, and bunions

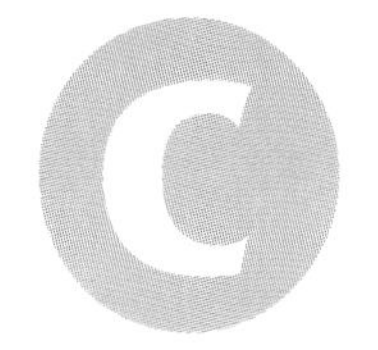

CALLUSES, CORNS, AND BUNIONS

The most common childhood foot problems are calluses, corns, and bunions. A callus is a thickened layer of skin that develops on the hands or feet. A corn is a thickened layer of skin that develops on a toe. Both are caused by repeated pressure or friction against the skin. A bunion develops when the fluid-filled pad known as a bursa that covers the joint at the base of the big toe becomes firm. This joint projects outward and the big toe turns inward. The bunion can become very painful when it repeatedly rubs against the inside of the child's shoe. The joint deformity itself may develop from pressure on the joint from tightly fitting shoes.

SIGNS AND SYMPTOMS Calluses and corns are hard, small, raised areas of skin that are usually round or oval. They may or may not be painful. A soft corn can develop on a child's toe in areas where perspiration and moisture collect. A bunion sometimes becomes inflamed and painful from irritation from tightly fitting shoes.

DIAGNOSIS AND TREATMENT Calluses and corns usually go away on their own if the source of pressure or friction is removed. For example, if your child's callus or corn developed because of poorly fitting shoes, give your child another pair of shoes that fit better and the callus or corn will disappear in a few weeks. Place an over-the-counter corn or callus pad on the hardened skin until the thickening goes away. Do not try to cut away the thickened skin; this may cause infection.

If you think that your child has a bunion, take the child to his or her doctor. The doctor will examine your child's toe and may take X-rays of his or her foot. If the bunion is small and in the early stages of development, the doctor will recommend that you buy your child wider shoes and tell you to apply pads to the bunion to protect the area. He or she may also recommend a special shoe insert or pad that will help prevent the deformity from getting worse. If the bunion gets bigger and causes severe pain, the doctor may recommend surgery.

CANCER

Normal cells in the body divide and produce new cells continually throughout life to replace old, dying cells. Cancer develops when cells that are abnormal in structure form and grow at an uncontrollable rate, producing a mass of tissue known as a tumor.

Although cancer is rare in children, about 10,000 children are diagnosed with cancer every

Most Common Cancers in Children

Cancer is rare in children, but the types of cancer that most often occur in children differ from those that occur in adults. The chart below shows the number of newly diagnosed cases of cancer per 100,000 children each year.

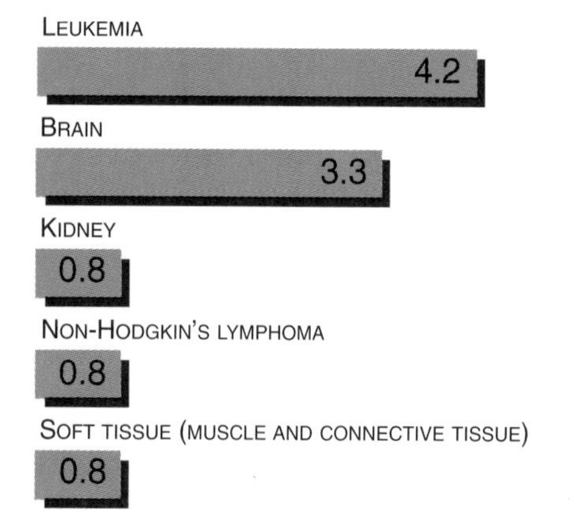

year in the United States. While cancers in adults frequently may be affected by environmental or lifestyle factors, such as smoking, cancers in children are not believed to be affected by the environment.

Children also tend to get different types of cancer than adults (see chart on page 444). The most common cancers in children are LEUKEMIA and LYMPHOMA, which affect a child's blood and lymphatic system; BRAIN TUMORS and NEUROBLASTOMA, which strike a child's brain and nervous system; WILMS' TUMOR, a cancer of the kidney; OSTEOGENIC SARCOMA, EWING'S SARCOMA, and RHABDOMYOSARCOMA, which attack bones or muscles; RETINOBLASTOMA, a cancer of the eye; and testicular cancer, which affects the testicles of young men over 14 years of age.

Cancer cells are malignant, meaning that they can invade and destroy surrounding tissue and organs. They can also break away from a tumor and spread to other parts of the body through the bloodstream or lymphatic system (part of the immune system). A malignant tumor that develops in one part of a child's body, such as the bone, is called the primary tumor. When cancer cells from the primary tumor spread to another part of the child's body to form new tumors, the new tumors are called secondary tumors.

What is cancer remission?

Remission is a temporary suspension of the symptoms of cancer and a return to good health during or after treatment, while a cure is a permanent halt to symptoms for at least 5 years after treatment. Doctors distinguish between two different kinds of remission:

- A complete remission is a complete stopping of the disease process. All the symptoms disappear, test findings return to normal, and the abnormal tumor cells are no longer detectable in your child's body. Even with a complete remission, your child will still need chemotherapy for months or even years after the remission occurs to prevent the cancer from recurring. For example, a child with leukemia must undergo chemotherapy for 2 to 3½ years after remission; a child with Wilms' tumor needs chemotherapy for up to 2 years.
- A partial remission is a partial stopping of the disease process. Some or most of the symptoms disappear, but your child still needs more cancer treatment.

SIGNS AND SYMPTOMS Different cancers can cause different symptoms, but some of the more common symptoms of cancer generally include a noticeable and sometimes painful lump in a child's arm or leg, lymph gland, or abdomen; frequent infections; a general feeling of tiredness; loss of appetite; weight loss; chronic fever; diarrhea; constipation; a constant cough or hoarseness; difficulty swallowing; HEADACHES; or easy bruising. But some types of cancer have no symptoms at all until they reach an advanced stage of development.

Many of these symptoms can indicate other diseases as well, but if you see that your child has any of these symptoms for longer than a week, take him or her to the doctor for a proper diagnosis. Make sure your child gets regular checkups so your doctor can detect any signs of disease in the early stages.

DIAGNOSIS A *biopsy* of any abnormal tissue is routine in cancer diagnosis. Blood and urine tests and X-rays can show the extent of the cancer's spread. Your doctor may also order laboratory tests of other body fluids for specific types of cancer.

If your doctor suspects your child has a certain type of cancer, he or she will refer your child to a cancer specialist (oncologist) for further evaluation. The specialist might use a number of the following diagnostic imaging techniques (examinations that take pictures of the inside of your child's body) to confirm the diagnosis:

- X-rays, the most common imaging exams, are taken by a machine that passes invisible electromagnetic waves through a specific area of your child's body and records the image onto film.
- *Computed tomography* (CT) combines an X-ray machine with a computer to produce a series of

Common side effects of cancer treatment

If your child is being treated for cancer, he or she may experience side effects from the treatment. Long-term side effects depend on the treatment method used, the location and severity of the cancer, and the age of your child. Ask your doctor exactly what kind of short-term and long-term effects your child can expect from the specific treatment used to manage his or her condition. Here are some of the common temporary side effects of various treatments:

- **Surgery** Your child will probably be in pain after any type of surgery, but he or she will receive medication to control it. The amount of time it takes your child to recover from surgery will depend on the surgery itself and on how sick your child is.
- **Radiation therapy** During therapy, your child may feel tired, lose his or her appetite, experience nausea or vomiting, have superficial skin burns, and lose hair where the radiation was applied. He or she might also get more infections than usual because radiation destroys white blood cells needed to fight infection. Radiation treatment does not hurt while your child is undergoing it.
- **Chemotherapy** Cancer cells replicate rapidly so the drugs used in chemotherapy are designed to kill cells that multiply quickly. But chemotherapy can also kill rapidly duplicating normal cells, such as the hair follicles, white blood cells, and cells in the intestine. The side effects of chemotherapy depend on the specific drugs used but, during treatment, your child may have no energy, develop anemia, have more infections than usual, bruise or bleed easily, lose his or her appetite, experience nausea and vomiting, and have sores in his or her mouth. The potential for nerve and organ damage also exists.
- **Biological therapy** Your child may develop symptoms of the flu (see page 231). He or she may also have red or purple spots on the skin and bruise easily. These effects usually disappear gradually after treatment ends.

These cancer therapies place a lot of physical stress on your child's body. To keep up your child's strength during treatment, proper nutrition is important, but a child undergoing radiation therapy or chemotherapy often loses his or her appetite. Ask your doctor or a dietitian for advice about ways you can ensure that your child consumes an adequate amount of food during his or her cancer treatment.

images of your child's body on a computer screen. CT scanning minimizes your child's exposure to *radiation*.

- *Radionuclide scans* measure radioactivity levels in targeted organs after your child is given a mildly radioactive substance by mouth or injection. Radiation exposure is low and can be less than that of a routine X-ray test.
- *Ultrasound* uses sound waves to create an image of organs inside your child's body.
- *Magnetic resonance imaging* (MRI) links a powerful magnet with a computer to make detailed cross-sectional images of your child's body without X-rays or other radiation.

Doctors use these imaging devices to find out how far the cancer has progressed.

TREATMENT Your child's treatment will depend on the type of cancer and how far it has progressed. Your child might have to have surgery to remove the tumor, or radiation, *chemotherapy*, biological therapy, or bone-marrow transplantation to combat the cancer:

- Radiation therapy focuses high-energy X-rays on the tumor or cancer cells to destroy them.
- Chemotherapy uses powerful drugs to kill cancer cells throughout a child's body.
- Biological therapy employs substances, such as interferon and interleukin, grown from human cells, to stimulate the body's natural defense system against infection and disease.
- Bone marrow transplantation uses bone marrow donated from a family member or unrelated person to replace a child's diseased bone marrow after he or she receives very strong doses of chemotherapy that destroy the child's own bone marrow.

Find out all you can from your child's doctor about how your child's specific treatment will be done and if you or your child need to follow any special measures, such as dietary restrictions, at home. All of these treatments represent powerful ways to fight childhood cancer, but they can also damage normal cells and tissues in your child's body and cause a number of unwanted side effects (see box on facing page). You will need to prepare yourself and your child for the discomforts caused by these side effects during the therapy period.

CANKER SORES

Canker sores are painful ulcers or open sores inside the mouth and on the lips. They can occur in children of any age, but most often first appear in children 10 years of age and older. The exact cause of canker sores is unknown, but they are believed to result from aggressive tooth and gum brushing, biting the inside of the mouth, emotional or physical stress, not getting enough vitamins and iron in the diet, dental work that injures the inside of the mouth, menstrual periods, changes in body hormones, or infection, especially with a virus.

SIGNS AND SYMPTOMS The first sign of a canker sore is a burning or tingling sensation on the lips, tongue, inside of the cheeks, back of the roof of the mouth, or gums. Then a small, red spot appears that opens into a sore. The sore turns white or yellow and becomes surrounded by a red halo. A canker sore can be quite painful, but the pain usually diminishes in 3 or 4 days. The pain may make it hard for your child to eat or drink some things. There may be only one or two sores in the child's mouth or a cluster of three or more. Sometimes the sores become covered by a thin, gray membrane just before healing. They usually heal on their own in 10 days to 2 weeks, but often return.

DIAGNOSIS AND TREATMENT If your child has canker sores, you will be able to recognize them by their appearance. You don't need to take your child to the doctor, but, if the sores get worse instead of better or last longer than 2 weeks, call the doctor. You should also call the doctor if the sores come back more than two or three times a year.

The sores should disappear within a couple of weeks without treatment. You can prepare a soothing mouthwash for your child by mixing a half teaspoon of salt in an 8-ounce glass of water. Have your child rinse with the wash three or four times a day. Tell him or her to avoid foods or drinks that could irritate the sores. Make sure your child brushes and flosses his or her teeth daily and gets regular dental cleanings to prevent mouth infections.

CARDIOMYOPATHY

Cardiomyopathy is a heart condition in which the heart muscle is weakened so badly that it cannot pump blood efficiently. Eventually, the condition can result in heart failure. The disease may be inherited and present at birth or it can develop later in life. In children, cardiomyopathy can be caused by viral or bacterial infections, a deficiency of certain vitamins or minerals, severe forms of MUSCULAR DYSTROPHY, RHEUMATIC FEVER, JUVENILE RHEUMATOID ARTHRITIS, LUPUS, severe anemia, or some genetic diseases. Sometimes the cause is unknown.

SIGNS AND SYMPTOMS The symptoms of the disease can be mild or severe. Cardiomyopathy can affect only a small part of a child's heart muscle or the entire heart. If the disease is mild and affects only part of the heart, the child may have no symptoms or only mild chest pain and a rapid heartbeat (see ARRHYTHMIAS). Extensive cardiomyopathy can cause congestive heart failure (see HEART FAILURE, CONGESTIVE), which is marked by a fast or irregular heartbeat, fatigue, breathing difficulties, swollen feet or ankles, a loss of appetite, lethargy, listlessness, irritability, grunting, and a persistent cough that sometimes produces bloody fluid from the lungs. Babies born with severe cardiomyopathy or children who develop cardiomyopathy later in life can die suddenly. Children who have this condition sometimes also develop an enlarged heart.

DIAGNOSIS If your child has symptoms of cardiomyopathy, the doctor will measure the electrical activity in his or her heart with an *electrocardiogram*. The doctor may also order an *ultrasound* of the heart, known as an *echocardiogram*, or X-rays of your child's heart and lungs.

TREATMENT If an underlying condition is causing your child's cardiomyopathy, the doctor will treat the condition. Otherwise, your child's doctor will treat the specific signs and symptoms of cardiomyopathy with drugs or other measures. Your child may need to be hospitalized for a few days for supportive care. In rare cases, if the disease is severe and cannot be treated successfully, your child may need a heart transplant.

CAT-SCRATCH FEVER

Cat-scratch fever is a relatively mild bacterial infection marked by swelling of the lymph nodes or glands (ADENITIS) near the site of a scratch from a cat. Kittens are more likely to transmit the disease than older cats.

SIGNS AND SYMPTOMS The lymph glands near the scratch become swollen and tender about 10 days after the scratch occurs and may stay swollen for months. Because children are often scratched on the arm or hand while playing with a kitten, the lymph glands in the armpits or just above the elbow are most likely to be affected. You may also notice a small pimple on the skin at the site of the scratch. Only about a third of infected children actually have a fever. Less common symptoms include loss of appetite and headache. Occasionally, the infected glands enlarge and begin to drain pus through an opening in the skin. In rare cases, a brain infection (ENCEPHALITIS) can develop.

DIAGNOSIS If your child has swollen lymph glands and has recently been scratched by a cat, he or she probably has cat-scratch fever. Your doctor will do a physical examination and will confirm the diagnosis by obtaining a positive skin test for the bacterium that causes the disorder. Sometimes a blood test or *biopsy* is done to identify the bacterium.

TREATMENT Most children recover fully in a few weeks or months without treatment. You can apply hot, wet cloths to the swollen lymph glands for 20 minutes three times a day to reduce tenderness and speed healing. Glands that are filled with pus may need to be drained with a needle by a surgeon. In rare cases, doctors treat the disease with antibiotics.

CELIAC DISEASE

Celiac disease is a digestive disorder in which a child has an allergy to gluten, a protein found in foods that contain wheat, rye, oats, and barley. The disease prevents the child's small intestine from absorbing certain nutrients needed for normal growth and development. Children with a family history of this disease are at increased risk of having the disorder.

SIGNS AND SYMPTOMS Symptoms develop as soon as the infant or child begins to eat foods containing gluten. He or she may look tired and pale, seem irritable, have a decreased or increased appetite, and get colds or the flu (see page 231) often. The infant may have a swollen abdomen and abdominal pain from excessive gas. He or she may have severe diarrhea or large, pale, foul-smelling stools. The inability to absorb nutrients causes weight loss, iron-deficiency anemia (see ANEMIA, IRON-DEFICIENCY), vitamin deficiency, and eventual stunting of growth. The diarrhea can lead to dehydration (see page 283) and serious illness. Symptoms continue as long as the child eats foods containing gluten.

DIAGNOSIS If your infant or child has symptoms of celiac disease, the doctor will order laboratory tests of your child's blood and stool. A diagnosis can be made by intestinal *biopsy.* If the child's condition improves after he or she begins consuming a gluten-free diet and gets worse with the reintroduction of gluten, the diagnosis will be confirmed.

TREATMENT The only way to treat celiac disease is to eliminate all foods that contain gluten from your child's diet, usually for life. Gluten is found in a wide variety of foods so you will need to consult with a dietitian to plan your child's diet. A broad range of gluten-free breads and other foods are available on the market. The child's symptoms will start to clear up within a few weeks of starting a gluten-free diet.

CEREBRAL PALSY

Cerebral palsy is a disorder of the nerves and muscles caused by damage to the motor (muscular movement) centers in the brain. Damage to the brain can arise from a lack of oxygen to the fetus during pregnancy, infection such as MENINGITIS, head injury, lead or other poisoning, malformation of the brain, CHROMOSOMAL ABNORMALITIES, substance abuse by the mother during pregnancy, premature birth, or low birthweight. The cause is unknown in half of all cases. Cerebral palsy is a lifelong disease, but it does not get worse as a child gets older.

SIGNS AND SYMPTOMS Children with cerebral palsy have problems controlling and coordinating their movements. Signs and symptoms can range from minimal to severe. An early sign in infancy is difficulty in breast- or bottle-feeding because the child lacks the muscle tone needed to suck properly. The growing child may have trouble sitting, crawling, walking, or forming speech sounds. Many infant reflexes (see page 38), which normally disappear by 3 to 4 months of age, linger in children with cerebral palsy, interfering with motor development. Many children with cerebral palsy develop unusual body postures from muscle stiffness and spasms in their arms and legs. They also may exhibit involuntary writhing motions, purposeless mouth and tongue movements, uncontrollable hand twisting and turning, and facial contortions. Seizures and deficits in hearing, vision, and speech sometimes afflict children with cerebral palsy. Many have a learning disability (see page 551) despite normal intelligence. About half of all children with cerebral palsy have some degree of MENTAL RETARDATION.

Children with cerebral palsy have high energy requirements because of their spastic, uncontrolled movements. A poor ability to suck or feed and high nutritional needs may lead to FAILURE TO THRIVE in children with cerebral palsy.

DIAGNOSIS If your child has any risk factors for cerebral palsy, your child's doctor will monitor him or her for proper muscle tone and reflexes at each office visit. The doctor will also check to make sure that your child has met the developmental milestones, such as crawling or walking, that are appropriate for his or her age. The doctor will be able to diagnose cerebral palsy through a physical examination and by talking with you about the child's development and ability to coordinate his or her movements. Blood and other laboratory tests, chromosomal testing, and *computed tomography* or *magnetic resonance imaging* may be able to help the doctor find out the cause of your child's cerebral palsy.

TREATMENT Children with cerebral palsy cannot be cured but they can improve their skills with special education, physical and occupational

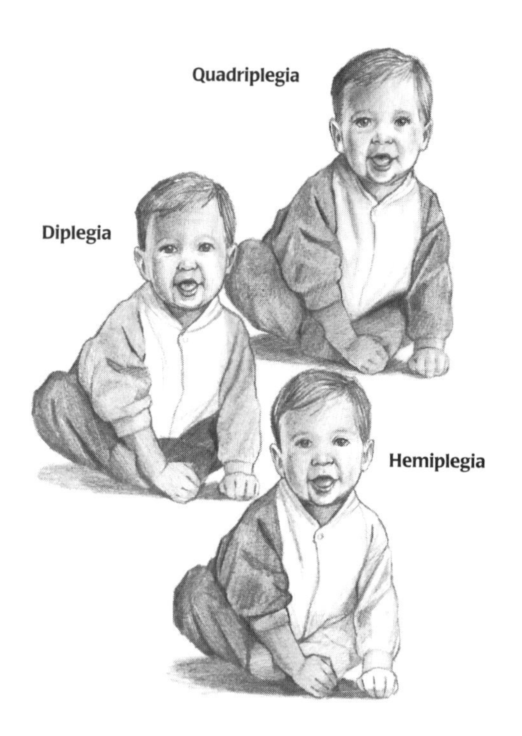

Three types of muscle weakness
Children with cerebral palsy cannot control their muscles to varying degrees and display spastic, uncoordinated movements. They can be affected in one of three ways. In a child who has quadriplegia (top), all four limbs are equally affected. A child with diaplegia (center) also has four affected limbs, but the legs are more affected than the arms. If a child has hemiplegia (bottom), he or she can control the arm and leg on one side of the body only. The other side is affected by cerebral palsy.

therapy, speech therapy, psychotherapy, and social services. Treating impairments in hearing, vision, and speech maximizes your child's ability to learn. Some affected children benefit from surgery to correct bone and joint deformities. Braces or wheelchairs can help support affected limbs and prevent involuntary movements. Doctors sometimes prescribe medications to control spastic movement. Some children who have cerebral palsy need tube feeding to maintain proper nutrition.

Many children with cerebral palsy live at home under the care of a loving, supportive family. Severely affected children often need care in an extended care facility. Ask your doctor or a social worker at your local hospital for the names of support groups or organizations that can give you information and guidance about caring for a child with cerebral palsy.

CHEST DEFORMITIES

Two common chest deformities occur in childhood—funnel chest, or pectus excavatum, and pigeon breast, or pectus carinatum. Both involve an abnormal formation of the sternum (breastbone) and rib cage. These chest deformities affect boys more often than girls, and they tend to run in families. For the most part, funnel chest and pigeon breast are cosmetic problems that have no serious effects on the child's health. As they get older, boys can develop muscles in the chest and girls develop breasts that help hide the deformities. Severe deformities can affect the child's self-image, and, in rare cases, they can also cause serious health problems.

TYPES OF CHEST DEFORMITIES The two types of chest deformities commonly occurring in childhood are funnel chest and pigeon breast.

Funnel chest A child with funnel chest has a sunken or caved-in chest because the distance between his or her breastbone and spine is abnormally short. Funnel chest is usually present at birth and is thought to develop while the fetus is in the mother's uterus. It has been linked to a CHROMOSOMAL ABNORMALITY known as TURNER'S SYNDROME. Funnel chest can also develop after birth in children with a GENETIC DISORDER known as MARFAN SYNDROME. It rarely causes any other health problems, but severe funnel chest in infants can cause frequent colds or PNEUMONIA. Children and adolescents with severe funnel chest may have breathing difficulty, chest pain, and frequent chest or respiratory infections. They may also have rounded shoulders, an abnormally curved or abnormally straight spine, and a potbelly.

Pigeon breast A child with pigeon breast has a breastbone that looks pushed out because the distance between his or her breastbone and spine is abnormally long. Pigeon breast usually develops in early adolescence (from 11 to 14 years old) in boys and somewhat earlier in girls. Pigeon breast can cause occasional tenderness and pain in the chest and sometimes emphysema, a lung disease that can produce shortness of breath and lead to respiratory or heart failure (see HEART FAILURE, CONGESTIVE).

DIAGNOSIS AND TREATMENT The doctor can diagnose chest deformities in your child during a physical examination. A chest X-ray, an *electrocardiogram*, and an *echocardiogram* may be needed to check for a serious problem caused by the deformity if your child is having chest pain or respiratory difficulty or if he or she cannot tolerate exercise. No treatment is necessary unless your child is embarrassed by his or her appearance or has severe health problems from the chest deformity. In such cases, cosmetic surgery to reposition the breastbone can improve the deformity and treat any health problems. Your child will need to be hospitalized for the surgery and may have to wear a chest brace for 6 to 8 weeks after surgery.

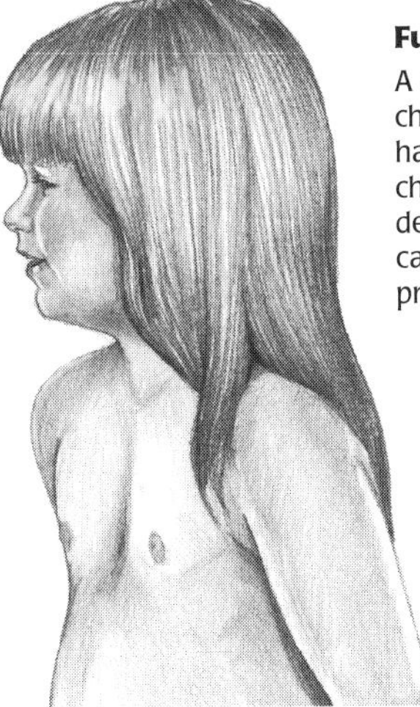

Funnel chest
A child with funnel chest appears to have a sunken chest. The mild deformity rarely causes any health problems.

CHICKENPOX

Chickenpox is a common, highly contagious childhood disease caused by a virus. Most children get chickenpox by the time they reach the age of 10 years. Since 1995, a vaccine has been available that can prevent the disease or lessen its severity. The vaccine is recommended for healthy children over 1 year of age who have not had the disease. Children can get chickenpox by direct contact with someone who has either chickenpox or shingles (an infection caused by the same virus) or by inhaling the virus from the air after a person with either disease sneezes or coughs. It is easily spread in schools and day-care centers, and from one child to another in the same household. It occurs most often in winter and early spring. Once a child has had the disease, he or she is immune to it for life, but the virus remains dormant in the child's body and can emerge later in life as shingles.

SIGNS AND SYMPTOMS Chickenpox is usually a mild disease in otherwise healthy children. Symptoms appear within 8 to 21 days after exposure to the virus. The disease starts with a mild fever and then a skin RASH that appears on the child's body and scalp. The rash begins as small, red spots but turns to fluid-filled blisters within hours. Over the next 3 or 4 days, the rash spreads to the child's face, arms, legs, and genital area. It can also appear in the mouth and throat and cause a dry cough. After 5 to 7 days, the blisters begin to dry up and turn to scabs. The child may also have chills, HEADACHE, a poor appetite, and be fussy or irritable. If the child scratches the blisters, they can become infected with bacteria that cause an infection called cellulitis. While healthy children usually have mild cases of chickenpox, children with LEUKEMIA and other diseases that weaken their immune systems (see IMMUNE DISORDERS), infants under 1 month old, and babies born to mothers who had chickenpox at the time of birth are at risk of getting more seriously ill. In some cases, the virus can cause PNEUMONIA and ENCEPHALITIS.

DIAGNOSIS AND TREATMENT If your child has chickenpox, you can usually treat him or her at home. Your child's doctor can probably diagnose the infection over the phone. If your child has a fever for more than 4 days, a temperature above 102°F, a cough or sore throat, or signs of cellulitis (red, warm, tender, and swollen skin), the doctor will probably want you to bring your child to the office for an examination. Make sure your child rests while he or she has symptoms of chickenpox. Applying calamine lotion and giving your child an oatmeal bath can help relieve the itching. To give an oatmeal bath, you can use a prepackaged oatmeal preparation or just put oatmeal in your child's bathwater. Sponge baths with lukewarm water can help keep the blisters from becoming infected. Keep your child's fingernails short and ask your child not to scratch the blisters. Place mittens or cotton socks on the hands of babies and young children to prevent them from scratching.

Give your child acetaminophen or ibuprofen (not aspirin) for fever and aches and pains. An older child can gargle with salt water to help soothe a throat that is sore from blisters. The doctor may prescribe antibiotics if your child has cellulitis or an antiviral drug called acyclovir, taken by mouth, if your child is at risk of developing a severe case of chickenpox, (for example, if your child is undergoing *chemotherapy)*.

Your child can spread the disease from 1 or 2 days before the rash appears until the blisters have fully scabbed, usually within 7 to 10 days. Keep him or her home from school or day care until all the blisters have turned to scabs. Notify your child's school or day-care center if your child has chickenpox so the staff can notify the parents of the other children. Children with immune disorders or cancer may require a special injection at the time of exposure to prevent chickenpox from developing or to minimize its consequences.

CHLAMYDIA

Chlamydia, the most common sexually transmitted disease (STD) in the United States, is a bacterial infection that can be acquired through vaginal or anal intercourse and sometimes through oral sex. If a pregnant girl or woman has chlamydia, she can pass the infection to the eyes and lungs of her newborn as the infant passes through the birth canal. Sexually active teenagers are at high risk of getting chlamydia.

Chlamydia is the leading cause of pelvic inflammatory disease (an infection of the female internal reproductive organs) and a major cause of urethritis (inflammation of the urethra, the tube through which urine passes from the bladder) in males. It can also cause scarring in a woman's fallopian tubes, leading to infertility (the inability to have children) and ectopic pregnancy (one that develops outside the uterus). More than 4 million Americans contract chlamydia through intimate sexual contact every year.

The most common sites of infection are the cervix (the neck of the uterus), urethra, uterus, fallopian tubes, ovaries, rectum, and epididymis (a long tube that transports sperm from the testicles).

SIGNS AND SYMPTOMS About 80 percent of women and up to 20 percent of men infected with chlamydia have no symptoms. In girls or women who have symptoms, the most common is an abnormal discharge from the vagina. Other symptoms can include pain or a burning sensation while urinating, irregular or excessive bleeding during the menstrual cycle, pain or sensations of pressure in the lower part of the abdomen, fever, or nausea. Males commonly have a white or clear discharge from the penis.

Other symptoms can include pain or a burning sensation during urination and painful testicles. A person who practices receptive anal intercourse may have rectal pain, painful bowel movements, bleeding from the rectum, and rectal discharge. In both sexes, the first symptoms appear about 7 to 21 days after infection.

Newborns who get chlamydia from their mother's infected birth canal can develop CONJUNCTIVITIS or PNEUMONIA. Conjunctivitis produces red, watery, swollen eyes, with pus forming in the eyes 3 to 20 days after birth. A newborn with pneumonia may have a dry cough that develops 3 to 16 weeks after birth.

DIAGNOSIS Many people with chlamydia have no symptoms, so they do not see a doctor in the initial stages of infection, although a number of different laboratory tests, using a sample of vaginal discharge in girls or women and a sample of secretions from the urethra in boys or men, can accurately diagnose chlamydia. The disease often occurs with other types of STDs, especially GONORRHEA and GENITAL WARTS, so, if your adolescent has chlamydia, he or she may also be tested for other STDs.

TREATMENT If diagnosed and treated promptly, the disease lasts only a short time and causes no complications. Doctors treat chlamydia with antibiotics taken by mouth for 1 to 2 weeks. Sometimes an antibiotic given in a single dose is sufficient to treat a chlamydia infection. During treatment, a girl should not use vaginal douches, which can spread infection up into the uterus. Infected people should not have intercourse until treatment is completed to avoid spreading the disease. The doctor will also want to treat the adolescent's sexual partner or partners. Your adolescent will need to return to the doctor 3 to 4 weeks after treatment for a follow-up laboratory test. Relapses occur in about 20 percent of people; a longer treatment period, up to 28 days, and possibly a different antibiotic will be needed to treat relapses.

How to prevent a chlamydia infection

Chlamydia is epidemic in the United States, especially among adolescents. Many infected adolescents have no symptoms of chlamydia infection, so they may not know they have the disease. Sexually active teenagers need to protect themselves from chlamydia infection. Here are some steps your son or daughter can take:

- Always use a latex condom each and every time you have sex. Natural animal skin condoms are not effective in preventing chlamydia. The spermicide nonoxynol 9 does not kill the bacteria that cause chlamydia.
- Before you have sex with a new partner, ask if he or she has any sexually transmitted diseases (STDs). But be aware that your partner may not be telling the truth. Your partner may not know if he or she is infected or may choose not to be honest for fear of sexual rejection. This means you must practice safer sex each and every time. Be aware that your risk of infection increases with the number of sexual partners. However, it only takes a single encounter to get an STD.
- See a doctor for a complete physical examination once a year and ask to be tested for chlamydia.

CHOLESTEROL ABNORMALITIES

Cholesterol abnormalities refer to high levels of cholesterol in a child's blood. Cholesterol is a fatty substance needed for normal body function. The liver makes cholesterol from certain substances in food, primarily saturated fats. The body also absorbs cholesterol directly from foods. High levels of cholesterol can build up in the child's blood vessels and put the child at increased risk of developing heart disease as an adult.

Some children are born with high levels of cholesterol in their blood because of inherited disorders that make their body incapable of processing cholesterol adequately. Others acquire high cholesterol levels by consuming a lot of foods rich in saturated fat and cholesterol, such as red meat, eggs, whole milk, and cheese. Still others have high cholesterol levels from certain diseases, such as diabetes (see DIABETES MELLITUS, TYPE I), that influence the breakdown of fats.

Cholesterol and fats move through a child's bloodstream as particles known as lipoproteins. Certain lipoproteins–the high-density lipoproteins or HDLs–protect against heart disease, while other lipoproteins–the low-density lipoproteins or LDLs–are harmful. A high proportion of LDLs in a child's blood increases the risk of heart disease.

SIGNS AND SYMPTOMS The primary sign of a cholesterol abnormality in children is a high level of cholesterol in the blood. Heart disease does not usually develop until adulthood.

DIAGNOSIS If your or your spouse's family has a history of heart disease before age 55 or either of you has high cholesterol levels, have your child's blood cholesterol levels tested before age 2.

TREATMENT If your child has high blood cholesterol and LDL levels, the doctor will place him or her on a diet that is low in saturated fat and cholesterol. If your child is overweight, the doctor may also recommend a low-calorie diet. Dietary changes are effective for children over the age of 2 years, but are not recommended for children under age 2. If changes in diet do not reduce your child's blood cholesterol levels by the time he or she reaches 10 years of age, the doctor may prescribe cholesterol-lowering medication.

CHONDRITIS, COSTAL

See Costal chondritis

CHROMOSOMAL ABNORMALITIES

Chromosomal abnormalities are errors in the number or makeup of *chromosomes* in the cells of a child's body that may result in GENETIC DISORDERS. These errors can occur during the formation of the mother's egg or the father's sperm, during the union of egg and sperm, or during cell division after fertilization.

Normally, when the mother's egg is fertilized by the father's sperm, 23 pairs of chromosomes are created containing genetic material from both the egg and the sperm. The chromosomes contain thousands of genes, which determine the specific physical and mental traits of the developing fetus.

Chromosomal defects can occur when an extra chromosome is present, if a chromosome is missing or broken, or if chromosomes unite in an abnormal way. DOWN SYNDROME is an example of a genetic disorder caused by the presence of an extra chromosome.

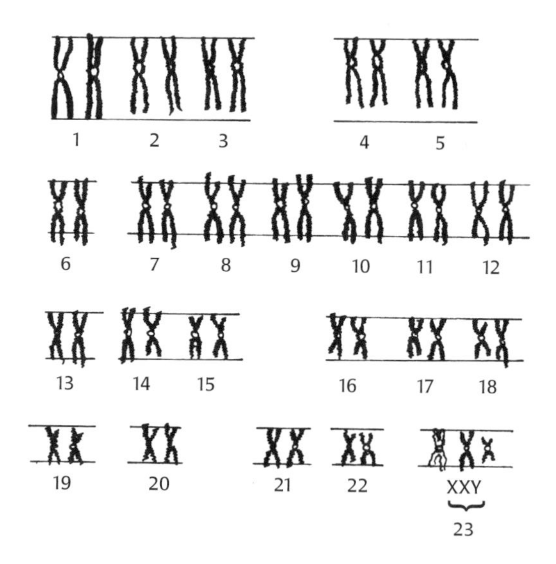

An extra X chromosome

A normal child has 23 pairs of chromosomes formed when the father's sperm unites with the mother's egg. A child with a chromosome abnormality is born with either an abnormal number of chromosomes or defective chromosomes. One possible chromosome abnormality is the presence of an extra X chromosome. In this illustration, the position of the extra chromosome indicates the condition known as Klinefelter's syndrome, which produces abnormal sexual development in males.

As a woman grows older and her egg cells age, she has a greater chance of having a child born with a chromosome abnormality, such as Down syndrome. The chances increase after age 35 and continue to rise as a woman ages.

SIGNS AND SYMPTOMS Chromosomal abnormalities can produce abnormal physical features, delays in growth and development, and MENTAL RETARDATION. The symptoms can be mild or severe. Some abnormalities can cause early death. Abnormal physical development of organs and bones can lead to such problems as heart or kidney disease. Almost any organ or part of the child's body can be affected. The child may also experience abnormal sexual development, behavioral problems, or learning disabilities.

DIAGNOSIS Doctors diagnose chromosomal abnormalities in a fetus using *amniocentesis* and by studying the cells of the fetus for abnormal chromosomes under a microscope. Your doctor may also use *ultrasound* to look for abnormal physical development in your fetus. Doctors use *chorionic villus sampling* to detect certain kinds of abnormalities, but the test cannot diagnose all types. After birth, your doctor will regularly check your child's physical and mental development for signs of disorders caused by chromosomal abnormalities.

TREATMENT Your child's treatment will depend on his or her specific physical abnormalities and mental disabilities.

CLEFT LIP AND CLEFT PALATE

Cleft lip and cleft palate are BIRTH DEFECTS in which a baby is born with an abnormally separated upper lip or palate (roof of the mouth) or both. The malformations appear in the early weeks of fetal development, long before the baby is born. In normal fetal development, the right and left sides of the lip and palate eventually grow together. About 1 in 700 babies are born with upper lips or palates that do not meet properly. About one third of the babies born with clefts have a family history of the defects. Clefts in the remaining two thirds may be caused by an external factor (such as exposure to alcohol and other drugs or to cigarette smoke before birth) or a genetic mutation.

SIGNS AND SYMPTOMS The cleft in a newborn's lip can range from a slight notch in the upper lip to a complete separation of the upper lip that extends into the baby's nose. The cleft can occur on one or both sides of the upper lip. The cleft in a newborn's palate can affect only a small portion of the back of the roof of the mouth or can extend from the front of the palate all the way to the back. Babies born with clefts may have difficulty with feeding, breathing, and speech development. Many babies born with a cleft palate develop ear infections (see pages 480) because of the malformation of the palate. The baby may also have HEARING LOSS and other birth defects, such as CLUBFOOT.

DIAGNOSIS Newborn babies are routinely checked for cleft lip and cleft palate. The defect is readily apparent at birth. The doctor will examine the infant immediately after birth to determine the extent of the defect.

TREATMENT A baby with one or both of these defects needs plastic surgery. He or she will receive care from a team of specialists, including a pediatrician, speech therapist, orthodontist, pediatric dentist, plastic surgeon, and otolaryngologist (a doctor who specializes in disorders of the ear, nose, and throat). If your baby is having trouble feeding before surgery, the dentist will make a device called an obturator that fits into the top of your baby's mouth to cover the cleft while he or she is eating. Occasionally, your baby may need to be fed through a tube placed in the nose or mouth that extends into his or her stomach. For long-term tube feeding, a tube may be

C

placed in the stomach through a small surgical incision in the baby's abdomen.

Surgical correction of a cleft lip is done as soon after birth as possible, usually when the baby is about 10 weeks old. After surgery, the doctor will prescribe medication to relieve any discomfort. The child's dressings will be removed in a day or two, and stitches will dissolve or be removed in about 5 days. Young infants sometimes need elbow restraints for a few weeks to prevent them from rubbing the affected area. Your baby will probably have a minimal scar.

Surgery for a cleft palate is more extensive than that done for a cleft lip, so the surgeon will wait until the baby is a little older and bigger, usually between 9 and 18 months old. After surgery, the baby will be in some pain for a day or two, but the doctor will prescribe medication to relieve the soreness. The baby will need to be fed fluids *intravenously* for a couple of days and may need elbow restraints for a few weeks. Follow the doctor's advice on feeding after the baby leaves the hospital.

To help prevent ear infections, an otolaryngologist may place a small plastic tube inside each of the child's eardrums at the time of cleft palate surgery. The tubes help air circulate across the eardrum and permit proper drainage of fluid. The plastic surgeon may recommend additional surgery when your child gets older to improve the appearance of his or her lip, palate, nose, and gums. Your child will also need care from an orthodontist (dentist who specializes in correcting irregularities of the teeth) to make sure his or her teeth are growing in properly. Your doctor may recommend speech therapy and regular hearing checkups.

CLUBFOOT

Clubfoot is a common BIRTH DEFECT that causes a newborn baby's foot and ankle to be twisted or turned out of shape. One or both feet may be affected. About 1 in 1,000 babies is born with clubfoot. It is more common in boys than in girls. The deformity occurs as the fetus is developing in the mother's uterus. Clubfoot, which is also called talipes equinovarus, tends to run in families. In rare cases, it is linked to other birth defects.

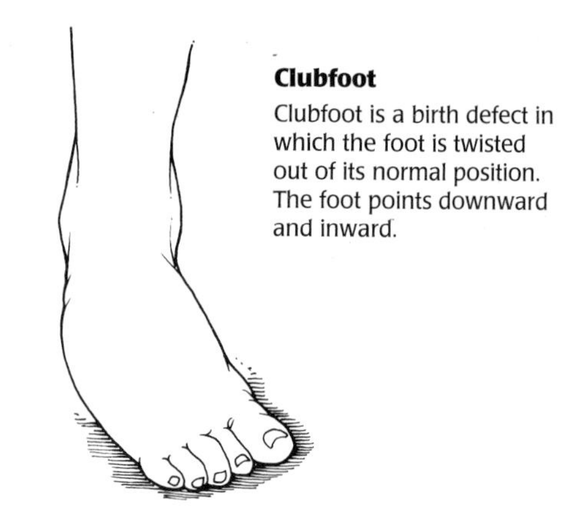

Clubfoot
Clubfoot is a birth defect in which the foot is twisted out of its normal position. The foot points downward and inward.

SIGNS AND SYMPTOMS The baby's foot usually twists inward and upward. If both feet are affected, the baby's toes point inward toward the toes of the opposite foot. Clubfoot is usually not painful, but affects the child's ability to stand and walk. Untreated, the affected foot cannot move normally and the child must walk on the sides or top part of the foot.

DIAGNOSIS AND TREATMENT If your child has clubfoot, the doctor will usually be able to diagnose it soon after birth during a physical examination and by taking X-rays of the affected foot. Once the deformity is diagnosed, the doctor will refer your child to an orthopedic (bone) specialist who will gently manipulate your baby's foot into a more normal position and then place a cast on the foot to keep it in place. The doctor will change the cast, moving your baby's foot closer and closer to a normal position, every few days at first and then every few weeks. The treatment begins soon after birth, often as early as the first week of life, and usually takes about 3 to 6 months. If the casting does not correct the problem, the doctor may recommend surgery to correct the deformity.

COARCTATION OF THE AORTA

Coarctation of the aorta is a BIRTH DEFECT (see HEART DISEASE, CONGENITAL) characterized by an abnormal narrowing of the aorta (the major artery leading away from the heart). The narrowing usually occurs just beyond the point where the aorta branches out to supply blood to different parts of the body. The narrowing causes blood flow in the aorta to increase before the narrowing and decrease after the narrowing. The child develops HIGH BLOOD PRESSURE in the upper portion of his or her body (the head, neck, upper part of the chest, and right arm) and low blood pressure in the lower part (the abdomen, groin, and legs), and the child's heart needs to work harder to supply blood to the body.

SIGNS AND SYMPTOMS The symptoms of this condition are most often present shortly after birth, but they may develop throughout childhood, up to adolescence. An affected infant may feed poorly, become inactive, and have poor skin color. The pulse in the groin area may be weak or absent and the infant could have a HEART MURMUR. An affected older child can experience dizziness, throbbing HEADACHES, cold feet or legs, weakness in the legs, or leg cramps after exercise. Older children can also have high blood pressure, a weak or absent pulse in the groin area, and a heart murmur. In severe cases, an infant or child can develop heart failure (see HEART FAILURE, CONGESTIVE).

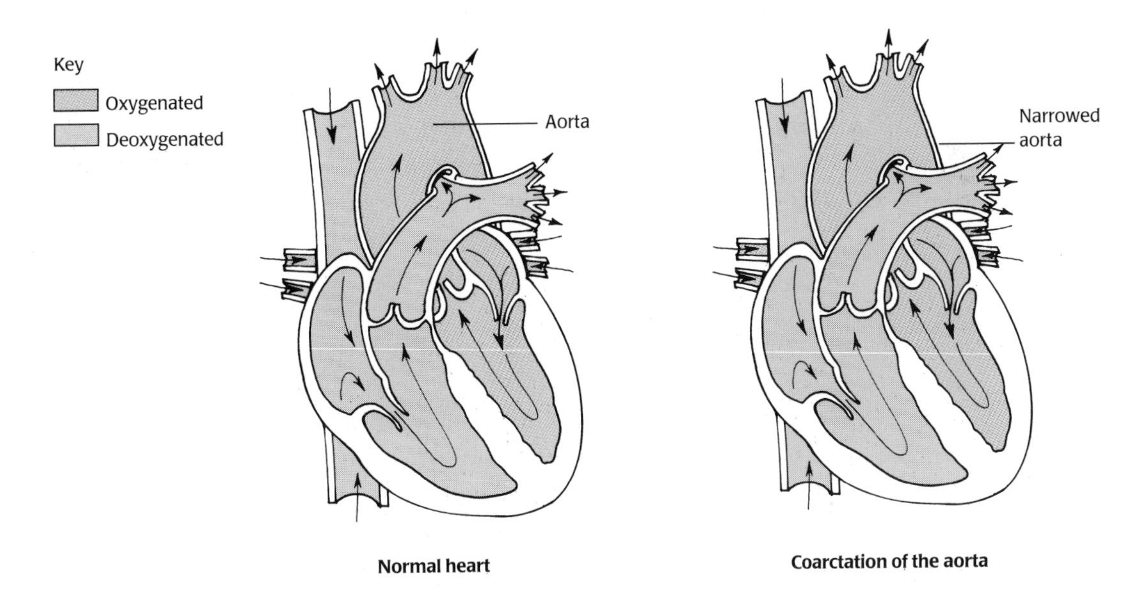

Constriction in the aorta

A baby born with coarctation of the aorta (right) has a narrowing in the aorta, usually just past the point where the blood vessel that supplies blood to the infant's head, neck, and right arm branches from the aorta. The constriction slows the flow of blood through the aorta beyond that point. The baby's head, neck, upper part of the chest, and right arm receive an adequate supply of blood, and the abdomen, groin, legs, and left arm receive a diminished supply. The baby's heart must then work harder to pump blood to these areas of the body.

DIAGNOSIS Quite often, the doctor discovers coarctation of the aorta during a baby's first examination by finding a weak or absent pulse at the groin. The doctor might also take the baby's blood pressure in different parts of the body to look for differences in pressure. The diagnosis can be confirmed by chest X-rays or *ultrasounds* of the child's aorta and heart.

TREATMENT Surgery can correct the narrowing; it is usually performed when the child is between the ages of 2 and 4, but may be done in infancy. Surgery relieves the symptoms quickly, prevents damage to the child's heart, and forestalls high blood pressure.

COLD SORES

Cold sores, also called fever blisters, are small, painful, fluid-filled blisters that erupt on the lips, gums, mouth, throat, and parts of the face. Cold sores are caused by infection with herpes simplex virus 1. The virus is spread by kissing or sharing eating utensils or through contact with an infected person who has an infection on the skin, a discharge from the eye, or a cold sore.

Once a child has the herpes simplex virus, he or she has it for life. The initial infection generally occurs between 6 months and 5 years of age. The virus may lie dormant inside nerves and then erupt months or years later in the mouth, on the face, and, in rare cases, in the eyes. Most children develop antibodies that keep the virus in check unless they are under stress, exposed to excessive sun or cold, or become ill; then the cold sores can develop.

SIGNS AND SYMPTOMS In the initial infection, cold sores will appear on the tongue, gums, back of the throat, and insides of the cheeks. The child will feel sick and have a high fever (101°F or higher), intense pain in the mouth, and difficulty swallowing. The child may also have headaches, a poor appetite, and foul breath and be irritable and restless at night. The glands in the neck may be tender and swollen. During recurrent infections, cold sores that look like small blisters surrounded by a tiny red ring will occur on the lips or face. The painful blisters fill with fluid, dry up, form a scab, and disappear in 7 to 10 days.

DIAGNOSIS You will probably be able to recognize cold sores on your own. Take your child to the doctor if the child develops an eye infection during the first infection, the fever continues for more than a week, the cold sores get worse after a week, or the child is weak and shows signs of dehydration (see page 283).

TREATMENT There is no cure for cold sores or herpes infection. Most cases clear up within 2 or 3 weeks without treatment. Applying cool, wet cloths for up to an hour at the first sign of tingling may help reduce the severity of the cold sores. Topical antiviral creams sometimes ease the pain and make the sores heal more quickly. While the blisters are present, your child is contagious so keep the child from kissing other people or sharing cups or utensils.

COLIC

See page 41

COLOR BLINDNESS

Color blindness is the inability to see certain colors or, in rare cases, any colors except shades of gray. This disorder is usually inherited and boys are affected much more often than girls.

SIGNS AND SYMPTOMS Children who are born color blind most often have trouble distinguishing the colors red and green or shades of red and green. Some children have difficulty seeing blue and yellow or shades of those colors. In rare cases, a child may be able to see shades of gray only. Inherited color blindness affects both eyes equally.

DIAGNOSIS You may not be able to detect color blindness in your child until he or she is old enough to talk and identify colors. Many pediatricians screen children for color blindness at age 3 or 4. If your child cannot distinguish colors correctly, the doctor will send him or her to an eye specialist who will test for color blindness by asking your child to identify numbers or shapes by color.

TREATMENT Color blindness cannot be treated, but your child can learn to compensate for it by memorizing colors by shape or position, such as the position of green and red lights on a traffic signal. Some children find it helpful to wear a special red contact lens on one eye.

CONGENITAL ADRENAL HYPERPLASIA

Congenital adrenal hyperplasia is a rare GENETIC DISORDER that is present at birth and affects the production of the hormone cortisol (also known as hydrocortisone) by the adrenal glands. Cortisol plays a role in the body's use of nutrients. Because of a genetic defect, the affected child is missing or deficient in an enzyme (a protein that speeds up chemical reactions in the body) that is needed for the production of cortisol. Many enzymes are involved in cortisol formation and any one of them can be absent or deficient. The decreased cortisol formation triggers an overproduction of male sex hormones (androgens). The absent or deficient enzyme can also cause the adrenal glands to decrease production of the hormone aldosterone, which is needed to properly balance the amount of salt in the blood.

SIGNS AND SYMPTOMS The overproduction of male sex hormones can cause newborn girls to have ambiguous genitalia. The clitoris enlarges to the size of a small penis and the external lips of the vagina (labia) may fuse to look like a scrotum. As they get older, these girls sometimes develop a deep voice and do not menstruate or have abnormal menstrual periods (see MENSTRUAL DISORDERS). Newborn boys may look normal at birth, but display signs of puberty long before the normal age, sometimes as early as 2 or 3 years of age. Their penis enlarges, their voice deepens, pubic hair appears, and their body becomes muscular.

A deficiency in aldosterone can cause a severe loss of salt from an infant's body, resulting in dehydration (see page 283), vomiting, and an abnormal heartbeat (see ARRHYTHMIAS). This condition occurs during the first few days of life. It can be life threatening and requires emergency medical treatment.

DIAGNOSIS Many states require newborn screening for the most common missing enzyme, so many affected children can be diagnosed and treated early, before symptoms appear. The doctor will diagnosis congenital adrenal hyperplasia in a child who has not been screened based on the child's symptoms and physical findings. The doctor will order blood, urine, and hormone level tests to detect the disorder and may also do an *ultrasound* of the child's adrenal glands. If your child is severely dehydrated and vomiting, take him or her to a hospital emergency department for immediate treatment no matter what has caused the dehydration. The signs of dehydration include pale, dry skin that looks loose; dry lips and tongue; a rapid heartbeat; sunken eyes; a lack of tears; a lack of energy; a sunken soft spot on the skull, if still present; and behavioral changes in extreme cases.

TREATMENT Children with congenital adrenal hyperplasia receive drugs that replace the deficient hormones, returning their hormone levels to normal and decreasing the androgen formation. They need to continue taking this medication for life. Baby girls with ambiguous genitalia need surgery to correct the appearance of their external reproductive organs. The reconstructive surgery is generally done when the child is between the ages of 1 and 3 years. With early treatment, the child attains normal sexual development and function.

CONJUNCTIVITIS

Conjunctivitis, commonly called pinkeye, is inflammation of the conjunctiva, the lining of the inside of the eyelids. Inflammation can also affect the whites of the eyes. Conjunctivitis is common in infants and children and is easily spread from child to child. Although frequently caused by bacteria, conjunctivitis can also be caused by viruses, allergies, an injury, or an irritating chemical or pollutant, such as a household cleaner or dust, that gets into a child's eye.

SIGNS AND SYMPTOMS If your child has conjunctivitis caused by bacteria, his or her eyes will burn or feel scratchy and painful, the eyelids may swell up, and a thick or crusty discharge will seep from the eyes and make the eyelids stick together, especially during sleep. Pinkeye caused by a virus produces similar symptoms, but the discharge will be more watery and the child will have the symptoms of a cold. Intense itching and tearing of the eyes occur when allergies or irritants cause conjunctivitis.

DIAGNOSIS The doctor will be able to diagnose conjunctivitis by the appearance of your child's eye. If the discharge from the eye is clear, the infection is probably caused by a virus. If pus is present, the infection is caused by bacteria.

TREATMENT Your child's doctor will prescribe antibiotic eyedrops or an antibiotic ointment for pinkeye caused by bacteria. Periodically wipe the edges of your child's eyelids clean using a clean, moist towel or cotton ball. The eye infection should begin to clear up in a couple of days with treatment. Conjunctivitis caused by a virus does not respond to treatment with antibiotics, but you can give your child over-the-counter eyedrops to soothe the irritation until the infection clears up on its own, which usually takes about 8 to 10 days.

To clear up conjunctivitis, make sure that your child avoids the irritants or allergies that bother his or her eyes. Antihistamines taken by mouth may relieve the itching or discomfort. Don't let other members of your family share washcloths or towels with your infected child or they could become infected as well.

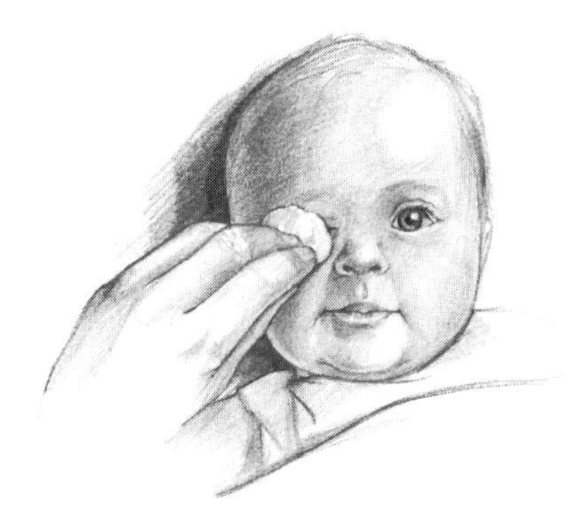

Cleaning an infected eye
When your baby has conjunctivitis, his or her infected eye produces a sticky discharge that causes the eyelids to stick together. To remove the discharge, wipe his or her eyes four or five times each day with a clean cotton ball soaked in cool water. Wipe gently down and away from your baby's nose. Always wash your hands before and after touching your baby's face.

CONTACT DERMATITIS

Contact dermatitis is an allergic irritation of the skin caused by direct contact with something to which your child's skin is sensitive. Substances that can trigger the blistery rash characteristic of contact dermatitis include rubber, nickel and other metals, hair dyes, cosmetics, antibiotics and other medications applied directly to the skin, chromates (compounds that contain the metallic element chromium), and plants such as POISON IVY. Certain chemicals, detergents, acids, fabrics, and soaps can also irritate your child's skin and cause contact dermatitis. Some substances, such as sunscreens, shaving lotions, and certain perfumes, cause contact dermatitis only if, after application, the child's skin is exposed to sunlight.

SIGNS AND SYMPTOMS The exposed skin becomes reddened with raised, scaly, small areas or BLISTERS that itch. The blisters may ooze with fluid and crust over, and the skin can become leathery, scaly, and raw. Sometimes the skin feels warm to the touch.

DIAGNOSIS Call your doctor if you see a red patchy or blistery rash on your child's skin. The doctor will ask you and your child about any irritating substances your child may have been in contact with. Your doctor may do a skin patch test to find out what substances your child may be allergic to and may also order a skin lesion *biopsy* to rule out other causes of the irritation.

TREATMENT Wash the area thoroughly with water to remove any irritants that may still be on the skin. Once your doctor identifies the irritant causing the dermatitis, he or she will tell your child to avoid exposure to the substance. Your doctor may recommend wet dressings and anti-itch or moisturizing lotions to soothe the itching. He or she may also prescribe an antihistamine to reduce the itching or a *corticosteroid* cream to treat the inflammation. The symptoms should clear up in 2 or 3 weeks.

CONVULSIONS

See Seizure disorders

CORNS

See Calluses, corns, and bunions

COSTAL CHONDRITIS

Costal chondritis is a relatively common inflammation (pain and swelling) of the cartilage that attaches a child's ribs to his or her breastbone. The inflammation can occur following an injury to the chest, strenuous physical activity, or a viral infection causing a cough or cold. Sometimes it occurs for no known reason.

SIGNS AND SYMPTOMS Your child may have pain and tenderness in his or her chest. The pain may be sharp, sudden, darting, and short-term or it may develop gradually as a dull ache that lasts hours or days. Pressure on the chest, sudden movements, and coughing make the pain more intense. Your child may feel pain in more than one area of the chest and even in his or her arm. He or she may also feel tightness in the chest. The discomfort usually lasts for only a few days.

DIAGNOSIS AND TREATMENT Unless the pain is intense or lasts more than a few days, you don't need to see your child's doctor for a diagnosis. If your child has mild pain in the chest, he or she should avoid activities that can put strain on or injure the ribs. You can give your child acetaminophen or ibuprofen (not aspirin) for the pain. If you take your child to the doctor, he or she will examine your child to make sure no other disorder is causing the pain.

CRADLE CAP

Cradle cap is a common childhood skin irritation that occurs on an infant's scalp and affects babies primarily in the first 3 to 6 months of life. Cradle cap is a harmless form of SEBORRHEIC DERMATITIS that does not affect your baby's overall health and usually clears up with treatment at home. The condition is caused by a buildup of oil and scaly skin on the scalp. As infants develop rapidly, oil glands under the skin produce large amounts of oil that can cause dead skin to stick to the scalp.

SIGNS AND SYMPTOMS At first, you will see dry scales of skin on your baby's scalp (see page 23). These scales become greasy yellow or brown patches of dead skin that can feel crusty. The crusty patches can cover your baby's entire scalp and even extend to his or her eyebrows and behind the ears. Your baby may temporarily lose some hair.

C

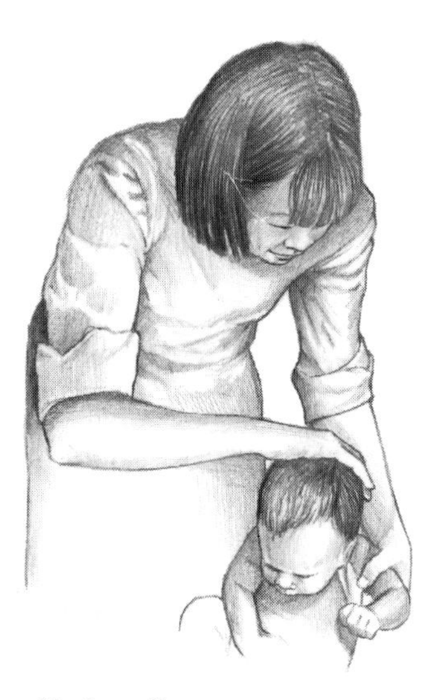

Getting rid of cradle cap
To get rid of your child's cradle cap, rub his or her scalp with unscented baby oil and leave it on overnight. The next day, wash your baby's scalp with a gentle shampoo and comb his or her hair to remove the scales.

DIAGNOSIS Your child's doctor will be able to recognize cradle cap from its appearance.

TREATMENT Rub unscented baby oil into your baby's scalp and leave it on overnight to loosen the scales. The next day, wash your baby's scalp and hair with a gentle shampoo and then comb his or her hair with a fine-tooth baby comb or gently scrub his or her scalp with a moist towel to get rid of the dead skin. Once you have treated your baby's cradle cap, keep his or her scalp clean with soap-and-water baths followed by thorough drying. The condition often returns, so apply baby oil to your child's scalp and wash his or her hair with shampoo frequently to keep the area clean and free of dead skin.

CROHN'S DISEASE

Crohn's disease is a chronic inflammation of the digestive tract—the mouth, esophagus, stomach, small and large intestines, and anus. Crohn's disease can occur anywhere along the digestive tract but most commonly affects the small intestine, especially where the small intestine meets the large intestine.

The inflammation extends deep into the walls of the intestine and can cause ulcers that penetrate the intestinal walls. Crohn's disease can begin in childhood—most frequently in the teenage years—and the symptoms can flare up from time to time throughout life. Children are sometimes more severely affected than adults. The cause of Crohn's disease remains unknown, although it tends to run in families.

SIGNS AND SYMPTOMS The classic symptoms of Crohn's disease are abdominal pain, diarrhea, and blood in the stool. Other symptoms of Crohn's disease include RECTAL PROLAPSE (protrusion of the rectum through the anus), weight loss, persistent fever, abdominal cramps, and frequent bowel movements. If the child loses a lot of blood, he or she can develop anemia (see ANEMIA, BLOOD-LOSS). Crohn's disease can also produce inflammation of the joints (arthritis), a rash, or growth retardation. Symptoms can range from mild to severe and tend to disappear and then flare up again periodically for months or years. Most cases are mild or moderate, but severe cases can cause disabling diarrhea and overwhelming abdominal pain.

DIAGNOSIS To diagnose Crohn's disease, the doctor will order blood and stool tests. A gastroenterologist (doctor who specializes in stomach and intestinal disorders) may look at your child's rectum and colon through an endoscope (a flexible tube) inserted through the child's anus. The doctor may take a small sample of tissue from the colon to examine under a microscope.

Your child may also undergo X-ray tests of various sections of the digestive tract to pinpoint the disease. The tests may include a *barium X-ray* study, in which an enema filled with barium, a chalky solution that helps reveal inflammation or ulcers on X-ray film, is placed in your child's rectum. If a barium X-ray

What is endoscopy?

If your child needs an endoscopic examination, the doctor will use a flexible viewing instrument called an endoscope with an eyepiece at one end that he or she will introduce into your child's body to visually examine the organs inside. An endoscope allows the doctor to actually see what is currently happening inside your child's body. The fiberoptic instrument is made of a thin plastic tube containing bundles of fibers. The doctor shines a light down one bundle of fibers to illuminate the part of the body being viewed. The light is reflected back along a second bundle of fibers and the image is magnified inside the eyepiece. The doctor can pass a variety of other instruments down the endoscope to take a sample of tissue or remove an abnormal growth. Some endoscopes even carry a miniature television camera that can record images of internal organs and display them on a screen.

Before having an endoscopic examination, your child will be lightly sedated but will not be completely unconscious during the procedure. The doctor may also give him or her a local anesthetic to reduce discomfort. Depending on the site of the examination, the doctor might pass the endoscope into your child's mouth and down his or her esophagus (the passageway that connects the mouth and the stomach), or insert the instrument into your child's anus and pass it into his or her intestines. During surgery, doctors sometimes use an endoscope, which is introduced through a small incision made in the body, to treat a digestive tract disorder.

After the examination, your child may feel a little light-headed until the anesthesia wears off. The examination itself is safe and painless although your child may be able to feel movement while the endoscope is inside his or her body. If your child is old enough to understand, the doctor will explain the procedure beforehand and tell your child how he or she will feel afterward. Assure your child that you will stay with him or her before and after the endoscopy so he or she can feel less anxious about the procedure.

of the stomach and upper intestinal tract is needed, your child will have to drink the barium so the doctor can take X-rays of the substance as it moves through the stomach and small intestine.

TREATMENT There is no cure for Crohn's disease, but medications can control the symptoms. Your doctor may prescribe sulfa (antibacterial) drugs, *corticosteroids*, antibiotics, and nonsteroidal anti-inflammatory drugs to control the inflammation that causes pain and diarrhea.

If your child has a severe flare-up of Crohn's disease, he or she may need to be hospitalized to get proper nutrition and rest. If drug therapy fails or your child develops serious complications, such as a blocked intestine or an abscess (a buildup of pus) in the intestine, he or she may need surgery to remove the diseased part of the intestine or to drain the abscess. Your child may need to take medication or be hospitalized periodically as the disease flares up throughout life. Some children also need psychiatric support to cope with the disease and its treatment.

CROSSED EYES

See Vision problems

CROUP

Croup is an infection of the upper airway around the voice box (larynx). It is usually marked by the presence of a dry, barking cough; a hoarse voice; and a low-grade fever. It is caused by cold or influenza (see page 231) viruses and commonly occurs in late fall and early spring. Croup is most common in children who are 6 months to 3 years old.

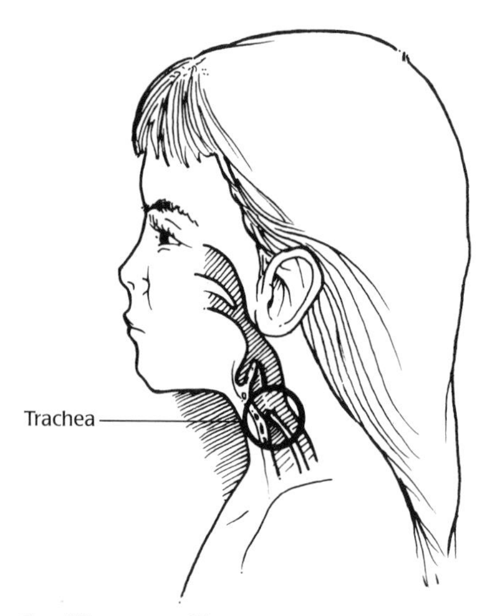

Swelling caused by croup
In a child with a mild case of croup, the trachea, or windpipe, is swollen, narrowing the air passage (circled area). The swelling causes the child to become hoarse and have difficulty breathing and produces a distinctive, barklike cough.

Signs and symptoms Two or 3 days after getting an infection in the nose and throat, the child's voice becomes hoarse. His or her throat also becomes sore as the laryngeal area swells. The child then develops a hacking cough that sounds like the barking of a seal or small dog. The cough often gets worse at night. The child may also have a fever and may gag and vomit. Breathing may become difficult. When the child inhales, he or she often makes a harsh, high-pitched noise known as stridor. Infants with croup are irritable and very tired and may lose their appetites. Most cases of croup are mild and symptoms improve in 3 to 5 days. For another week or two, the child may continue to have a dry cough. Getting another infection can cause the symptoms of croup to recur. The symptoms of croup are the worst in children under 3 years old.

Diagnosis The doctor will examine your child, monitor his or her breathing patterns, and listen for the distinctive cough. He or she will also order X-rays of your child's neck to look for a narrowing of the air passages, which can differentiate croup from the more serious epiglottitis. Your child will also be examined to make sure he or she has not inhaled a foreign object or contracted an infectious inflammation of the trachea. If your child has a fever higher than 103°F, extreme restlessness, drooling, or pale blue skin, or if he or she seems to be using the neck, chest, and abdominal muscles to breathe, take him or her to a hospital emergency department immediately.

Treatment Most cases of croup are mild and can be treated at home, although you and your child may be frightened by the sound of the cough. Place a humidifier in your child's room to help open his or her airways. Some parents find it helpful to turn on the hot water in the shower and sit with their child in the steam-filled bathroom; the child should begin to feel better in 20 to 30 minutes. Give your child plenty of fluids or ice pops to prevent dehydration (see page 283). Keep your child home from school or day care until he or she feels better. If your child does not respond to home treatment in 3 to 5 days or if the condition gets worse, call the doctor. He or she may give your child a breathing treatment with a drug called epinephrine or *corticosteroids.* If your child needs to be hospitalized, he or she will be given humidified oxygen in a tent or through a mask.

Cushing's syndrome

Cushing's syndrome is a rare disorder caused by an excessive amount of *corticosteroid* hormones in the body. It can be caused by abnormal functioning of the child's pituitary gland (a pea-sized gland at the base of the brain) or Cushing's disease, which is caused by a tumor in the pituitary gland that causes the adrenal glands to release too much of the hormone cortisol (also called hydrocortisone). Prolonged use of corticosteroids, prescribed for the treatment of certain diseases, such as JUVENILE RHEUMATOID ARTHRITIS and ASTHMA, can also cause Cushing's syndrome.

SIGNS AND SYMPTOMS Cushing's syndrome initially accelerates growth but, left untreated, can eventually retard growth. It produces a characteristic round, red, moon-shaped face. Affected children also develop a large abdomen, a barrel chest, thin arms and legs, a hump between the shoulders, thin skin, body hair, and ACNE. They BRUISE easily and can have purple stretch marks on their abdomen, chest, and thighs. Puberty may be delayed and girls can develop MENSTRUAL DISORDERS and a masculine appearance. HIGH BLOOD PRESSURE can also occur.

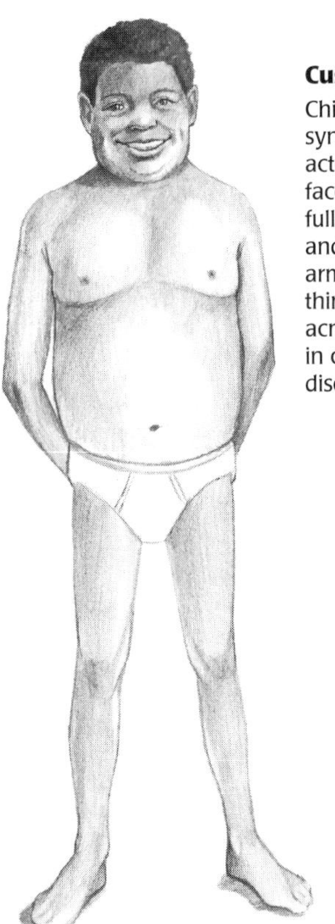

Cushing's syndrome
Children with Cushing's syndrome have a characteristic moon-shaped face. Their bodies are full around the waist and chest, but their arms, legs, and hips are thin. Facial hair and acne are also common in children with the disorder.

DIAGNOSIS If your child has symptoms of Cushing's syndrome, the doctor will probably refer him or her to an endocrinologist (a doctor who specializes in the treatment of hormonal disorders) who will test the hormone levels in your child's blood and urine. The doctor or endocrinologist may also do an *ultrasound* or *computed tomography* (CT) of your child's adrenal and pituitary glands. *Magnetic resonance imaging* or CT of your child's brain may also be needed to evaluate the pituitary gland.

TREATMENT If long-term use of corticosteroids has caused your child's Cushing's syndrome, the doctor will recommend gradually reducing the drugs your child takes and substituting another medication for them, if possible.

A tumor in the pituitary or adrenal glands requires surgery. The surgeon will remove the tumor, if possible, but may have to remove the pituitary or adrenal glands themselves. If the glands are removed, your child will need to take hormone replacement drugs for life. *Radiation* and *chemotherapy* to shrink a pituitary tumor are possible alternatives to surgery. With treatment, your child's chances of a full recovery are good, unless the adrenal tumor is found to be cancerous. There is also a chance that the tumor or tumors may recur after surgery.

CYSTIC FIBROSIS

Cystic fibrosis is an inherited GENETIC DISORDER that causes persistent lung and digestive problems. To inherit the disease, a child must have two parents who are each carriers of the defective gene that causes cystic fibrosis. The child inherits one defective gene from each parent. Parents can carry a defective gene for cystic fibrosis and not know it because carriers have no symptoms of the disease. A carrier has one defective gene and one normal gene and the normal gene prevents symptoms in carriers. Children of parents who are carriers of the defective gene have a 25 percent chance of having cystic fibrosis, a 50 percent chance of being a carrier but not having the disease, and a 25 percent chance of not having the disease and not being a carrier. The disease causes the lining of the airways leading to the lungs to produce excess mucus (a thick, sticky fluid) that clogs the lungs and makes the child vulnerable to chronic lung infections. Cystic fibrosis also causes the child's pancreas (the organ that secretes insulin) to fail to produce the pancreatic enzymes that help digest food.

More than 50 percent of children with cystic fibrosis survive into their 20s or 30s. Many variations of the disease occur and some adults live into their 40s and beyond. Early diagnosis and aggressive management to delay the onset of lung damage greatly improve survival.

Signs and symptoms Infants with cystic fibrosis may display symptoms right after birth or may not show them until months or years later. An infant may delay passing meconium (newborn stool) for more than 48 hours after birth, but, more typically, the infant or child has foul-smelling stools that are pale and greasy. He or she may not absorb enough nutrients from food (see MALABSORPTION), may lose weight, and could fail to thrive (see FAILURE TO THRIVE). The child may seem out of breath and have a constant cough that produces thick mucus. The child may also have frequent bouts of PNEUMONIA, BRONCHITIS, and REACTIVE AIRWAY DISEASE. Males can become infertile (unable to produce sperm). The child's growth can be stunted because of chronic MALNUTRITION and lung disease. The child may have salty-tasting sweat and be more prone to dehydration (see page 283) than other children. Children with cystic fibrosis may also have nasal polyps (abnormal growths in the nose) or rectal prolapse (protrusion of the lining of the rectum out of the anus). A long-term complication of cystic fibrosis is diabetes mellitus (see DIABETES MELLITUS, TYPE I) caused by damage to the pancreas.

Diagnosis and treatment To diagnose cystic fibrosis, the doctor will order a sweat test, which can detect an abnormally large amount of chloride in your child's sweat. The doctor may also order chest X-rays, a stool analysis, an analysis of your child's mucus, and a test that measures the amount of a protein known as trypsinogen in the

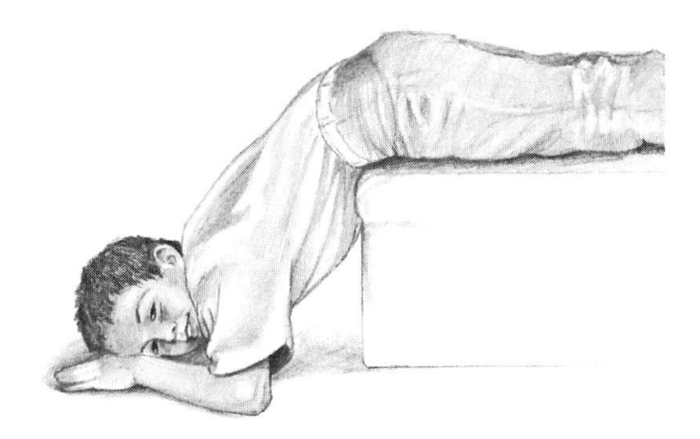

Postural drainage

Postural drainage allows a child with cystic fibrosis to drain mucus from his or her lungs by lying in various positions. Gravity pulls the mucus toward the throat so the child can cough it up and spit it out.

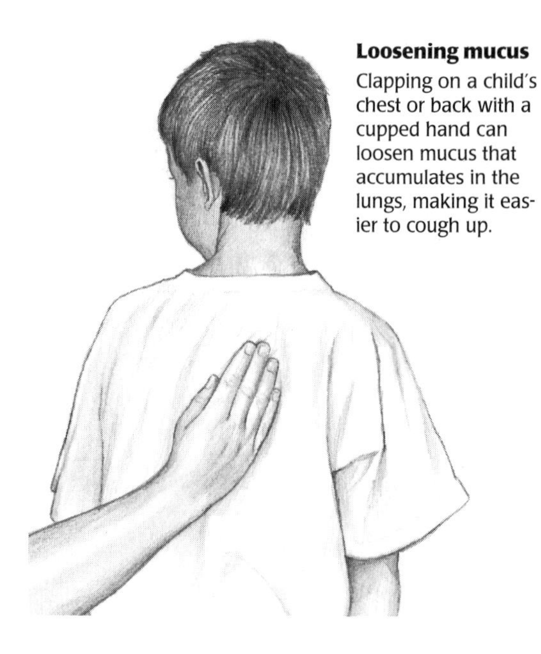

Loosening mucus

Clapping on a child's chest or back with a cupped hand can loosen mucus that accumulates in the lungs, making it easier to cough up.

blood. Doctors can use *amniocentesis* to test for the genetic defect causing cystic fibrosis before birth, although the test is not 100 percent accurate.

The doctor will prescribe pancreatic enzyme powders or pills that your child will need to take with every meal to help digestion. Vitamin and nutritional supplements and a diet rich in calories and proteins will improve your child's overall health. Your child may also need to take antibiotics for lung infections, decongestants, and bronchodilator drugs that open up the airways congested by mucus. At home, you can use chest clapping (gentle pounding and pressing of the child's chest with a cupped hand) and postural drainage (positioning your child so that mucus drains from his or her lungs) to help loosen the mucus. Good respiratory care and nutrition improve the long-term health of children with cystic fibrosis.

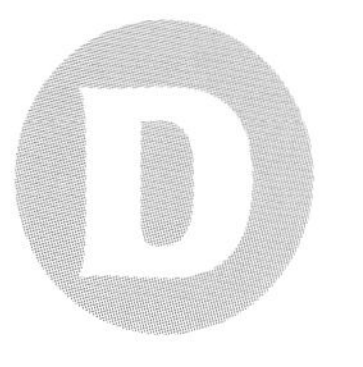

DEAFNESS

See Hearing loss

DENTAL PROBLEMS

See Teeth development problems

DEPRESSION

Depression is an emotional state marked by deep sadness, boredom, irritability, and hopelessness. It can bring on weight loss, sleep disturbances, fatigue, poor self-esteem, poor concentration, and thoughts of suicide. Like adults, children often become unhappy for short periods in reaction to unfortunate or disruptive life events but, when a child's sadness lasts for more than 2 weeks or interferes with the child's normal activities, it can indicate a serious depression. Among children, adolescents are the most prone to depression, although infants and younger children can also become depressed. The causes of childhood depression vary. It can be triggered by a family or individual tragedy, such as divorce of the parents; a death, serious illness, or DRUG AND ALCOHOL ABUSE in the family; or sexual or physical abuse (see page 326). Less dramatic events, such as moving to a new house or city, can also cause depression. Teenagers sometimes become depressed when breaking up with a boyfriend or girlfriend.

Depression can be produced by certain drugs, including alcohol and barbiturates. Long-term illnesses, such as diabetes (see DIABETES MELLITUS, TYPE I), commonly cause children and teens to become depressed. Depression is also linked to some mental and emotional disorders, such as BIPOLAR DISORDER, LEARNING DISABILITIES, and OBSESSIVE-COMPULSIVE DISORDER.

SIGNS AND SYMPTOMS Depressed children of any age have certain common symptoms of depression, including extreme irritability, rebellious behavior, lack of interest in activities the child used to enjoy, and noticeable changes–such as losing weight or trouble sleeping–in normal eating and sleeping habits. Other symptoms depend on the child's age and stage of development. Infants and toddlers may grow abnormally slowly or not gain enough weight (see FAILURE TO THRIVE) or fail to progress in language and movement skills (see DEVELOPMENTAL DELAY). Infants may show little expression and may appear to have no attachment to their parents. Some throw up and reswallow their food after feedings (see RUMINATION).

Young children who have not yet started school can wet their beds (see BED-WETTING) or soil their clothing with stool (see ENCOPRESIS). They may be aggressive, reckless, or destructive at play and even become preoccupied with death and suicide. School-age children often perform poorly in school and may be slow to develop social skills. Self-esteem may fall. Affected children sometimes withdraw from family and friends or even steal or lie.

Depressed adolescents feel sad, anxious (see ANXIETY), or emotionally empty. They may be constantly bored or have difficulty concentrating. Some withdraw from family and friends, have low self-esteem and extreme feelings of guilt, begin abusing alcohol or other drugs, lose interest in their appearance, and do unusually poorly in school. They may be obsessed with death and threaten to commit suicide. Lying, stealing, and running away from home are all possible symptoms of depression.

Diagnosis Your child's doctor will do a thorough physical examination and order a battery of tests to determine if there are any underlying physical causes, such as HYPOTHYROIDISM or anemia, for your child's symptoms. The doctor will also ask you and your child questions about your family relationships, whether either parent has a serious illness or abuses alcohol, and whether any other relatives have ever suffered from depression. He or she will also try to find out if your child is under extreme stress or whether he or she has undergone a traumatic event recently. The doctor may refer your child to a psychiatrist or psychologist for a complete evaluation.

Treatment The usual treatment for depression is individual or family psychotherapy or both. In severe cases, your child's doctor or a psychiatrist may prescribe antidepressant medications, although their effectiveness has not been proven in children or teens. If your child or teenager attempts suicide, he or she will need to be hospitalized for treatment. The length of treatment depends on the severity of the depression. Children with mild cases of depression may be better in a month or two after beginning treatment. Those with more severe cases may require long-term psychotherapy for months or years.

Dermatomyositis

Dermatomyositis is inflammation of the skin and muscles. It is a chronic disease, meaning that it can affect a child for life, with alternating periods of flare-up and relief. Dermatomyositis most commonly affects children between the ages of 5 and 12. The condition is thought to be an AUTOIMMUNE DISORDER, in which the body's natural defense mechanisms begin to attack the body's own tissues. Dermatomyositis can develop after infections, drug reactions, or vaccinations. The cause is unknown.

Signs and symptoms The first signs of the disease are fatigue and muscle weakness, especially in the child's thighs and shoulders. Typically, the child has difficulty keeping up with others and may ask to be carried more and more. He or she tires easily when climbing up and down stairs or when lifting things above his or her shoulders. The child's muscles may ache and be tender to the touch. A RASH usually develops on the child's face, particularly over the nose and cheeks. His or her eyelids become discolored and purple. The child may also have a red, scaly rash or tiny bumps on his or her elbows, knuckles, and knees. Other signs include a general feeling of ill health, shortness of breath, weight loss, and a low fever.

Diagnosis If the doctor suspects that your child has dermatomyositis, he or she will order blood tests to look for unusual levels of certain muscle proteins in the blood. The doctor may also order an electromyograph test and a nerve conduction velocity test, which measure electrical activity in the child's muscles and nerves. Both tests can be quite painful because the doctor needs to insert a large needle into the child's muscle and cannot use an anesthetic because the drug would alter the test results. The doctor may also recommend a *biopsy* of your child's skin or muscle tissue. Your child may be referred to an immunologist (a doctor who specializes in treating disorders of the immune system) for treatment.

TREATMENT Your child will need to begin taking *corticosteroids* by mouth or by injection. These drugs reduce the inflammation in your child's skin and muscles. The duration of medication will depend on your child's case. Some complications of corticosteroid therapy can include high blood pressure, effects on growth, and CUSHING'S SYNDROME. Discuss these and other possible side effects with your doctor. If your child's condition does not improve adequately, the doctor may prescribe other drugs that suppress your child's immune system. These drugs, as well as corticosteroids, might make your child more susceptible to infection.

Your child will also need physical therapy to maintain muscle movement while his or her muscles are healing and then to strengthen the muscles after the inflammation has been reduced. With treatment, your child's chances for a complete recovery are good. Some children are left with persistent muscle weakness. A small percentage may need to use a wheelchair. In severe cases, a child could die if the disorder affects his or her lungs and other vital organs.

DEVELOPMENTAL DELAY

Developmental delay means that a child under 5 years of age has not achieved the physical, intellectual, and social development that is normal for his or her age. A child's development proceeds in a predictable fashion, with key milestones, such as sitting up, walking, and talking, occurring within set ranges of time in a child's life. Between birth and age 5, children constantly change and develop their skills in four areas: movement, language, intellect, and sociability. Children vary in the pace at which they develop these skills, but the variations lie within defined limits. For more information about developmental milestones and how to stimulate your child's development as he or she grows, see chapters 1 through 5.

When children shows signs of delay, it may be because they have HEARING LOSS or VISION PROBLEMS that need to be recognized and treated before they can catch up with their peers. But children who are delayed in most areas of development probably have a more general problem, such as limited intelligence, lack of proper stimulation, or a disease that affects development. Whatever the cause, the sooner parents and doctors recognize the problem and treat it, the better off the child will be developmentally.

If your child was born prematurely, keep in mind that he or she may achieve developmental milestones later than other children by roughly the amount of time he or she was born prematurely. For example, if your child was born 1 month early, he or she may begin walking a month later than a child who was born full term. Premature babies should catch up to their peers by age 2.

MOVEMENT SKILLS Motor or movement skills include the ability to sit, crawl, walk, grasp and hold objects, and stack blocks. Your doctor will be able to tell you the approximate age at which your child should achieve these motor skills (see page 100).

For example, a child who can't sit independently by 7 or 8 months of age or walk by 18 months is probably delayed in motor development. Of all the developmental skills, motor skills are the least connected to intelligence. If your child has delayed motor skills, a physical cause, such as SPINA BIFIDA or CEREBRAL PALSEY, is more likely than a mental cause.

Children with motor delay sometimes have other, related delays that contribute to the motor delay. For example, children who are delayed in skills involving hand-eye coordination may have a visual impairment affecting their ability to see and grasp objects. A lack of stimulation in the child's environment can cause a delay in motor skills.

LANGUAGE SKILLS A child's ability to master a language in a few short years is astounding. But language development also follows a predictable pattern. Your child's language development may be delayed if he or she does not begin to babble ("ba ba, da da") by 9 months of age or if he or she speaks fewer than three understandable words by 18 months. Your child should be able to speak two words together by age 2, speak in sentences by age 3, and be almost fully understandable by age 4. A 4-year-old should be able to use prepositions and a 5-year-old should be able to speak in short, grammatically correct sentences.

Deafness is the leading cause of delayed language development in children. Other causes include lack of verbal stimulation at home, a family history of delayed speech, and damage to the muscles and organs involved in speech.

INTELLECTUAL SKILLS Parents may find it difficult to detect intellectual impairment in their child because mild forms of delayed mental abilities are hard to spot. Early signs of delayed intellectual development include a child's failure to repeat an action that evokes a response, such as smiling, by 4 months of age. An infant should look for dropped objects by 7 months and hidden objects by 1 year.

A 2-year-old should be able to recognize and categorize things that are similar (such as animals or cars). By age 3, a child should be able to recognize shapes and colors, and count to 10. A 4-year-old can recognize symbols and draw circles and faces. Five-year-olds can draw stick figures and write their own name.

Inherited disorders, such as FRAGILE X SYNDROME and DOWN SYNDROME, can cause delayed intellectual development. Exposure to infections before or after birth, or an injury in early infancy or childhood are examples of things that can adversely affect a child's intellectual development.

SOCIAL SKILLS A young child's loving and nurturing relationship with his or her parents is the key to social and emotional development. Although each child has his or her own individual temperament, social skills too develop in a predictable pattern that you can follow.

Your child should develop a social smile by 3 months of age and should be laughing by 4 to 5 months of age. Be concerned if your child maintains little or no eye contact with you and refuses to be comforted by you. Other red flags include extreme aggression, lack of interest in people, and repetitive movements.

One cause of delayed social and emotional development is a lack of the right kind of interaction between child and parents. To develop your child's social skills, make sure your child receives plenty of affection, social stimulation, and varied experience, plus consistent guidelines on acceptable ways of behaving.

DEVIATED NASAL SEPTUM

The nasal septum is a wall that divides the inside of the nose into two parts. The nasal septum is made of bone at the back of the nose and cartilage near the tip of the nose. A deviated nasal septum is one that is crooked or out of line. A baby can be born with a deviated septum, but, more frequently, a child gets a deviated septum after receiving a blow or other type of injury to the nose.

SIGNS AND SYMPTOMS Sometimes, the deviation is not noticeable and causes no symptoms. In other cases, a child may have a crooked nose and difficulty breathing because the deviation obstructs the flow of air. An affected child may have chronic nasal drainage, especially during a cold, and be prone to SINUSITIS (inflammation of the sinus cavities). The child's voice may also have a nasal quality.

DIAGNOSIS AND TREATMENT In most cases, the deviation is small, causes no major problems, and needs no treatment. But, if the child has difficulty breathing or chronic nasal congestion, take him or her to the doctor for an evaluation. The doctor may recommend surgery in adolescence to permit unobstructed breathing and relieve symptoms.

DIABETES INSIPIDUS

Diabetes insipidus is a rare hormonal disorder that affects the kidneys and causes an excessive loss of water through the urine. A child with this condition either lacks a hormone known as antidiuretic hormone or has a kidney disorder in which the kidneys fail to respond to the hormone. Antidiuretic hormone, which is produced by the pituitary gland (a pea-sized gland at the base of the brain), causes the kidneys to reabsorb water. The child's pituitary gland may fail to produce antidiuretic hormone because of an infection, surgery, a BRAIN TUMOR, or a head injury. In rare cases, this disorder can be inherited (see GENETIC DISORDERS).

SIGNS AND SYMPTOMS Diabetes insipidus causes a child to urinate copiously, up to 40 pints of urine in 24 hours. He or she also becomes excessively thirsty and drinks a lot of water to replace the water lost through urination. Affected infants who are not given enough water and children who have a faulty thirst mechanism can become severely dehydrated because they don't get enough water to replace the water lost. Some of the signs of dehydration (see page 283) are dry lips and a dry tongue, a lack of tears, dizziness, confusion, a fast heartbeat, and eventually coma (unconsciousness).

DIAGNOSIS If your child has signs of severe dehydration, take him or her to a hospital emergency department immediately for diagnosis and treatment, no matter what the cause. If your infant or child has other symptoms of diabetes insipidus, take him or her to the doctor. The doctor will order blood and urine tests and hormone analyses to pinpoint a diagnosis. In some cases, an affected child may need to be hospitalized for a test known as a water-deprivation test, to assess his or her body's reaction to being deprived of water.

TREATMENT For an infant, the doctor may recommend that you dilute the baby's formula with water and keep records of how much urine your baby passes every day. If your child lacks antidiuretic hormone, the doctor will prescribe a synthetic substitute for the hormone inhaled as a nasal spray. If your child has a kidney disorder that prevents the kidneys from responding to the hormone, the doctor will place your child on a salt-free diet and prescribe other medication to control the condition. In either case, your child will need to take medication for life. You will need to make sure that your child drinks enough water to avoid dehydration.

DIABETES MELLITUS, TYPE I

Type I diabetes mellitus is a hormonal disorder in which a child's pancreas, a small gland in the abdomen just behind the stomach, is unable to produce the hormone insulin. The body needs insulin to absorb glucose, a sugar in digested food that serves as the body's main fuel. The pancreas normally releases insulin in response to glucose levels in a child's blood. When blood glucose levels are high after a meal, the pancreas secretes insulin to allow cells to absorb glucose from the blood. When blood glucose levels fall after the glucose is absorbed, the pancreas stops releasing insulin. Unlike in type II diabetes mellitus (adult type), in which the body's response to insulin is diminished, in type I diabetes mellitus the pancreas is unable to release any insulin.

Type I diabetes is also called insulin-dependent diabetes mellitus or, inaccurately, juvenile-onset diabetes because it can occur at any age, up to about age 35. However, it is most common in children between the ages of 10 and 16 years. The disorder tends to run in families. Medical researchers believe that a viral infection triggers a response in a susceptible child's immune system (the body's natural defense system against infections) that damages the child's pancreas, leaving it unable to produce insulin (see AUTOIMMUNE DISORDERS).

SIGNS AND SYMPTOMS Without insulin, the glucose in a child's blood rises to abnormally high levels. The kidneys are unable to reabsorb the extra glucose, causing extra water and glucose to be in the urine; this results in excessive urination. Excessive urination causes the child to become extremely thirsty. The child also becomes hungry because his or her body needs increased energy. Despite the increased appetite, the child loses weight, becomes weak, and has a general feeling of ill health. Some children experience nausea and vomiting. If the condition goes untreated and the child does not drink sufficient quantities of water, he or she will develop dehydration (see page 283). Acid levels rise in the child's body, causing confusion, changes in consciousness, and vomiting. Without treatment, the child can fall into a diabetic coma and die within a few days or weeks.

DIAGNOSIS The doctor can diagnose type I diabetes mellitus by testing your child's blood and urine for elevated glucose levels. The urine will also be checked for ketones, a by-product of food metabolism produced when glucose is not available. In some cases, along with urine testing for glucose, the blood test for the glucose level is done after an overnight fast or 2 hours after a meal.

TREATMENT Your child will need to take daily injections of insulin for life and the doctor will start the insulin injections soon after diagnosis. Giving your child just the right amount of insulin is important. The doctor will explain how insulin works in the body and will tell you the signs to look for that signal low blood sugar levels (see HYPOGLYCEMIA), which could be caused by giving too much insulin. An overdose of insulin causes irritability, confusion, tremors, sweating, and fainting. Too little insulin can cause the symptoms of diabetes to recur. It may take weeks to adjust the dosage to meet your child's needs and lifestyle. Your child may be hospitalized initially for treatment of his or her symptoms and to determine the proper insulin dosage. After your child is released from the hospital, you will have to give your child the daily insulin injections yourself. When your child is about 10 or 11 years old, he or she can begin administering the injections, under your supervision. By adolescence, he or she can assume complete responsibility for the injections. The doctor will show you and your child how to inject the insulin just under the skin, using a needle and syringe. He or she will also teach you how to check your child's blood for glucose using blood sugar monitoring strips and how to monitor your child's urine glucose levels. You can buy home test kits over the counter for this purpose. You will need to test your child's blood glucose levels every day, usually before meals and before a bedtime snack. Check your child's urine for

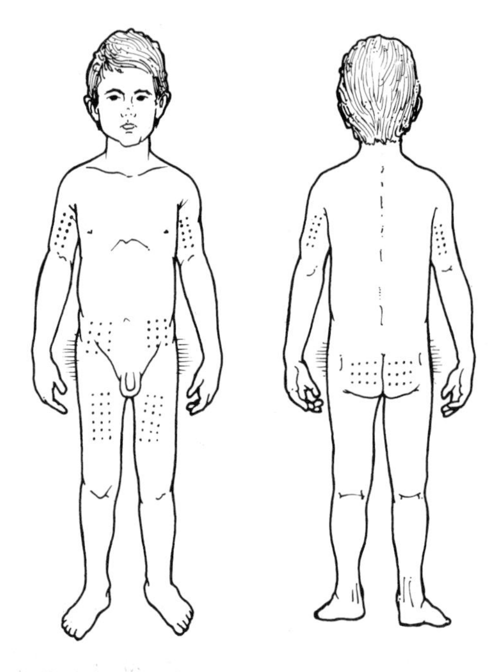

Insulin injection sites

If your child has type I diabetes, he or she needs daily injections of insulin. Rotate the injection sites frequently to reduce the chances of injury to your child's tissues; such injury could affect the absorption of insulin into the body. Injection sites you can use include those in your child's arms, lower abdomen, thighs, and buttocks.

Controlling type I diabetes

To control your child's diabetes and avoid the effects of too much or too little insulin, you will have to teach your child to follow a fairly strict regimen. Your child will need insulin injections and a special diet. The doctor will refer your child to a dietitian who can plan a diet with the right balance of carbohydrates, fats, and protein. The dietitian will recommend that your child eat three meals and three snacks at about the same time each day to keep his or her blood glucose levels steady. He or she should also carry a sugary snack, such as a candy bar, juice, or hard candies, at all times to eat right away in case any of the symptoms of low blood sugar, such as sweating, dizziness, trembling, and irritability, appear. You should also have a glucagon kit in your home in case your child's glucose level becomes too low. Glucagon is a hormone that reverses the effects of insulin and elevates the blood glucose level.

Your child also needs to exercise regularly to control his or her blood glucose levels and insulin requirements. Exercise also helps burn off excess fat and calories so your child can maintain his or her ideal weight. Notify your child's school, family, and friends of his or her condition so they can recognize the signs of too much or too little insulin. Your child should always wear a medical identification tag in case of an emergency.

D

ketones or glucose when his or her blood glucose levels go over a certain level or when he or she is sick. Your child will also need a special diet and exercise program to keep his or her diabetes in check (see box).

Long-term complications of diabetes mellitus include kidney disease, nerve damage, and impaired vision. An affected child is prone to developing hardening of the arteries and other heart diseases (such as HIGH BLOOD PRESSURE) later in life.

Good foot care is important for diabetic children because the disease can damage nerves and blood vessels in the feet. Small cuts and scrapes can easily become infected, increasing the chances of gangrene (tissue death) in severe cases. Instruct your child to put on clean cotton socks every day, change damp shoes and socks promptly, keep toenails short (see page 536), and wash and dry his or her feet thoroughly. Check your child's feet every day for cuts and scrapes.

It may be difficult for you to accept that your child has a chronic disorder that needs daily management. Learn as much as you can about diabetes so you can help your child keep his or her blood sugar levels steady. Join a support group of other parents with diabetic children and encourage your child to participate in group activities with other diabetic children. With treatment, diet, and self-monitoring, your child can expect to live a long and normal life.

DIPHTHERIA

Diphtheria is a serious, life-threatening bacterial infection that is spread through coughing or sneezing and affects a child's mouth, throat, nose, or skin. Once a leading cause of death among infants and children, diphtheria is now an extremely rare illness in the United States, thanks to an immunization program against diphtheria that began in the late 1940s.

SIGNS AND SYMPTOMS One type of diphtheria attacks the nose and throat, producing a thin, gray membrane of tissue that covers the throat and can interfere with swallowing and breathing. Two to 4 days after infection, a sore throat, slight fever, chills, and swollen glands in the neck follow. A second type of diphtheria that affects the skin causes scabs, sores, or pimples that may be swollen, red, and painful. Unchecked, the diphtheria bacteria produce a powerful poison that spreads through the child's body, ultimately causing PNEUMONIA, paralysis, heart failure, or suffocation.

Diagnosis If you see symptoms of diphtheria in your child, take him or her to your doctor who will order a throat *culture* and blood tests to confirm the diagnosis.

Treatment A confirmed case of diphtheria is a medical emergency. Your doctor will hospitalize and isolate your child to prevent spreading the disease. Your child will receive a diphtheria *antitoxin,* which neutralizes the poison, and antibiotics to fight the bacteria. The child may need bed rest for 2 or 3 months if the poison has spread throughout the body. Everyone in your household in contact with your sick child may be contagious. If family members have already been immunized, they will be given a booster shot. If not, they will receive antibiotics.

Down syndrome

Down syndrome is a common inherited BIRTH DEFECT caused by a CHROMOSOMAL ABNORMALITY. Children with Down syndrome have an extra chromosome (chromosome number 21) in the cells of their bodies. The extra chromosome may exist on its own or be abnormally attached to another chromosome. A baby with Down syndrome is born with mental impairment and characteristic physical traits. These children have a life expectancy that is at least 15 to 20 years less than unaffected children. Most do not survive beyond age 55, although some adults with Down syndrome have lived into their 80s. Women who conceive children after age 35 are at higher risk of having a baby with Down syndrome than are younger women.

Signs and symptoms The symptoms of Down syndrome can vary from mild to severe. Infants with Down syndrome have poor muscle tone, and their movements appear floppy. Children with Down syndrome have eyes that slope upward at the outer corners and ears that are small and folded over slightly at the top. Their facial features tend to be small, especially their mouths, which make their tongues look large and protruding. The back of their head and the bridge of their nose are flat. They have short necks, small hands, and short fingers. Many are small for their age and exhibit delays in physical and mental development.

All children with Down syndrome have some degree of MENTAL RETARDATION, with below-normal IQs ranging from 30 to 80. Up to half of these children are born with heart defects (see HEART DISEASE, CONGENITAL). They may also have HEARING LOSS and VISION PROBLEMS. Intestinal obstruction can also occur shortly after birth. Down syndrome children tend to get LEUKEMIA, PNEUMONIA, and ear infections (see page 480) more often than other children.

Diagnosis The unusual physical characteristics of Down syndrome children are apparent at birth. Your doctor will confirm the diagnosis with blood

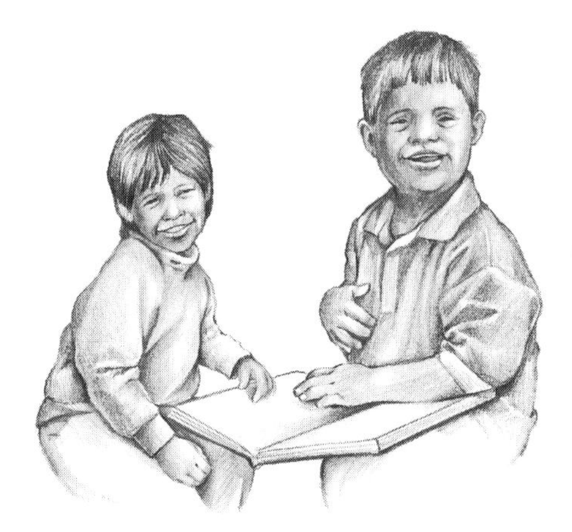

Children with Down syndrome

A child with Down syndrome usually gets along well with others. Affected children (such as the child on the right) tend to be friendly, affectionate, and good-natured. They can be active and loving members of the family.

Living with Down syndrome

If your child has Down syndrome, he or she can learn to do most of the things that other children do, including walking, talking, dressing himself or herself, going to school, and possibly even holding a job when he or she gets older. But your child will take longer to learn these skills and will need special education and training. Many children with Down syndrome can learn to read and write, and some can eventually join mainstream classrooms while receiving special education. Those who don't find a job after finishing school often enter special state-sponsored jobs programs.

In rare cases, people with Down syndrome get married. Having children is risky because a woman with Down syndrome has a 50 percent chance of having a child with Down syndrome. Men with Down syndrome usually cannot father a child.

Severely retarded children with Down syndrome may need to live in extended-care facilities when they become adolescents or adults if they can't be cared for at home. Others may live at home, attend school, and grow up to live relatively independent lives.

tests that detect the extra chromosome. Down syndrome can also be detected in a fetus before birth through *amniocentesis* or *chorionic villus sampling* (see Genetic testing, page 498). A blood test given during pregnancy that shows a low level of a protein know as alpha-fetoprotein will alert your doctor to the need for genetic testing. A family history of Down syndrome and a mother's advanced age may prompt a doctor to advise genetic testing.

TREATMENT There is no cure and no method of prevention for Down syndrome. A Down syndrome child needs the same basic medical care as any other child. Your child's doctor will treat any complications of Down syndrome as they arise. Children with Down syndrome are at increased risk of spinal instability in the neck region. They should have an X-ray of the neck between 1 and 2 years of age, and then once every 3 to 5 years to make sure the spine is stable, especially before any gymnastic activity. Work with your doctor to learn about the special educational needs of your Down syndrome child and how these needs can be met in your community. Genetic counseling (see page 497) can enable you as a prospective parent to understand the risks of having a child with Down syndrome.

D

DRUG AND ALCOHOL ABUSE

Drug and alcohol abuse means the overuse or misuse of alcohol and other drugs to such an extent that the behavior causes physical, psychological, or social problems. The reasons children and teens start using drugs and alcohol vary but include peer pressure, curiosity, escapism, rebelling against authority, or mood alteration. Drugs and alcohol can become physically and emotionally addictive and can cause changes in mood and behavior, serious health problems, and even death. Children are more likely to abuse drugs and alcohol if they have a family history of drug or alcohol abuse; feel that they do not fit in with their peers; are naturally defiant, aggressive, or impulsive; have parents who often fight, are absent a lot, or are too strict or lenient; have suffered sexual abuse (see page 326) or started having sex at an early age; have low self-esteem; or have friends who abuse alcohol or other drugs.

Children in grammar school and early adolescence sometimes use chemical inhalants to get high because the substances are legal and easy to obtain. Some of the commonly used inhalants include airplane glue, hair spray in aerosol cans, whipped cream in aerosol cans, gasoline, cleaning fluids, liquid correction fluid, and paint thinner. Inhalants and alcohol are known as "gateway" drugs because they introduce the child to the feeling of getting high and can lead to the use of drugs such as marijuana, cocaine, amphetamines, barbiturates, heroin, or LSD.

Signs and symptoms Drug and alcohol abuse can cause many physical signs and symptoms, depending on the substance used. Bloodshot eyes, dilated or constricted pupils, disorientation, confusion, weight loss, hallucination, dizziness, difficulty sleeping, irregular heartbeat (see ARRHYTHMIAS), and rapid breathing may occur. Drug and alcohol abuse can also delay or stop physical or mental growth in children and adolescents. Substance abuse leads to other types of risky behavior, such as reckless driving, injuring others, and having sex without adequate protection against sexually transmitted diseases or pregnancy (see page 185). Children may perform poorly in school and can become involved in criminal acts, such as theft, to obtain the money for drugs.

Diagnosis and treatment As soon as you notice any signs of drug or alcohol abuse in your child or teenager, get help from your child's doctor or a drug abuse counselor. The earlier you seek help, the better your child's chances are for recovery. If you notice any of these symptoms in friends of your child, talk to your child about his or her own use of drugs and alcohol. Should your child become dizzy, confused, hallucinate, have difficulty breathing, develop an irregular heartbeat, or become unconscious, take him or her to an emergency department immediately.

Once addicted, your child will need counseling in a special program for drug and alcohol dependence run by a hospital or drug treatment center. Children can usually be treated on an *outpatient* basis, but your child may need to be hospitalized or admitted to a residential treatment center if outpatient treatment fails. Most outpatient programs include group therapy with other children or teens. Family therapy is sometimes necessary to find out and work through the causes of substance abuse.

Recovery may be slow and the process painful, depending on how much your child has abused drugs and alcohol. Relapse is possible. Your child will need your constant support and encouragement throughout his or her treatment. For tips on helping your child resist drugs and alcohol, see page 196.

Dwarfism

Dwarfism is a group of disorders marked by extremely short stature (see HEIGHT PROBLEMS). The condition can be inherited but, in 80 percent of all cases, the parents are of average height and there is no family history of dwarfism. Dwarfism can be caused by defects in bone formation, growth hormone deficiency, or inability of the body to respond to the hormones responsible for growth.

Signs and symptoms Children with abnormalities caused by cartilage, connective tissue, or bone malformation are recognizable at birth. The child is disproportionately small, with short, deformed arms and legs; a comparatively long body; and a large head. The forehead may be prominent or bulge out. Some children have HYDROCEPHALUS. The child's nose may be turned up, the jaw protrude, and the eyes be deep-set. He or she may have prominent buttocks from a curvature of the spine and have an abdomen that appears comparatively long. He or she has small hands and feet and stubby fingers and toes.

Some affected babies die at birth or in early infancy. Children who survive grow to about 4 feet with disproportionate features. They may have DEVELOPMENTAL DELAY in motor (movement) skills, such as crawling and walking. They also have frequent ear infections (see page 480). Some of these children may have speech problems in early childhood, but the problems usually disappear by the time they go to school. Most have normal intelligence and will lead independent lives in adulthood. Children with growth hormone problems may not stop growing until they are about 2 years old.

Diagnosis and treatment A doctor will usually be able to diagnose disproportionate dwarfism in a child at birth or shortly after. Sometimes a diagnosis can be made before birth using an *ultrasound.* An affected child may need physical therapy and a spinal brace in early childhood. Surgery to correct bowing of the legs may be needed during adolescence. All ear infections need to be treated with antibiotics immediately to prevent HEARING LOSS. Many affected children live a normal life span.

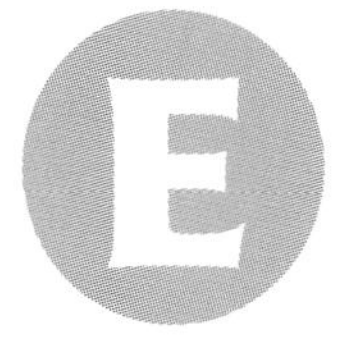

EAR ABNORMALITIES, CONGENITAL

Congenital ear abnormalities are malformations of the outer, middle, or inner ear that are present at birth. These malformations can develop before birth or from an injury during birth. They can affect both the appearance and function of a newborn's ears.

The outer part of the ear connects to a canal or tube that leads to the eardrum, a thin membrane that vibrates when hit by sound waves. Three small bones in the middle ear pass the sound waves on to another thin membrane, the inner ear membrane. Structures in the inner ear turn the vibrations into electrical impulses that travel through a nerve to the brain. The structures of a fetus's inner ear develop during the first half of its 9-month gestation period, but the structures of the middle and outer ear are still growing at birth.

Congenital ear abnormalities range from ears that stick out to damage to the inner structures of the ear that can affect a baby's hearing (see HEARING LOSS). Damage to the structures of the ear can be inherited (see GENETIC DISORDERS) or can occur from an injury at birth; from maternal infections during pregnancy; or from exposure to radiation, alcohol and other drugs, or certain antibiotics before birth.

SIGNS AND SYMPTOMS Malformations of the outer ear include ears that stick out or are abnormally small or low-set. In rare cases, a baby may be born with no external ear. Other visible abnormalities include an extremely narrow or no ear canal or abnormally large earlobes. Structural abnormalities of the ear canal or middle and inner ear can produce mild to total hearing loss. The first sign of hearing loss may be when the baby fails to turn his or her head or move his or her eyes in response to your voice or other sounds (see page 71). The hearing-impaired infant may not be able to make simple sounds or babble at the proper time.

DIAGNOSIS The doctor will be able to detect abnormalities of the outer ear in a newborn during a physical examination. If your baby has unusually shaped or positioned ears or signs of hearing loss, talk to your doctor. He or she may refer you to an otolaryngologist (an ear, nose, and throat specialist) for an assessment. The otolaryngologist will examine your child's ears with special viewing instruments and order tests of your baby's hearing.

TREATMENT The doctor or otolaryngologist will try to determine the exact cause of your baby's hearing loss or ear abnormalities and recommend appropriate treatment. Structural abnormalities in the inner ear usually cannot be treated. Malformed outer ears can sometimes be corrected by cosmetic surgery. If your baby has some hearing loss, he or she may need a hearing aid or a cochlear implant (see page 510). Your child may also need speech and language therapy and special education classes in school. The sooner you have your baby treated for hearing problems, the better, because hearing loss can affect language development and school performance.

EAR INFECTIONS

See page 480

EATING DISORDERS

See Anorexia nervosa; Bulimia; Obesity; Overeating

ECZEMA

See Atopic dermatitis

ENCEPHALITIS

Encephalitis is an inflammation of the brain most commonly caused by a viral infection. The most common virus that causes encephalitis is herpes simplex virus 1, which also causes COLD SORES. Encephalitis can also be caused by the virus that causes MUMPS; the coxsackievirus, which causes HAND-FOOT-AND-MOUTH DISEASE; and the human immunodeficiency virus, which causes AIDS. In warm weather, mosquitoes carry a virus that can cause encephalitis in children and adults. Bacteria, a fungus, parasites, and other microorganisms (for example, those causing tuberculosis or syphilis) can also cause encephalitis. In rare cases, encephalitis can arise as a complication of other viral diseases, such as MEASLES or CHICKENPOX or from ingestion of a poison, such as lead. Often the membranes that surround the brain, known as the meninges, also become inflamed.

SIGNS AND SYMPTOMS Children with mild cases of encephalitis may have no symptoms or only mild symptoms, such as a fever, HEADACHES, and a general feeling of ill health. More serious cases of encephalitis can produce significant swelling of the brain, resulting in unconsciousness, seizures, vomiting, personality changes, paralysis on one side of the body, difficulty speaking and remembering things, double vision, and disorientation. If the meninges are affected, the child may have a stiff neck and his or her eyes may become very sensitive to light. Severe cases can be fatal.

DIAGNOSIS If your child has symptoms of encephalitis, take your child to the doctor immediately. The doctor may order *magnetic resonance imaging* or *computed tomography* of your child's brain, an electroencephalogram (a test that measures the electrical activity of the brain), and blood tests. To determine the type of infection and its cause, the doctor will take a sample of the fluid surrounding the child's brain and spinal cord and send it to a laboratory for analysis. In rare cases, a brain *biopsy* may be needed to identify the cause of encephalitis.

TREATMENT If encephalitis is left untreated, a child can fall into a coma. If your child is diagnosed and treated before falling into a coma, the chances of recovery are good. Encephalitis caused by the herpes simplex virus is treated with an antiviral drug, such as acyclovir, given *intravenously* for about 10 days in a hospital. Treatment for other types of encephalitis depend on the cause. Permanent brain damage or death sometimes occurs in infants and younger children who get encephalitis, but older children usually recover slowly in 2 to 3 weeks without complications. Mild cases may come and go without being identified.

ENCOPRESIS

Encopresis is a disorder in which a child over the age of 4 years involuntarily passes feces into his or her underwear. The condition can occur either before or after toilet training. Encopresis results from chronic constipation that builds up large amounts of hard stool in the child's bowel that becomes difficult or painful to pass. Causes of encopresis include opposition to or fear of toilet use, decreased sensation in the rectum, excessive activity (the child won't sit still long enough to use the toilet), or stress.

SIGNS AND SYMPTOMS A child with encopresis finds it painful to have a bowel movement.

Although the child is constipated, he or she often passes watery stools that leak around the hard stool built up in the bowel. The child may feel embarrassed around other people because the frequent soiling causes a foul odor.

DIAGNOSIS The doctor will examine a child with symptoms of encopresis for signs of an underlying disorder. The doctor will feel your child's abdomen to check for hard stools in the bowel. He or she may also perform a rectal examination to check for hard stools.

TREATMENT The doctor may recommend that you give your child enemas or rectal suppositories for several days to clear the bowel. Stool softeners may be prescribed for a month or two and then are gradually withdrawn when the child establishes a regular bowel routine. You need to encourage your child to move his or her bowels on a regular schedule every day, usually after meals. Give your child a high-fiber diet and plenty of liquids to soften the stools so that he or she can pass them painlessly.

If your doctor suspects that stress has caused your child's encopresis, be sensitive to your child's feelings and try to help him or her through the situation by encouraging him or her to talk about it. Try not to overemphasize toilet training. Your child should outgrow this problem with treatment. About 30 percent of affected children have an underlying emotional problem, so the doctor may refer your child to a child psychiatrist or other mental health professional.

ENDOCARDITIS

Endocarditis is an infection of the valves in the heart or the lining of the heart caused by bacteria or a fungus. This rare heart infection most often occurs in children with heart defects present at birth; previous rheumatic heart disease; defective, scarred, or artificial heart valves; and previous endocarditis or heart surgery. It can also occur in young people who inject drugs with dirty needles.

The main source of infection is bacteria that has invaded the bloodstream (BACTEREMIA) during dental or other types of surgery or diagnostic procedures performed on the heart, nose and throat, urinary tract, or intestines. The bacteria lodge in the heart and damage the heart valves and lining. Infected blood clots form on the heart valves and can dislodge and travel through the bloodstream to the brain, lungs, kidneys, or spleen. Untreated, endocarditis can cause permanent damage to the heart, brain, and other organs; heart failure; and death.

SIGNS AND SYMPTOMS Endocarditis produces fever, unusual fatigue, loss of appetite, shortness of breath, headache, chills, night sweats, aching joints, and a general feeling of ill health. The symptoms may develop slowly or suddenly. If they develop slowly, the child may have a fever for weeks before other symptoms occur. Eventually, small, dark lines (called splinter hemorrhages) appear under the child's fingertips. Infected blood clots on the child's heart valves can cause a heart murmur (an abnormal sound heard in the heart). The child may also develop a rapid or irregular heartbeat as the disease progresses. The spleen may enlarge and the child's feet and legs may become swollen.

DIAGNOSIS Your doctor will ask if your child has a history of heart disease or heart deformities and will perform a thorough physical examination. To identify the source of infection, the doctor will order a series of blood *cultures.* An erythrocyte sedimentation rate test that measures the amount of inflammation in the heart valves, a *complete blood cell count,* and a urine test will also be done to check for infection. The doctor may also order X-rays of the heart and lungs, an *electrocardiogram* (which measures the electrical activity of the heart), or an *echocardiogram* (an image of the heart made with sound waves, or *ultrasound*).

EAR INFECTIONS

After colds, ear infections are the most common childhood illness. By age 3, four out of five children have had at least one ear infection, but most of these infections clear up with antibiotic treatment. Ear infections are most common between the ages of 6 months and 1 year. Then they occur less and less frequently and usually stop when the child reaches about 5 years of age. Some children have a tendency to develop frequent ear infections that, even when treated, can lead to complications such as hearing loss. Extended hearing loss during the years when a child is learning to talk can cause delays in speech and language development.

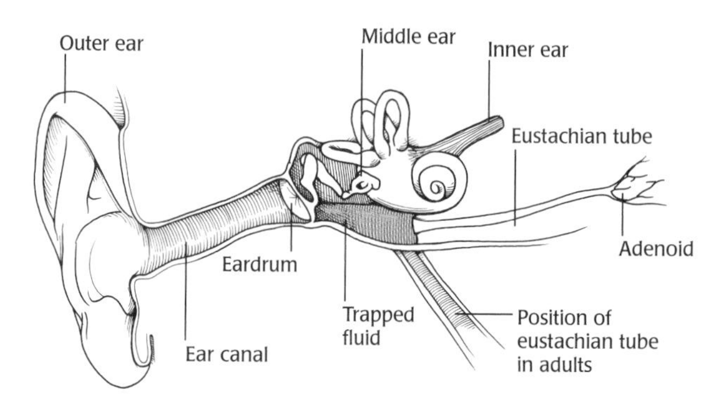

How do ear infections develop?

A child's ear has three main parts—the outer, middle, and inner ear. A channel called the eustachian tube connects the middle ear to the back of the child's throat and nose. When a child has a nose or throat infection, a cold, or an allergy, the eustachian tube can become blocked, causing fluid to build up in the middle ear (shaded area). A child's eustachian tubes are more prone to blockage because they are smaller and more horizontal than those of adults, making drainage more difficult. The backed-up fluid in the middle ear can become infected by bacteria or, more rarely, by a virus, causing the eardrum to swell and the ear to become painful. This type of ear infection is called otitis media, which means middle ear infection.

Is your child at risk?

The following factors can raise a child's chances of developing ear infections:

- Being in a group child care setting, which increases exposure to other children's germs, causing more frequent upper respiratory infections.
- Being around people who smoke, because exposure to secondhand smoke increases the risk of respiratory infections and respiratory tract inflammation.
- Having previous ear infections, especially before the first birthday.
- Having a family history of frequent ear infections (in siblings or parents).
- Being bottle-fed rather than breast-fed. Breast milk provides some increased immunity against ear infections. Also, if a bottle-fed child is given a bottle while lying down, formula can pool in the back of his or her throat, causing congestion and blocking adequate drainage of the eustachian tubes, the tubes that connect the child's throat and ears.
- Being a boy or Native American or Inuit. For unknown reasons, these groups tend to have more middle ear infections.
- Having a cleft palate, a skull or throat malformation, or Down syndrome, all of which change the anatomy of the eustachian tubes.
- Having a weakened immune system from an inherited or congenital (present at birth) defect, from drugs that suppress the immune system, or from a disease such as AIDS.

You can reduce some of these risk factors. For example, you can breast-feed your child, bottle-feed him or her sitting up, keep him or her away from tobacco smoke, and reduce his or her risk of colds and other respiratory infections by keeping his or her hands and face clean.

Symptoms

It's important to be able to recognize the symptoms of an ear infection so that you can get medical treatment for your child quickly. Your child's doctor will decide whether you should bring the child in and what kind of treatment he or she will need. Call the doctor when you first notice the following symptoms:

- **Pain** A young child may pull on his or her ear or become fussy and irritable, especially during feedings or bedtime.
- **Fever** The temperature might range from 101°F to 104°F.
- **Fluid draining from an ear** The fluid could be yellow or white and may be tinged with blood or have a bad odor.
- **Difficulty hearing** Fluid buildup in the middle ear can interfere with the transmission of sound to the brain. Hearing loss could linger after the infection has cleared up if fluid remains in the ear.
- **Dizziness or ringing in the ears** Older children may feel dizzy or hear ringing in the ear.

Telltale signs of ear pain

Your young child may not be able to tell you that his or her ear hurts, so be alert for telltale signs. The pain may cause the child to tug on his or her ear or become more fussy and irritable than usual.

How are ear infections treated?

To avoid potential problems such as hearing loss, ask the doctor to examine your child whenever he or she has any symptoms of an ear infection. If the doctor diagnoses an ear infection, he or she may recommend one or more of the following treatments:

- Antibiotics can kill the types of bacteria that usually cause ear infections. If your doctor prescribes an antibiotic, follow his or her instructions closely and give your child the entire prescription (see page 278). Otherwise, some of the bacteria might remain and cause another infection. Avoid over-the-counter cold medications (decongestants or antihistamines); they don't help clear up ear infections.
- Pain relievers such as acetaminophen or ibuprofen can reduce pain and discomfort. Never give your child aspirin because it has been linked to a life-threatening condition called Reye's syndrome (see page 609).
- Warm, damp cloths placed against the child's ear can help relieve pain. Don't use compresses while your child is sleeping or if the child is under 12 months of age because of the risk of a burn.

E

What if my child has frequent ear infections?

For children who get more than three ear infections in 6 months, doctors sometimes prescribe a low-dose antibiotic taken each day for 1 to 6 months. This treatment carries some risk. Taking antibiotics in this way may promote the growth of bacteria that are resistant to antibiotics (see page 278). You and your doctor should discuss the risks and benefits involved in this type of treatment.

Another treatment for persistent or recurring ear infections is a surgical procedure called tympanostomy, in which tiny tubes are placed in the eardrum to drain fluid from the middle ear. A tympanostomy tube can restore hearing and relieve pain and can prevent fluid from reaccumulating and causing another ear infection. Like any surgical procedure, tympanostomy carries some risk. In addition to the risks of general anesthesia, the tubes sometimes cause scarring or leave a hole in the eardrum.

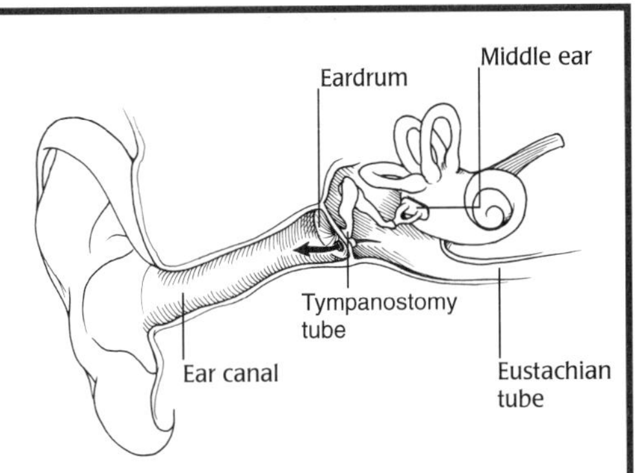

How are the tubes put into my child's ear?

A small slit is made in each of the child's eardrums and fluid is suctioned out of the middle ear. A small plastic tube is placed into each slit. The tubes stay in place from 6 to 18 months and either fall out or are removed by the doctor.

Antibiotics before surgery

Children who have heart disease that was present at birth, a defective heart valve, a heart murmur, or a history of endocarditis are at increased risk of endocarditis during any type of surgery, tooth extractions, or even tooth cleanings. Be sure to tell your doctor and dentist if your child has had any of these conditions and request that he or she be given antibiotics before any procedure that involves cutting into the body so that endocarditis can be prevented. Your child should also wear a medical identification necklace or bracelet that describes his or her medical condition to alert medical personnel in an emergency. The tag explains that he or she should be given antibiotics before any surgery.

TREATMENT Your doctor will probably put your child in the hospital and administer antibiotics *intravenously*. The child will have to remain on antibiotics for 2 to 6 weeks, depending on the type of bacteria causing the endocarditis. Your child may receive the antibiotic therapy in the hospital the entire time or possibly under your care at home. Some children may require surgery to replace infected heart valves.

Once the child returns home, he or she will need to rest until fully recovered. Encourage your child to flex his or her legs often, to prevent blood clots from forming in the veins, if he or she has been in bed for a long time . When your child regains strength, he or she can resume normal activities. Your child will receive follow-up care from your doctor to prevent a relapse of the condition.

ENTEROCOLITIS

See Necrotizing enterocolitis

EPILEPSY

See Seizure disorders

ERYTHEMA MULTIFORME

Erythema multiforme is a severe skin RASH that occurs most often in children over 3 years of age. Most cases do not affect a child's overall health and clear up with treatment, but some cases can have serious complications. The rash sometimes appears as a reaction to certain drugs, including penicillin, sulfa (antibacterial) drugs, and drugs used to treat convulsions. It can accompany viral infections, especially COLD SORES or bacterial infections such as STREP INFECTIONS in the throat. Other possible causes include vaccinations, exposure to *radiation*, or pregnancy. At least half of all cases have no known cause.

SIGNS AND SYMPTOMS The main symptom is a rash made up of red spots that itch. Some spots look like a bull's eye, with red rings around a pale center, but the redness does not extend as far as it does in LYME DISEASE. The rash occurs mainly on a child's arms and legs but sometimes breaks out on the entire body, including the face. The rash sometimes becomes raised, like HIVES.

A child with erythema multiforme may also have a sore throat, muscle aches, fever, diarrhea, and HEADACHES. Erythema multiforme can progress to a more serious form of the condition known as Stevens-Johnson syndrome, in which mucous membranes in the mouth, eyes, digestive tract, and genitals become red and swollen and develop open sores. If Stevens-Johnson syndrome remains untreated, it can spread throughout the body and cause your child to go into shock (see page 678), a dangerous condition characterized by dizziness or fainting, vomiting, pale skin, weakness, rapid breathing and heart rate, and very low blood pressure.

DIAGNOSIS Your child's doctor will probably be able to diagnose erythema multiforme from a physical examination. He or she will order a *biopsy* of tissue from an open sore to find out if the condition has progressed to Stevens-Johnson syndrome.

TREATMENT Your child's doctor will treat erythema multiforme brought on by drugs or infections by discontinuing drug treatment or treating the underlying infection. The doctor may also prescribe *corticosteroids* to reduce the inflammation and antihistamines to relieve itching. You can place warm, moist cloths on the rash and on surrounding areas to soothe the irritation. The rash should clear up in 2 to 4 weeks but could recur.

If your child's condition has progressed to Stevens-Johnson syndrome, he or she will have to be admitted to the hospital so the doctor can administer fluids *intravenously* and give pain medication. A child with Stevens-Johnson syndrome is at increased risk of bacterial infection of the skin because of the open sores produced by the disorder, so your child's doctor will closely watch him or her for signs of infection.

EWING'S SARCOMA

Ewing's sarcoma is a cancer of the bones that most frequently occurs in children and adolescents between the ages of 10 and 20. Boys are twice as likely to get Ewing's sarcoma as girls. It most commonly affects a child's pelvis, upper arm bone, thighbone, shinbone, rib bones, spinal vertebrae, or shoulder blades.

Ewing's sarcoma may occur in only one spot or spread from one spot to other parts of the body, most often to a child's lungs, other bones, or the bone marrow (the tissue inside bone in which blood cells are manufactured). This form of childhood cancer may also recur after it has been treated. Recurrent Ewing's sarcoma can reappear in the bone where it first occurred or in other parts of the child's body.

SIGNS AND SYMPTOMS Pain and tenderness in the affected bone are the most common signs of Ewing's sarcoma. The pain may be severe or dull and could either come and go or be continuous. The area around your child's bone might swell up and feel warm to the touch. Very rarely, a fever and weight loss accompany the other symptoms.

Your child may have trouble sleeping at night because of the pain. If the cancer occurs in your child's legs or arms, he or she may have difficulty walking or moving his or her affected limbs.

DIAGNOSIS Call your child's doctor if your child experiences any pain or tenderness in his or her bones. As with all cancers, the sooner Ewing's sarcoma is diagnosed and treated, the better are your child's chances of surviving.

Your child's doctor will examine your child's arms and legs for warmth, tenderness, swelling, or a lump. If the doctor suspects cancer, he or she will refer your child to a cancer specialist (oncologist) for diagnosis. Cancer specialists typically use X-rays to detect Ewing's sarcoma. The specialist may also do a surgical bone *biopsy* to determine the exact nature of the cancer. During this procedure, the surgeon will look at the bone and take a sample for testing. Your child will be under general anesthesia (see page 292).

Your child may also have to undergo *computed tomography* so the oncologist can find out if the cancer has spread to other parts of his or her body. To detect any new cancers, the doctor may also do a *radionuclide scan*, in which a trace amount of radioactive substances called radionuclides are injected into your child's vein. The radionuclides emit a small amount of radiation that is detected by a special kind of camera, which produces an image of your child's bone structure on a screen.

TREATMENT Your child will receive combination therapy—surgery, *chemotherapy*, and *radiation*—to treat his or her Ewing's sarcoma. Your child's chances of surviving the disease depend on where the cancer is located, how long it has developed, and whether it has spread. With combination therapy and early treatment, many children who get the disease survive for 5 years or longer.

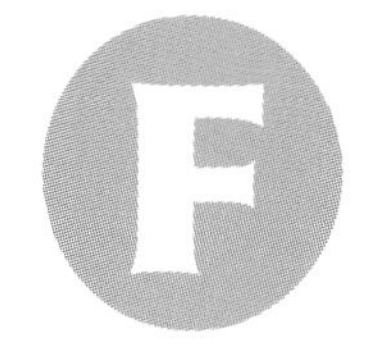

FACIAL DEFORMITIES, CONGENITAL

Congenital facial deformities are malformations of a baby's facial features that are present at birth. A large number of congenital deformities that develop before birth can affect a baby's face and head. Some are inherited (see GENETIC DISORDERS), while others occur as a result of damage to the fetus. Some occur spontaneously during fetal development without a known cause. The most common congenital facial deformities are CLEFT LIP AND CLEFT PALATE, in which a newborn has an abnormally separated upper lip, palate (roof of the mouth), or both.

TYPES OF FACIAL DEFORMITIES Facial deformities can affect the look and shape of a newborn baby's mouth, lips, jaws, cheekbones, nose, eyes, and forehead. Most of these malformations are rare.

Hemifacial microsomia This is a congenital deformity in which an infant is born with small facial features on only one side. The deformity can affect the entire side of the baby's face or just certain parts, such as the jaws, cheekbone, facial muscles, and ear.

Dysostosis Dysostosis is a congenital deformity that affects a baby's skull and face (known as craniofacial dysostosis) or face and jaws (known as mandibulofacial dysostosis). In craniofacial dysostosis, the skull joins together abnormally, causing one part of the child's skull or face to grow out of proportion to the rest of the head or face. Other facial features are affected as well. The eyes may be spaced far apart with a downward slant to the eyelids, one eye may turn out, the lower jaw may protrude beyond the upper jaw, or the lower lip may stick out. The face and hands of a fetus develop at the same time, so the baby may also have deformities of his or her hands and feet, such as webbed fingers or toes.

In a baby with mandibulofacial dysostosis, the face and jaws are affected. The baby may have a large nose that looks like a beak, deformed ears (see EAR ABNORMALITIES, CONGENITAL), flat cheeks, a large mouth, and a lower jaw that recedes under the upper jaw. The baby may also have HEARING LOSS from the ear abnormalities.

Ocular hypertelorism and hypotelorism These congenital deformities affect the sockets of a baby's eyes. Ocular hypertelorism means that the eye sockets are set too far apart, while ocular hypotelorism means that they are set too close together. The shape of the eye sockets may be unusual and the baby may have crossed eyes or other eye abnormalities (see VISION PROBLEMS).

Encephalocele Encephalocele is a congenital deformity in which an infant's brain actually protrudes out from the skull into a sac or pouch in the forehead or elsewhere on the head. It can cause the baby's eye sockets to be set far apart and widen the bridge of the nose.

DIAGNOSIS The doctor will be able to detect congenital facial deformities during a routine examination. The baby will be referred to an otolaryngologist (ear, nose, and throat specialist) who will examine the child and order diagnostic tests that can include X-rays, *computed tomography*, and hearing tests. For an encephalocele, your child will be referred to a neurosurgeon for evaluation and treatment.

TREATMENT Depending on the specific deformity and its symptoms, an affected child may need treatment from a variety of specialists. Many facial deformities can be corrected or at least improved by surgery. It is best to have corrective surgery done early in the child's life. The child may need a series of operations over months or years to correct the facial deformities, and the operations can involve taking bone and other tissue from other parts of the child's body to reconstruct the face. In addition to surgery, the child may need care from an orthodontist (a dentist who specializes in misalignment of the teeth), eye care from an ophthalmologist (an eye specialist), and speech therapy if the child has any hearing loss. If you have a child with congenital facial abnormalities, you should seek genetic counseling (see page 497) before having any more children.

FAILURE TO THRIVE

Failure to thrive refers to infants and children who do not grow at the expected rate for their age and sex. It most often affects children under 5 years of age, especially those under age 2. Inadequate nutrition or insufficient emotional stimulation from parental neglect, poverty, inexperience at child rearing, abuse (see page 323), or rejection of the child can cause failure to thrive. The condition can also be caused by an underlying disease or by disease combined with neglect. Children born prematurely or with a physical deformity that affects their ability to feed, such as CLEFT LIP AND CLEFT PALATE, may fail to thrive. Infants born to mothers who smoked, drank alcohol, or used street drugs such as cocaine during pregnancy may also fail to thrive. The condition can also occur in children adopted from a developing country, especially if they have been institutionalized in an orphanage.

Chronic diseases or disorders that can cause failure to thrive include DOWN SYNDROME, diabetes (see DIABETES MELLITUS, TYPE I), congenital heart disease (see HEART DISEASE, CONGENITAL), SICKLE CELL ANEMIA, CEREBRAL PALSY, a long-term infection, and diseases that affect the ability to absorb food, such as CYSTIC FIBROSIS and CELIAC DISEASE.

Poverty, ignorance, inexperience in raising children, stress, and drug and alcohol addiction can affect a parent's ability to provide adequate physical nourishment and emotional stimulation to a child. If a parent rejects, withdraws from, or is hostile or violent toward the infant or child, the child may fail to thrive.

SIGNS AND SYMPTOMS Affected children are underweight for their age and sex, may have a smaller head size, and may be shorter than normal (see page 238). Their rate of growth is slowed or negligible. They may also have DEVELOPMENTAL DELAY or be unusually thirsty, urinate frequently, and have particularly bad-smelling stools. They may also throw up partially digested food and chew it and swallow it again (see RUMINATION). In extreme cases, children with the condition may look limp and have pale or dry skin. If emotionally neglected, some may bang their heads or rock back and forth constantly to stimulate themselves. Others may be extremely or inappropriately clingy to caregivers. Children who fail to thrive because of a chronic disease also exhibit the symptoms of that disease.

DIAGNOSIS If your child does not seem to be growing at the expected rate, the doctor may diagnose failure to thrive during a routine examination. Your child's doctor will weigh and measure your child and compare the findings with the measurements on standard growth charts (see page 239) and your child's previous measurements. He or she will also evaluate your child for delayed development. You will need to give your child's doctor a thorough family history of any diseases or emotional problems in the family, such as child abuse. The doctor will order various tests, including blood, urine, and stool tests, to rule out any underlying disease or infections that could cause the delayed growth. If your infant is not thriving, your child's doctor may observe you or your partner and your infant during feedings to try to determine if the problem lies in the way your infant is being fed or the way your infant is taking in food. A nutritional evaluation to determine your child's caloric intake may also be required.

TREATMENT Your child needs to start feeding properly right away. Infants will get an enriched formula with extra calories to maintain normal growth. Older children receive solid foods that are rich in calories, vitamins, and minerals. Your child will usually be treated on an *outpatient* basis with frequent doctor visits to monitor growth. In some cases, hospitalization is necessary to evaluate or treat the child who is not thriving. If the cause of your child's condition is a social or economic problem at home, the doctor may involve a social worker or mental health professional to help you work through the problem. If the failure to thrive is caused by an underlying physical disorder, the doctor will prescribe the appropriate treatment for that disorder.

FEBRILE SEIZURES

Febrile seizures are convulsions (sudden, uncontrolled body movements) and loss of consciousness caused by a rapidly rising fever. They occur in 3 to 5 percent of all children, most often between the ages of 6 months and 5 years. Boys tend to get them more often than girls, and they are more likely to occur in children with a family history of febrile seizures. About one third of children who have a febrile seizure have at least one more, usually within a year of the first one. Children who get a febrile seizure under 1 year of age are more likely to have recurrent febrile seizures. But children who get febrile seizures in infancy do not have an increased risk of a SEIZURE DISORDER (such as epilepsy) or developmental problems later in life.

SIGNS AND SYMPTOMS The child first gets a fever that rises quickly, usually from an infection. Then the child loses consciousness and begins to twitch and jerk uncontrollably. The child may also lose control of urinary or bowel functions. Febrile seizures can last as long as 15 minutes. When the child regains consciousness, he or she may be tired and irritable and want to sleep for several hours. While a febrile seizure is frightening to observe, it usually does not harm the child unless it affects breathing.

DIAGNOSIS The doctor will probably want to examine a child who has had a febrile seizure to find out what caused it. He or she may also order tests of the child's blood, urine, and spinal fluid to rule out MENINGITIS.

TREATMENT If you see your child having a seizure, try to ease him or her to the ground so that he or she does not fall. Remove nearby objects that might hurt the child. When the seizure stops, place your child on his or her side and make sure your child can breathe. If the seizure lasts for more than 5 minutes, or your child has bluish lips or skin, call an ambulance and get your child to a hospital emergency department.

When your child is awake, try to reduce the fever by giving him or her ibuprofen or acetaminophen and a sponge bath with lukewarm water. Keep your child cool; do not cover him or her in heavy blankets or clothing. After the seizure, take your child to see the doctor. Make a note of the details so you can tell the doctor how high your child's fever was, how soon the seizure began after the fever rose, how long the seizure lasted, and whether your child slept after the seizure. Your doctor will treat an infection with appropriate medication.

FETAL ALCOHOL SYNDROME

Fetal alcohol syndrome is a group of BIRTH DEFECTS found in children born to women who drink alcohol during pregnancy. Alcohol enters the fetus's bloodstream through the mother's placenta, producing physical and intellectual abnormalities in the fetus. The more alcohol a pregnant woman drinks, the more serious are the defects. Constant use of alcohol during pregnancy is more dangerous than occasional use, but no known safe level of alcohol consumption exists for pregnant women.

SIGNS AND SYMPTOMS Newborns with fetal alcohol syndrome rarely have the symptoms of withdrawal from alcohol, such as restlessness, spasms, and twitching. Instead, they have feeding difficulties, poor sleeping habits, irritability, and increased sensitivity to sound. Infants born with fetal alcohol syndrome have certain common facial (see illustration) and other characteristics. Most have MENTAL RETARDATION and delays in speech and language skills, coordination, and motor (movement) skills (see DEVELOPMENTAL DELAY). Affected infants and toddlers are sometimes clumsy and hyperactive. Their growth is usually retarded and they may have heart defects (see HEART DISEASE, CONGENITAL), a small brain, cleft palate (see CLEFT LIP AND CLEFT PALATE), or a dislocated hip (see HIP DISORDERS). Most are short for their age (see HEIGHT PROBLEMS), a problem that persists for life. A school-aged child with fetal alcohol syndrome maintains some of the physical characteristics of infants with fetal alcohol syndrome although the features may become less obvious with time. He or she may have LEARNING DISABILITIES and be developmentally delayed. Affected children are often inattentive and hyperactive, have a short memory span, and develop irregular sleep patterns. Adolescents with the disorder may be socially withdrawn, extremely unhappy, and have behavior problems and inappropriate emotional responses.

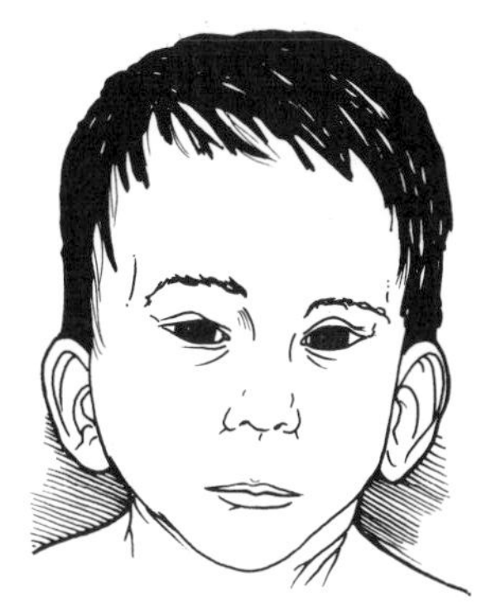

Characteristic features of fetal alcohol syndrome

An infant with fetal alcohol syndrome typically has a small head with narrow, wide-set eyes, thin lips without a vertical groove above the middle of the upper lip, a wide space between the nose and lips, and protruding ears that are set low on the head.

DIAGNOSIS AND TREATMENT There is no specific medical test for fetal alcohol syndrome. A diagnosis is made on the basis of the child's physical features and the mother's history of alcohol use. Diagnosing an older child may be more difficult. If your child has fetal alcohol syndrome, he or she will require medical treatment for his or her specific physical or mental defects. For example, your child may need heart surgery for heart defects, plastic surgery for a cleft palate, or bone surgery for a hip dislocation. In addition, your child may need physical therapy, speech and language therapy, occupational therapy, and special education.

FIFTH DISEASE

Fifth disease, also called erythema infectiosum, is a common childhood infection caused by a virus that produces a RASH on the child's cheeks, arms, and legs. It occurs frequently among elementary school children, usually in winter and spring, and spreads when a child who has the disease coughs or sneezes into the air. The infection can spread most easily from 3 days to 2 weeks before the rash appears, so children usually are exposed to fifth disease without knowing it. The disease is not contagious when the rash is present.

SIGNS AND SYMPTOMS Many children with fifth disease have no symptoms at first. Others develop a mild fever (101°F), fatigue, irritability, body aches, and mild cold symptoms for 3 or 4 days. The rash appears in three stages. First, a bright red rash appears on both cheeks, which look like they have been slapped. A day or two later, a lacelike, blotchy rash that itches appears on the upper arms and legs and spreads to the buttocks and trunk of the child's body. This rash can last from 3 to 24 days. Then the rash begins to fade, but can reappear if the child's skin becomes irritated.

Adolescents who get fifth disease sometimes develop mild pain and swelling in their joints, especially the knuckles, wrists, and knees. The joint pain can last from several days to a few months, but has no lasting effects. Adolescents with fifth disease often do not develop a rash. If you or your adolescent is pregnant and has been exposed to fifth disease, call your doctor because fifth disease can cause miscarriage or anemia in the fetus.

DIAGNOSIS You may be able to recognize the characteristic rash of fifth disease on your own (see page 24). Your child's doctor will be able to diagnose it from its appearance. Healthy children who get fifth disease do not usually need to be seen by a doctor because they recover on their own. But a child who has a blood disorder, such as SICKLE CELL ANEMIA or hemolytic anemia (see ANEMIA, HEMOLYTIC), or a child with cancer needs to be seen by a doctor because he or she is at increased risk of anemia.

TREATMENT Fifth disease is a mild and harmless condition and most children need no treatment. Oatmeal baths can help relieve itching. You can buy oatmeal bath products over the counter. Simply empty the packet into a bathtub full of water and have your child sit in the tub for a while. If your adolescent has joint pains, offer acetaminophen or ibuprofen for the pain and swelling. Call your doctor if your child's fever rises, the joint pains get worse, or he or she has a chronic blood disorder.

FLAT FEET

Flat feet (also known as flatfoot) refers to a condition in which a child's feet do not have a visible arch. The soles of the feet rest flat on the ground. Because young children's arches have not yet formed and because they retain a fat pad on the bottom of their feet to stabilize them for walking, young children often look as if they have flat feet. But, by the time a child reaches the age of 5 or 6 years, the arch should be apparent, although about one child in seven never develops an arch. Flat feet are not painful and create no problems for the child, as long as his or her feet are flexible. In very rare cases the feet may be rigid and difficult to move. Rigidity can indicate that bones in the child's foot have fused together or that the child has an underlying disease, such as JUVENILE RHEUMATOID ARTHRITIS or CEREBRAL PALSY.

DIAGNOSIS AND TREATMENT Your child does not need medical treatment for flat feet. But, if your child complains of pain in his or her feet or ankles, take the child to the doctor for an evaluation. The doctor will examine your child's feet and may order foot X-rays. Doctors no longer think that children with flat feet benefit from wearing special corrective shoes. If your child has a rigid foot or foot pain, the doctor may refer him or her to an orthopedic (foot) specialist for further evaluation and treatment.

FOOD ALLERGIES

See Allergies to food

FOOD POISONING

Food poisoning occurs when a person eats food or drink contaminated with certain types of bacteria or viruses. Infants and children are at increased risk of food poisoning and of developing serious complications because their immune systems—the body's main weapon against infection—may not yet be fully developed.

The main sources of bacteria that cause food poisoning are raw or undercooked meat, chicken, turkey, fish, eggs, or shellfish; unpasteurized or contaminated milk, cheese, and other dairy products; or the skin of unwashed fruit.

The specific bacteria responsible for food poisoning include salmonella, staphylococcus, Escherichia coli (commonly known as E coli), Campylobacter species, shigella, clostridium, Listeria species, and Bacillus cereus. Shellfish can become contaminated by either bacteria or viruses. The most common types of viruses that cause food poisoning are Norwalk virus and rotavirus, which contaminate shellfish in water containing human excrement. Children can also get food poisoning if they come into contact with people or pets–dogs, cats, turtles, lizards, birds, chickens, ducks, or iguanas–infected with bacteria.

Most children get better on their own without serious complications, but food poisoning caused by certain bacteria can be serious. Infection with E coli can cause a life-threatening disease called HEMOLYTIC-UREMIC SYNDROME, which destroys red blood cells and causes the child's kidneys to fail. Salmonella infection can produce severe dehydration, which can be fatal to infants. BOTULISM food poisoning is life-threatening to infants and children.

SIGNS AND SYMPTOMS The main symptoms of food poisoning are diarrhea, stomach cramps, and nausea or vomiting that last for 2 or 3 days. Your child may or may not have a fever. Sometimes the child's stool will be bloody. Excessive diarrhea and vomiting can cause your child to become dehydrated (see page 283), with a dry mouth, reduced tear production, dark-colored urine, or less frequent urination than normal. In extreme cases, the child could go into shock (see page 678) and collapse. Severe food poisoning can also produce breathing problems.

Symptoms of food poisoning can develop within 1 to 8 hours of eating contaminated foods, although symptoms sometimes take up to 5 days to develop. Mild cases of food poisoning can cause diarrhea two or three times a day, while severe cases can bring about watery diarrhea every 10 to 15 minutes.

How to prevent food poisoning

Food becomes contaminated with bacteria when it is improperly handled, refrigerated, and stored. Here are some tips for handling food safely:

- Make sure that meat, poultry, seafood, and eggs are cooked thoroughly (above 140°F) to kill the bacteria; do not serve foods that are raw or undercooked.
- Wash knives and cutting boards used to cut up raw meat or poultry in hot, soapy water.
- At a picnic or barbecue, keep hot foods hot and cold foods cold. Refrigerate leftovers promptly.
- Always wash your hands after using the bathroom and before preparing food. Make sure your children wash theirs as well.
- Throw out old food, food that smells bad, and food in bulging tin cans or in containers with leaky tops.
- Store refrigerated raw meat no longer than 3 days and poultry no longer than 2 days.
- Defrost foods in the refrigerator to keep bacteria from growing. In a pinch, use the microwave and then cook the food immediately.
- Don't refreeze frozen foods that you have defrosted; cook them immediately or throw them away.
- Wash fruit before eating it.
- Don't place cooked food onto a plate used for raw food.

DIAGNOSIS Parents can usually recognize the symptoms of food poisoning in their children. You should take your child to the doctor if the symptoms persist for 3 days or more or if symptoms get worse with treatment. Your doctor will examine your child and ask you when the symptoms started and what the child ate. He or she may also take a stool *culture* for signs of bacterial infection. Your doctor may put a child with severe diarrhea and vomiting in the hospital to prevent dehydration.

TREATMENT Most cases of food poisoning are not serious and clear up within a few days. Give your

FRACTURES

A fracture is a partial or complete break in a bone. Children can fracture their bones during a fall, while playing sports, or in a motor vehicle collision. Fractures can also occur during child abuse. The bones that children are most likely to break include the collarbone and the bones in the arms, wrists, hands, legs, feet, and nose. Fractures can be either closed or open. In a closed fracture, the broken bone does not penetrate the skin. In an open, or compound, fracture, the broken bone breaks through the skin, damaging surrounding nerves, blood vessels, and tissue. Open fractures are more serious and carry a high risk of infection.

What are the signs of a fracture?

The signs of a fracture vary depending on the location of the affected bone and the nature and extent of the injury. Fractures can cause pain, swelling, tenderness, immobility, and, sometimes, bruising in the area around the bone. The bone may also look deformed. A fracture in the ribs or nose can cause difficulty breathing. A fracture in the spine can cause numbness or paralysis in the back, arms, legs, or neck.

If you think your child has a fracture, see page 672 for first-aid procedures and then take your child to the doctor.

Doctors use X-rays to confirm that a child's bone has been fractured and to determine the location, type, and extent of the injury. X-rays also help doctors prescribe the most effective treatment.

Types of fractures

Bones can break or crack in various patterns, depending on the direction and force of impact. Here are some of the most common types of fractures and how they are treated.

- **Transverse fracture** Transverse fractures are breaks straight across a bone that usually arise from a direct blow or angled force. Doctors treat them by immobilizing the bone in a cast.
- **Spiral fracture** Spiral fractures, which usually affect arm or leg bones, often occur during child abuse when someone violently twists a child's limb. The bone can break through the skin and damage surrounding nerves and blood vessels. Spiral fractures are treated with immobilization in a cast or, sometimes, with traction (the application of tension to a bone to align and immobilize it) or surgery.
- **Comminuted fracture** A comminuted fracture, in which the bone splinters into three or more pieces, is usually caused by a high-impact injury or direct blow. Comminuted fractures are sometimes difficult to treat because the pieces of bone need to be carefully repositioned.
- **Greenstick fracture** In a greenstick fracture, a long arm or leg bone snaps or buckles on only one side, usually from a severe blow or jarring force. Greenstick fractures are common in children because a child's bones are more pliable than an adult's. Doctors treat this type of fracture by immobilizing the bone in a cast.

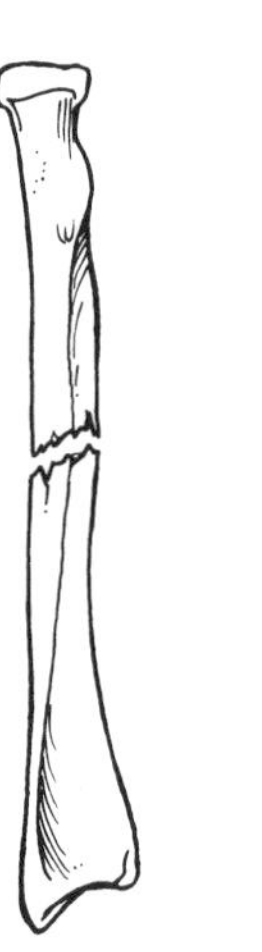

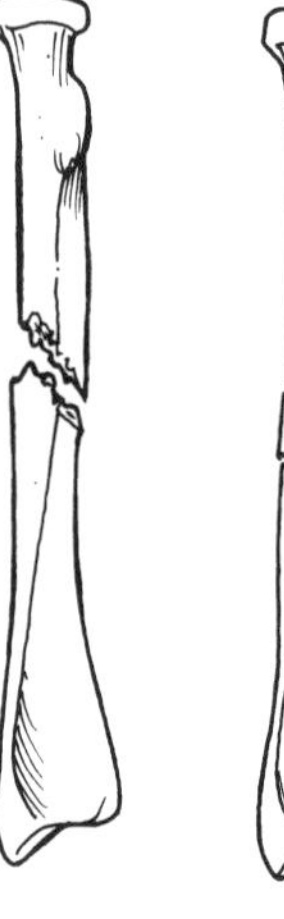

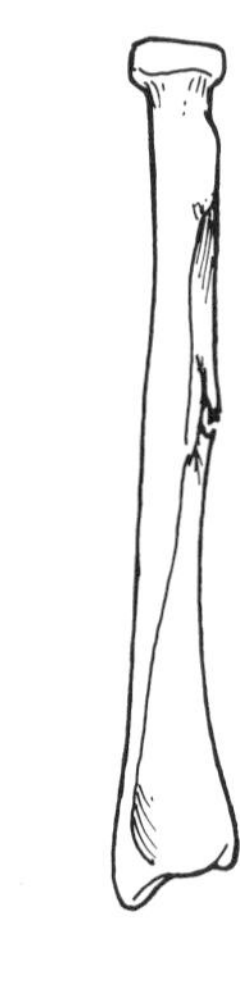

Transverse fracture | Spiral fracture | Comminuted fracture | Greenstick fracture

How do doctors treat fractures?

Treatment depends on the type of fracture and the bone that has been broken—for example, a fractured finger or toe can be splinted or taped to the adjoining digit while a fractured femur (thighbone) or pelvis may need traction. In general, however, doctors realign the broken or fragmented bone and then immobilize it so it can heal properly. Fractures in growth plates (the areas near the ends of bones where growth occurs) need especially careful treatment because improper healing can result in arrested growth or deformity of the affected limb.

Doctors can realign fractures from the outside (with casting, traction, splinting, taping, or manipulation by hand) or from the inside (using pins, plates, wires, or screws). Casting is the most common way to immobilize broken bones in children. Fractures heal more quickly in children than in adults, usually in about 3 weeks, depending on the bone and the severity of the injury.

If the broken bone does not heal properly, the child may need surgery.

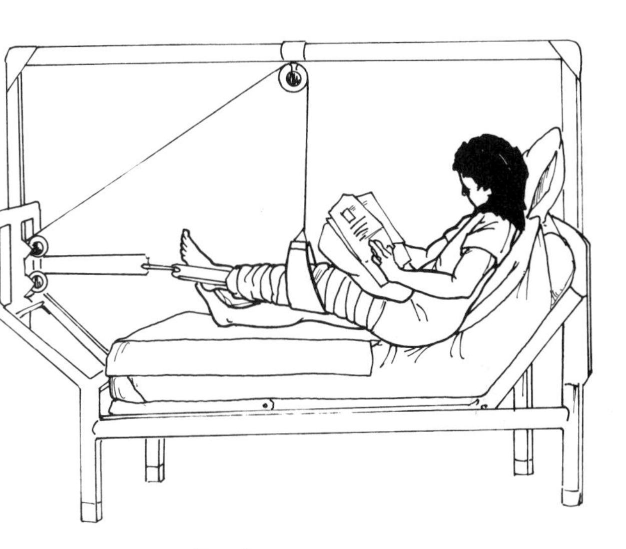

Traction

Doctors treat some fractures, such as those in the thighbone and lower leg, with traction, which puts tension on the bone to align it, allowing the broken ends to grow together correctly. Traction is usually done in the hospital.

When your child has a cast

Most casts are still made from plaster, but newer plastic casts are more lightweight and permit clearer X-ray pictures. Before your child leaves the hospital with a cast, the doctor or a nurse will teach you how to care for it at home. A child's activities are usually limited for about 8 weeks while the broken bone heals. Severe fractures often require long-term physical therapy and rehabilitation. Follow these home care guidelines when your child has a cast:

- Keep the cast clean and dry. Cover it with a plastic bag or plastic wrap when your child bathes or showers. If the cast gets wet, call the doctor.
- Check the skin around the edges of the cast for irritation, rubbing, or blistering. The skin should be clean and dry.
- Use a cotton-tipped swab and rubbing alcohol to cleanse the skin under the edges of the cast and between the toes or fingers. Don't use lotions, oils, or powders because residue can build up and cause skin irritation.
- Don't poke sharp or small objects down inside the cast to relieve itching; they could cause skin irritation and interfere with blood circulation.
- Frequently check for good blood circulation. Make sure the fingers or toes are pink, not blue or white. The tips of the fingers or toes should turn white when you pinch them and return to normal color when released; the skin should feel warm.
- For the first 48 hours after the injury, raise the arm or leg with the cast above heart level to prevent or reduce swelling.
- If your child notices any swelling, numbness, or tingling; blood or fluid leaking from the cast; or an unusual odor, call the doctor. A cracked cast or one that seems loose or starts slipping off should also be reported to the doctor.

child plenty of liquids, especially clear broth or bouillon, and make sure the child rests. To replace fluids and electrolytes (essential salts) lost through diarrhea and vomiting, give the child over-the-counter oral electrolyte maintenance solutions or sports drinks until the diarrhea stops. After the child is able to keep liquids down, give him or her soft, bland foods, and then gradually return to a normal diet. Avoid giving your child dairy products while he or she is sick.

You can help relieve stomach cramps by placing a hot-water bottle on the child's stomach or abdomen. Give your child acetaminophen or ibuprofen (not aspirin) to reduce fever. Do not give your child antidiarrhea medications because they will slow the recovery process. Your doctor will usually not prescribe antibiotics for food poisoning, except in special cases. Keep the child away from other family members to prevent spreading the infection.

Fractures

See page 490

Fragile X syndrome

Fragile X syndrome is an inherited GENETIC DISORDER that causes a range of mental impairments in infants and children. It is the most common inherited type of mental retardation. The disorder is passed from parent to child, but the parent is usually only a carrier of the gene that causes the disease and has no symptoms of the disorder.

The defective gene is located on the X chromosome (see CHROMOSOMAL ABNORMALITIES). Fragile X syndrome is so named because the defect causes the affected part of the chromosome to become narrow and look fragile. Male infants and children get this disorder much more frequently than females and develop more severe symptoms. When the mother is the carrier of the disease, her sons are at risk of getting fragile X syndrome. Her daughters are at risk of becoming carriers and could develop a mild form of the disease. A father who is a carrier of the gene cannot transmit it to his sons but can pass it to his daughters, who become carriers. The daughters can develop moderate symptoms of the disease if they inherit the gene from their mother.

Signs and symptoms Features characteristic of fragile X syndrome may be evident at birth but they are more commonly seen after the child reaches puberty. These features include large ears, a long face, strabismus (crossed eyes or walleye), a prominent jaw and forehead, enlarged testicles in males, and loose finger joints. The features are usually more subtle in girls.

Most boys with this disease have some degree of mental impairment, ranging from lower-than-normal intelligence to severe MENTAL RETARDATION. The IQs of affected boys decline during childhood, and their mental impairment may grow worse with age. About 20 percent of affected boys have symptoms similar to those of AUTISM, such as poor social interaction, avoidance of direct eye contact, hand-biting, and hand-flapping. About 30 percent of girls who carry the gene are mentally retarded to some degree.

Diagnosis If your child's doctor knows that you or your partner has a history of fragile X syndrome in your family, he or she will order a blood test that can identify your child as either a carrier of fragile X syndrome or one who is directly affected by the disease. Results of the blood test take several weeks to obtain.

Treatment No treatment exists for fragile X syndrome, although your child may receive medication for behavior problems and special education for learning disabilities caused by the disease. Prospective parents with a history of this condition should receive genetic counseling (see page 497) before conceiving a child.

Frostbite

See page 680

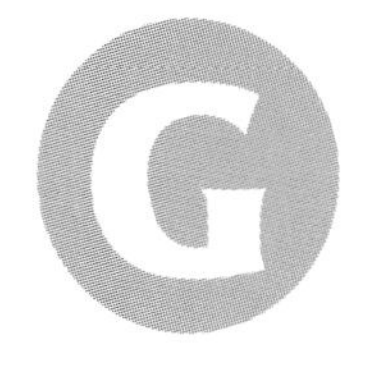

GALACTOSEMIA

Galactosemia is a rare inherited INBORN ERROR OF METABOLISM. Infants with this disorder lack an enzyme (a protein that speeds up a chemical process) that helps the body use galactose (milk sugar) for energy. Galactosemia generally appears in the first few days of a newborn's life after he or she drinks breast milk or formula. Higher than normal levels of galactose and its by-products build up in the infant's blood and damage the child's liver, brain, kidneys, and eyes if he or she is not diagnosed and treated right away. Both parents must be carriers of the disease for a child to inherit it.

SIGNS AND SYMPTOMS The earliest signs of the disease include JAUNDICE, enlargement of the liver, and vomiting. The baby may also be irritable, fail to gain weight, have diarrhea, and get serious infections. If the newborn does not get treatment, he or she may vomit blood, have poor eyesight because of cataracts (clouding of the lens of the eye), or show signs of MENTAL RETARDATION.

DIAGNOSIS Your doctor will order blood and urine tests to detect the disease in your child. Many states have laws requiring that all newborns be tested for galactosemia.

TREATMENT If your child has galactosemia, he or she will need to follow a diet that is free of milk and other foods that contain galactose or lactose (the milk sugar that galactose is derived from) for life. You will have to stop breast-feeding and begin feeding your child a special galactose-free milk. With early treatment, many symptoms of galactosemia can be reduced and your child's weight gain, growth, and development can be improved.

You should seek genetic counseling (see page 497) to find out what your chances are of having another child with galactosemia. If you become pregnant again, your doctor may recommend that you follow a galactose-free diet during your pregnancy to make your body as normal an environment for your fetus as possible.

GASTROENTERITIS

Gastroenteritis is an inflammation of the stomach and intestines, caused by infection with a virus, bacteria, or parasites. The infection can be spread by eating contaminated food or by sharing food with someone who is infected. It can occasionally be spread through coughing or sneezing. Frequent hand washing helps to prevent transmission of the infection. Children under age 5 tend to get more serious cases of gastroenteritis.

SIGNS AND SYMPTOMS The symptoms, which can range from mild to severe, include nausea, vomiting, and diarrhea. The infant or child may also have stomach or abdominal cramps or pain, a fever, weakness, and appetite loss. Babies may also become irritable.

Most cases of gastroenteritis are mild and disappear in 2 to 5 days. Newborns and infants under 18 months of age are at risk of severe illness from excessive vomiting, diarrhea, and dehydration (see page 283). The signs of dehydration include a sunken soft spot, dry mouth, sunken eyes, decreased tear production, refusal to eat, decreased urination, irritability, and weakness.

DIAGNOSIS Call the doctor if your child begins vomiting and has diarrhea. The doctor will ask what your child has eaten recently and if anyone in the family is sick. He or she may also take blood tests and stool samples.

TREATMENT Mild cases of gastroenteritis can be treated at home with plenty of rest and clear fluids until symptoms disappear. Give your child fluids containing sugar and salt, such as flat soft drinks, broth, or ice pops. Avoid milk and other dairy products because they are hard to digest. Juice may make the diarrhea worse. Once your child can keep the fluids down, give him or her small amounts of bland food, such as bananas, rice, apple sauce, plain toast, or crackers. Resume a normal diet as your child's condition improves. If your infant has signs of gastroenteritis and you are breast-feeding, you can continue breast-feeding or give him or her a commercial rehydration solution that you can buy over the counter. Don't give your child an over-the-counter antidiarrhea medication because it decreases the natural movement of the intestines and could affect your child's ability to flush the infection from his or her system.

If your infant or child can't keep fluids down or has signs of serious illness, such as dehydration, take him or her to a hospital emergency department for treatment. Your child will receive fluids *intravenously* at first, and then by mouth, as he or she recovers.

GASTROESOPHAGEAL REFLUX AND HIATAL HERNIA

Commonly called heartburn or acid indigestion, gastroesophageal reflux is the flow of acidic stomach contents back up into a child's esophagus (the muscular tube that connects the mouth to the stomach). A muscle at the bottom end of the esophagus controls the passage of food from the esophagus to the stomach and prevents the stomach contents from flowing back into the esophagus. Children with gastroesophageal reflux have a weak or poorly functioning muscle. Many children with this disorder also have a hiatal hernia, in which part of the stomach slides up through the diaphragm, the muscle that separates the chest cavity from the abdomen.

Gastroesophageal reflux may be more common in infants and children than previously thought. Some infants are probably born with the condition. In other infants and children, overfeeding or lying flat immediately after eating may contribute to the condition's frequency. Certain foods and liquids seem to worsen gastroesophageal reflux, including spicy foods, chocolate, drinks that contain caffeine, carbonated drinks, and alcohol. In older children and teenagers, smoking and being overweight or pregnant are also risk factors.

SIGNS AND SYMPTOMS Gastroesophageal reflux is a painful, burning sensation that begins in the chest behind the breastbone and moves up toward the neck. Many children experience an acidlike or bitter taste if the stomach contents flow all the way back into the mouth. Children may also vomit, cough, belch, and feel pain when swallowing.

Infants with gastroesophageal reflux often vomit after eating. They may also have coughing episodes and difficulty breathing from inhalation of the stomach contents or become irritable from the burning discomfort. In rare cases, an infant may have more severe symptoms, such as FAILURE TO THRIVE. Infants usually outgrow gastroesophageal reflux in the first year of life.

Hiatal hernia can produce symptoms similar to gastroesophageal reflux–heartburn or belching–or no symptoms at all.

DIAGNOSIS Your doctor may use X-ray studies to diagnose gastroesophageal reflux. Your child will be asked to drink a liquid containing barium sulfate, which will be traced on X-ray film as it moves through the child's digestive tract. The test is painless and the liquid passes out of the body easily. The doctor may also use a pH probe, a long, thin instrument placed into your child's mouth and down his or her esophagus to measure acid levels in the esophagus over 24 hours. It may cause brief, mild discomfort when it is inserted. Another instrument used to diagnose gastroesophageal reflux is an endoscope, a narrow, flexible tube inserted through the mouth into the esophagus. Using an endoscope (see page 463), a doctor can visually examine the lining of your child's esophagus while the child is sedated. The doctor may also take a *biopsy* through the endoscope to confirm the diagnosis.

TREATMENT Gastroesophageal reflux and hiatal hernia are treated with dietary and lifestyle changes and possibly also with medication prescribed by your child's doctor. Reflux is more likely to occur when your child is lying flat. If your infant has this disorder, position him or her upright in your arms or prop your baby up with a large pillow under the head of the mattress for about 30 minutes after feeding. You could also lay your baby down on his or her right side after feeding to help the food stay down. The doctor may recommend that you give your baby a formula thickened with rice cereal that will not flow back easily. Be sure to burp your infant several times during and after meals.

Children should avoid caffeine-containing foods and drinks because they can relax the muscle that prevents the stomach contents from flowing back up, causing reflux. They should not eat right before going to bed at night. Allow 2 or 3 hours between meals and bedtime. Raise the head of your child's bed 4 to 6 inches so that his or her head is elevated. If your child is overweight, the doctor will probably recommend a reducing diet.

If these treatments do not work, the doctor may prescribe medication to reduce stomach acid, to speed the emptying of food from the stomach to the intestine, or to tighten the muscle at the junction of the esophagus and the stomach. These drugs are usually effective at controlling symptoms. If not, surgery may be needed to prevent reflux and to repair the hernia.

GAUCHER'S DISEASE

Gaucher's disease is a rare inherited INBORN ERROR OF METABOLISM that affects a child's central nervous system, producing a decline in mental and physical functioning. A child with Gaucher's disease cannot produce enough of a protein needed to break down a certain body fat. When the fat accumulates, symptoms of the disease appear. Most commonly occurring in Jews of Central and Eastern European descent (Ashkenazi Jews), the disease can take three forms, first appearing in infancy, childhood, or adulthood. Only one form can affect a given family.

SIGNS AND SYMPTOMS When it occurs in infants, the disease causes a swollen abdomen from spleen and liver enlargement, mild anemia, strabismus (see VISION PROBLEMS), inability to swallow, and a characteristic bending backward of the infant's head. The infants frequently get seizures, and most die by the time they reach 2 years of age.

In the form occurring in childhood known as juvenile Gaucher's disease, affected children have poor coordination, decreased sensation and muscle function, abnormal eye movement, and behavior changes. Mental function gradually deteriorates. Gaucher's disease also affects bone marrow production and destroys bone.

DIAGNOSIS Doctors can diagnose Gaucher's disease before a child's birth using amniocentesis. If your infant or child has symptoms of Gaucher's disease, your doctor may take a sample of the fluid inside your child's bone marrow (tissue inside the cavities of bones in which blood cells are manufactured). The doctor will withdraw the fluid from the bone with a needle and have the fluid analyzed. Your child's doctor may also do a blood test or a liver *biopsy* to check the level of the deficient protein.

TREATMENT To treat Gaucher's disease, doctors replace the child's missing protein with a synthetic one or with one taken from the blood of a human placenta (the organ that connects a fetus's blood supply to the mother during pregnancy) or from healthy bone marrow. In rare cases, the child's spleen is surgically removed if there is a danger that the spleen could rupture.

GENETIC DISORDERS

Genetic disorders are conditions that can be passed from parent to child through the genetic material known as DNA, which is contained in human cells. The conditions cause abnormal physical or mental characteristics.

Genes contain the genetic information that determines every human physical and mental trait, from eye color to intelligence. Children inherit most genetic disorders from one or both of their parents. Sometimes, however, normal genes mutate (change) as cells divide, or become altered by environmental factors and cause a genetic disorder that is not inherited. Once the child has a mutant gene, he or she may pass it on to his or her own children. Other types of genetic disorders are caused by CHROMOSOMAL ABNORMALITIES.

If you or your partner have a family history of any type of genetic disorder, you should seek genetic counseling (see page 497) and genetic testing (see page 498) before having children.

TYPES OF GENETIC DISORDERS Genetic disorders fall into several categories depending on the number and type of mutant genes a child inherits from his or her parents.

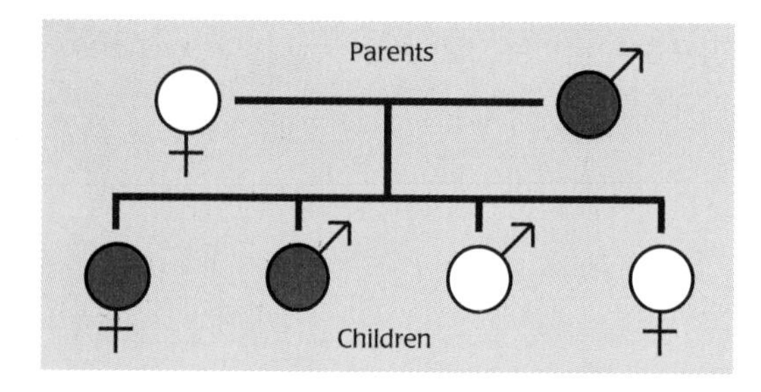

Dominant inheritance
If a person inherits an abnormal gene from either parent, that person will be affected by the genetic disorder. Each of the person's children has a 50 percent chance of inheriting the abnormal gene and getting the disorder.

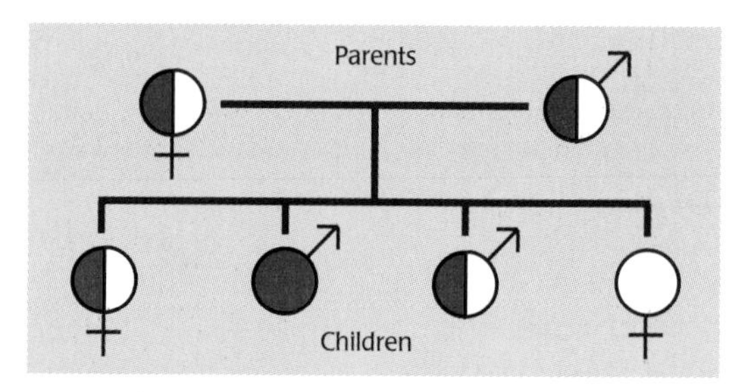

Recessive inheritance
In recessive inheritance, each parent is a carrier—he or she carries an abnormal gene but does not have the disease. Each of their children has a 1 in 4 chance of inheriting the disease, regardless of sex.

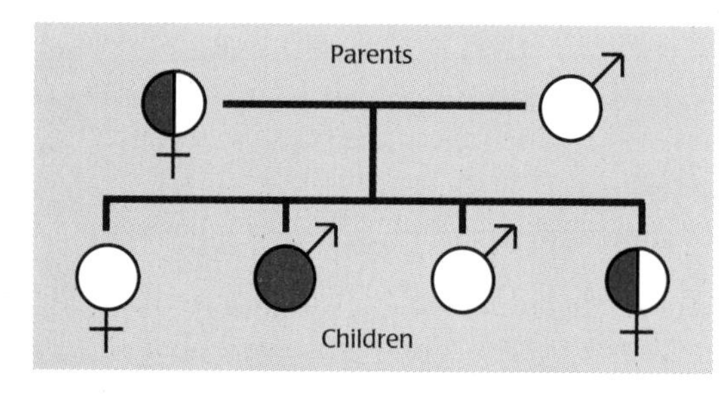

X-linked inheritance
A disease caused by one abnormal gene on the X chromosome affects only male children. Each son of a female carrier has a 50 percent chance of inheriting the genetic disorder. Each daughter has a 50 percent chance of becoming a carrier.

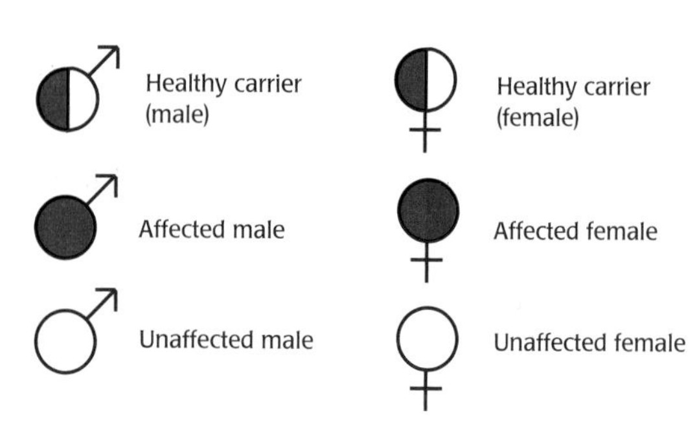

Genetic counseling

Genetic counseling can help you and your partner understand and identify your chances of passing on GENETIC DISORDERS, BIRTH DEFECTS, and physical or emotional traits to your children. Genetic counselors explain how inherited traits are passed from parents to children and help families learn how to care for children with inherited problems. You should consider genetic counseling if you have experienced any of the following circumstances:

- You have a family history of genetic disorders or birth defects.
- You have just had a baby who was diagnosed at birth with a genetic disorder or birth defect.
- You already have a child with a genetic disorder or birth defect.
- You have been told by your doctor that you may be at risk of having children with birth defects or genetic disorders.
- You are a woman over age 35 who is pregnant or planning to become pregnant (you have a higher risk of having children with CHROMOSOMAL ABNORMALITIES, such as DOWN SYNDROME).
- You have had a baby who died as an infant or you have had two or more miscarriages.
- You have been exposed to toxic chemicals, high doses of radiation, or other environmental factors that might pose a risk of having children with birth defects.
- You are planning to have children with a person who is a close blood relative, such as a first cousin.

The genetic counselor will ask you for information about your family's medical history. He or she will want to know what diseases—heart disease (see HEART DISEASE, CONGENITAL), diabetes (see DIABETES MELLITUS, TYPE I), other genetic disorders, or MENTAL RETARDATION—run in the family. The counselor will also ask about your personal history, such as your diet, health problems, activities, livelihood, and ethnic background, because these factors could all have a bearing on your health. Based on this information, the counselor will tell you what genetic traits or disorders you may be likely to pass on and the chances your children have of inheriting these genetic conditions or of being born with birth defects. Your counselor may also refer you to a doctor for a physical exam and special genetic testing (see page 498).

For more information on counseling resources, contact your local chapter of the March of Dimes or the March of Dimes Birth Defects Foundation, 1275 Mamaronek Ave, White Plains, NY 10605.

Dominant gene disorders A dominant gene carries a human trait that will determine a characteristic in a child no matter what other type of gene is found in the matching *chromosome.* For example, the gene that determines brown eyes is a dominant gene. If a child inherits a gene for brown eyes from his or her father and a gene for blue eyes from his or her mother, the child's eyes will be brown. The same is true for a genetic disorder, such as MARFAN SYNDROME, which is carried on a dominant gene. A child who receives the gene for Marfan syndrome from either parent will get the disease. If only one parent carries the gene for the disorder, then each of the children has a 50 percent chance of inheriting the gene (see illustration on previous page).

Recessive gene disorders A recessive gene will determine a characteristic in a child only if both parents contribute recessive genes for that trait. For example, the gene that determines blue eyes is a recessive gene. If a child inherits recessive genes for blue eyes from both parents, the child's eyes will be blue. Recessive genes for genetic disorders work in the same way. If a child receives a recessive gene for a genetic disorder, such as SICKLE CELL ANEMIA or CYSTIC FIBROSIS, from both parents, then the child will have that disease. If both parents have a recessive gene for a genetic disorder, then each of their children has a 25 percent chance of inheriting the disorder.

Genetic testing

We all inherit chromosomes from our parents, and some of the chromosomes we inherit may contain defective, altered, or missing genes. Genetic testing is a way to identify children and adults who have BIRTH DEFECTS, CHROMOSOMAL ABNORMALITIES, INBORN ERRORS OF METABOLISM, or other GENETIC DISORDERS that can be passed from parent to child. Most genetic testing involves taking samples of blood or other body fluids for analysis. Genetic testing is available for such diseases as PKU, CYSTIC FIBROSIS, TAY-SACHS DISEASE, and SICKLE CELL ANEMIA and can be done for the following purposes:

- **Screening of newborns** Blood samples are taken from most newborns 24 hours after birth and sent to a laboratory for analysis (see page 223).
- **Looking for carriers** Some people carry the genes for disease and can pass the genes and the disease on to their children. Genetic testing can identify these carriers.
- **Testing of pregnant women** Use of *amniocentesis* (analysis of the cells inside the fluid surrounding the fetus), *chorionic villus sampling* (analysis of the tissue surrounding the sac that envelopes the fetus), or *ultrasound* (scanning of the fetus with high-frequency sound waves) to detect genetic defects in the fetus.

Be aware that genetic testing is not 100 percent accurate because geneticists have discovered only some of the genetic pattern responsible for certain diseases. Ask a geneticist how reliable the screening is for the specific disease you need to be tested for. If you are considering genetic testing for any reason, you should also consider getting genetic counseling (see page 497) to help you understand what the tests mean and to help you make decisions about parenting based on the test results. If your child is affected by a genetic disorder, genetic counseling can also help you find out how to care for him or her.

Single-gene disorders Most genetic disorders in children are caused by a single, recessive gene. A child will not inherit these disorders unless both parents contribute a gene for the disease. Examples of single-gene recessive disorders are cystic fibrosis and PKU. In a few single-gene disorders, the responsible gene is a dominant one. That means a child will get the disease if he or she inherits the dominant gene from only one parent.

X-linked gene disorders Certain single-gene disorders are caused by a gene located on the X chromosome, which carries the genes that determine the sex of a child. A defective gene located on an X chromosome causes what is known as an X-linked or sex-linked genetic disorder. For example, to inherit the disease HEMOPHILIA, a child must receive the defective gene on an X chromosome from the mother along with a Y chromosome from the father. The child will be a boy and have the disease.

Multiple-gene disorders Other diseases, such as ALLERGIES and diabetes, are inherited through more than one gene. These conditions often run in families and occur in varying forms and at different times of life.

Carriers If either parent carries only one recessive gene for a single-gene disorder, then that parent is a carrier of the disease but does not have the disorder. For example, if a man who is color-blind has children with a woman who has normal genes for color vision, their children will not be color-blind, but all of their daughters will be carriers of the color-blindness gene. The only way that the child of a carrier can get the disease is if both parents pass on the same defective gene or if a carrier mother passes an X-linked genetic disorder to her son. Blood tests can identify carriers of such genetic disorders as hemophilia, beta-THALASSEMIA, sickle cell anemia, and TAY-SACHS DISEASE. Carriers should seek genetic counseling before having children.

GENITAL HERPES

Genital herpes is an infection of the genitals and surrounding areas caused by the herpes simplex virus and characterized by painful blisters and open sores on the genitals. It is transmitted through sexual contact with an infected person but it can also be passed from an infected mother to her newborn as the infant passes through the birth canal. The disease is most easily spread when the blisters or sores are visible, but it can also spread when there are no signs of disease. Sexually active teenagers are at high risk of contracting genital herpes.

Herpes simplex virus 2 causes about 90 percent of genital herpes infections. The remainder are caused by herpes simplex virus 1, which also causes the blisters commonly known as COLD SORES around the mouth. There is no cure for the herpes virus. Once a person is infected, he or she has the virus for life. The virus stays in the body in a dormant state after the initial outbreak and may cause frequent, repeated outbreaks of blisters and sores. The new outbreaks can be triggered by sexual intercourse, menstruation, stress, exposure to the sun, or other infections.

Genital herpes transmitted to an infant at birth is life threatening because the baby's immune system may not be able to fight off the infection. The disease can also be life threatening to a transplant recipient or anyone with cancer, AIDS, or a human immunodeficiency virus (HIV) infection, or other diseases that weaken the immune system, the body's main defense against infection.

SIGNS AND SYMPTOMS One half to two thirds of infected people have no initial symptoms. Those who do have signs of a first infection develop flu-like symptoms (see page 231) with a low-grade fever, headaches, muscle pain, and a tingling sensation in the genitals. These symptoms are followed by the appearance of groups of painful blisters on the genitals and surrounding areas (the lips of the vagina, the anus, the cervix, and the head of the penis). The blisters spread, break open, and then scab over, generally healing within 3 weeks. The fluid in the blisters spreads the infection. New crops of blisters form in the second week of infection, causing the glands in the genital area to swell. Other symptoms include pain during urination and, in girls or women, a discharge from the vagina.

Mild symptoms eventually develop in people who have no initial symptoms. Most people experience outbreaks of blisters in the first year after infection and these outbreaks may continue after the first year. New outbreaks are often preceded by itching, tingling, or pain in the genitals 2 to 48 hours before blisters appear at the site of the first outbreak. Repeated outbreaks are usually less severe than the first outbreak and not all people have repeated outbreaks.

DIAGNOSIS To confirm a diagnosis of genital herpes, your child's doctor will do a thorough physical examination for signs and symptoms of the disease. Doctors sometimes *culture* the infected fluid contained in the herpes blisters but cultures for herpes are not always accurate. The doctor may also take a scraping from the base of the blister to confirm the diagnosis. Results are available in 1 day.

TREATMENT Your doctor may prescribe a drug called acyclovir to fight the herpes simplex virus. The drug is usually taken by mouth. It is also available in a cream form that can be spread on the infected area, but the cream is much less effective than the pill. Acyclovir taken by mouth reduces the spread of the virus, eases the pain of the blisters, speeds healing, and shortens the length of the outbreaks, but it does not kill the virus. Other drugs are available, but acyclovir is the most effective.

Your adolescent can take acetaminophen or ibuprofen to ease the pain. Placing a lukewarm or cool cloth on the infected area or taking warm baths can also soothe the pain. Wearing loose-fitting cotton clothing helps avoid irritation.

How to avoid spreading genital herpes

Adolescents who have genital herpes should take the following steps to avoid spreading the infection.

- Wash your hands after touching the herpes blisters or sores because, during an initial outbreak, you could spread the infection to other parts of your body.
- Pat infected areas dry rather than wiping them to avoid spreading the infection to other areas.
- Don't engage in sexual activity while the blisters and sores are visible or are healing.
- Use a latex condom during all sexual activities, even oral sex.
- Use a sperm-killing cream or jelly in the vagina that contains nonoxynol 9 (check the label) in addition to a condom during sex.
- Tell your sexual partner or partners about your infection so they can watch for signs of infection.
- Be aware that having sex with more than one partner increases your risk of infection, but remember that it only takes a single encounter to get a sexually transmitted disease.
- If you ever get pregnant, tell your doctor that you have had herpes so precautions can be taken to prevent infection of the baby at birth.

GENITAL WARTS

Genital warts are a common sexually transmitted disease caused by infection with the human papillomavirus. The virus enters through microscopic tears in the outer layers of skin during intercourse. The virus can become dormant and remain in the body for life. An infected person spreads the disease most easily when warts are present, but he or she can also transmit it while the virus is dormant. Human papillomavirus can also be passed from an infected mother to her newborn as the infant passes through the birth canal.

Genital warts most frequently occur in young people between the ages of 15 and 30 who have more than one sexual partner. Genital warts have been linked with abnormal Pap smears (see page 255) and cancer of the cervix (neck of the uterus), vulva (the external female genitals), penis, and anus.

SIGNS AND SYMPTOMS Most people infected with the virus that causes genital warts have no symptoms. Others develop warts on their external and internal sex organs–the vulva, vagina, cervix, penis, and anus. The warts look like soft, flesh-colored growths that can be pointed, flat, or raised, or look like tiny cauliflowers. They vary in size, are usually painless, and can appear in clusters or one by one. The symptoms usually appear 1 to 4 months after exposure. Some girls or women also have a bloody or unusual vaginal discharge.

Infants infected at birth can develop warts as well as a serious throat infection known as either juvenile laryngeal papillomatosis or recurrent respiratory papillomatosis. The infection causes hoarseness and breathing difficulty in the first several years of life.

DIAGNOSIS Genital warts located in the internal female genitals may be especially difficult to see. To detect them, the doctor may place a diluted vinegar solution on the skin around the genitals that turns the warts white and makes them easier to find. Doctors diagnose children with symptoms of juvenile laryngeal papillomatosis using a test known as DNA hybridization or the Southern blot test, which detects the particular markers of the DNA (deoxyribonucleic acid) found in the virus that causes genital warts.

TREATMENT There is no cure for the viral infection that causes genital warts. Your doctor can remove the warts by freezing them with liquid nitrogen, applying a chemical called podophyllum, using a laser, or exposing the warts to an electric current. More than one treatment may be needed because the warts are so small and difficult to detect. Girls or women who have a history of human papillomavirus should have a Pap smear (see page 255) every 6 months for a year because the virus can produce abnormal changes in the tissue of the cervix that could, if left untreated, lead to cervical cancer. If these Pap smears are normal, testing done once each subsequent year will be sufficient.

Sexually active adolescents should always use a latex condom during sexual activity and should be aware that limiting their sexual partners can help prevent the spread of genital warts. Adolescents should always use condoms, but condoms may not prevent the spread of genital warts because the warts can grow on areas not covered by a condom.

Infants infected at birth need to be monitored for symptoms for several years. Doctors remove any growths in infants surgically or with a laser. Pregnant women who have genital warts large enough to interfere with vaginal delivery may be offered cesarean (surgical) delivery.

GERMAN MEASLES

German measles, also known as rubella, is a contagious infection caused by a virus. It most commonly occurs in children, although adults can also get it. It is spread when an infected person coughs, sneezes, or breathes the virus into the air. The infection can also spread from an infected pregnant woman to her fetus. Outbreaks of German measles occur most often in spring. Children are usually immunized against this disease when they are 12 to 15 months old and again at 4 to 6 years of age. They generally receive the vaccine along with the vaccines for MEASLES and MUMPS. Women in their childbearing years who have not had German measles or have not been vaccinated against it should receive the vaccine at least 3 months before they plan to get pregnant.

SIGNS AND SYMPTOMS About 2 to 3 weeks after exposure, most children get mild symptoms that include a fever up to 101°F, an itchy RASH that begins on the child's face and spreads all over the body, and swollen glands behind the ears and in the neck. The rash may last for up to 3 days and the fever for 1 to 5 days. The disease is most dangerous to a developing fetus during the first 4 months of gestation. The fetus could be stillborn or the baby could be born with such BIRTH DEFECTS as deafness (see HEARING LOSS); MENTAL RETARDATION; and heart, liver, and eye defects.

DIAGNOSIS AND TREATMENT Your child's doctor can diagnose German measles from the appearance of the rash itself and with blood tests. Most children need no treatment except rest and plenty of fluids. You may give your child acetaminophen (not aspirin) for the fever and calamine lotion to soothe the itchy rash. Your child can spread the infection from 1 week before he or she gets the rash until 1 week after the rash disappears. Recovery takes about a week.

GIARDIASIS

Giardiasis is an intestinal illness caused by a common parasite transmitted through the stool of infected humans, wild animals, and pets. It is a growing problem in day-care centers, where children can catch the parasite from infected children who do not wash their hands after using the toilet or from day-care workers who fail to wash their hands after changing diapers. Food prepared by an infected person can also carry the parasite. Once the parasites enter the body, they multiply in the small intestine and are excreted in stool .

Parasite-infected stool from animals and humans can contaminate lakes, streams, and reservoirs both in the United States and in foreign countries. Children and adults can then get giardiasis after drinking the untreated water or by eating raw food that was washed in untreated water. Treated city water supplies are generally safe from giardiasis.

G

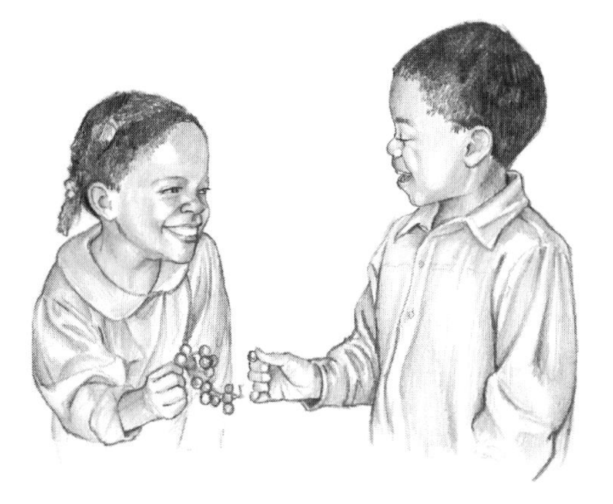

Preventing the spread of giardiasis
Giardiasis can spread when children share contaminated toys or food. The best way to prevent transmission of giardiasis is to make sure your child washes his or her hands after using the toilet.

SIGNS AND SYMPTOMS Mild to severe diarrhea is the major symptom of giardiasis. Other symptoms include belching, gas, bloating, stomach cramps, and indigestion. Intestinal gas has the odor of rotten eggs. Some children get diarrhea that lasts for weeks or months and lose weight. An infected child usually does not have a fever.

Symptoms take from 1 to 3 weeks to develop. Many children infected with the parasite have no symptoms at all but can still pass giardiasis on to others. The infectious stage can last from 3 weeks to a few months after infection.

DIAGNOSIS Your child's doctor will do a complete physical examination and will ask about the circumstances surrounding the child's illness. Be sure to tell your doctor if your child is in day care or has recently been on a camping trip or to a foreign country.

Your doctor will confirm a diagnosis of giardiasis with a stool sample, which may have to be repeated several times over a week or two because early tests sometimes come back falsely negative. Your doctor may also order a blood test called an enzyme-linked immunosorbent assay (ELISA) to detect giardiasis. In the rare event that these tests do not confirm the diagnosis, your doctor may need to examine the contents of your child's small intestine using a tube inserted through the child's mouth.

TREATMENT Your doctor may treat your child for giardiasis solely on the basis of the physical exam and interview because the initial stool tests can be unreliable. To treat giardiasis, your doctor may prescribe an antiparasite medication called metronidazole, which should be taken by mouth daily for 5 to 10 days. The drug can cause nausea and vomiting. Your doctor may prescribe another medication if your child is pregnant. Children with only mild symptoms usually are not given any medication unless the child's school requires documented proof of treatment. In extreme cases, when diarrhea causes dehydration (see page 283), your doctor may hospitalize your child and replace his or her fluids *intravenously.*

At home, make sure your child gets plenty of liquids. Keep an infant or young child away from others as much as possible to prevent spreading the illness and keep your child home from day care or school until he or she has recovered.

GIGANTISM

See Height problems

GLAUCOMA

Glaucoma is an eye disease in which fluid inside the eye does not drain properly, causing increased pressure inside the eye. The increased pressure damages the nerve and blood vessels leading to the eye and can cause partial or total loss of vision. Glaucoma is a common eye disease in adults over 60, but it is rare in children. Children can be born with the disease (congenital or infantile glaucoma) or develop it in early childhood (juvenile glaucoma).

SIGNS AND SYMPTOMS Glaucoma causes a child's eyes to be unusually sensitive to light. The eyelids close suddenly and the eyes tear excessively. Other symptoms include enlarged or cloudy corneas (the outer covering of the eye) and pain or redness in the eyes. Vision may be blurred. The child may also see colored halos around lights and lose his or her peripheral (side) vision.

DIAGNOSIS If your child has symptoms of glaucoma, or if the doctor sees evidence of it during a physical examination, the doctor will send the child to an eye specialist (ophthalmologist) who will measure eye pressure with a test known as tonometry. The ophthalmologist will also examine the inside of your child's eyes for damage and will test for any loss of vision.

TREATMENT The faster glaucoma is diagnosed and treated, the better the outcome for your child. Early treatment can not only control the symptoms but also prevent total BLINDNESS in most cases. The doctor may recommend surgery or laser treatment to reduce the pressure inside your child's eyes. With or without surgery, your child will receive eyedrops or pills to reduce the pressure.

GONORRHEA

Gonorrhea is a bacterial infection of the reproductive organs, throat, and rectum transmitted during sexual contact with an infected person. Newborn infants can also become infected when they move through the birth canal of an infected mother.

The disease most often occurs in sexually active young people between the ages of 15 and 30 years who have multiple sex partners; one quarter of people infected with gonorrhea are between the ages of 10 and 19 years. A child who gets gonorrhea before reaching puberty is usually a victim of sexual abuse.

In a boy or man, the bacteria usually infect the urethra (the tube through which urine and semen pass). The bacteria primarily infect the cervix (the neck of the uterus) or the urethra in women and girls who have reached puberty. Girls who have not reached puberty usually become infected in the vagina (the muscular canal that leads from the uterus to the outside of the body) or vulva (external female genitals). Both sexes can become infected in the throat and rectum through oral and anal sexual activity. Infected newborns usually develop eye infections (CONJUNCTIVITIS). Infected children and adults can also develop eye infections by touching their eyes after touching the infected parts of their bodies.

SIGNS AND SYMPTOMS In males, symptoms include frequent and painful urination and a thick, greenish yellow discharge from the penis. Most boys and men experience symptoms of gonorrhea about 2 to 7 days after infection. Most girls or women infected in the cervix or urethra have either no symptoms or mild and easily missed symptoms, such as a swollen vulva or an unusual discharge from the vagina. Girls and women infected in the vagina or vulva may not have any symptoms or may have a thick, greenish yellow discharge from the vagina; itching in the vagina; pain in the vulva; or painful urination.

Gonorrheal eye infections produce a greenish yellow pus in the eyes. People who are infected in the throat may or may not have a sore throat. A gonorrheal infection in the rectum may cause some rectal pain, especially during a bowel movement, or an unusual, cloudy discharge from the rectum. People with gonorrhea may also develop arthritis.

DIAGNOSIS Children who have symptoms of gonorrhea should go to a doctor or a clinic for sexually transmitted diseases. The doctor will ask the child about sexual activity and sexual partners and will do a physical examination.

Complications from untreated gonorrhea

Unchecked, the bacteria that cause gonorrhea can spread to other parts of the body and cause serious complications:

- A newborn with untreated gonorrhea infection can have gonorrhea-related eye infections that can cause scarring of the eyes and even blindness.
- In females, the bacteria can spread from the vagina to the lining of the uterus and the fallopian tubes (that convey eggs to the uterus), causing abnormal menstrual bleeding and infertility (the inability to have children).
- In males, the bacteria can spread from the penis to the prostate gland (a gland that secretes the fluid that becomes part of the semen) and the epididymis (a tube that stores sperm from the testicles), causing the testicles to enlarge. Urination can become difficult, and the boy or man can become impotent.
- In infected people of both sexes and all ages, untreated gonorrhea can spread through the bloodstream and cause serious infections in the blood (SEPTICEMIA), joints (see ARTHRITIS, SEPTIC), heart (ENDOCARDITIS), spinal cord and brain (MENINGITIS), and many other parts of the body.

Sexually active girls who have no symptoms may be screened for gonorrhea during a routine gynecologic exam (see page 172).

Your doctor will order cultures of any discharge from the reproductive organs, throat, eyes, or rectum, along with a blood test to check for other sexually transmitted diseases. The doctor will also examine other areas on the body for possible infection.

People with gonorrhea typically have other sexually transmitted diseases, such as CHLAMYDIA and SYPHILIS as well, so your doctor will also test for these diseases. The human immunodeficiency virus (HIV), which causes AIDS, is also sexually transmitted, so the doctor may recommend an HIV test.

By law, a doctor must report to the proper authorities any suspected cases of child abuse. The child may have to be interviewed by the doctor or a social worker to find out how he or she became infected with gonorrhea.

TREATMENT Gonorrhea is easily treated with antibiotics, given either in pill form (cefixime) or by injection (ceftriaxone sodium). Eye infections are treated by irrigation of the eye with salt water and by ceftriaxone injected into a vein or muscle. Newborns are routinely treated with injections of penicillin given *intravenously* or ceftriaxone for confirmed gonorrhea-related eye infections.

You will have to bring your infant, child, or teenager to the doctor after treatment for a follow-up examination to make sure that the treatment was effective. People infected with gonorrhea should suspend all sexual activity until repeated testing shows the infection has cleared up after 7 to 14 days of treatment. The doctor will also want to test and treat your child's sexual partner or partners.

Left untreated–or if treatment is delayed–gonorrhea can have serious complications, including blood poisoning such as SEPTICEMIA, septic arthritis (see ARTHRITIS, SEPTIC), ENDOCARDITIS, MENINGITIS, BLINDNESS in infants, and infertility.

GUILLAIN-BARRÉ SYNDROME

Guillain-Barré syndrome is a form of nerve damage that causes muscle weakness, loss of sensation, and loss of normal reflexes. The symptoms begin in the leg nerves and travel up the body to affect the abdominal, chest, arm, and facial muscles. Sometimes the muscles that control breathing are also affected. Most cases of Guillain-Barré syndrome follow an infection by a virus. In rare cases, the syndrome can occur after a child receives an immunization.

SIGNS AND SYMPTOMS About a week or two after a child has had an infection or immunization, he or she begins to feel weakness in the legs and feet, often with tingling and numbness. The weakness spreads quickly up to other parts of the child's body. The muscle weakness can progress to paralysis that lasts for weeks or months. Weakness in the chest and facial muscles can cause breathing difficulty. The child breathes with effort, becomes anxious, and his or her skin turns bluish. Facial muscle weakness can cause speech problems and difficulty swallowing.

DIAGNOSIS If your child has symptoms of Guillain-Barré syndrome, take him or her to the doctor immediately. The doctor will perform a thorough physical examination and will order a *lumbar puncture* and an electromyography examination (a test that measures the speed of nerve impulses) to diagnose the condition.

TREATMENT Your child will need to be hospitalized so that he or she can be monitored closely for evidence of respiratory (breathing) failure. In severe cases, your child may need a breathing tube and may have to be placed on a ventilator (breathing machine). Your doctor may recommend plasmapheresis (a procedure in which your child's blood plasma is withdrawn and replaced with donated plasma) to cleanse the plasma of antibodies to the virus that caused the disorder. After treatment, your child may also need intensive physical therapy to improve muscle strength weakened by nerve damage.

Most children recover completely without permanent damage. Recovery can take as little as 2 or 3 weeks or as long as a year or more, depending on how severe the condition is. Some children have permanent muscle weakness. Having the disease does not confer immunity, so a child can get the disease again, although recurrence is rare.

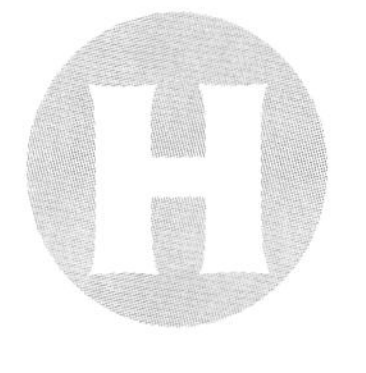

HAIR PULLING

See Alopecia

HAND-FOOT-AND-MOUTH DISEASE

Hand-foot-and-mouth disease is a mild viral infection that causes painful sores in the mouth and throat and a blistery rash on the hands and feet. The illness usually occurs in children under age 10. It is prevalent among children in day-care centers and nursery schools, and most commonly occurs in summer and early fall.

Infected children can spread the virus when they fail to wash their hands after going to the bathroom. They can also transmit it by coughing or sneezing or when they put their hands or toys in their mouths or touch the fluid inside the blisters and then touch another person.

SIGNS AND SYMPTOMS Within 5 days of infection with the virus, your child may develop a sudden fever with temperatures from 100°F to 103°F, a sore throat, and a runny nose. Blisters (see page 24) then appear in the mouth and throat, break open, and become open sores. Eating becomes painful and your child may lose his or her appetite. In rare cases, the child could become dehydrated. Small blisters and a painful rash may also develop on the palms of the child's hands; the soles of the feet; in between the fingers and toes; or on the thighs, groin, and buttocks. The symptoms are relatively mild, complications are rare, and the child usually recovers within 10 days, although the virus may remain in the stool for several weeks.

DIAGNOSIS Your child's doctor will be able to diagnosis the disease based on the symptoms.

TREATMENT Make sure your child drinks plenty of fluids. Give him or her cold foods, such as ice cream, to numb the pain in the mouth, and acetaminophen for fever. Keep your child home until the fever and sores disappear. Don't let the child share eating utensils.

HAY FEVER

Hay fever, which is also called allergic rhinitis, is the inflammation and irritation of the thin, moist tissue–known as the mucous membrane–lining the nose. It is an allergic physical reaction to pollen produced by trees, grasses, and weeds. Hay fever can also be triggered by dust, mold, and other tiny substances spread in the air. Hay fever is a common ALLERGY in children. Many children get seasonal hay fever from inhaling the pollen from trees in the spring, from grass in the summer, and from weeds in the summer and fall. Other children have hay fever all year round from dust, mold, and other air-borne particles.

SIGNS AND SYMPTOMS The most common symptoms of hay fever are nasal congestion, sneezing, and an itchy and runny nose. The child may frequently rub his or her nose. Breathing becomes difficult, and the child may snore at night (see SNORING). The child's eyes also become itchy, as well as watery and red. When mucus from the back of the nose drips into the throat, the child may begin to cough. HEADACHES, earaches, and HEARING LOSS can also occur. Other symptoms include breathing through the mouth and the temporary loss of smell and taste. These symptoms can last for days or months.

DIAGNOSIS To diagnose hay fever, the doctor will give your child a skin test. The doctor will inject a small amount of a suspected irritant into the child's skin or apply it on top of the skin to see if the skin reacts to the substance. The doctor may also analyze a small sample of the mucus from your child's nose to determine the cause of your child's hay fever. A blood test known as a radioallergosorbent test (RAST) is often helpful in detecting *antibodies* to specific substances.

TREATMENT Once your child's doctor has identified the specific cause of the hay fever, your child must try to avoid that substance. On days when the pollen count is high, your child may need to stay inside in an air-conditioned house with the windows shut so that he or she can breathe air that has had most of the pollen filtered out of it. Keep your home as free of dust as possible to minimize the effects of a dust allergy and keep your child out of damp basements and away from damp leaves if he or she has a mold allergy. To avoid the buildup of mold, clean humidifiers and vaporizers frequently. Follow your child's doctor's advice on avoiding other possible allergens.

Your child's doctor may prescribe an antihistamine or you may be able to give your child an over-the-counter antihistamine to treat his or her sneezing and itchy and runny nose. Always talk to your child's doctor first before giving your child nonprescription medications because they can make your child sleepy and cause other side effects. You may be able to give your child decongestants for a stuffy nose, but only for a short time because, when they wear off, decongestants can make symptoms worse with continued use. Your child's doctor may also prescribe inhaled *corticosteroids* to reduce any swelling in your child's nasal passages. A drug called cromolyn sodium that is inhaled as a nasal spray might be prescribed to reduce allergic reactions, especially in young children. In addition, the doctor may give your child allergy shots once a week to desensitize him or her to allergens.

HEADACHES

Pain in the head from a headache is common in children. Headache is most often a mild, temporary pain caused by a bump on the head, too much or too little sleep, too much sun, or worry about school. Headaches are also a frequent symptom of other illnesses, ranging from a mild cold to severe infections or a BRAIN TUMOR. The pain itself can come from pressure on or injury to the skull, brain, blood vessels, or membrane lining the brain (the meninges). The skin on the scalp, the blood vessels in the scalp, or the muscles in the head and neck can also become painful.

Ear infections (see page 480), SINUSITIS, colds or influenza (see page 231), STREP INFECTION, and ALLERGIES are some common illnesses that cause headaches. Dieting and skipping meals can also produce headaches. Use of alcohol and prescription or nonprescription drugs, such as birth-control pills or diet pills, can result in headache pain. MIGRAINE is the most common headache that is unrelated to other disease or injury in children. A migraine is a throbbing headache usually on one side of the head that can last for an hour or more; children who get migraines often have a family history of this type of headache. Tension headaches—a dull ache caused by stress or ANXIETY—are more common in adults.

SIGNS AND SYMPTOMS A child who gets a headache from an illness or injury will have a combination of symptoms that indicate the underlying problem. Children under age 3 cannot tell you that they have a headache. Children with migraines have pounding, throbbing pain in the front of the head that can occur on one or both sides. Episodes of migraines can occur repeatedly over a lifetime. The headaches last an hour or more. The child looks pale and may lose his or her appetite or feel nauseous. Some children experience an aura—bright flashes of light, blurred vision, and black holes or blind spots—in one or both eyes just before the pain begins. The child may vomit (see page 284) during the aura. Children with migraines are tired and irritable, have abdominal pain, and appear confused and withdrawn. Toddlers experience a type of migraine known as paroxysmal vertigo, in which the child has a dizzy feeling of spinning or whirling that happens suddenly and disappears in minutes.

Tension headaches cause a constant dull ache on both sides of the child's head, along with muscle tightness in the neck and scalp. The child may be tired and weak, nauseous, and unusually sensitive to light and sound. The child's appetite may be poor and he or she may have trouble sleeping. Tension headaches can persist on and off for months.

DIAGNOSIS AND TREATMENT If your child has a headache that you suspect might be from a disease or injury, take him or her to the doctor for diagnosis and treatment. Call the doctor immediately if your child is awakened at night by a headache or if he or she vomits; shows changes in behavior, coordination, or vision; or loses consciousness. Your child's doctor will do a thorough physical examination and may order *computed tomography* or *magnetic resonance imaging* of your child's head to test for the presence of a brain tumor.

If your child has symptoms of a migraine, encourage your child to sleep or at least lie quietly in a dimly lit room to relieve the symptoms. See your child's doctor for a definite diagnosis. He or she may prescribe medication that can either help prevent the migraines from occurring or relieve the pain. Ask the doctor if your child should take over-the-counter pain relievers, such as acetaminophen or ibuprofen. For tension headaches, your child should rest in a dark room and try to sleep. Offer your child a light meal. Encourage him or her to talk about what is causing the tension and try to help your child change the way he or she reacts to stress. You can also give your child an over-the-counter pain reliever, such as acetaminophen or ibuprofen (but not aspirin).

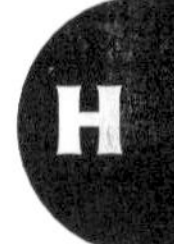

HEAD, NECK, OR SPINE INJURIES

Injuries to the head, neck, or spine can take many forms. Most children get minor head injuries while playing or during sports. But, when children injure their head, they can also injure their neck and spine. Simply falling backward can injure the head, neck, and spine. If, after a fall or bump on the head, your child has no pain in the neck or spine and gets up right away, it's likely that no serious harm has been done. But you should watch your child closely over the next day or two for signs of more serious injury. Call the doctor if your child is bleeding; has changes in mental alertness or behavior; has numbness, tingling, or decreased feeling; or cannot use some part of his or her body.

The most frequent cause of serious head, neck, and spine injuries is an automobile collision. Other common causes are playing sports, falls, and biking injuries. Serious injuries to a child's head, neck, or spine can have devastating consequences, including brain damage, paralysis, and death.

SIGNS AND SYMPTOMS Symptoms of different injuries can vary and overlap. Here are descriptions of frequent symptoms of each type:

- **Head injuries** Injuries to the head can cause minor cuts, bumps, BRUISES, deep cuts, open wounds, and skull fractures (see page 490). A head injury can also produce internal bleeding and brain damage. Immediate physical signs occurring after a head injury include a severe HEADACHE, bleeding from the scalp, blurred vision, vomiting, weakness, stumbling, seizures, pupils of different sizes, and blood or a clear fluid draining from the ears or nose. Other signs can occur 2 days or more after the injury, including fatigue, a persistent headache, dizziness, unusual sensitivity to sound and light, vomiting, and difficulty sleeping and speaking. Mental and behavioral signs that can occur immediately after a head injury include loss or a diminished level of consciousness, drowsiness, memory loss, and confused speech. Depending on the severity of injury, the child may also have difficulty concentrating, start falling behind in school, have difficulty remembering things, get easily upset or angry, show moodiness, be impatient, and lack interest in his or her usual activities. These symptoms can occur days or weeks after the injury.
- **Spinal injuries** Injuries to the bones that surround the spinal cord (vertebrae) can cause severe pain and swelling at the site of injury. Spinal cord injuries can cause weakness, paralysis, loss of bladder and bowel control, severe back pain, numbness or tingling in the arms or legs, and difficulty walking. Spinal cord injuries that occur below the neck can cause weakness, loss of feeling, and complete paralysis below the level of the injury, especially in the legs. Injuries to the spinal cord that occur in the neck can cause weakness, loss of feeling, and complete paralysis below the neck. In some children, breathing may become difficult because of injury to the nerves controlling breathing. The higher the injury on the spinal cord, the more extensive the symptoms.
- **Neck injuries** A child's neck can also be injured by being twisted to one side or being whipped backward by a sudden or forceful blow (whiplash). Such injuries can cause stiffness or pain in the neck, dizziness, headache, nausea, and vomiting.

DIAGNOSIS If your child has signs of serious injury to the head, neck, or spine, don't move the child yourself unless he or she is in further danger. Keep your child's head, neck, and spine as still as possible. Do not remove a helmet your child may be wearing. Call an ambulance to take your child to a hospital emergency department immediately. A doctor will assess the extent of your child's injuries with X-rays, *computed tomography*, and *magnetic resonance imaging*.

TREATMENT Your child's treatment will depend on the type and extent of injury he or she sustained. The doctor will treat any external injuries, such as deep cuts, right away. Depending on what your child's diagnostic studies reveal, he or she may need surgery to stop internal bleeding, repair severe skull fractures, or treat spinal injuries. Your child may require either a collar or brace to support an injured neck or spine or a body splint to immobilize any fractured vertebrae so they can heal. Traction, which aligns the injured bones by placing tension on the spine, may also be needed. Healing can take months.

An injured child may also need physical therapy to regain movement after treatment for head or spinal cord injuries. He or she may also need to use crutches or a wheelchair. Individual and family counseling may be necessary to help your child and your family adjust to any permanent physical or mental disabilities your child may have sustained from the injury. For information on how to prevent injuries to your child's head, neck, or spine, see page 299.

HEARING LOSS

Hearing loss refers to a partial or complete inability to hear sounds. A hearing loss can be temporary or permanent and can occur in one or both ears. Complete, permanent hearing loss in both ears is rare, and it is usually congenital (present at birth).

Sound waves travel from a child's outer ear down the ear canal to the eardrum, a thin membrane that vibrates when the sound waves hit it. Vibrations from the eardrum travel to the child's middle ear where three tiny bones vibrate and cause another membrane, the inner ear membrane, to vibrate. The vibrations pass to the inner ear, where they are turned into electrical impulses that travel through the acoustic nerve to the child's brain.

Among children, the most common reason for a temporary hearing loss is a middle-ear infection (see page 480) that causes a buildup of sticky fluid in the middle ear. The fluid interferes with the transmission of sound waves through the ear. About a fourth of all children starting school have some hearing loss from a middle-ear infection that they have had in the past.

There are two major types of hearing loss–conductive and sensorineural. Conductive hearing loss means that something interferes with the transmission of sound waves from a child's outer ear to his or her inner ear. This type of hearing loss may be caused by a blockage in the ear from fluid or earwax, damage to the eardrum, or damage to one of the three bones that make up the middle ear.

Sensorineural hearing loss means that sound waves that reach the inner ear cannot be transmitted to the child's brain because of damage to the structures of the inner ear or to the nerve that sends messages to the brain. A child may be born with this type of hearing loss or develop it later in life. Congenital sensorineural hearing loss is rare.

Damage to the inner ear can be inherited, can occur before or at birth, or can develop later in life from exposure to loud noises, viral infections, or certain drugs–especially some types of antibiotics. A tumor on the acoustic nerve or an infection such as bacterial MENINGITIS can damage the nerve.

SIGNS AND SYMPTOMS Hearing loss can range from mild to complete. In an infant, the first sign of hearing loss may be the baby's failure to turn his or her head and move his or her eyes in response to a voice or other sounds. The infant may not begin to form sounds or babble words at the proper time. For an infant with complete hearing loss, learning to speak is possible but quite difficult.

In addition to difficulty hearing sounds, an affected child may also have a ringing in the ears, pain in the ears, or dizziness and loss of balance. He or she may constantly turn only one ear toward a voice or sound or often ask people to repeat what they are saying. The child may have trouble carrying on a conversation. A child with complete hearing loss cannot hear any sounds. The child may sense sound-wave vibrations from physical objects, such as floors or walls, and may be able to hear very loud sounds, but he or she cannot hear normal speech, so learning to speak is seriously affected.

DIAGNOSIS Take your child to the doctor if you notice any signs of hearing loss in your child because impaired hearing can seriously affect his or her speech development and school performance. The doctor will probably refer your child to an otolaryngologist (an ear, nose, and throat specialist) who will examine your child's ears and order hearing tests.

TREATMENT If your child has a buildup of earwax that is causing hearing loss, the doctor or specialist will remove it. The doctor will treat an infection in the ear with antibiotics. A buildup of fluid in the ear may require surgical drainage. A perforated eardrum that has caused hearing loss can heal on its own. However, if it doesn't, your child may need surgery to repair the perforation. Your child may need a hearing aid (see illustration below) if his or her hearing loss is serious. In some cases of sensorineural hearing loss, the doctor may recommend a cochlear implant (see illustration at right). Your child may also require speech therapy, lipreading education, sign language training, and special education classes at school.

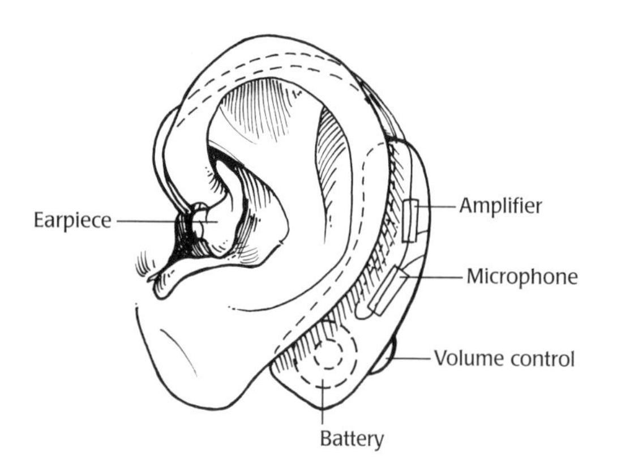

How a hearing aid works

A hearing aid is a battery-operated electronic device that can help improve a child's hearing. A hearing aid amplifies sound by collecting sound waves with a microphone and transforming them into an electric current. The amplifier increases the current and conveys it into an earpiece that converts the current back into louder (amplified) sound. A child can adjust the volume of the sound by turning a tiny knob on the device.

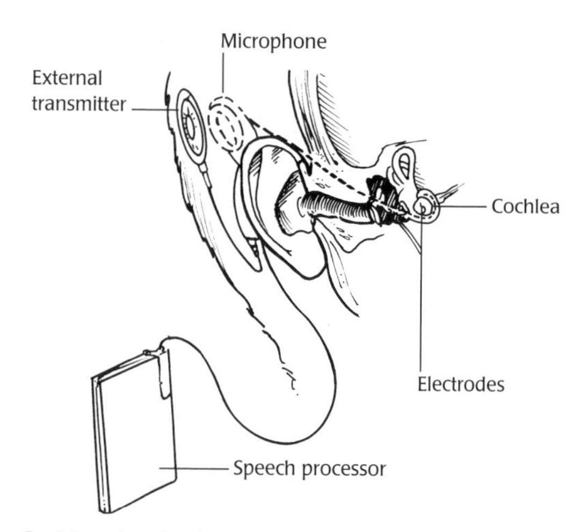

Cochlear implants

A cochlear implant is an electronic device that is surgically implanted in the inner ear to help a child with profound sensorineural hearing loss (nerve deafness) better distinguish speech. Sounds in the environment are picked up by a small microphone worn above the ear, then sent to a speech processor (worn under clothing or at ear level) that converts sounds to electronic signals. These signals go to an external transmitter behind the ear and then to an implanted receiver/stimulator (not shown), which sends the signals to the cochlea (a structure in the inner ear that changes sound vibrations into nerve impulses). The cochlear implant does not amplify sound, as a hearing aid does, but provides sound information by stimulating nerve fibers.

HEART DISEASE, CONGENITAL

Congenital heart disease is the term used to describe one or more defects, present at birth, in a newborn baby's heart or in the blood vessels connected to the heart. The defects develop at various stages in the growth of the fetus. Although the defects are present at birth, they may not be discovered or diagnosed until later in the child's life. Congenital heart disease is the most common BIRTH DEFECT.

Among the most common forms of congenital heart disease are COARCTATION OF THE AORTA, HYPOPLASTIC LEFT HEART SYNDROME, PATENT DUCTUS ARTERIOSUS, SEPTAL DEFECTS, aortic or pulmonary stenosis (see STENOSIS, AORTIC AND PULMONARY),

Risk factors for congenital heart disease

While scientists don't know exactly what causes congenital heart disease, they do know that some environmental and genetic factors affecting the parents have been shown to increase a newborn's risk of a heart defect. These factors include:

- **Chronic illnesses, such as diabetes (see DIABETES MELLITUS, TYPE I) and PKU, in the mother** If you have a chronic disorder, seek a doctor's advice on controlling the condition before you become pregnant.
- **A case of GERMAN MEASLES in the first 3 months of pregnancy** Women should be tested for immunity to German measles before becoming pregnant.
- **Use of alcohol and certain drugs during pregnancy** Such drugs include an acne medicine known as isotretinoin, lithium, and some medications for SEIZURE DISORDERS. Stop drinking alcohol and seek a doctor's advice about the use of any drug before or during pregnancy.
- **Inherited factors** Heart defects can run in families and may be related to other birth defects, such as DOWN SYNDROME. Parents with a family history of heart defects should seek genetic counseling (see page 497) before having children.

TETRALOGY OF FALLOT, TRANSPOSITION OF THE GREAT ARTERIES, and VALVE ABNORMALITIES. These defects are discussed in detail in individual entries. Most of these heart defects either obstruct the flow of blood through a baby's heart, producing inadequate blood flow to the body, or cause the blood to flow through the baby's heart abnormally, depriving the body of essential oxygen in some cases. No one knows for sure what causes most cases of congenital heart disease, but a number of factors have been linked to this type of birth defect (see box above).

SIGNS AND SYMPTOMS The symptoms of congenital heart disease may begin at birth or later in childhood. Newborns and infants with congenital heart disease look pale, feed poorly, and become irritable and lethargic. The most common initial sign is cyanosis, which means that the baby's skin turns bluish. Cyanosis occurs because the baby's heart cannot pump enough blood or because the heart is circulating blood that does not contain sufficient amounts of oxygen. If the cyanosis is severe enough and lasts a long time, the tips of the infant's fingers and toes can become thick and club-shaped.

An affected baby may also have breathing problems, typically shortness of breath and rapid breathing (more than 60 breaths per minute). The baby may grunt and wheeze and flare his or her nostrils. The breathing difficulties and cyanosis can worsen when the infant cries, feeds, or has a bowel movement. The infant can also have difficulty feeding, which can result in poor weight gain. In severe cases, the newborn or infant may also sweat excessively while feeding, and have RESPIRATORY DISTRESS SYNDROME, FAILURE TO THRIVE, and congestive heart failure (see HEART FAILURE, CONGESTIVE).

An affected older child may be tired, weak, and short of breath in response to stress or while exercising strenuously. The child may need to stop and squat down to make it easier to breathe (see illustration on page 647). He or she may also have fainting spells, especially during exercise.

Chest pain in an otherwise healthy child is another sign of congenital heart disease. Other findings include an irregular heartbeat (see ARRHYTHMIAS), a HEART MURMUR, and dizziness. In severe cases, the child can die suddenly of heart disease.

DIAGNOSIS If your child has any symptoms of congenital heart disease, the doctor will thoroughly examine your child and listen to his or her heart with a stethoscope to detect a heart murmur, irregular heartbeat, or other signs of congenital heart disease. To pinpoint the diagnosis, your doctor will need to order other examinations, including a chest X-ray, *electrocardiogram, echocardiogram,* or *cardiac catheterization.*

H

TREATMENT If your child has congenital heart disease, the doctor will refer him or her to a heart specialist (cardiologist). In some cases, the cardiologist prescribes medications, rest, or oxygen to control the child's symptoms over the short term, or even indefinitely. Some defects, such as ventricular septal defect, sometimes disappear on their own without treatment. If your child has severe disease, he or she may need to be hospitalized for treatment.

In many cases, a child requires surgery to correct the defect or replace a defective heart valve. Doctors have become quite skilled at performing heart surgery in infants and children, so the chances are good that surgery will be successful. In 3 to 6 months after surgery, your child should be able to resume full activities and even participate in sports. Infants usually grow and develop normally after successful surgery.

HEART FAILURE, CONGESTIVE

Congestive heart failure is a condition in which a child's heart pumps insufficient amounts of blood to his or her body. The heart does not actually fail or stop, but it does become too weak to circulate enough blood through the child's body. As a result, blood backs up in other organs, especially in the child's lungs and liver. Some children are born with heart defects (see HEART DISEASE, CONGENITAL) that can cause congestive heart failure. Other children develop congestive heart failure from diseases, such as ENDOCARDITIS, RHEUMATIC FEVER, CARDIOMYOPATHY, and HIGH BLOOD PRESSURE, that they acquire after birth.

SIGNS AND SYMPTOMS A baby with congestive heart failure is slow to feed and requires frequent feedings. He or she may breathe rapidly and sweat excessively while feeding. The infant may have problems gaining weight, be irritable, cry a lot, have puffy eyes, and have a persistent cough. Children with congestive heart failure are very weak and tired. They may not be able to engage in strenuous exercise and they often wheeze or cough when exercising. They may have swelling and pain in the abdomen, be short of breath when resting, flare their nostrils, have a chronic cough, have swollen legs or ankles, develop a rapid or irregular heartbeat, sweat excessively, and have a swollen liver. The child's skin may be pale and cool, especially in the hands and feet. A HEART MURMUR and blood pressure changes may also be present.

DIAGNOSIS If your child has symptoms of congestive heart failure, see the doctor immediately for diagnosis and treatment. The doctor will probably order X-rays of your child's chest and abdomen and order an *electrocardiogram* or an *echocardiogram*. These diagnostic studies are painless. The doctor will also order blood tests and a urine analysis. Some affected children need a procedure known as *cardiac catheterization*, in which a thin tube is threaded through a vein in your child's leg into his or her heart to monitor blood pressure inside the heart. The doctor may also infuse dye into the tube and watch the movement of the dye through the heart using an X-ray machine, to assess blood flow and detect any defects. The procedure is done using local anesthesia and causes little discomfort. Your child may have to stay overnight in the hospital for the procedure.

TREATMENT Using these tests, the doctor will try to find out the underlying cause of your child's congestive heart failure and then treat the cause. If your child has a structural defect, such as a valve abnormality or COARCTATION OF THE AORTA, in his or her heart, the child may need surgery to correct the defect. If an infection is causing the heart failure, your child will receive antibiotics, usually *intravenously*, while in the hospital. He or she may also receive medications to treat other underlying diseases.

Your child will need to rest in bed with his or her upper body elevated. All physical activity must be curtailed until the symptoms are controlled by medication or surgery. He or she may also need to take diuretics to rid the body of excessive fluid and heart medication to regulate the heartbeat and heart function. Your child may need to take antibiotics before any future dental work or surgery to reduce the risk of a possible heart infection.

HEART MURMUR

A heart murmur is an extra sound produced by the heart, caused by blood passing through abnormal holes in the heart or through partially blocked vessels or valves. Sometimes the sound is caused by the normal closing of heart valves—known as functional (or innocent) murmurs. The sound is most often heard in children and teenagers, but can also occur in infants. Most heart murmurs are functional, but sometimes they indicate a serious underlying heart condition or disease, such as a congenital heart defect (see HEART DISEASE, CONGENITAL) or RHEUMATIC FEVER.

SIGNS AND SYMPTOMS There are two normal heart sounds, which you can hear by placing your ear to your child's chest. One sounds like a "lubb" followed by one that sounds like a "dubb" at a higher pitch. A heart with a murmur produces an extra sound, sometimes described as a "swishing" sound. Some children have more than one murmur. A heart murmur can rarely be heard without an instrument called a stethoscope placed on the chest.

Many newborns have a heart murmur in the first 2 days of life, as the heart is converting from fetal to human circulation and complete closure of the ductus arteriosus occurs (see PATENT DUCTUS ARTERIOSUS). Heart murmurs can occur in children anytime during childhood. They may be more distinct after exercise or when a child has a fever. They can come and go, or remain permanently.

DIAGNOSIS A doctor usually detects a heart murmur while using a stethoscope to listen to your child's heart during a routine physical examination. Your child's doctor, or a heart specialist known as a cardiologist to whom your child may be referred, can judge whether or not the murmur is harmless (medically called functional or innocent) by simply listening to your child's heart. If the quality or type of murmur is in doubt, the doctor will order additional tests, such as a chest X-ray, an *electrocardiogram*, or an *echocardiogram* (an *ultrasound* of the heart).

TREATMENT A harmless heart murmur requires no treatment. There is no reason to become overprotective of your child or to limit his or her activities. Most such murmurs disappear in time. If your child has an underlying heart defect or disease that is causing the murmur, then the doctor will treat your child accordingly with observation, medication, or surgery. Children who have a heart murmur may need to take antibiotics before dental work or surgery to prevent a possible infection of the heart.

HEAT STROKE

See page 679

HEIGHT PROBLEMS

Height problems refer to height that is either unusually short or unusually tall for a child's age. Height is generally determined by the genes children inherit from their parents. Short children usually have short parents (or at least one short parent) and tall children usually have tall parents. Sometimes a child's height is affected by a disorder of the pituitary gland, a pea-sized gland located at the base of the brain that secretes growth hormone (see PITUITARY DISORDERS). The pituitary is sometimes called the master gland because it regulates the activities of other glands in the body. The pituitary gland also produces a number of other hormones, in addition to growth hormone. There are two main types of height problems that can occur in childhood—tall stature (gigantism) and short stature (dwarfism).

SIGNS AND SYMPTOMS In gigantism, a tumor on a child's pituitary gland can cause the gland to produce an excessive amount of growth hormone during childhood or adolescence. Pituitary tumors are usually benign (unable to spread to surrounding tissue). But, left untreated, the tumor can destroy the pituitary gland and cause death early in adult life.

The main sign of tall stature in a child is abnormal overall growth. The child attains an unusually tall height and his or her bones, muscles, and organs grow proportionately large, but the child's sexual development may be delayed. He or she may continue to grow even after reaching adulthood. Symptoms that mimic those of a BRAIN TUMOR, such as HEADACHES, vomiting, and VISION PROBLEMS, can occur. If the child develops a pituitary tumor after his or her arms and legs have stopped growing, he or she will instead develop acromegaly, an enlargement of the skull, feet, hands, and jaw. He or she may also have a large nose, enlarged ears, and a husky voice. It is common for gigantism and acromegaly to occur simultaneously. In rare cases, a child can grow very tall from a disorder, such as MARFAN SYNDROME, that is unrelated to the pituitary gland.

In dwarfism, a pituitary tumor can also cause the pituitary gland to produce too little growth hormone, resulting in an abnormally short child. Pituitary dwarfism differs from dwarfism caused by skeletel or connective tissue disorders, which produce abnormal proportions of the child's body in addition to short height. The signs of pituitary dwarfism are retarded growth or no growth at all, abnormally short height, delayed or no sexual development in adolescents, headaches, excessive thirst, excessive urination, and HYPOGLYCEMIA. The retarded growth may begin in infancy and can continue throughout childhood. Dwarfism can also be caused by a damaged or missing pituitary gland, an inability to respond to growth hormone, deficiencies or unresponsiveness to other hormones needed for growth (see HYPOTHYROIDISM), infection, and certain diseases (chronic kidney failure [see KIDNEY FAILURE, CHRONIC], CYSTIC FIBROSIS, DOWN SYNDROME, and TURNER'S SYNDROME). Poor nutrition and emotional or physical abuse can also result in retarded growth.

DIAGNOSIS The doctor will measure your child's growth at each well-child visit and compare it to the measurements of children his or her age on a standard growth chart. The doctor may also order X-rays of your child's bones, blood tests to measure growth and other hormone levels, and *computed tomography* or *magnetic resonance imaging* of your child's head to look for abnormalities in the pituitary gland.

TREATMENT If your child has a pituitary tumor, he or she will need surgery, medication, or *radiation* to remove or destroy the tumor. Your child may also need to take drugs that lower growth hormone levels or hormone therapy to replace the missing growth hormone. If your child's height problem is caused by another type of disorder, the doctor will treat your child accordingly. If your child's dwarfism is inherited, you and your child should seek genetic counseling (see page 497).

HEMANGIOMA

A hemangioma is a birthmark that can appear anywhere on a baby's face or body at birth or within a few weeks of birth. Hemangiomas are made up of blood vessels clustered together under the skin that are visible at the surface. Hemangiomas can also occur internally and can appear later in life after an injury to the affected area. Hemangiomas are more common in female babies and premature infants. There are two main types of hemangiomas–strawberry birthmarks and cavernous hemangiomas.

SIGNS AND SYMPTOMS Strawberry birthmarks are slightly raised, bright red, and lie close to the surface, while cavernous hemangiomas are larger, more bluish, and lie deeper under the skin.

Strawberry birthmark hemangiomas begin as a slightly discolored spot on the skin and then grow rapidly in size, some up to 2 or 3 inches in diameter, in the first 8 months of life. After that, they usually stop growing and turn pink-gray. Then they begin to shrink away slowly over the next 6 to 12 months, although this process could take up to 5 years.

Cavernous hemangiomas can grow up to 5 to 8 inches or more and can take from 5 to 9 years to shrink. Many disappear almost completely, but often leave a faint mark on the skin.

Newborns usually have only one hemangioma, but may get two or three. It is rare to get more. Such birthmarks are usually painless but in rare cases, if they grow or shrink at an unusual rate, they can form open sores and become infected. If hemangiomas appear on an infant's eyelids, mouth, nose, or rectum, or on the genitals of girls, they can interfere with normal vision, feeding, breathing, or other body functions. Some cavernous hemangiomas may consume the platelets (cells needed to clot wounds) in your child's blood and bleed from within, causing anemia.

DIAGNOSIS Your doctor will examine your baby's birthmark carefully to confirm the diagnosis of hemangioma and will decide whether it needs treatment.

TREATMENT In most cases, doctors leave hemangiomas untreated so they can shrink on their own. If your child has a hemangioma on his or her eyelids or on another area that can interfere with normal function or appearance, he or she may need treatment with oral or injected *corticosteroids* or laser surgery, done by a dermatologist (a doctor who specializes in disorders of the skin), to reduce the size of the birthmark. The drugs might be taken by mouth or injected directly into the hemangioma. Your child may feel some pain while receiving laser treatment. Ask your doctor if he or she thinks your child needs to have any pain medication before the laser treatment. Hemangiomas that have developed after infancy may require surgical removal.

HEMOLYTIC-UREMIC SYNDROME

Hemolytic-uremic syndrome (HUS) is a rare but serious and life-threatening kidney disease that causes rapidly progressing kidney failure, anemia, and other organ damage from abnormal internal blood clotting. It usually occurs in children under 10 years of age, especially those under 5 years old. Seventy-five percent of all children who develop HUS have been infected by a specific type of the intestinal bacteria Escherichia coli (E coli) known as E coli 0157:H7. Children are infected from eating undercooked chicken or beef or contaminated dairy products or fruit.

Children can also become infected with the bacteria by direct contact with the feces of other people who have the bacteria in their stool. Person-to-person spread of E coli is a particular problem in day-care centers, where infected children may not wash their hands after using the toilet, or day-care workers may not wash their hands after changing the diapers of infected infants.

In an infected child, the bacteria release a *toxin* that spreads through the bloodstream and causes clotting, leading to kidney failure and damage to other organs. Destruction of red blood cells causes anemia. Some children die of kidney failure or of damage to their brain, heart, liver, or intestines. Others survive but have permanent kidney, brain, or intestinal damage. In rare cases, HUS can recur.

SIGNS AND SYMPTOMS A child first develops stomach cramps and diarrhea that turns bloody in a day or two. Some children also become nauseous and start vomiting. A slight fever may or may not be present. Within 2 days to 2 weeks, symptoms of weakness, irritability, rapid heartbeat, rapid breathing, pale or yellow skin, and less frequent urination develop. More severe symptoms, such as kidney failure, stroke, coma, seizures, or intestinal rupture may follow.

DIAGNOSIS If the doctor suspects your child has an E coli 0157:H7 infection, he or she will request a stool *culture* to screen for the bacteria. Then the doctor will closely watch your child for signs—such as pale skin, decreased urination, and increased blood pressure—of HUS. Your doctor will also order blood and urine tests to rule out other infections and to help monitor your child's anemia and kidney function.

TREATMENT No specific treatment for HUS exists but a child with the disorder will be hospitalized so his or her symptoms can be treated. The child will receive fluids *intravenously*, high blood pressure medication, and a high-calorie, high-carbohydrate diet that is low in protein. Dialysis treatments (see page 545) may be necessary to remove waste from the child's blood if kidney failure occurs. The doctor may also order blood transfusions and immune globulin (a protein that helps suppress the destruction of red blood cells and platelets) given intravenously. Sometimes doctors use a technique called plasmapheresis to treat HUS. In this procedure, a machine withdraws the child's blood, removes particles that can damage the blood cells, and reinfuses the blood into the child. In general, most children with HUS who receive prompt treatment do well in the long run, but the outcome depends on how severe the disease was in the beginning and how the child responds to treatment.

If your child is in day care, he or she will not be able to return to the day-care center until two stool cultures show no evidence of infection.

HEMOPHILIA

Hemophilia is an inherited BLEEDING DISORDER caused by the deficiency of a clotting protein in the blood, producing extensive or prolonged bleeding. There are two types of hemophilia—A and B. A child with hemophilia A is deficient in clotting factor VIII, while a child with hemophilia B, which is much less common, lacks clotting factor IX.

The vast majority of hemophiliacs are boys. The disease occurs only rarely in girls, but girls can be carriers of the condition, passing it on from one generation to the next. A male hemophiliac passes the disease gene to his daughters (who become carriers) but not to his sons. His unaffected daughters then pass the disease to some of their sons, while some of their daughters become carriers.

SIGNS AND SYMPTOMS The symptoms of hemophilia usually do not appear until the child begins to crawl and walk, when bleeding inside the joints occurs and cuts and scrapes fail to stop bleeding. Hemophilia sometimes produces excessive bleeding that can be external (from the skin) or internal (inside the body). A fall can cause internal bleeding into the brain or deep bruises on the child's skin. The seriousness of the bleeding can vary from child to child and from family to family; it depends on the amount of clotting factor present in the child's blood. Children with mild hemophilia usually have fewer complications from bleeding.

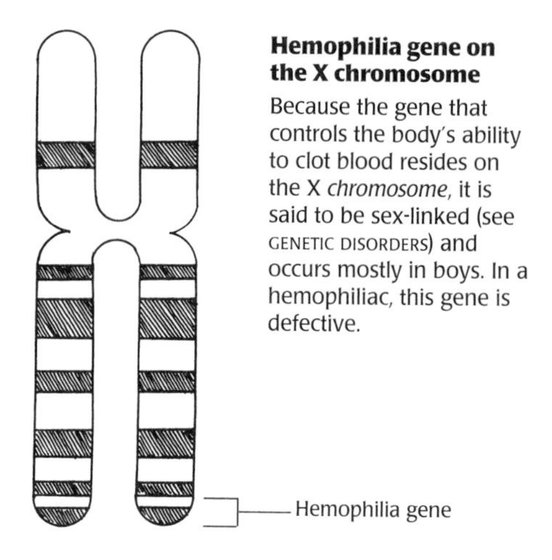

Hemophilia gene on the X chromosome

Because the gene that controls the body's ability to clot blood resides on the X *chromosome*, it is said to be sex-linked (see GENETIC DISORDERS) and occurs mostly in boys. In a hemophiliac, this gene is defective.

Even minor cuts and tooth extractions can cause long periods of bleeding. The child may also develop sudden NOSEBLEEDS and have blood in his urine. While he is bleeding, he may have swollen legs or arms and swollen, painful joints, especially his ankles, knees, or elbows. Left untreated, recurrent bleeding inside a joint can cause permanent joint damage, making movement difficult. Bleeding into the muscles after an injury can cause anemia. By the time an affected child is old enough to go to preschool, he can learn to recognize serious bleeding in his joints by a tingling sensation inside the joint, followed by swelling, pain, a sensation of warmth, and difficulty moving the joint.

DIAGNOSIS If your child's doctor suspects that your son has hemophilia, he or she will take a family history (see page 224) to determine if hemophilia runs in your family, although 20 to 30 percent of hemophiliacs have no family history of the disease. To confirm the diagnosis, your doctor will test your child's blood to find out if his factor VIII or factor IX level is abnormally low.

TREATMENT Your son's doctor will control his bleeding by replacing the missing clotting factor *intravenously*. The doctor may teach you and your child to give injections of factor VIII or factor IX at home to prevent further bleeding and to minimize organ or tissue damage when an injury occurs and your child begins to bleed. Your child will still need to go to a hospital for injections of the clotting factor if he is injured severely, bleeding excessively, or has suffered a head injury.

As a hemophiliac, your child needs to avoid sports that involve physical contact, such as football and basketball, but he or she can still participate in such activities as swimming, biking, running, and walking in moderation. Your child should also avoid taking aspirin and ibuprofen or drugs that contain them because they may increase bleeding.

In the past, hemophiliacs were at risk of becoming infected with the human immunodeficiency virus (HIV), the virus that causes AIDS, from blood transfusions and infusions of factor VIII or IX. The current use of genetically engineered factor VIII or IX and more effective blood-screening methods for HIV have substantially reduced that risk. If your child has hemophilia, talk to your doctor about the current risk of HIV transmission through blood transfusion.

It is important to seek treatment for your child at the first signs of hemophilia because the earlier the treatment, the less chance of excessive bleeding, anemia, or permanent damage to the brain, muscles, and joints. Hemophilia cannot be cured, but with proper treatment, your child can lead a nearly normal life. Anyone with a family history of hemophilia should receive genetic counseling (see page 497) before having children.

HEPATITIS

Hepatitis is an inflammation of the liver caused by a number of different viruses and characterized by flulike symptoms and occasionally jaundice (yellowing of the whites of the eyes and the skin). Children usually get hepatitis from a virus carried in human stool or in contaminated food or drink. The virus enters the body through the child's mouth and spreads to the liver through the bloodstream. Certain medications and toxic substances, such as alcohol, can also cause hepatitis.

TYPES OF HEPATITIS There are at least seven major types of hepatitis—types A, B, C, D, E, F, and G—defined by the specific virus that invades the liver. Children are most likely to get hepatitis A. The usual means of transmission is through food or liquids handled by an infected person. Hepatitis A can also be spread in water contaminated by sewage.

The hepatitis B and C viruses are spread through direct contact with the blood, semen, or other body fluids of infected people, usually through sexual activity or after being stuck with a needle contaminated by hepatitis-infected blood. The B and C viruses can also pass from an infected mother to her newborn as the infant goes through the birth canal.

Children—especially those age 5 years and under—who live with someone infected with the hepatitis B or C viruses are at risk of contracting these types of hepatitis. Infants and children infected with the hepatitis B or C viruses may develop chronic (repeatedly occurring or long-term) hepatitis, which can lead to cirrhosis (scarring of the liver), liver failure, or liver cancer.

Less is known about the hepatitis D, E, F, and G viruses. Type D appears to be the most serious, but it only causes disease when the hepatitis B virus is also present. As medicine continues to discover new viruses, the list of hepatitis viruses will probably grow.

SIGNS AND SYMPTOMS The symptoms of hepatitis usually begin with fever, headache, an upset stomach, vomiting, loss of appetite, sore muscles and joints, fatigue, and weakness. These symptoms can last from several weeks to several months. A few days or weeks later, the child's urine may darken, the stool may become light or whitish in color, and the child may become jaundiced, although jaundice is rare in children. Most children who get hepatitis B or C have no symptoms. If symptoms do develop, they are usually milder in children than in adults.

DIAGNOSIS If your child has been exposed to someone with hepatitis or has any of the characteristic symptoms, take the child to your doctor. To rule out other possible illnesses and confirm a diagnosis of hepatitis, the doctor will order tests of your child's blood, urine, stool, and liver function. In severe and chronic cases of hepatitis, a liver *biopsy* may be needed to confirm the diagnosis and assess the level of damage to the liver.

TREATMENT There is no effective medication to treat hepatitis. In most cases, you can care for your child at home without getting hepatitis yourself. Make sure he or she gets plenty of rest. If the child can't keep down solid foods or has lost his or her appetite, offer broth and juices until the child can eat again. Give plenty of fluids to drink. Your doctor may also recommend giving the child vitamins. Never give anyone with hepatitis anything that contains alcohol.

While the child is sick, provide separate or disposable eating and drinking utensils to avoid spreading the disease to other family members. Make sure the child washes his or her hands after using the toilet and before meals. Ideally, he or she should use a separate bathroom. If you have an infant with hepatitis, be sure to wash your own hands after changing diapers and before preparing or eating food. If your child has severe nausea and vomiting, your doctor may place him or her in the hospital to treat dehydration (see page 283) with fluids given *intravenously*, and to provide a special diet.

Your child can resume normal activities as soon as he or she feels strong enough. Keep the child out of school or day care and away from other people—especially children—as much as possible for at least 1 week after his or her symptoms begin or until any jaundice goes away. In severe cases, the child may have to be kept away from others for up to 6 weeks.

If your child has been exposed to someone with hepatitis A but has no symptoms, tell your doctor. The doctor may give the child a shot of gamma globulin, a protein that can help reduce the severity of symptoms or prevent them from developing. A child who lives in a household with a known carrier of the hepatitis B virus or one who was born to a hepatitis-infected mother may receive a vaccine against hepatitis B in a series of three injections. Doctors now routinely give newborns, infants, children, and teens the hepatitis B vaccine to protect them against the disease.

HEREDITARY SPHEROCYTOSIS

See Spherocytosis, hereditary

HERNIA, DIAPHRAGMATIC

Diaphragmatic hernia is a condition present at birth in which the abdominal organs protrude into the chest cavity through a defect in the diaphragm, the muscle that separates the abdomen from the chest. The displaced abdominal organs press against the lungs. The condition is life threatening because the baby's lungs can't grow to their full size to sustain normal breathing.

SIGNS AND SYMPTOMS The most common symptom of diaphragmatic hernia is breathing difficulty shortly after birth. The infant breathes rapidly and begins to turn blue from lack of oxygen. The child's abdomen is flat or sunken because the abdominal organs are in the chest cavity.

DIAGNOSIS If your newborn has difficulty breathing, the doctor will order a chest X-ray. If a diaphragmatic hernia is present, the lungs will look small and the abdominal organs will be visible inside the chest cavity on the X-ray film.

TREATMENT Your baby will be placed on a ventilator (a machine to help him or her breathe) and he or she will need emergency surgery to correct the diaphragmatic hernia. A surgeon will reposition the child's abdominal organs into his or her abdomen and repair the defect in the diaphragm. Your child may need to be placed on a ventilator or a heart-lung machine again after surgery to keep the lungs functioning. If the defect was severe or if the lungs have not grown sufficiently, surgery may not correct the problem and the baby may not survive.

HERNIA, INGUINAL

An inguinal hernia is the projection of part of the small intestine into the groin through a defect in the abdominal wall. Inguinal hernias are very common in boys, but can also occur in girls. The disorder can appear in early infancy or later in childhood.

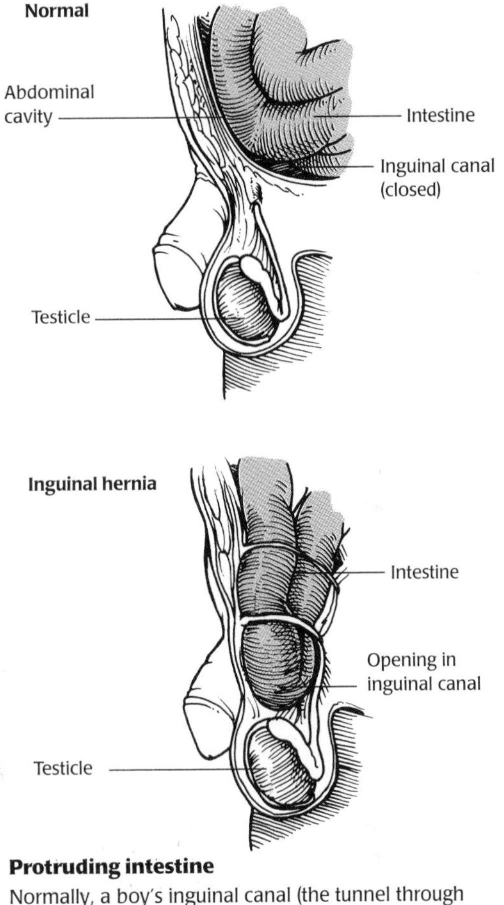

Protruding intestine

Normally, a boy's inguinal canal (the tunnel through which the testicles descend into the scrotum) closes before birth (top), keeping the intestine inside the abdominal cavity. An inguinal hernia (bottom) occurs when part of the intestine protrudes through an opening in the inguinal canal.

SIGNS AND SYMPTOMS A child with an inguinal hernia gets a lump or swelling in the groin area when crying or trying to pass stool, or while exercising (in older children). Some mild tenderness may also be present around the swelling. If the intestine becomes trapped (strangulated) in the abdominal wall, its blood supply can be cut off. A strangulated hernia causes intense pain and swelling in the groin area. If the intestine becomes obstructed, the child will vomit and his or her abdomen will distend.

Diagnosis If your child has a lump near the groin, take him or her to the doctor, who will be able to diagnose an inguinal hernia during a physical examination of the area.

Treatment Most inguinal hernias can be pushed back into the abdomen in the doctor's office. If the hernia is strangulated or has caused an intestinal obstruction, the child will need emergency surgery. Surgical correction of the hernia needs to be done promptly after diagnosis, especially in infants. Simple hernias can be surgically corrected on an *outpatient* basis, but, if the hernia is strangulated or the child is an infant, he or she will have to stay in the hospital after surgery. During the operation, a surgeon will reposition the intestine in the abdomen and repair the defect in the abdominal wall. The surgeon will want to see the child within 10 days to 2 weeks after surgery for a follow-up examination. The child can resume normal activities shortly afterward.

Hernia, umbilical

An umbilical hernia is the protrusion of part of an infant's small intestine through a defect in the abdominal wall around the navel. The defect occurs because the baby's abdominal wall muscles have not yet completely grown together. Umbilical hernias occur most frequently in newborns, especially in premature infants. They are more common in African-American infants.

Signs and symptoms A soft bulge appears around the baby's navel, especially when the baby cries. The baby usually does not feel any pain or discomfort.

Diagnosis A doctor can diagnose a newborn's umbilical hernia from its swollen appearance.

Treatment Most babies with umbilical hernias do not need treatment because the defect usually heals on its own in 3 to 5 years, sometimes sooner. If the hernia enlarges within 2 years after birth, or if the baby experiences pain, discomfort, and difficulty feeding, he or she may need to undergo surgery to repair the hernia.

Herpes, genital

See Genital herpes

Hiatal hernia

See Gastroesophageal reflux and hiatal hernia

High blood pressure

High blood pressure means that a child's blood pressure is higher than normal for his or her age. The medical term for high blood pressure is hypertension. A child's blood pressure normally rises in response to physical activity or stress, but a child with hypertension has elevated blood pressure even at rest.

In adults, normal blood pressure is about 120/80 and high blood pressure is 140/90 or higher. Children have much lower normal blood pressure readings than adults (see page 232), and the normal readings rise steadily from infancy through adolescence, when blood pressures level off to the adult readings. So normal blood pressures in children vary according to their age.

The numbers used to record blood pressure represent two measurements. The first is a measure of the heart's peak blood pressure as it pumps blood out to the body, known as systolic blood pressure. The second is a measure of the heart's blood pressure at rest, when the heart is filling up with blood, known as diastolic blood pressure.

There are two main types of high blood pressure: primary hypertension and secondary hypertension. Primary hypertension is a disease of unknown cause that generally lasts a lifetime. It is the most common type in adolescents and adults. Secondary hypertension is high blood pressure caused by an underlying disease.

Children under 12 are more likely to have secondary hypertension, most often because of an underlying kidney disease, such as NEPHRITIS, or kidney disorders leading to kidney failure (see KIDNEY FAILURE, ACUTE and KIDNEY FAILURE, CHRONIC). Other causes of secondary hypertension in children include COARCTATION OF THE AORTA, NEUROBLASTOMA, HYPERTHYROIDISM, LUPUS, burns, and drug use.

High blood pressure is a lot less common in children than in adults. But children who do get it are at risk of developing heart, kidney, and nervous-system diseases in adulthood. Hypertension seems to run in families. Children who are overweight are at a high risk of developing hypertension.

SIGNS AND SYMPTOMS Children with primary hypertension usually have no noticeable signs or symptoms, other than higher-than-normal blood pressure measurements. Children with secondary hypertension usually exhibit the signs and symptoms of the underlying disease. Signs of severe hypertension include HEADACHES, seizures, VISION PROBLEMS, shortness of breath, and fatigue.

DIAGNOSIS If your child has symptoms of severe hypertension, bring him or her to the doctor immediately. Doctors usually discover hypertension that produces no symptoms using an inflatable blood-pressure cuff during a physical examination (see page 233). If your family has a history of hypertension, tell the doctor so that he or she can check your child's blood pressure in infancy. If your child has hypertension, he or she will require regular blood pressure checkups and examinations for any symptoms of other diseases.

Once high blood pressure has been diagnosed, the doctor may order blood and urine tests to help detect any underlying disease. The doctor may also order a cholesterol test to assess your child's risk of developing heart disease later in life (see CHOLESTEROL ABNORMALITIES). Your child may also have to undergo other tests, such as a chest X-ray, an *ultrasound* of the heart known as an *echocardiogram*, or an *electrocardiogram*, which is a measurement of electrical activity in your child's heart. These tests are painless. Depending on the test results, the doctor may refer your child to another doctor who specializes in heart or kidney disorders.

Lowering your child's blood pressure

If your child has high blood pressure, the doctor will probably ask you to make changes in your child's diet and lifestyle as the first line of treatment. The following list describes some of the most common guidelines. Always check with your child's doctor before initiating any of these changes.

- Limit the amount of salt your child eats. Not all children are affected by salt, but eating a lot of salty foods can raise blood pressure in some children. Read labels for salt (sodium) content and don't add salt when cooking.
- Make sure your child gets enough potassium, calcium, and magnesium in his or her diet. These minerals can help lower blood pressure. Potassium is found in potatoes, bananas, spinach, squash, bran cereals, apricots, prunes, raisins, tomatoes, cantaloupe, and navy beans. Magnesium-rich foods include green vegetables, shellfish, and whole-grain foods. Milk, cheese, fish, and greens are high in calcium.
- If your child is overweight, he or she should lose weight. Even a 5 percent weight loss can help lower your child's blood pressure.
- Make sure your child exercises regularly. Set a goal of at least 30 minutes of exercise a day, three or four times a week. Good exercises include walking, jogging, biking, and swimming.

TREATMENT Most cases of hypertension in children are mild and are treated with changes in diet and lifestyle (see box above). If diet and lifestyle changes do not lower your child's blood pressure, the doctor may prescribe antihypertension medication. If your child's hypertension is caused by an underlying disease, he or she may need medication or surgery. Once the underlying cause of secondary hypertension is treated, your child's blood pressure may become normal. If your child has primary hypertension, he or she may require treatment for life.

Hip disorders

Hip disorders in children include congenital (present at birth) hip dislocation, avascular necrosis of the femoral head, and slipped capital femoral epiphysis. Also, an infection such as septic arthritis (see ARTHRITIS, SEPTIC) can damage a child's hips, and toxic synovitis (see SYNOVITIS, TOXIC) can cause the hips to become inflamed.

Types of hip disorders A number of different disorders can affect a child's hip.

Congenital hip dislocation This disorder (also called developmental dysplasia of the hip) can be present at birth or develop in early infancy. The head of a newborn baby's thighbone (femur) does not fit properly into the hip socket. The bone may lie completely out of the socket or it may be easy to dislocate out of the socket by moving the child's leg.

Avascular necrosis of the femoral head Bone cells in the head of the thighbone begin to die because of a poor blood supply. An injury to the blood vessels that supply the femur or a disease, such as SICKLE CELL ANEMIA, can cause avascular necrosis. Taking *corticosteroids* for a prolonged time can also eventually result in avascular necrosis; if your child has been prescribed corticosteroids, discuss their use with your child's doctor.

Slipped capital femoral epiphysis The upper growing end (epiphysis) of the thighbone has slipped into an abnormal position. While the thighbone is growing, the epiphysis becomes separated from the rest of the bone by cartilage and the bone weakens. The disorder is rare and is related to the effects of growth hormone on the bone during early puberty. It most often occurs in overweight children between the ages of 11 and 13 years. Also, a sports injury or a fall can knock the epiphysis out of its normal position.

Signs and symptoms Congenital hip dislocation in a newborn may be hard to detect. One of the infant's legs may be difficult to move or the fat folds around one thigh may not look the same as the folds around the other thigh. After about 3 months of life, the baby's hips do not line up and one leg appears shorter than the other. It may be difficult to spread the baby's legs to change a diaper. As the child gets older and begins to walk, he or she may have a limp and lurch to one side, because the hip is dislocated and the length of the legs is not equal.

Avascular necrosis can cause pain and stiffness in the affected thigh. The child may also limp and have limited range of motion in the hip joint.

A child with a slipped capital femoral epiphysis walks with a limp and usually has pain in his or her knee. The child's leg may turn outward and he or she may have difficulty moving the affected thigh and hip in their full range of motion.

Diagnosis and treatment Early diagnosis and treatment of congenital dislocation of the hip shortly after birth is the best way to prevent complications, such as leg length discrepancy, limping, pain, and SCOLIOSIS, later in life. The doctor will examine your baby's hips at each well-child visit. He or she will check carefully for dislocation. The baby is at increased risk of congenital dislocation of the hip if this disorder runs in your family, if the baby was born in the breech (feet first) position, or if she is a girl. If the doctor is able to dislocate the hip during the examination, or notices a misalignment in the child's skin folds or leg length, he or she will refer your child to an orthopedist (a doctor who specializes in disorders of the bones and joints).

The specialist will move your baby's femur back into its proper place by hand and put a special harness (known as a Pavlik harness), a splint, or a brace on the child's legs to keep the bones in place. For babies up to 3 months old, the specialist will probably use a harness to position the thighbone and correct the problem. The specialist may recommend surgery if your infant has a bone deformity, if your child's hip dislocation was not treated early, or if the harness does not work.

To diagnose avascular necrosis, the doctor may use a *radionuclide scan, magnetic resonance imaging,* or X-ray tests. He or she will prescribe drugs to reduce pain and swelling and physical therapy to maintain the full range of motion in your child's hip. Surgery may also be needed to correct avascular necrosis. If your child's necrosis is in the early stages of development, the doctor may recommend an operation called a core decompression, in which a surgeon removes some of the dying bone and grafts new bone in its place. In advanced stages, the entire hip joint may need to be replaced. In one form of the disease, known as LEGG'S DISEASE, the disorder will run its course and blood supply to the head of the thighbone will be restored on its own.

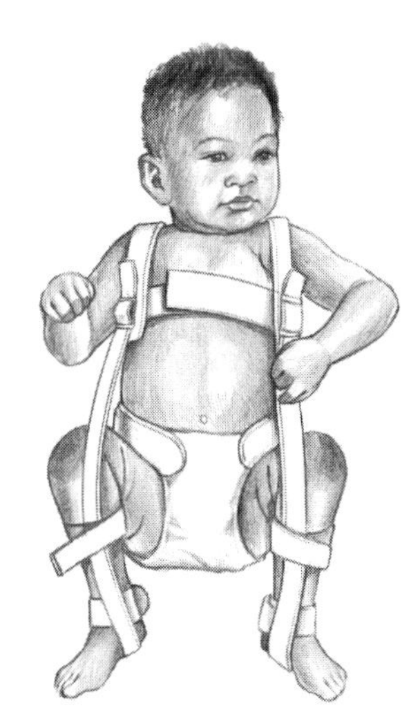

The Pavlik harness

Once a child's thighbone is back in its proper position, the doctor can use a Pavlik harness to keep the baby's thighbone in place until the hip joint forms properly. The harness is usually used for babies up to 3 months old.

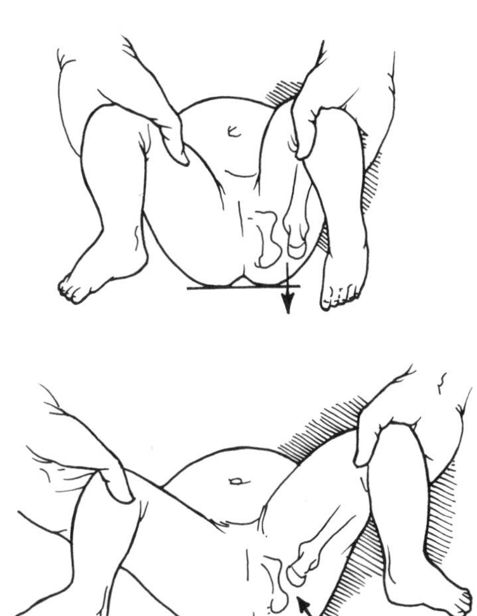

Treating a congenital hip dislocation

In a child born with a hip dislocation, the head of the thighbone has dislocated out of its socket (top). To treat this disorder, the doctor will manually maneuver the baby's thighbone back into its proper place in the infant's hip (bottom).

Surgery may be necessary to correct a slipped capital femoral epiphysis. A surgeon will move your child's slipped epiphysis back into place and keep it there using metal pins.

HIRSCHSPRUNG'S DISEASE

Hirschsprung's disease is a BIRTH DEFECT in which the nerve cells that control bowel movements are missing from the lower part of an infant's large intestine (colon). This defect causes the colon to narrow and block the passage of stool. The disorder affects boys more often than girls, and it tends to run in families. It sometimes appears in children who have other disorders, such as DOWN SYNDROME. In rare cases, the disease affects the entire colon.

SIGNS AND SYMPTOMS Constipation is the hallmark symptom of Hirschsprung's disease. The intestinal contents accumulate and cause the abdomen to distend. Babies born with Hirschsprung's disease cannot pass meconium (the thick, green feces passed by a newborn). The infant develops an intestinal obstruction, loses interest in feeding, and begins vomiting. The infant may develop a fever if the intestines become infected.

Some infants with this disease pass meconium normally and do not develop symptoms until after discharge from the hospital. Then they become constipated and bloated, begin vomiting, and have gas and a poor appetite. Affected infants may develop enterocolitis, an inflammation and infection of the intestines marked by fever, abdominal pain, and vomiting.

If symptoms appear later in infancy, the child usually has alternating symptoms of constipation, diarrhea, and poor bowel control. Older children experience constipation, pain in the abdomen, belching, the passing of gas, and an enlarged abdomen. When the child has a bowel movement, the stools smell very bad and are shaped like a ribbon.

Diagnosis If your infant or child has symptoms of Hirschsprung's disease, see your doctor for an evaluation. If your child seems to have symptoms of enterocolitis, take him or her to a hospital emergency department right away for emergency treatment.

The doctor will perform a rectal examination using his or her finger to check for an absence of stool in the rectum. The doctor may also order X-rays of the child's abdomen and a *barium X-ray* study to look for a narrowed colon. A test called a manometric study may also be needed. The normal urge to defecate arises when the child feels pressure in the colon from stool or gas. A manometric study measures the response of the muscle around the anus to pressure in the rectum with an instrument called a manometer. To confirm the diagnosis of Hirschsprung's disease, the child may have a tissue sample taken from his or her rectum to check for the absence of nerve cells.

Treatment A child with Hirschsprung's disease needs surgery to remove the segment of colon that is not working, but this operation is usually not performed until the child is at least 6 months old. Just before the surgery, the infant may need to have a tube placed down his or her nose into the stomach to withdraw stomach contents and gas or a tube placed into his or her rectum to remove stool from the colon to prevent intestinal obstruction. He or she will also need antibiotics and fluids given *intravenously* if enterocolitis has occurred. During surgery to remove the affected part of the child's colon, the surgeon may have to perform a temporary colostomy to rest the bowel. In a colostomy, the normal part of the colon is disconnected from the affected part and pulled through the baby's abdominal wall so that stool can empty into an external bag attached to the baby's abdomen. Later, the colostomy is reversed and the remaining part of the colon is joined to the child's rectum so the child can defecate normally.

The outlook is very good for children who have surgery to correct this defect. The child's bowel movements become nearly normal as they grow and mature. In rare cases, children experience loss of bowel control or constipation after surgery.

HIV

See AIDS

Hives

Hives are raised, itchy areas on the skin that arise in reaction to some substance to which your child is sensitive. In response to this irritant, your child's body releases a substance called histamine. Histamine, in turn, causes the small blood vessels underneath the skin to leak blood plasma and swell the skin. A variety of things in a child's environment can stimulate the release of histamine and cause hives, including certain foods, medications, temperature, emotional stress, insect bites, and infections.

What causes hives?

A number of common factors in your child's environment can cause hives to develop. Read over the following list and then think about the things your child comes into contact with during his or her day to help your doctor find out what may be causing your child's hives.

- **Foods** The most common foods that cause hives are nuts, eggs, shellfish, milk, and cheese. Some food additives and preservatives can also trigger hives.
- **Medications** Almost any over-the-counter or prescription drug can cause hives in some children, including vitamins, painkillers, aspirin, codeine, antacids, eyedrops, douches, laxatives, antibiotics, tranquilizers, sedatives, and diuretics (drugs that cause water loss from the body).
- **Weather** Children can get hives from exposure to cold, sunlight, and heat.
- **Exercise** Sweating and vigorous exercise can trigger hives.
- **Strong emotion** Emotions—such as anger, stress, or embarrassment, which raise the temperature of the skin—can cause hives.
- **Insect bites** Stings or bites from bees, wasps, hornets, yellow jackets, and fire ants can produce hives.
- **Infections** Infections caused by bacteria, viruses, and fungi can cause hives. In children, nose and throat infections are common triggers of hives.

Hives can be either acute (occurring suddenly) or chronic (long-term), depending on how long they last and how often they occur. An acute case of hives commonly lasts 3 to 5 days (but may last up to 6 weeks), while a chronic case of hives can last for years. The cause of chronic hives is often harder for a doctor to determine than the cause of acute hives, although emotional stress; exposure to sunlight, cold water, or cold temperatures; and a type of yeast infection called candidiasis are known causes of chronic hives.

SIGNS AND SYMPTOMS Hives (see page 23) consist of pink swellings on the skin called wheals that usually arise suddenly, last a few hours to a few days, and then fade away. New swellings of hives can develop as the old ones fade. The wheals have flat tops and clearly defined edges. They usually itch when they are developing but they can also sting or burn. The wheals can occur on any area of the body and range in size from a pencil eraser to a plate. Single wheals sometimes join together to form larger swellings called plaques. Hives around the lips, eyes, or genitals can cause excessive swelling known as angioedema.

Hives caused by reactions to foods can develop right after eating or up to 2 hours later. Those appearing after exposure to sun swell up in minutes and fade in an hour or two. Wheals caused by anything that raises the body's temperature, such as sweating, heat, strong emotions, or sunlight look like tiny bumps with a red or white halo around them and itch intensely. Accompanying symptoms can include headaches, excessive production of saliva, and stomach cramps.

Hives sometimes lead to anaphylaxis, a life-threatening form of shock triggered by an allergic reaction. Anaphylaxis causes a runny nose, wheezing, pale skin, low blood pressure, and cold sweats. If not treated, anaphylaxis can cause a coma or cardiopulmonary arrest (stopping of the heart and breathing).

DIAGNOSIS Your doctor will examine your child and ask you and your child about things he or she has recently been exposed to that could have brought on the hives. To rule out infections or an autoimmune disease (a condition caused by the body's natural defenses turning against the body itself), your child's doctor might order blood tests and a urine test (urinalysis). Your child may also get allergy testing (skin patch or blood tests) to find out if he or she has allergies.

TREATMENT The best way to manage hives is to avoid the substances that trigger the outbreaks. Your doctor can prescribe antihistamines taken by mouth for hives that do not fade right away. If antihistamines alone don't work, they can be supplemented with *corticosteroids*, such as prednisone, also taken by mouth. Antihistamines work best when taken regularly to prevent new wheals from forming. Your child could become drowsy from the antihistamines; your doctor may be able to prescribe antihistamines that don't cause drowsiness.

To treat a child whose eyes or lips are badly swollen, the doctor may inject epinephrine (a form of adrenaline) into the child's arm or leg. The swelling will gradually go down. Your child will probably be extremely uncomfortable from the itching. To reduce his or her discomfort, place cool, wet cloths over the affected areas and apply calamine lotion onto the skin.

If your child shows signs of anaphylaxis or has difficulty breathing, call your doctor immediately and get your child to an emergency department as quickly as possible because anaphylaxis can be life threatening. Children with food allergies should always carry a portable premeasured dose of epinephrine with them in case they accidentally eat something they are allergic to. Those who have food allergies and asthma should seek immediate medical attention if they ever eat something they are allergic to.

HODGKIN'S DISEASE

See Lymphoma

HUMAN IMMUNODEFICIENCY VIRUS

See AIDS

HYDROCEPHALUS

Hydrocephalus is the excessive buildup of the normally occurring cerebrospinal fluid inside a child's brain. Tissues lining the ventricles (cavities) of a child's brain produce fluid that bathes and cushions the brain and spinal cord. The thin membranes, known as the meninges, that surround the brain normally reabsorb the fluid, but, if too much fluid is produced or it cannot be reabsorbed, excessive fluid accumulates, causing hydrocephalus.

An infant can be born with blocked passageways in the brain, causing hydrocephalus. A child can also develop hydrocephalus after a head injury, bleeding in the brain, an infection in the brain, or a BRAIN TUMOR. Hydrocephalus can also arise from a brain malformation caused by a condition such as SPINA BIFIDA.

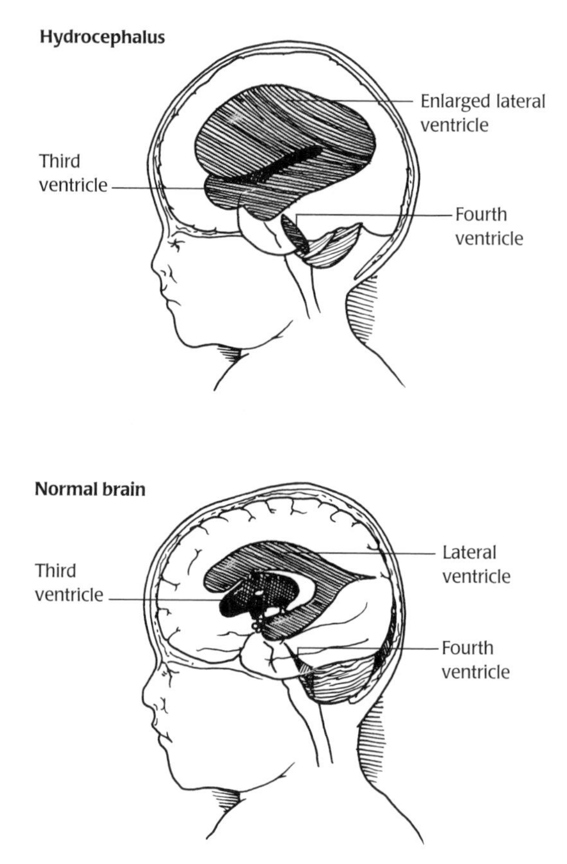

Child with hydrocephalus

In a child with hydrocephalus, the ventricles or cavities in the brain become filled with excess cerebrospinal fluid. The ventricles enlarge (top) and create pressure on the skull to expand. Compare the enlarged ventricles to those of a normal child (bottom).

SIGNS AND SYMPTOMS A baby born with hydrocephalus may have a normal-sized or enlarged head. After birth, the head grows rapidly from the buildup of fluid. The infant may be irritable or lethargic, have a poor appetite, vomit, and be unable to look up. The baby's skull bones may be separated or the soft spot may be enlarged. If the baby's hydrocephalus is not treated, it can cause brain damage, seizures, or DEVELOPMENTAL DELAY or it can be fatal.

When hydrocephalus occurs later in childhood, pressure builds up within the brain because the child's skull is too rigid to expand. The child begins vomiting and has HEADACHES, poor coordination, mental deterioration, and language problems. Left untreated, the elevated pressure can be fatal.

DIAGNOSIS During your child's routine well-baby visits, the doctor will measure your baby's head circumference (see page 243) and check it against a chart of normal measurements for your child's age. An abnormally large head or a rapidly growing head will alert the doctor to the possibility of hydrocephalus. The doctor will order *computed tomography, magnetic resonance imaging,* or an *ultrasound* of your child's head to diagnose the condition and help determine the cause.

TREATMENT The usual treatment for hydrocephalus is surgical placement of a shunt (a small plastic tube) in the ventricles of the child's brain to drain the excess fluid away from the brain into the child's abdomen. In some cases, the doctor may need to treat only the underlying cause of the hydrocephalus or simply prescribe medication for the hydrocephalus. A series of *lumbar punctures,* in which a needle is inserted into the meninges (the membranes that surround the brain and spinal cord) near the lower spine to withdraw fluid, may be enough to remove the excess fluid. The child might also need surgery to remove the obstruction in the ventricles.

HYPERACTIVITY

See Attention disorders

HYPERTENSION

See High blood pressure

HYPERTHYROIDISM

Hyperthyroidism is a hormonal disorder in which a child's thyroid gland overproduces thyroid hormones, which regulate growth and metabolism (the rate at which nutrients and chemicals break down or build up in the body). The thyroid gland is a butterfly-shaped organ that wraps around the windpipe just below a child's Adam's apple. The most common cause of hyperthyroidism is Graves' disease, an AUTOIMMUNE DISORDER that enlarges the thyroid gland, causing overproduction of the thyroid hormones. Hyperthyroidism can also be caused by nodules (small lumps of tissue) on the thyroid gland.

SIGNS AND SYMPTOMS Children with mild hyperthyroidism may have no symptoms at all. In more serious cases, the overproduction of thyroid hormones causes restlessness, hand tremors (shaking), a large appetite accompanied by weight loss, and a rapid heartbeat. The child may also display changes in behavior. Other symptoms include a goiter (an enlargement of the thyroid gland) and

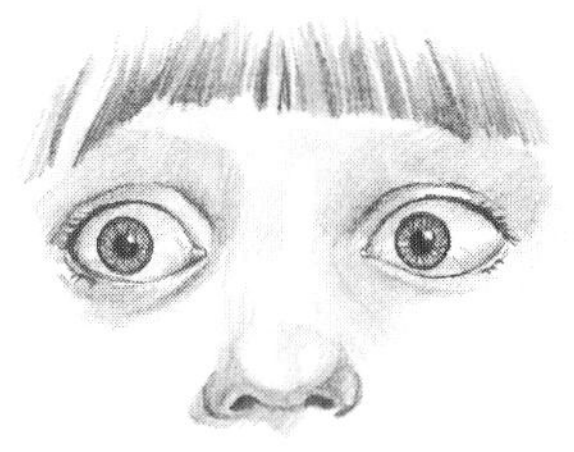

A sign of hyperthyroidism
Children with hyperthyroidism have characteristic bulging eyes. This symptom, called exophthalmos, is caused by a swelling of the tissues around the child's eyes. The swelling pushes the child's eyeballs forward, forcing the eyelids open and exposing a large part of the front of the eyes. The child appears to be staring.

eyes that appear to bulge out. The child may also be weak, tired, and intolerant of heat, sweat a lot, and have frequent bowel movements. Adolescent girls may have irregular periods (see MENSTRUAL DISORDERS). Affected children can also experience what doctors call a thyroid storm, in which the child has fever, high blood pressure, a rapid heartbeat, and behavior changes. This condition is an emergency requiring immediate medical treatment.

DIAGNOSIS The doctor can diagnose the disorder by taking blood tests and analyzing your child's hormone levels. He or she may also order a *radionuclide scan* or an *ultrasound* of the thyroid. In rare cases, the doctor may also order *magnetic resonance imaging.* This scan is needed to check for a possible disorder of the pituitary gland in the brain (see PITUITARY DISORDERS). The pituitary gland regulates the activities of all the other glands in the body.

TREATMENT The usual treatment for hyperthyroidism is medication to suppress the overproduction of thyroid hormones and to reduce your child's thyroid gland to normal size. Your child will need to take this medication for 3 to 5 years, and the doctor will monitor your child's progress carefully during that time. If medications do not work or if your child has nodules on his or her thyroid gland, the doctor may recommend surgery to remove part or all of the thyroid gland. An alternative to surgery is giving your child radioactive iodine in capsule form. The thyroid absorbs the radioactive iodine, which destroys your child's thyroid tissue. Surgery and iodine therapy can cause HYPOTHYROIDISM in some children, however. Your child would then have to take replacement thyroid hormone for life. With treatment, most of your child's symptoms should disappear, but, in some cases, the hyperthyroidism returns. Children with hyperthyroidism become fatigued easily and often need a high-calorie diet. Schedule rest periods at home and at school and provide five or six moderate meals per day.

HYPOGLYCEMIA

Hypoglycemia is the medical term used to describe an abnormally low level of sugar, also known as glucose, in a child's blood. Glucose comes from the sugars in foods, and the body stores it in the liver. Blood glucose is essential for life, especially for brain functioning, growth, and energy. Newborns can become hypoglycemic if they are premature, small for their age, or born to a mother with diabetes mellitus (see DIABETES MELLITUS, TYPE I), a disease that affects blood-glucose levels. Children can develop hypoglycemia if they have not eaten enough food, for example, after fasting overnight, or if they are not getting enough carbohydrates (a form of sugar) in their diet. Fasting hypoglycemia most often occurs in children between 2 and 6 years of age who are thin, active, and have a poor appetite.

Children with diabetes mellitus can also develop hypoglycemia if they take too much insulin for their diabetes or if they miss a meal, eat too few carbohydrates, or are overly active. Insulin is a hormone produced by the pancreas (a gland in the abdomen, behind the stomach) that regulates blood-glucose levels. In children with type I diabetes mellitus, the pancreas fails to produce insulin.

Deficiencies of certain enzymes (proteins that speed up chemical processes in the body), infections, and other diseases can also cause hypoglycemia. In rare cases, children and adolescents can develop hypoglycemia if they drink alcohol (accidentally or intentionally). Deficiencies in the pituitary, thyroid, or adrenal glands can also produce hypoglycemia. It can also occur in children who have a tumor on the pancreas, which secretes insulin.

SIGNS AND SYMPTOMS Newborns and infants with hypoglycemia may have no physical symptoms. If symptoms do occur, the child may look pale, breathe quickly, have a weak or high-pitched cry, feed poorly, appear limp, have cyanosis (a bluish color to their skin), or vomit. Older children with hypoglycemia can appear jittery, irritable, and confused. They roll their eyes, look listless, and have frequent HEADACHES. They may also experience trembling, weakness, drowsiness, cold sweats, blurry or double vision, and speech problems. If the condition progresses untreated, affected children can develop seizures or fall into a coma.

DIAGNOSIS The doctor will diagnose hypoglycemia by measuring the glucose levels in your child's blood. He or she may also order urine and hormone analyses for the diagnosis. To make sure that the hypoglycemia does not recur, the doctor will try to find out the underlying cause of the condition. Infants born to diabetic mothers and those who are small or large at birth should have their blood glucose levels checked promptly after birth and often thereafter so hypoglycemia can be diagnosed and treated with frequent feedings. The child's hypoglycemia usually resolves within 24 hours. Children with diabetes who take insulin can monitor their blood-glucose levels with a commercially available home test kit. If your child has a seizure or lapses into a coma, take him or her to a hospital emergency department immediately for treatment.

TREATMENT To counteract your child's hypoglycemia, the doctor will give him or her glucose, either by mouth or *intravenously*. If your child has hypoglycemia and becomes unconscious, he or she will need to be given an infusion of a glucose solution intravenously or an injection with the hormone glucagon, which raises blood-sugar levels. If your child is diabetic, the doctor will recommend that he or she always carry sugary snacks, such as a candy bar, juice, or hard candies, or glucose tablets so that he or she can take them whenever symptoms appear. Your child's insulin dosage may also need to be adjusted.

Children who get hypoglycemia should avoid fasting for long periods of time. If your child develops hypoglycemia, make sure he or she eats a balanced diet. The doctor may recommend that your child eat small meals frequently throughout the day and have a bedtime snack. Your child should avoid foods such as candy that contain simple sugars because they raise the blood glucose levels rapidly. Foods that contain complex sugars, such as bread and fruit, help the body maintain a more constant blood sugar level. Your adolescent should avoid drinking alcohol.

HYPOPLASTIC LEFT HEART SYNDROME

Hypoplastic left heart syndrome is a heart defect (see HEART DISEASE, CONGENITAL) in which a baby is born with inadequate development of the left side of the heart. The baby's left ventricle (the pumping chamber), left atrium (the receiving chamber for blood from the lungs), aorta (the main blood vessel from the heart), and the valves in the left side of the heart are poorly formed. As a result, the right side of the infant's heart must do the job of both sides in circulating blood through the child's body. Within days after birth, the baby's heart begins to fail. Without immediate treatment, the child usually dies within a week.

SIGNS AND SYMPTOMS A newborn with hypoplastic left heart syndrome may look healthy at first, but soon becomes weak and short of breath, has difficulty feeding, and may turn very pale or blue. His or her pulse is weak, and the child may have signs of congestive heart failure (see HEART FAILURE, CONGESTIVE), such as excessive sweating, a swollen abdomen, and difficulty breathing. The doctor may detect a HEART MURMUR. The child's heart fails and then stops within days of birth because of poor blood circulation.

DIAGNOSIS AND TREATMENT If signs and symptoms develop in the hospital nursery, the doctor can usually diagnose the problem with a chest X-ray, *echocardiogram*, or *electrocardiogram*. If your baby has signs of this disease after he or she goes home, take him or her to a hospital emergency department immediately for diagnosis and treatment.

The doctor will stabilize the infant with heart and blood pressure medication given *intravenously*. The baby will need surgery within days to reconstruct the left side of his or her heart. The initial operation is followed by a second operation in 12 to 18 months. Your child will require medication between the two operations, including antibiotics to prevent infection and medications to stabilize heart function and blood pressure. The doctor will keep a close watch on your baby's progress. If this two-stage surgery fails to correct the heart defect or if surgery is not advisable because of the severity of the disorder, the doctor will probably recommend a heart transplant to save your child's life, if a suitable donor can be found.

HYPOSPADIAS

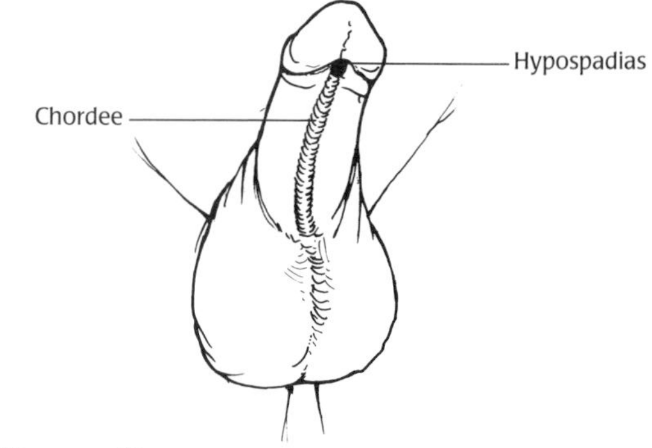

Hypospadias
A common site of hypospadias, an abnormal placement of the opening of the urethra, is just under the head of the penis. Hypospadias can also occur closer to the head of the penis, anywhere along the shaft, at the base of the penis, in the scrotum, or between the scrotum and the anus. Many boys also have a fibrous band of tissue known as a chordee, which pulls the penis downward.

Hypospadias is a BIRTH DEFECT in which a boy's urethra (the tube that carries urine from the bladder) opens on the underside of his penis. About 1 in 300 boys are born with this defect.

SIGNS AND SYMPTOMS The location of the opening can vary from just below the tip of the penis to anywhere down the shaft and scrotum. In rare cases, the opening lies between the genitals and the anus and the child's true gender may be considered ambiguous, especially if the doctor cannot locate the child's undescended testicles (see TESTICLE AND SCROTUM DISORDERS). Boys born with hypospadias sometimes also have a chordee (a fibrous band of tissue that pulls the penis down) or undescended testicles. Often the boy has a normal-looking opening at the tip of his penis that does not function.

DIAGNOSIS If your son has this condition, the doctor will be able to detect it at birth during a physical examination.

TREATMENT The usual treatment for hypospadias is surgery to create a working opening for the urinary tract at the tip of the boy's penis and to straighten a penis that has been pulled down by a chordee. A newborn with hypospadias should not be circumcised because the surgeon will use the foreskin to repair the abnormality. The operation is usually done when an infant is between 6 and 12 months of age. Surgery will allow your son to urinate normally and will promote normal sexual functioning in adulthood.

HYPOTHERMIA

See page 670

HYPOTHYROIDISM

Hypothyroidism is a hormonal disorder in which a child's thyroid gland underproduces thyroid hormones, which regulate growth and metabolism (the rate at which nutrients and chemicals break down or build up in the body). The thyroid gland is a butterfly-shaped organ that wraps around the windpipe just below the child's Adam's apple. The hormones it produces are essential to life. Hypothyroidism can be congenital (present at birth) or acquired (developing later in life). Congenital hypothyroidism develops before birth because of the abnormal development of the thyroid gland. Acquired hypothyroidism most commonly develops in children between the ages of 11 and 14 years as a result of another disease, usually an AUTOIMMUNE DISORDER, that damages the child's thyroid gland.

SIGNS AND SYMPTOMS Infants and children with mild hypothyroidism may have no signs or symptoms at all. Infants born with hypothyroidism often have a poor appetite and develop difficulty swallowing milk or formula within weeks of birth. The infant's growth may be retarded, making the baby's legs and arms shorter than normal in relation to the rest of his or her body. He or she may also have DEVELOPMENTAL DELAY, affecting both motor skills–such as sitting, crawling, and walking–and intellectual skills. His or her movements may be slow. The infant may have a flat nose with wide-set eyes, a large, protruding tongue that makes it hard for the baby to close his or her mouth, and cool skin from a slow heart rate and poor blood circulation.

Children with acquired hypothyroidism often develop a goiter (enlarged thyroid gland) because the thyroid works harder to produce enough thyroid hormone. They may have slow growth, low energy, weak muscles, muscle cramps, fatigue, poor concentration, flaky or coarse skin, a husky voice, and hair loss. Weight gain is common. Their sexual

The endocrine system

Your child's endocrine system is a network of glands, organs, and tissues that releases hormones that control many body functions, including growth, sexual development, and metabolism (the rate at which nutrients and chemicals break down or build up in the body). The endocrine system is made up of the following organs:

- The **hypothalamus**, a small region in the center of the brain, regulates the pituitary gland.
- The **pituitary gland**, at the base of the brain, stimulates other glands to release hormones. It affects growth, reproduction, and the fluid balance.
- The **thyroid gland**, just below the Adam's apple, releases hormones regulating metabolism and body temperature.
- The **parathyroid glands**, on top of the thyroid gland, secrete a hormone that controls blood calcium levels.
- The **adrenal glands**, which sit on top of the kidneys, release hormones that govern many cell activities, respond to stress, and control the level of salts in the body.
- The **pancreas**, located just behind the stomach, releases hormones, including insulin, that regulate the body's use of sugar, fats, and proteins.
- The **ovaries** produce female sex hormones.
- The **testicles** produce male sex hormones.

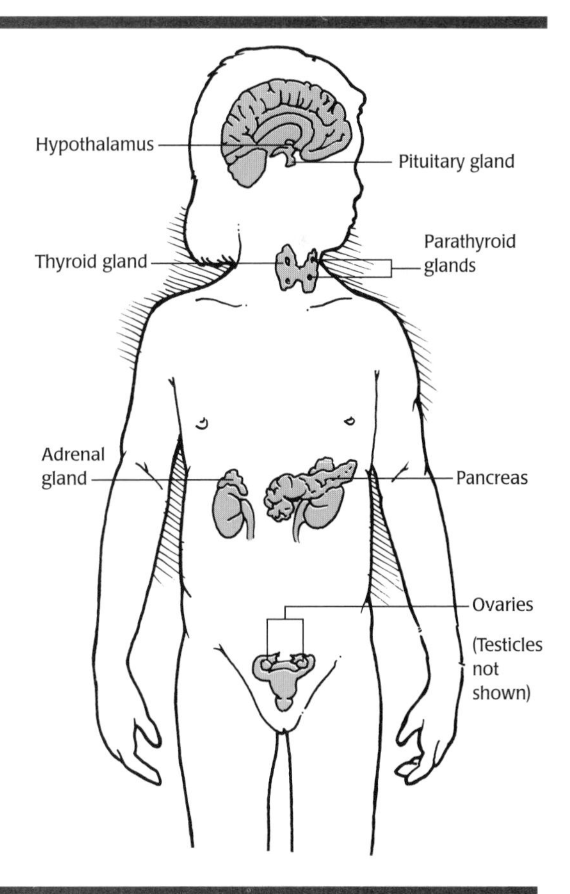

development may be delayed or their sexual function impaired. In its most severe form, hypothyroidism can cause a child to go into a coma.

DIAGNOSIS The doctor will diagnose this disorder by taking blood tests and measuring the thyroid hormone levels in your child's blood. He or she may also order other blood tests to determine the exact cause of the hypothyroidism. In rare cases, *magnetic resonance imaging* of your child's head may be needed to look for signs of a pituitary tumor (see BRAIN TUMOR). Newborn screening tests are done shortly after birth to detect congenital thyroid abnormalities before symptoms develop.

TREATMENT The doctor will treat your child's hypothyroidism with medication that replaces the thyroid hormones your child's body is missing. Your child will have to take these hormones every day for life. The doctor will also treat the underlying cause of the hypothyroidism with whatever measures are appropriate. With treatment, your child will begin to grow and develop normally within 2 to 4 months of beginning treatment, and his or her energy level and mental abilities should also return to normal. Some children grow rapidly to make up for their formerly slow growth and development and these children may need vitamins to supplement the growth spurt.

IMMUNE DISORDERS

Immune disorders are acquired diseases or inherited defects that impair the immune system, the body's natural defense against infection. The immune system combats foreign matter–such as viruses or bacteria, cancer cells, transplanted organs, or mismatched blood products–that has entered the body. Certain acquired disorders–such as MALNUTRITION, LEUKEMIA, and AIDS–damage the immune system and cause it to malfunction. Inherited defects–such as severe combined immunodeficiency disease (a deficiency in two disease-fighting components of the immune system), agammaglobulinemia (the absence of a protein essential to the immune system called gamma globulin), and SICKLE CELL ANEMIA–prevent the immune system from developing and functioning normally.

The immune system is made up of organs–including the tonsils, adenoids, lymph nodes, lymphatic vessels, thymus, and spleen–as well as tissue such as bone marrow and specialized cells located throughout the body. Each part of the immune system contributes to the development or activation of white blood cells that help fight infection. Some of these white blood cells, known as lymphocytes, travel to the thymus where they become specialized infection-fighting cells known as T lymphocytes. The T lymphocytes–also called T cells–attack and destroy invading infectious organisms, other foreign particles, and some cancer cells. Other lymphocytes, known as B lymphocytes (or B cells) also fight infection by creating *antibodies* that attack invading microorganisms, such as viruses and bacteria. The antibodies remain in the body, ready to attack an invader the next time it strikes.

A child's immune system is immature at birth. As the child is exposed to infectious organisms, his or her body develops more and more antibodies and a stronger immune system, so the ability to fight off disease grows as the child matures. Children with immune disorders have a weakened or poorly functioning immune system that cannot fight invading organisms. They get frequent infections, often with life-threatening consequences.

SIGNS AND SYMPTOMS Most childhood immune disorders are inherited, and symptoms can appear right after birth. Children with these disorders are vulnerable to a wide variety of infections, including colds, CHICKENPOX, MUMPS, MEASLES, mononucleosis (see MONONUCLEOSIS, INFEC-

TIOUS), PNEUMONIA, and MENINGITIS. They may be irritable, pale, weak, and constantly sick. These children commonly have swollen glands and may also have a swollen liver or spleen. They may also have frequent RASHES or BLISTERS, skin sores, a rapid heartbeat, CONJUNCTIVITIS, and diarrhea. An affected child may have a number of illnesses at once.

Children with immune disorders do not respond well to treatment and may have an adverse reaction to vaccines made up of live viruses, such as the vaccines for POLIO, mumps, measles, GERMAN MEASLES, or chickenpox. Because the immune system is weakened, recovery from illness takes a long time. The child may never recover completely. Because the immune system extends throughout the body, an immune system disorder can affect many body systems and be life-threatening.

DIAGNOSIS If your child has been constantly sick since infancy and never seems to recover or has other signs and symptoms of an immune system disorder, the doctor will order blood tests to look for infection and to check the levels of T lymphocytes, B lymphocytes, immunoglobulins, and other white blood cells. The doctor may also analyze your child's stool samples and urine for infection and will take X-rays to look for internal complications.

TREATMENT Some children outgrow an immune disorder and regain a fully functioning immune system. In others, symptoms are mild and cause only occasional illness. Your child's doctor will treat infection with therapy, such as antibiotics, when possible. Drugs such as interferon can help your child's immune system fight off infections. All illnesses must be treated aggressively. In severe cases, a child may need a bone marrow transplant in which healthy, matching bone marrow from a donor, usually a brother or sister, is given to the child *intravenously* after the child's own defective marrow is destroyed by drugs or *radiation.* Severe immune disorders can be fatal.

IMPERFORATE ANUS

Imperforate anus is a BIRTH DEFECT in which a baby is born without an anus, the external opening of the rectum (the lower end of the large intestine). The opening is covered over with skin, or the internal canal leading from the baby's rectum to the anus fails to develop before birth.

SIGNS AND SYMPTOMS Without an anus, the newborn cannot have a bowel movement. A greenish bulge of skin or a dimple may be visible where the anus should be. The child may also have an abnormally developed urinary tract. If the baby has an anus, but it is not connected to the rectum, he or she may have symptoms of an abdominal obstruction, such as vomiting and abdominal distention.

DIAGNOSIS If your child is born with an imperforate anus, your doctor will be able to detect the defect by physical examination shortly after the baby is born.

TREATMENT The baby will need surgery to correct the defect. If your infant's anus is covered by skin, a surgeon will remove the skin. After surgery, the surgeon may need to enlarge your baby's anus during a procedure known as anal dilatation, using a finger or a special device to widen the anus.

If your baby's rectal canal failed to develop, he or she will need reconstructive surgery to create an anus and connect it to the rectum. Before anal surgery, your infant may need to have a temporary colostomy to clear the collected stool from his or her intestines. A colostomy is an operation in which a surgeon pulls part of the baby's large intestine through an incision in the abdomen so that stool can empty into an external bag attached to the baby's abdomen. After anal surgery, the chances are good that your baby will develop normal bowel control within a few years. About 80 percent of affected children are toilet trained by age 4.

IMPETIGO

Impetigo is a skin infection caused by streptococcal or staphyloccocal bacteria. The infection causes a RASH that occurs on the face, arms, or legs of affected infants and children. Impetigo occurs most often in summer when cuts, scrapes, or insect bites allow the bacteria to invade a child's skin. The infection is very contagious. Children frequently spread impetigo by scratching at an insect bite or rash and then touching other parts of their body or other children.

SIGNS AND SYMPTOMS Children usually become infected around the nose and mouth first. Impetigo (see page 23) caused by streptococcal bacteria begins as a red rash with tiny BLISTERS that grow into pimples and then form into itchy sores. The sores are soon covered by a yellowish-brown scab, and pus sometimes drains from them. Impetigo caused by staphylococcal bacteria produces small sores that grow to blisterlike rings with a crusty center.

DIAGNOSIS Your child's doctor can diagnose impetigo based on the appearance of the rash.

TREATMENT Your child's doctor will prescribe antibiotics to treat impetigo. Mild impetigo can be cleared up by applying a prescription antibiotic ointment. More severe cases require antibiotic pills taken by mouth. Your child's sores should heal in about a week without any scarring, although mild, red discoloration may remain for several weeks. Healing begins 3 days after treatment. When the sores heal, they get dry, scab over, and begin to fade.

Before applying the antibiotic ointment on your child's skin for the first time, thoroughly wash the affected areas with soap and water. The sores may bleed a little, but that is nothing to be alarmed about. After applying the ointment, cover the sores with bandages.

To prevent your child from spreading the infection, keep his or her fingernails short, wash your child's hands often with antibacterial soap, cover the open sores with a bandage, and caution your child against scratching or picking at the sores. Use separate towels, washcloths, and bed linen for your child so the infection does not spread to other family members. If you are using an antibiotic ointment on your child's impetigo, your child can stay in school or day care as long as the sores are covered by bandages or clothes.

INBORN ERRORS OF METABOLISM

Inborn errors of metabolism are GENETIC DISORDERS that prevent a child's body from metabolizing (processing) certain components of food, such as proteins, fats, or carbohydrates, in a normal way. The seriousness of the child's condition depends on the specific disorder and can range from mild to life threatening.

Examples of inborn errors of metabolism include GALACTOSEMIA, GAUCHER'S DISEASE, and PKU. All of these disorders are caused by defects in a single gene in the child's cells.

SIGNS AND SYMPTOMS In newborns, the initial physical symptoms of an inborn error of metabolism can include a poor appetite, vomiting, a lack of interest in activities, jitteriness, poor muscle tone, JAUNDICE, seizures, and FAILURE TO THRIVE. Other physical symptoms in infants and children can include ALOPECIA, red spots on the child's retina (the membrane that lines the back of the eye), cataract (cloudy lens in the eye), a swollen abdomen from an enlarged liver or spleen, abnormal bone growth, and poor muscle coordination.

Inborn errors of metabolism can also cause mental impairment or MENTAL RETARDATION in infants and children.

DIAGNOSIS To diagnose an inborn error of metabolism and rule out other diseases with similar symptoms, your child's doctor will take blood, tissue, or urine samples and send them to a labora-

Inborn errors of metabolism: What to do in an emergency

If your child has an inborn error of metabolism, he or she can become ill very easily after eating certain foods. In extreme cases, your child could even lapse into a coma and die. Act quickly in an emergency:

- Stop feeding your child any kind of food or liquid.
- Call the doctor and get your child to the emergency department of a hospital immediately.
- Tell your doctor or the emergency department doctors what your child ate and drank before becoming ill, what type of medication he or she takes, and the medicine's dosage.
- Make sure the doctors know what disease your child has and his or her symptoms.

tory for analysis. Every state in the United States requires testing of all newborns for PKU and HYPOTHYROIDISM shortly after birth. Many states also screen newborns for galactosemia.

TREATMENT Doctors treat most inborn errors of metabolism with a special diet that eliminates the foods that the child cannot tolerate. Some children need to stay on the diet for life and may need to take medication that helps correct his or her nutritional imbalances. Working with a dietitian, the doctor will monitor the affected child as he or she grows older to see if the diet needs to be changed. Some children with certain inborn errors of metabolism, such as a UREA-CYCLE DISORDER, may need liver transplantation. Additional treatment depends on the specific disorder.

INFECTIONS IN NEWBORNS

A number of infections can be present in newborn infants, including a group of infections caused by viruses and parasites known as TORCH syndrome—toxoplasmosis, GERMAN MEASLES, cytomegalovirus, and GENITAL HERPES. Bacterial infections, such as listeriosis and group B streptococcus infections, can also affect newborns, as can sexually transmitted diseases such as SYPHILIS. The organisms causing these infections are transmitted from mother to fetus during pregnancy or at birth as the newborn passes through the birth canal.

TOXOPLASMOSIS Toxoplasmosis is an infection caused by a parasite called Toxoplasma gondii. The parasite can be found in raw or undercooked meat, raw eggs, and raw goat's milk. It can be transmitted by contact with cat feces or insects that have been in contact with cat feces. A pregnant woman who is exposed to the parasite can pass the infection to her fetus through the placenta. If a woman has toxoplasmosis early in pregnancy, she can have a miscarriage or stillbirth. Infected newborns can develop eyesight-threatening infections, HEARING LOSS, MENTAL RETARDATION, LEARNING DISABILITIES, SEIZURE DISORDERS, or HYDROCEPHALUS. Some newborns with severe infections may have JAUNDICE, an enlarged liver and spleen, or a RASH. Severe infections can cause death in the first few days of life. Doctors use blood tests to diagnose the infection. Infected newborns are treated immediately after birth with two drugs, pyrimethamine and sulfadiazine, to help reduce or prevent complications.

CYTOMEGALOVIRUS Cytomegalovirus is a common newborn infection caused by a member of the herpes family of viruses. It is spread by close contact with an infected person through kissing, sexual intercourse, or touching infected body fluids, such as urine and blood. Fetuses can be infected at birth or before and babies can be infected through breast milk. Most newborns infected with cytomegalovirus have mild infections and no symptoms. Some have more serious and life-threatening problems, such as PNEUMONIA, an enlarged liver and spleen, and anemia (see ANEMIA, HEMOLYTIC). These newborns can later develop a variety of disabilities, including mental retardation, hearing loss, DEVELOPMENTAL DELAY, and VISION PROBLEMS. Doctors use blood and urine tests to diagnose cytomegalovirus. Infected newborns who show signs of the disease receive an antiviral medication called ganciclovir and supportive care.

Genital herpes Newborns can contract genital herpes, a sexually transmitted infection caused by the herpes simplex virus. When transmitted from an infected woman to her fetus or newborn, the virus can produce life-threatening complications in the baby. Initial symptoms in a newborn include eye infections and sores on the skin or in the mouth. If the herpes infection does not spread, the infant can develop normally, but the infection sometimes spreads to the brain and internal organs, causing seizures, BLINDNESS, hearing loss, mental retardation, CEREBRAL PALSY, liver damage, and even death. Infected newborns are usually treated with antiviral drugs, such as acyclovir or vidarabine. If the infection has not spread beyond the infant's skin, eyes, and mouth, the drugs can be effective. Once the infection has spread farther, the drugs become less effective and the baby usually requires treatment in a neonatal intensive care unit.

Listeriosis Listeriosis is an infection caused by the Listeria species bacteria, found in soil and water. Pregnant women can get the infection by eating contaminated vegetables, unpasteurized cheese, or undercooked meat and pass the bacteria to their fetus before or during birth. The woman may not have any symptoms. An infected newborn can develop pneumonia, SEPTICEMIA, or MENINGITIS, all of which could be fatal. Listeriosis can also cause miscarriage. The infection can be detected in pregnant women and newborns with certain blood tests. Doctors prescribe antibiotics to treat the disease.

Group B streptococcus Many women have group B streptococcus bacteria inside their vagina and can infect their fetus before or during birth. An infected newborn's symptoms can include difficulty breathing and the baby could develop either pneumonia shortly after birth or meningitis in early infancy. The child needs to be hospitalized so he or she can receive fluids *intravenously* and be given assistance with breathing. The doctor will prescribe antibiotics to treat the infection.

Ingrown toenails

An ingrown toenail is a condition in which the edge of a child's toenail grows into the skin of the toe or the skin of the toe grows over the edge of the toenail. It is usually caused by trimming the nail incorrectly, wearing tight-fitting shoes, or abnormally curved toenails.

Signs and symptoms The area where the skin covers the nail is red, swollen, and painful. The skin may become infected and filled with pus. An ingrown toenail usually occurs on a child's big toe, but can occur on any toe.

Diagnosis You will probably be able to recognize an ingrown toenail on your own. If you think your child has an ingrown toenail, take him or her to the doctor for treatment.

Treatment You can help relieve your child's pain at home by soaking his or her toe in warm

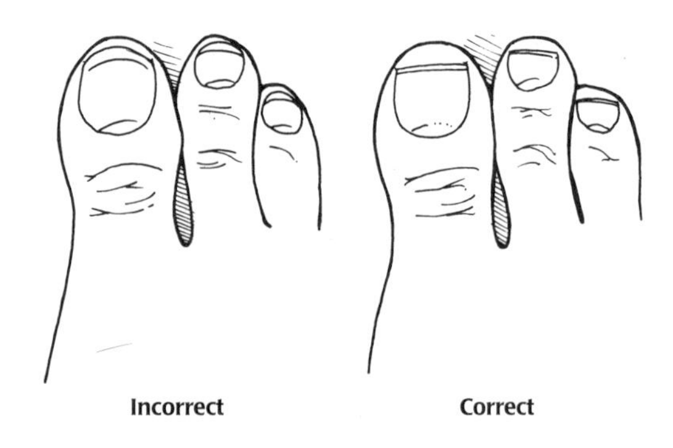

How to cut a child's toenails

Improper cutting of a child's toenails can cause an ingrown toenail. Instead of trimming your child's toenails on a curve (left), cut the nails straight across (right) so that the nail cannot grow into the skin around it.

water four or five times a day and then covering the nail with gauze. Make sure your child does not wear tight-fitting shoes that could aggravate the problem. If he or she develops an infection, the doctor will prescribe an antibiotic to be applied directly to the skin or taken by mouth. If necessary, your child's doctor may cut away the edge of the nail after applying a local anesthetic on the skin. He or she will also drain any pus at the site.

You can help prevent an ingrown toenail from returning by cutting your child's toenail (or teaching him or her to cut the toenail) straight across instead of on a curve or at an angle. That way, the nail will have no jagged edges that could cut into the skin around your child's toe. Keeping the feet clean and not trying to remove ingrown toenails yourself will help prevent infection.

INTESTINAL OBSTRUCTION

Intestinal obstruction is the partial or complete blockage of a child's small or large intestine. The blockage prevents food and feces from passing through the intestines and is life threatening if not treated promptly. The problem can be congenital (present at birth) or can develop during childhood.

TYPES OF INTESTINAL OBSTRUCTION A variety of digestive system disorders can cause intestinal obstruction.

Pyloric stenosis This congenital disorder creates a blockage at the lower outlet of the stomach, known as the pylorus, that empties into the small intestine. The muscle surrounding the pylorus thickens, obstructing the passage of food into the small intestine. The disorder usually occurs between the first 2 and 8 weeks of life and mainly affects boys. Symptoms include vomiting, dehydration (see page 283), body chemical imbalances, and malnourishment. Surgery is required to open the pylorus.

Intestinal atresia Infants born with intestinal atresia have an intestinal obstruction because part of the small or large intestine is either missing or underdeveloped.

Intestinal stenosis This partial blockage of the intestine results from a congenital narrowing of a segment of the small or large intestine.

Surgical adhesions When a child has any kind of abdominal surgery, he or she can develop bands of scar tissue, known as adhesions, inside his or her abdomen. The adhesions can wrap tightly around the intestines and cause obstruction.

Paralytic ileus A child's intestine can become paralyzed after infection or surgery and lose the ability to move food and feces to the rectum. The paralyzed intestine distends as it fills with fluid, food, and air.

Volvulus A loop of the child's intestine can twist around itself, causing an obstruction known as a volvulus. A congenital malformation of the intestines, MECKEL'S DIVERTICULUM, or adhesions can cause a volvulus to occur.

Tumors A tumor or abdominal mass that grows in or on the wall of the intestines, whether cancerous or not, can cause intestinal obstruction.

Other disorders Certain diseases and disorders can also cause intestinal obstruction, including CROHN'S DISEASE, HIRSCHSPRUNG'S DISEASE, IMPERFORATE ANUS, INTUSSUSCEPTION, and hernias (see HERNIA, DIAPHRAGMATIC and HERNIA, INGUINAL).

SIGNS AND SYMPTOMS The symptoms of intestinal obstruction vary according to the location of the obstruction and whether it is partial or complete. Cramps and pain in the abdomen are common symptoms when the small intestine is involved. The pain may be sharp, widespread, or constant, or it may come and go. Nausea and vomiting may also occur. The vomit commonly contains a green liquid called bile, a fluid secreted by the liver. The vomit can also contain blood or fecal matter. The child may also have a fever.

Pain and distention (swelling) in the abdomen are more likely to indicate an obstruction in the large intestine. The child may be unable to pass stools or even gas. Diarrhea can be a symptom of partial obstruction. The child may also become irritable, restless, lose his or her appetite, become dehydrated (see page 283), and lose weight from an intestinal obstruction.

DIAGNOSIS If your child has any of these symptoms, take him or her to the doctor right away. The doctor can make a diagnosis based on the information you give him or her and a physical examination. He or she may need to order X-rays of your child's abdomen to confirm the diagnosis and pinpoint the location of the obstruction. Your child's doctor may also order blood tests to help diagnose the cause of the obstruction.

TREATMENT Immediate treatment is essential. Your child will not be able to eat normally until the obstruction is relieved, so nourishment will be given *intravenously* in the hospital. Initially, the doctor will insert a flexible tube down your child's nose into his or her stomach to remove gas and the contents of the stomach and intestines mechanically. Surgery will be necessary to correct the obstruction. Normally, after surgery, you can expect your child's full recovery. He or she will be home from the hospital within a week.

INTRAVENTRICULAR AND PERIVENTRICULAR HEMORRHAGE

Intraventricular or periventricular hemorrhage is bleeding that occurs in the brain of a premature infant. The bleeding varies in severity and occurs in (intra-) or around (peri-) the fluid-filled spaces, called ventricles, inside the brain. It can result from an injury at birth or afterward that increases the pressure inside the blood vessels in the baby's head. It can also be caused by rapid changes in the infant's blood volume, high or low blood pressure, or severe lung disease. The bleeding occurs because the infant's developing brain contains tiny blood vessels that can easily break open. The risk of hemorrhage depends on the severity of the prematurity or illness. Infants at the greatest risk are those who weigh less than 2¼ pounds or are younger than 28 weeks of age at birth. About 2 percent of cases occur in full-term infants (37 weeks or older) because of an injury at birth.

SIGNS AND SYMPTOMS The most common symptoms are slowed or absent reflexes, poor muscle tone, excessive drowsiness or sleepiness, and sleep apnea (see SLEEP DISTURBANCES). A premature infant may begin to develop symptoms within the first few hours or days of life or after the first week. The infant's condition may suddenly get worse on the second or third day of life. Additional symptoms–such as pale or blue skin, jaundice, muscle twitches, seizures, paralysis, shock, apnea, a slow heartbeat, or unconsciousness–can also occur. The child can then go into shock (see page 678). The head circumference may increase rapidly; HYDROCEPHALUS can occur in 2 to 4 weeks from the beginning of the bleeding.

DIAGNOSIS Your child's doctor can diagnose intraventricular or periventricular hemorrhage with an *ultrasound* or *computed tomography*. The infant may also need a *lumbar puncture* and blood tests.

TREATMENT There is no specific treatment for intraventricular or periventricular hemorrhage, but your child's doctor will treat any symptoms your baby displays. For example, if your child has seizures, the doctor will prescribe anticonvulsant drugs. To treat shock, your child's doctor will give him or her blood transfusions, fluids, or medications. Hydrocephalus will probably require the surgical placement of a small plastic tube called a shunt into the ventricles of the baby's brain. The shunt directs the fluid to the child's abdomen and drains the excess fluid away from his or her brain. An affected child may have to undergo a series of lumbar punctures to relieve pressure in the fluid-filled cavities in the brain. The outcome depends on the severity of the bleeding in the brain. Profuse bleeding can lead to CEREBRAL PALSY, MENTAL RETARDATION, HEARING LOSS, VISION PROBLEMS, or death.

INTUSSUSCEPTION

Intussusception is an intestinal disorder in which a segment of a child's intestine folds in on itself, like a retracting telescope. It most commonly occurs in children 6 to 24 months of age, but can develop in other age groups as well. When the intestine folds into itself, it becomes partially or completely blocked and cannot digest food or absorb nutrients (see INTESTINAL OBSTRUCTION).

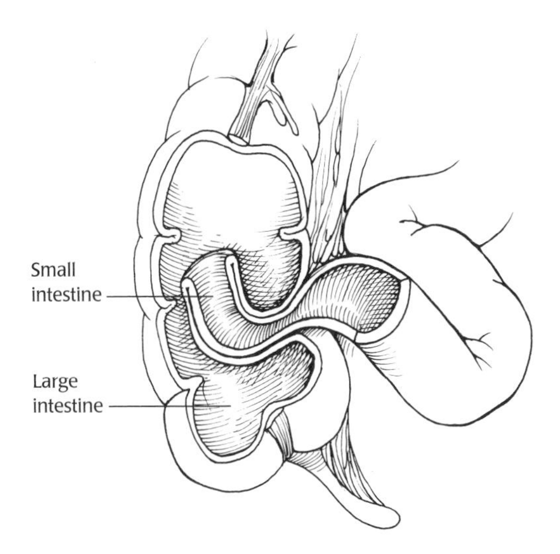

Intussusception
The intestine of a child with intussusception folds or telescopes in on itself. The disorder occurs most often in young children, and the small intestine usually telescopes into the large intestine.

Intussusception must be diagnosed and treated promptly or the baby could develop complications, such as dehydration (see page 283), shock, intestinal rupture, or even death.

SIGNS AND SYMPTOMS An infant or toddler who has intussusception experiences sudden abdominal pain, along with irritability or lethargy, and looks very ill. The child begins vomiting because the stomach and intestinal contents cannot move through the intestinal tract. The child's stool may look normal initially or the child may have only diarrhea, but then the stool becomes the consistency of currant jelly because inadequate blood flow in the intestines causes the tissue to die and then bleed. Sometimes a hard mass can be felt in the child's abdomen. The baby may also have a fever.

DIAGNOSIS If your infant or toddler has symptoms of intussusception, take the child to the doctor right away. The doctor will perform a physical examination, including a rectal examination to check for the presence of a mass, tenderness, or blood in the stool. A barium enema will be done to confirm the diagnosis. The doctor will introduce liquid barium into your child's rectum through a rubber tube and film the barium with X-rays as it moves through your child's large intestine to locate the site of the intussusception. The test is not painful. Traditional abdominal X-rays may also be done to rule out other causes of the obstruction.

TREATMENT A barium enema X-ray can also be used to treat this condition. The pressure used to send the barium through the intestines sometimes reduces or eliminates the intussusception. If the barium treatment fails, your child will need surgery to unfold the intussusception and remove any diseased intestine. Intussusception is one of the most common causes of emergency surgery among children under age 2. Your child should recover fully and be able to come home from the hospital within a week after surgery.

IRRITABLE BOWEL SYNDROME

Irritable bowel syndrome is a digestive disorder in which a child's colon (large intestine) passes or pushes along partly digested food too rapidly or too slowly.

SIGNS AND SYMPTOMS Irritable bowel syndrome can cause diarrhea or constipation, or a combination of both. It can also cause temporary abdominal pain or cramps that sometimes go away when the child has a bowel movement or passes gas and belches. Some children do not experience pain but have diarrhea first thing in the morning or around mealtime.

The symptoms may disappear for a while, but usually return periodically throughout life, often at times of stress, such as when the family is moving or the child is facing exams in school. Certain foods and beverages, such as chocolate, caffeinated foods and drinks, fatty foods, alcohol, and red meat, can make irritable bowel syndrome symptoms worse.

DIAGNOSIS If your child has diarrhea or constipation, or both, take him or her to the doctor for a diagnosis. The doctor will have to rule out other diseases that could cause your child's pain or irregular bowel habits.

TREATMENT The best treatment for irritable bowel syndrome is a change in your child's diet. Keep track of the foods your child eats before the symptoms flare up and then eliminate those foods from his or her diet. Your child needs to eat foods high in fiber—whole-grain breads, fruits, vegetables, cereals, and bran—and drink plenty of water.

Minimize stress in your child's life as much as possible. Plan both regular exercise and regular rest periods for your child to help relieve anxiety and stress. Encourage your child to talk about things he or she finds stressful. In extreme cases, the doctor may refer your child for counseling so he or she can learn how to manage stress.

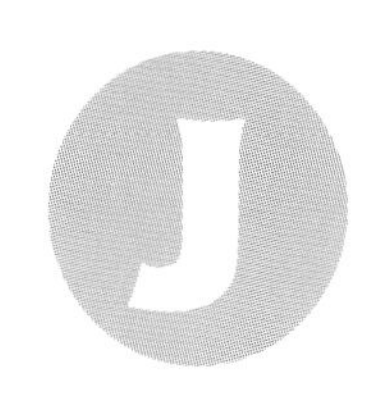

JAUNDICE

Jaundice is a yellowing of the skin and the whites of the eyes caused by an increase of bilirubin in the blood (see page 39). Bilirubin is a yellow pigment in bile (a fluid produced by the liver) that is produced as old red blood cells die. The liver normally filters bilirubin from the blood and sends it to the gallbladder until it is released into the intestines or absorbed into the bloodstream for disposal as waste. When too much bilirubin builds up in the blood, the excess amount goes into the layer of fat beneath the skin, producing a yellow tinting of the skin and whites of the eyes. The buildup of bilirubin is usually caused by a damaged or diseased liver or by excessive destruction of red blood cells.

Jaundice is common in newborn babies. It develops in the first few days of life because the baby's immature liver cannot filter out all the bilirubin being produced. A component of breast milk can also interfere with the baby's ability to handle bilirubin. Jaundice in newborns is usually not a serious condition and generally goes away without treatment within a week or two. In children and adults, jaundice usually signals an underlying disease, such as HEPATITIS, BILIARY ATRESIA, SICKLE CELL ANEMIA, hemolytic anemia (see ANEMIA, HEMOLYTIC), and hereditary spherocytosis (see SPHEROCYTOSIS, HEREDITARY).

SIGNS AND SYMPTOMS Yellowing of the skin and eyes may be accompanied by a loss of appetite, loss of energy, itchy skin, constipation, dry skin, and a bitter taste in the mouth. Other symptoms of jaundice in children include unusually dark urine, light or putty-colored stool, and tenderness in the upper right abdomen, where the liver is located.

DIAGNOSIS You will be able to best tell whether your child has jaundice if you look at his or her skin in natural daylight. If the skin or whites of his or her eyes look yellow, call your child's doctor. The doctor will order blood tests to check the levels of bilirubin, red blood cells, and liver enzymes in your child's blood. He or she will also test your child's blood for infection and take samples of your child's urine and stool.

To find out the exact cause of your child's jaundice, the doctor may have to do an *ultrasound* or a special X-ray of your child's liver and bile ducts. A liver biopsy may also be needed. Tests for thyroid disease and CYSTIC FIBROSIS may also be needed because these conditions sometimes produce jaundice.

TREATMENT To correct the jaundice, your child's doctor will need to treat the underlying cause, although mild jaundice in a newborn may not require any treatment. If your newborn's jaundice is more serious and does not clear up on its own, he or she may require phototherapy (light therapy). Phototherapy will probably be done in your home, with daily monitoring of your infant's bilirubin levels by a visiting nurse. The nurse will place your newborn under a blue or white fluorescent lamp that radiates ultraviolet B light. The light changes the bilirubin so that it passes into the baby's bloodstream and can be passed out in the urine. Phototherapy also promotes bowel movements, which clear bilirubin from the intestine. The nurse will check your baby's weight and feeding pattern every day to make sure he or she is tolerating the light treatment. While undergoing light therapy, your baby will have to wear eye covers to protect his or her eyes. Sometimes phototherapy blankets can be used in the home to deliver light therapy.

If you are breast-feeding your jaundiced child, you may have to give your baby either more breast milk or supplemental formula for a few days to help the baby pass more stool, clearing out the bilirubin, until the baby's liver has a chance to mature. Dangerously high levels of bilirubin in your baby's blood may require an exchange transfusion–replacement of your baby's entire blood supply with fresh blood from a donor. Your baby's doctor will carefully monitor his or her reaction to the exchange transfusion.

JUVENILE RHEUMATOID ARTHRITIS

Juvenile rheumatoid arthritis is a persistent inflammation of a child's joints and internal organs that can last for months or years. The disease begins before the child turns 16 years of age, most often between the ages of 2 and 5 years and 9 and 12 years. There are three types of juvenile rheumatoid arthritis. The most common form, called pauciarticular (meaning "few joints"), affects four or fewer of the child's joints, usually the knees, ankles, or elbows. The second most common form, called polyarticular (meaning "many joints"), affects five or more of the child's joints, including the small joints in the fingers and hands. The least common form, called systemic (meaning "throughout the body"), affects not only the child's joints but also the internal organs.

The causes of juvenile rheumatoid arthritis are not clear, but the disease is thought to be triggered by an infection that occurs in a child who is predisposed to developing arthritis. As an AUTOIMMUNE DISORDER, juvenile rheumatoid arthritis stimulates the child's immune system, the body's natural defense mechanism against infection, to attack the body's own tissue.

SIGNS AND SYMPTOMS The disease may periodically flare up and subside. It causes swelling, pain, heat, and stiffness in the joints and sometimes redness of the skin covering the inflamed joints. An early sign is often stiffness in the child's joints the first thing in the morning. The child may hold the sore joint still in a bent position because moving it is painful. Holding the joint still can cause the surrounding muscles to become weak and stiff and the tissues connecting the muscles to the bones–the tendons–to tighten and shorten, causing deformity of the joint. Inflammation that lasts a long time can damage the surface of the bone, producing pain when the joint is moved and limiting movement. Juvenile rheumatoid arthritis can affect the growth of the child's bones. Bones in the affected joints can become bigger or smaller than normal. The disease can also affect the child's appetite, resulting in weight loss or gain.

The eyes of children with pauciarticular arthritis are sometimes inflamed. If left untreated, the eye inflammation can affect the child's vision and even cause BLINDNESS. Children with polyarticular arthritis may have a low-grade fever and lumps on an affected joint because of pressure from shoes, chairs, or other objects. Children with systemic arthritis may have a high fever and chills that start in the late afternoon or evening and last a few hours. They may also have a RASH, swollen glands, an enlarged liver or spleen, and an overall feeling of ill health.

Diagnosis and treatment Juvenile rheumatoid arthritis can be difficult to spot because the child may not complain of pain or show any other signs. If your child limps or favors one arm, leg, or hand over another or has other characteristic symptoms, the doctor will take blood tests and X-rays of the affected joint. The doctor will recommend or prescribe medications–such as aspirin, ibuprofen, other anti-inflammatory drugs, or, in severe cases, *corticosteroids* or methotrexate–to relieve the symptoms. He or she may also prescribe gold therapy, in which your child would receive weekly or monthly injections of gold into a muscle. Your child will also need physical therapy and a regular exercise program to keep his or her joints from becoming stiff. He or she may need to wear splints to maintain joint position.

In rare cases, your child's doctor may recommend surgery to correct or replace a damaged joint. Joint replacement surgery, in which your child's arthritic joint is replaced by an artificial one, is usually reserved for older children with severely damaged joints. In most cases, this disease disappears by the time the child becomes a young adult. Some children are left with permanent joint damage and some continue to have arthritis into adulthood.

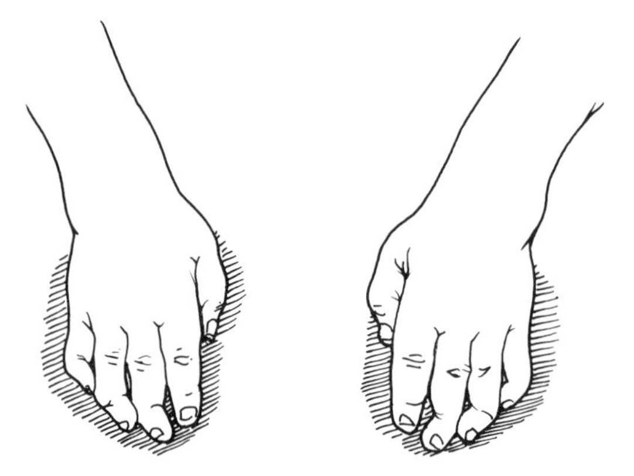

Telltale signs of juvenile rheumatoid arthritis
The wrists and knuckles of a child with juvenile rheumatoid arthritis become stiff and swollen. The fingers show a "swanlike" deformity in which the first knuckle of the finger bends inward.

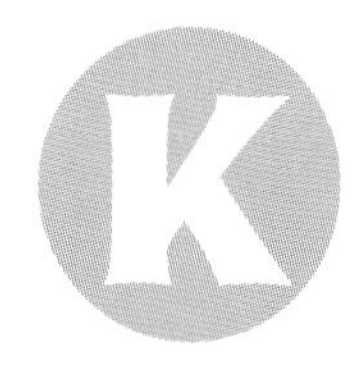

Kawasaki disease

Kawasaki disease is a rare condition that affects various parts of the body and causes inflammation of the lining of the blood vessels, especially the coronary arteries. It occurs almost exclusively in children under age 5 and especially in children between the ages of 1 and 2 years. The disease affects mainly boys and is most common among children of Asian descent. Researchers suspect that a bacteria or virus may be the cause, but no specific organism has been found. The disease occurs more often in winter and spring.

SIGNS AND SYMPTOMS The disease begins with a high fever that tends to spike up and down several times a day for 5 days or more. The child's temperature can range from 104°F to 107°F. The fever does not respond well to treatment with acetaminophen or ibuprofen and the child becomes very irritable and then develops a RASH all over the body. Other symptoms of Kawasaki disease are swollen glands in the child's neck, red eyes, swollen eyelids, dry or cracked lips, and swelling and redness of the tongue and throat. After a few days, the child's palms and soles become red, swollen, and painful. In a couple of weeks, the skin in those areas begins to peel. The child may complain of a headache, abdominal pain, joint pain, and a stiff neck.

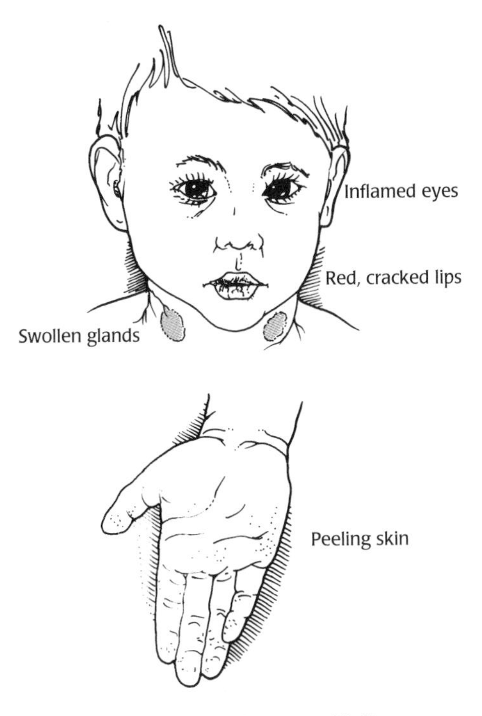

Physical characteristics of Kawasaki disease

A child with Kawasaki disease has several telltale physical characteristics, including inflammation of the eyes; red, cracked lips; and swollen glands in the neck (top). The skin on the palms of the hands peels and is red, swollen, dry, and painful (bottom). The child also has a fever that lasts longer than 5 days.

The child's condition may seem to improve without treatment after 2 weeks, but this phase of the disease is misleading. At this point, the disease begins to affect the vessels that supply blood to the heart and the heart itself. The child may develop a fast or irregular heartbeat (see ARRHYTHMIAS). The coronary arteries can become inflamed, causing an aneurysm (a ballooning out of the vessel), which can threaten the child's life if the vessel gets blocked or bursts.

DIAGNOSIS The doctor will look for the signs and symptoms of Kawasaki disease and will order blood and urine tests, an *electrocardiogram* to detect arrhythmias, an *echocardiogram* to detect any aneurysm, and a chest X-ray to evaluate the child's heart. If the entire group of symptoms—a fever lasting more than 5 days, swollen glands, inflammation of the eyes, cracked lips, body rash, and swollen hands—occurs with no apparent cause, doctors diagnose Kawasaki disease.

TREATMENT Early recognition and treatment of Kawasaki disease brings the best results. An affected child is hospitalized and given a blood product called gamma globulin *intravenously*. After one treatment, the child's condition should begin to improve in 2 or 3 days. Some children require a second injection of gamma globulin before their condition improves. Children with Kawasaki disease are treated with aspirin for a total of 8 weeks—high doses for 2 weeks and reduced doses thereafter. With successful early treatment, recovery should be complete. About 1 to 2 percent of children with this disease die of heart complications.

KIDNEY FAILURE, ACUTE

Acute kidney failure is the sudden inability of a child's kidneys to function. The kidneys normally filter waste products and water from the child's blood, turn them into urine, and keep body fluids and salt in balance. When the kidneys fail to work properly, waste products build up in the child's body and cause a number of problems. Acute kidney failure usually arises from an underlying disease or injury. With proper treatment, most acute kidney failure can be cured with no lasting effects, but untreated it can lead to long-term kidney failure, or death. Acute kidney failure occurs in people of all ages but is more common in adults than in children. The underlying causes of the disease fall into three main categories:

- **Kidney damage** The kidneys can be damaged by such diseases as NEPHRITIS, HEMOLYTIC-UREMIC SYNDROME, and LEUKEMIA; by a URINARY TRACT INFECTION; by exposure to toxic chemicals; and by certain medications, including anticancer medications.
- **Reduced blood flow** Severe burns, excessive bleeding, congestive heart failure (see HEART FAILURE, CONGESTIVE), blood poisoning (see SEPTICEMIA), and other diseases that affect blood flow can cause a sudden drop in the flow of blood to the kidneys, resulting in kidney failure.
- **Blocked flow of urine** The ureters (the tubes that carry urine from the kidneys to the bladder) and the urethra (the tube that carries urine from the bladder to the outside of the body) can become blocked by a malformation present at birth, injury, a tumor, blood clots, or kidney stones (see URINARY TRACT DEFECTS AND OBSTRUCTION).

SIGNS AND SYMPTOMS In most cases, a child will show signs of the underlying disease or injury before symptoms of acute kidney failure appear. The main symptom of kidney failure is a decreased urine output or none at all. In time, the child becomes weak and sick to the stomach. He or she may also vomit, be short of breath, have diarrhea, and lose his or her appetite. The child might also become drowsy and confused, have seizures, get unexplained bruises on his or her body, develop high or low blood pressure, or even lapse into a coma. Many affected children look puffy from fluid retention and gain excessive weight.

DIAGNOSIS If your child has symptoms of acute kidney failure, call the doctor and get your child to a hospital emergency department immediately. The doctor will order blood and urine tests to determine how well your child's kidneys are working. He or she will also try to identify the underlying cause of your child's acute kidney failure through a thorough physical examination, and laboratory and X-ray tests. A kidney *biopsy* may also be needed.

TREATMENT The doctor will treat the underlying cause of your child's acute kidney failure as soon as it is identified. Possible treatments include blood transfusions given *intravenously,* infusion of fluids and salts, surgery to correct kidney obstruction, and drug therapy for heart disease or infection. Your child may also need temporary kidney dialysis (see page 545) until his or her kidneys begin working again. The doctor will prescribe a special diet that is high in carbohydrates and low in salt and protein to help your child's kidneys recover. Your child may have to restrict his or her intake of fluids and will stop taking any drugs identified as the cause of the acute kidney failure.

KIDNEY FAILURE, CHRONIC

Chronic kidney failure is the slow, gradual loss of kidney function. The kidneys normally filter water and waste products from the blood, turn them into urine, and keep body fluids and salt in balance. As chronic kidney failure develops, waste products begin to build up in the child's body and the kidneys become less and less able to filter them out. Chronic kidney failure develops over months or years, not suddenly, as in acute kidney failure (see KIDNEY FAILURE, ACUTE). It arises from diseases that progressively damage the child's kidneys, such as chronic NEPHRITIS, chronic URINARY TRACT INFECTIONS, LUPUS, diabetes (see DIABETES MELLITUS, TYPE I), and urinary tract obstruction (see URINARY TRACT DEFECTS AND

OBSTRUCTION). Malformations of the kidneys or urinary tract present from birth and inherited kidney disorders can also cause chronic kidney failure.

SIGNS AND SYMPTOMS This disease can progress for years without symptoms. Initial symptoms are usually mild and include HEADACHE, fatigue, and a general lack of interest in things. The child's growth and physical development may be impaired. He or she may look pale and have a puffy face, a white tongue, and bad breath. At first, the child may begin to urinate more often than usual, but eventually, as the disease gets worse, he or she urinates less frequently than normal. Muscle cramps can develop as well as numbness, tingling, and burning in the child's legs and feet. The child may have pain in his or her bones, joints, and muscles. He or she may also have nausea, diarrhea, and appetite loss. Fluid retention produces swollen ankles and legs, and a swollen face and abdomen.

The child may begin to have mental confusion, and be drowsy, anemic, and short of breath. He or she might develop HIGH BLOOD PRESSURE and congestive heart failure (see HEART FAILURE, CONGESTIVE). Eventually, an affected child enters the final stage of kidney failure known as end-stage renal disease. At this stage, the child's kidneys are no longer able to support life and the child will die without dialysis (see box below) or a kidney transplant (surgery done to replace a diseased kidney with a healthy, donated kidney).

DIAGNOSIS To diagnose chronic kidney failure, your child's doctor will order blood, urine, and other tests needed to identify the underlying cause of the kidney failure. These tests may include a needle *biopsy* of your child's kidneys and X-rays or *ultrasounds* of your child's kidneys, abdomen, ureters, urethra, and bladder.

TREATMENT Once the doctor has identified the cause of your child's illness, he or she will treat

Dialysis for kidney failure

Dialysis takes over the normal functions of the kidneys in a child whose kidneys fail to work properly. A child may need dialysis for only a short time or for a long period, depending on the cause of his or her kidney failure and whether the cause can be completely cured. Some children are placed on kidney dialysis until a donated kidney becomes available for transplantation. There are two types of dialysis: peritoneal dialysis and hemodialysis.

Peritoneal dialysis is the type more commonly used to treat children. This type of dialysis uses a child's own body to filter out waste products and water instead of a machine. The child must have a small tube called a *catheter* implanted in the wall of his or her abdomen that serves as a port for the dialysis solution. The solution is infused from a plastic bag through a tube inserted into the catheter. The solution flows into the child's abdomen and must remain there for several hours while blood vessels inside the membrane that lines the abdomen filter water and waste products from the child's blood into the solution. Then the solution is allowed to drain out into another plastic bag. This procedure must be done five or six times a day, but it can be done at home, in a hospital, or at a dialysis center.

Hemodialysis uses a machine that filters a child's blood to remove excess waste products and water. A young child must first undergo a minor operation so the surgeon can place a shunt (a plastic tube) in his or her arm or leg. The shunt connects an artery to a vein and allows access to the bloodstream. Older children may have the vein surgically connected directly to the artery without a shunt. The child is then connected to the dialysis machine by tubes that pass the child's blood through a filter in the machine that removes waste products from the blood. The procedure takes about 4 hours and must be done at a special dialysis center three times a week.

the underlying disease and try to stop the progression of the kidney failure. Possible treatments include surgery and drug therapy. Better control of diabetes may slow kidney damage from this disorder. Your child may need short-term dialysis until the underlying cause has been treated, or long-term dialysis and a kidney transplant if the illness has progressed to end-stage renal disease.

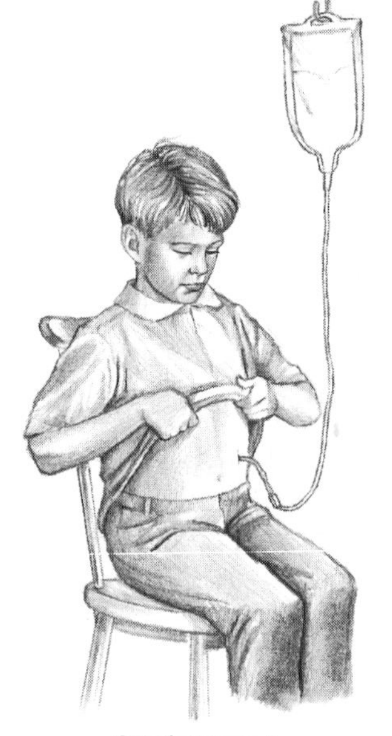

Solution flows in

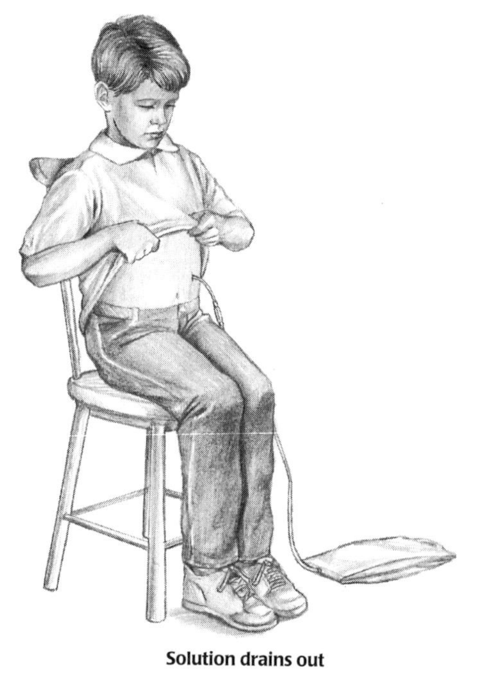

Solution drains out

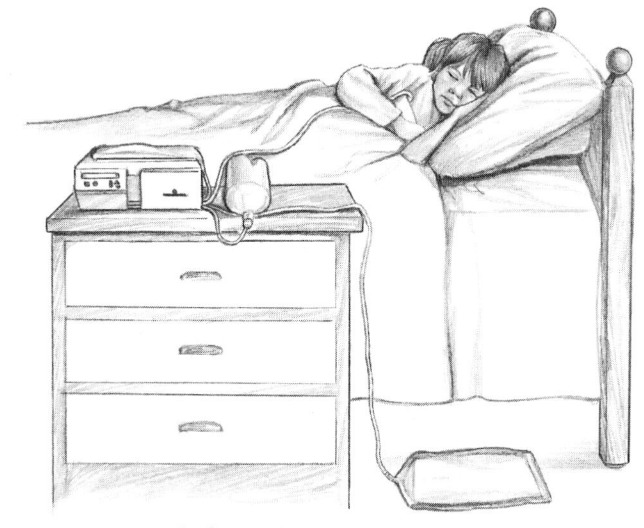

Cycling solution in and out at night

Peritoneal dialysis at home

Peritoneal dialysis makes use of the child's own body instead of a dialysis machine. The dialysis solution is infused into the child's abdomen (top left) and remains in place for several hours as the child goes about his or her activities. The small blood vessels in the peritoneum, the membrane that lines the abdominal cavity, filter waste products and water from the blood into the dialysis solution. Then the solution containing the waste and water drains out of the body (top right) and a fresh supply of solution is infused into the child's abdomen.

At night, a child can undergo peritoneal dialysis as he or she sleeps (left). Dialysis solution is infused into the child's abdomen and, after the waste products and water are filtered out, the solution drains into a plastic bag on the floor. The process is regulated by a machine that cycles the solution.

Klinefelter's syndrome

Klinefelter's syndrome is a CHROMOSOMAL ABNORMALITY that affects only boys and makes them unable to produce sperm. A boy acquires Klinefelter's syndrome when he inherits an extra X *chromosome*. The extra X chromosome also affects the boy's ability to produce the male sex hormone testosterone. About one male baby in 1,000 is born with this disorder.

Signs and symptoms A child with Klinefelter's syndrome grows tall and thin, and has a feminine body build and a small penis and testicles. At puberty, affected boys begin to develop breast tissue that may continue to grow throughout adolescence. Adolescents have normal erections and ejaculations, but their semen does not contain sperm, so they are infertile. They usually have only minimal facial hair. Some affected boys may have learning problems or MENTAL RETARDATION. They may also be shy, immature, and have low self-esteem.

Diagnosis Doctors can detect this inherited abnormality in a fetus through chromosomal analysis (see Genetic testing, page 498). During childhood, the child's physical features will prompt his doctor to test for Klinefelter's syndrome that has previously gone undetected.

Treatment If the boy's breasts become so large that they cause embarrassment, they may be surgically corrected. When a boy with Klinefelter's syndrome reaches 12 to 13 years of age, he will need a yearly blood test to measure his testosterone levels. If his hormone levels are low, he will have to get monthly injections of a synthetic form of testosterone to bring his physical and sexual development to a normal level. The testosterone will not give him the ability to make sperm, so he will always be infertile. As the boy gets older, he may need more frequent injections. If you have a son with Klinefelter's syndrome and are thinking about having more children, you should get genetic counseling (see page 497). Your son should also have genetic counseling to help him understand his genetic makeup and to help him cope with his infertility.

Knee injuries

Knee injuries can affect any of the bones, cartilage, muscles, ligaments, or tendons that comprise a child's knee. Three bones meet to form the knee–the kneecap (patella), thighbone (femur), and shinbone (tibia). These bones are stabilized by ligaments and tendons, which are strands of tissue that attach to bones or muscles. Cartilage is firm, flexible tissue that covers and cushions the ends of bones.

Children commonly injure their knees during play or sports. Stopping and starting, twisting and turning, and jumping and running all bring pressure on the knee and can lead to injury. Some of the most common knee injuries among children

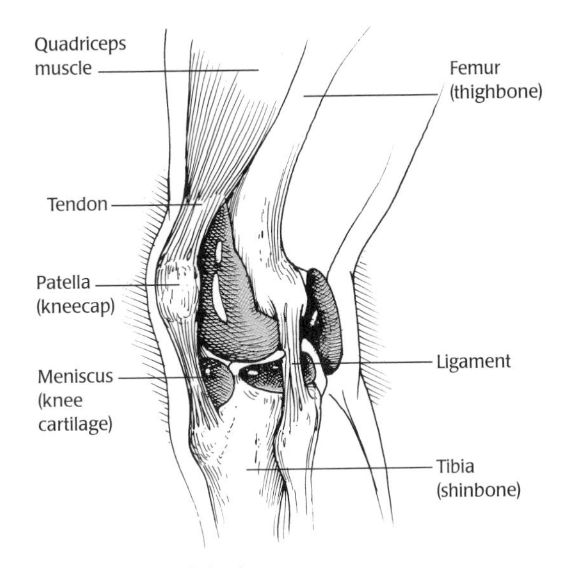

Common knee injuries

Injury to the complex structure of the knee can easily occur during sports or while your child is running or playing. Common knee injuries include torn or sprained ligaments, dislocation of the kneecap, bone fractures (see page 490), and torn cartilage.

are torn or sprained ligaments, dislocation of the kneecap, and fractures (see page 490). Adolescents frequently tear the C-shaped cartilage in the knee known as the meniscus.

SIGNS AND SYMPTOMS Common signs and symptoms of knee injuries include swelling, pain, tenderness, a popping sound heard at the time of injury, limping, and limited movement of the knee. If the child's kneecap is dislocated, it can be seen on the outside of the knee joint. The child may also be able to move the kneecap from right to left. If the meniscus is torn, the child's knee may either lock or give way frequently.

DIAGNOSIS To diagnose the specific knee injury, the doctor or emergency department physician will examine the knee and will observe the movement of the knee by maneuvering the knee into various positions. He or she may also order X-rays of the knee. If your child is in extreme pain or has signs of a dislocated kneecap, take him or her to a hospital emergency department for treatment. Try to minimize movement of the injured knee.

TREATMENT If your child's knee injury is mild, causing only minor pain and swelling, you can treat it at home by putting an ice pack or towel filled with ice directly on the injured area. Place a pillow under your child's knee and raise the leg and knee above his or her heart. Don't let your child walk on or move the injured knee until it has healed.

For more serious injuries, the doctor may refer your child to an orthopedic (bone) specialist for treatment. The specialist will place an elastic bandage, cast, or knee immobilizer (a removable device that keeps the knee from moving) on your child's knee, depending on the type and severity of the injury. The doctor will also recommend a pain reliever. Your child may have to walk on crutches until the injury heals. Your child needs to stay off the knee until the pain and swelling go down, which may take several days or weeks. Then he or she can slowly begin to resume normal activities until the movement in the knee returns to normal. He or she may also require physical therapy. For severe injuries, surgery may be necessary. With successful treatment, your child's knee should heal completely.

KNOCK-KNEES

Knock-knees are knees that touch because of an inward curving of the legs. If the knees touch when a child's feet and ankles are apart, he or she has knock-knees. Knock-knees are a normal part of development, most commonly occurring between the ages of 2 and 6 years. Knock-knees help children maintain balance while they are learning to walk. Overweight children are more likely to develop knock-knees than are children of average weight. In most cases, the position of the knees will become corrected over time. Knock-knees can also be caused by an underlying condition, such as rickets (a vitamin D deficiency that causes softened bones), a fracture (see page 490) of the leg bones, or JUVENILE RHEUMATOID ARTHRITIS.

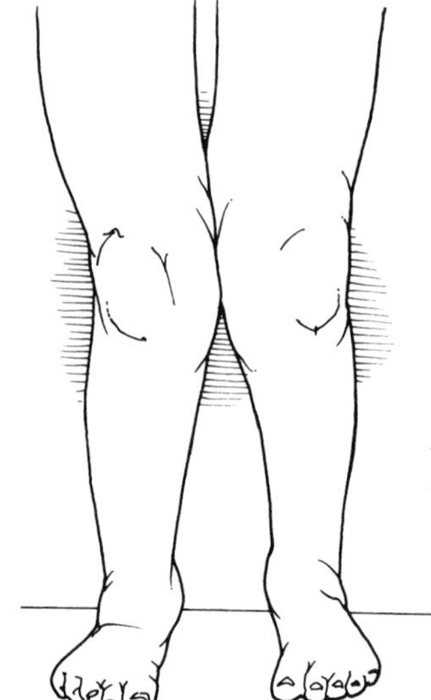

Knock-knees
Knock-knees help young children maintain their balance while they are learning to walk. Knock-knees are a normal part of development for most children. The knees usually return to a normal position as the child grows older.

DIAGNOSIS AND TREATMENT The doctor will do a thorough physical examination to rule out any underlying cause of knock-knees and may take X-rays of the child's legs and knees. Most doctors adopt a wait-and-see attitude toward knock-knees and do not recommend any treatment initially. If the child has an underlying disease, the doctor will recommend treatment appropriate for the specific problem. If the child does not grow out of knock-knees by the time he or she reaches 8 to 10 years of age, the doctor may recommend braces that the child can wear overnight to reposition the knees, or special shoes to correct the knee problems. If these treatments do not work, the child may need surgery to straighten his or her legs.

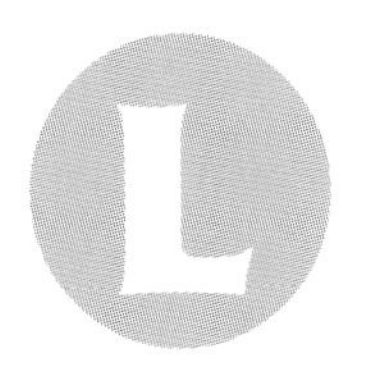

LACTOSE INTOLERANCE

Lactose intolerance is an inherited or acquired inability to digest a sugar known as lactose found in milk and milk products. The intolerance results from the shortage of an enzyme, known as lactase, that is produced in the small intestine. The enzyme lactase is necessary for the digestion of lactose. Some premature infants have temporary lactose intolerance because their immature bodies have not yet started to produce the lactase enzyme. Most often, children develop intolerance to lactose after they are 5 years old, when their small intestines begin to produce less lactase. In rare cases, children are born with permanent lactose intolerance. Other diseases or infections that affect the intestines, such as AIDS, CELIAC DISEASE, or GASTROENTERITIS can also cause lactose intolerance in children. Children of certain ethnic groups—Native Americans or those of Asian, African, or eastern European ancestry—are more likely than others to have lactose intolerance.

SIGNS AND SYMPTOMS The undigested lactose moves into the child's large intestine where it ferments, produces acids and gases, and interferes with water reabsorption. As a result, the child develops abdominal pain, watery diarrhea, a bloated abdomen, gas, vomiting, and cramplike abdominal pain. The child with significant lactose intolerance can be irritable, lose weight, be dehydrated, and fail to thrive (see FAILURE TO THRIVE).

DIAGNOSIS The doctor will ask you detailed questions about your child's eating habits and will do a thorough physical examination to rule out any other disorders. He or she will advise you to eliminate foods that contain lactose—for example, breast milk and cow's milk, cheese, ice cream, other dairy products, bread, salad dressings, and soups—from your child's diet and see if the symptoms get better. Symptoms that return when you reintroduce the lactose-containing foods confirm the diagnosis.

TREATMENT The usual treatment for lactose intolerance is a diet free of foods that contain lactose. Some children can consume limited amounts of foods that contain lactose without having symptoms. For example, children with lactose intolerance can usually eat fermented dairy foods, like yogurt, without any effects. You will need to help your child find out how much lactose he or she can tolerate through trial and error. Lactose-free milk and formulas are available for infants and young children. You can also buy lactase enzymes in liquid form that reduce the amount of lactose in milk. Chewable lactase tablets and capsules are also available to help your child digest other foods that contain lactose. Your child may need calcium supplements if he or she needs to avoid dairy products, which are a major source of calcium.

LARYNGITIS

Laryngitis is a mild inflammation of the vocal cords (larynx). It is usually caused by a viral infection, such as a cold, and produces hoarseness. Laryngitis can also be caused by a bacterial infection, ALLERGIES, overuse of the voice, laryngeal polyps (see POLYPS, LARYNGEAL), damage to the larynx from surgery, or irritation from smoking, secondhand smoke, or excessive use of alcohol. Laryngitis can occur anytime in infancy and childhood, but most often affects children from 3 months to 5 years of age. Children get laryngitis more frequently in the cold and flu seasons–late fall, winter, and early spring.

SIGNS AND SYMPTOMS An infant with laryngitis often sounds hoarse when he or she cries. An affected older child sounds hoarse, may only be able to whisper, and may even lose his or her voice. The child might feel a tickle in the back of his or her throat, have a SORE THROAT, and find it difficult to swallow. Laryngitis is often accompanied by a dry cough, low fever, fatigue, and a general feeling of ill health. The symptoms usually last a week or two and then disappear. If your child has difficulty breathing and a high fever, he or she may have a more serious illness, such as CROUP or epiglottitis, a rare but serious infection of the epiglottis (the flap of cartilage that covers the windpipe when swallowing to prevent choking on food).

DIAGNOSIS AND TREATMENT You will be able to recognize laryngitis by the hoarse sound of your child's voice. You can treat your child's laryngitis at home. Have your child drink a lot of liquids such as tea and juice, and avoid anything that might irritate his or her voice box–such as talking. He or she may or may not need to rest in bed, depending on the other symptoms. Place a humidifier or vaporizer in your child's room to humidify the air. Hot, steamy showers also help soothe the voice box. You can give your child over-the-counter pain relievers or cough syrup to relieve his or her discomfort, but avoid giving mouthwashes or gargles that contain alcohol because they can dry the throat. If the symptoms get worse, or if your child has difficulty breathing and a high fever, call the doctor for further advice.

LEAD POISONING

Lead poisoning is overexposure to the metal lead that causes illness. The lead enters the child's body through the mouth or lungs. Lead can be found anywhere in our environment–in air, soil, water, leaded gasoline, lead-based paint, plumbing in older houses, pottery glazes, lead crystal, batteries, and pewter containers. Since 1975, new cars have been required to use unleaded gasoline, and manufacturers have stopped using lead solder to seal the seams of food cans. House paint has been lead-free since 1978. Lead pipes are no longer used for plumbing, and lead solder is no longer used to seal plumbing joints. As a result, levels of lead in food and water are the lowest they have been in modern history. But children can still be exposed to lead or get lead poisoning in a variety of ways. The most common source of exposure is chewing on or swallowing paint chips or dust from lead-based paint on the walls, doors, windowsills, or furniture of houses painted with lead-based paint. Children can also be exposed to lead from inhaling air that is polluted with lead from automobiles or industry or by inhaling dust from the lead-based paint in older homes. They can also transfer soil or dust contaminated with lead from their hands to their mouth. Children also tend to suck on items such as miniblinds that may be covered with lead-based paint. A developing fetus will be exposed to lead through the placenta if the mother has been exposed to lead.

The human body cannot differentiate lead from other minerals–such as calcium, iron, or zinc–so it easily absorbs lead into the bloodstream. Children absorb proportionally more lead than adults do because of their smaller size. If a child is exposed to large amounts of lead daily, the metal will leave the bloodstream and be deposited in other parts of the body, such as the bone, brain, or kidneys (see KIDNEY FAILURE, ACUTE), where it can cause further damage.

SIGNS AND SYMPTOMS Children with mild lead poisoning may have no symptoms. When symptoms do appear, they include muscle aches, constant fatigue, irritability, indifference, drowsiness, poor concentration, abdominal discomfort, HEADACHE, vomiting, or weight loss. Children with lead poisoning are frequently anemic (see ANEMIA, IRON-DEFICIENCY) because of poor nutrition. Children with severe lead poisoning may develop swelling and inflammation of the brain, known as lead encephalopathy. They have symptoms of MENTAL RETARDATION, hyperactivity (see ATTENTION DISORDERS), abnormal behavior, seizures, confusion, BLINDNESS, and loss of consciousness. Severe lead poisoning can be fatal.

DIAGNOSIS You should have your child's blood screened for lead when he or she is between the ages of 6 months and 6 years (see page 236). Most states recommend a lead screening by 1 year of age and again at 2 years. Many preschools and kindergartens require children to take a lead test before entry. A blood test is the usual method of detecting lead exposure. Your child's doctor may also X-ray your child's abdomen and the bones of his or her arms or legs to detect any lead deposits. If lead poisoning is diagnosed (levels of over 10 micrograms per deciliter of blood; see page 236), your child's doctor may notify city or state officials to take paint and dust samples from your home and soil samples from around your house and test them for lead contamination.

TREATMENT The most important treatment is to prevent further exposure. In some cases, the doctor may prescribe chelating agents, which bind to the lead and carry it out of your child's body in urine. These agents may be taken by mouth or be given *intravenously* or by injection into a muscle. Your child's doctor may also prescribe a diet high in iron, calcium, zinc, and protein. In severe cases of lead poisoning, your child may need to be hospitalized to be treated with chelating agents, nutritional supplements, and other medications. Any complications–such as seizures or kidney disease–will also be treated.

After treatment, your child's environment must be completely lead-free. The long-term outlook depends on the extent of your child's exposure and how early he or she was treated. A child with severe lead poisoning will need to be treated for any complications caused by lead exposure and may need long-term follow-up care and psychological evaluation for possible brain injury from lead poisoning. The doctor will also closely keep track of the child's blood lead levels and order blood counts to monitor anemia. For ways to prevent lead poisoning, see page 302.

LEARNING DISABILITIES

Learning disabilities are a group of disorders that affect a child's ability to read, write, speak, listen, reason, or do math. Learning disabilities are thought to be caused by the way a child's brain handles information. These disabilities occur mainly in children with average or above-average intelligence but may be related to emotional or physical problems, such as HEARING LOSS, VISION PROBLEMS, MENTAL RETARDATION, or DEVELOPMENTAL DELAY.

Certain risk factors predispose a child to developing learning disabilities, including a family history of learning disabilities, premature birth or low birthweight, head injuries, stress placed on a baby before or after birth (such as a pregnant woman's illness, DEPRESSION, or DRUG AND ALCOHOL ABUSE), a brain infection (see MENINGITIS), or treatment for cancer.

TYPES OF LEARNING DISABILITIES A learning disability affects a child's ability to speak, read, write, do math, distinguish time and place, remember, interpret input from the senses, or pay attention.

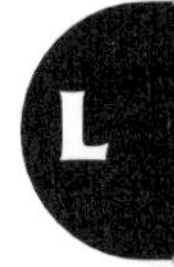

Reading problems Children with the reading disability known as dyslexia have difficulty reading letters, numbers, sentences, or paragraphs. An affected child may reverse or misread letters or words–for example, mistaking a "b" for a "d," reading "was" instead of "saw," or reading a "6" as a "9." This difficulty reflects not a vision problem but the way his or her brain processes visual information.

Writing problems Children with a writing disability known as dysgraphia have difficulty forming letters correctly and writing within an allotted space. They may turn in messy papers, have poor handwriting skills, and have difficulty finishing written tests. Turning in written assignments on time becomes a challenge because writing neatly takes extreme effort. Affected children may take a long time to copy material from a blackboard.

Language problems Children with a language disability have difficulty understanding and speaking words and sentences. They often ask parents or teachers to repeat instructions or other information. They may have difficulty expressing themselves in language–for example, by using the wrong words for an idea or scrambling the words in a sentence. When telling a story, they may get the sequence of events mixed up.

Math problems Children who have a math disability known as dyscalculia fail to grasp the basic concepts of math and have much more difficulty calculating or solving math problems than other children their age. Such children may be talented in other academic areas, such as English or history.

Problems with time and place Some children have trouble learning the concepts of time and direction. For example, they may confuse tomorrow with today or next week. Or they may have difficulty understanding the concept of direction, not knowing which way to go and often getting lost.

Memory problems Children with memory disabilities can have trouble remembering classroom assignments, days of the week, multiplication tables, and even their own address and phone number. When telling a story, they may forget where they are in the story.

Sensory problems Children with a sensory problem known as sensory integration dysfunction have problems interpreting sensory input. For example, they may not be able to learn the rules to a game or what the symbols mean on dice. Some of these children are overly sensitive to the environment, limiting their ability to become socialized.

Attention problems Children who have ATTENTION DISORDERS may have trouble focusing or concentrating their attention. They may be impulsive and easily distracted. Such children fail to finish

Early signs of learning disabilities

Different children develop learning skills at different rates but your child may have a learning disability if he or she displays any of the following early warning signs:

- At age 2½, your child does not speak in sentences.
- You cannot understand more than half of what your 3-year-old is saying.
- Your 5-year-old cannot distinguish shapes and sizes.
- Your 5-year-old cannot tie his or her shoes, hop, manipulate a button, or cut paper.
- Between ages 3 and 5, your child is unable to sit still while you read him or her a short story.
- Your 5- to 6-year-old has difficulty learning the names of letters, numbers, and colors or has problems understanding rhymes in songs and stories.
- Your 5- to 6-year-old cannot quickly name items belonging to a particular group, such as different types of animals.

school assignments or chores at home. They may not pay close attention to instructions or details and often make careless mistakes in school.

DIAGNOSIS AND TREATMENT Learning disabilities are lifelong problems that may not become evident until a child enters school. You can look for early warning signs of learning disabilities in your child (see box on page 552) and your child's doctor or teachers may also detect symptoms of learning disabilities. The doctor will thoroughly examine your child for physical problems and may refer you and your child to specialists–such as speech, language, eye, and hearing specialists; mental health professionals; or a neurologist–for a complete evaluation of your child's physical and mental status.

If your child has a learning disability, he or she may need special education or tutoring, speech and language therapy, and medication. You will need to work with your child's teachers and doctors to develop the best approach to the disability. Children with learning disabilities may have low self-esteem and fear going to school. Help your child feel good about himself or herself. Offer plenty of love and support and emphasize your child's strengths.

LEGG'S DISEASE

Legg's disease is a form of the hip disorder avascular necrosis (see page 522) in which the blood supply to a child's thighbone (femur) is blocked, causing the upper end of the bone to die over a 1- to 3-week period. The blood supply can become obstructed from an accidental blow to the bone, an infection, or an unknown cause. The blood supply replenishes itself 6 to 12 months after the initial injury and new bone replaces the dead bone within 2 to 3 years. The body heals itself through a process known as creeping substitution of bone.

Legg's disease occurs most often in children between the ages of 3 and 10 years, and it is much more common in boys than in girls. Usually only one leg is affected. However, in about 10 percent of cases, both legs are affected by the disease.

SIGNS AND SYMPTOMS Constant pain in the thigh or knee and a limp are the most common initial symptoms. The child may have difficulty walking and have limited range of motion in the affected hip. The child's hip may also be stiff, and his or her thigh muscles may be tender or weak.

DIAGNOSIS AND TREATMENT If your child has symptoms of Legg's disease, the doctor will examine the way your child walks and stands and move his or her hips into various positions. He or she may order X-rays of the hip and a *radionuclide scan* to help make a diagnosis. The doctor will probably refer your child to an orthopedic (bone) specialist. Your child's body will eventually heal itself, so the doctor will simply protect your child's leg from further injury and stress until it heals by advising your child to stay off the leg as much as possible and to get plenty of rest, especially in the initial stages of healing. The specialist may also put a brace on your child's leg to keep it in position. Some children need to first be put in traction (see page 491) for a few days and then be put in a brace. Children with severe forms of the disease may need corrective surgery.

LEUKEMIA

Leukemia is a cancer that affects a child's white blood cells. It is the most common form of childhood cancer. White blood cells are produced in a child's bone marrow. Normally, as new white blood cells develop, an equal number of old ones dies. When a child has leukemia, his or her body produces large numbers of abnormal white blood cells that don't work very well but live longer than normal white blood cells.

These abnormal white blood cells interfere with the child's ability to fight off infection. They can also spread throughout the bloodstream and affect the child's organs, especially the lymph glands, liver, spleen, and brain. They can also hamper the body's production of red blood cells (which carry oxygen to the tissues) and platelets (blood cells needed for blood clotting and the control of bleeding).

There are two general types of leukemia–acute and chronic. Acute leukemia refers to the abnormal production of immature white blood cells, while chronic leukemia is the abnormal production of mature white blood cells. Almost all childhood leukemias are acute and occur in children under age 10, especially those between the ages of 2 and 5. Acute leukemias are grouped by the types of white blood cells they affect–lymphocytes (acute lymphocytic leukemia) or granulocytes (acute myelogenous or granulocytic leukemia).

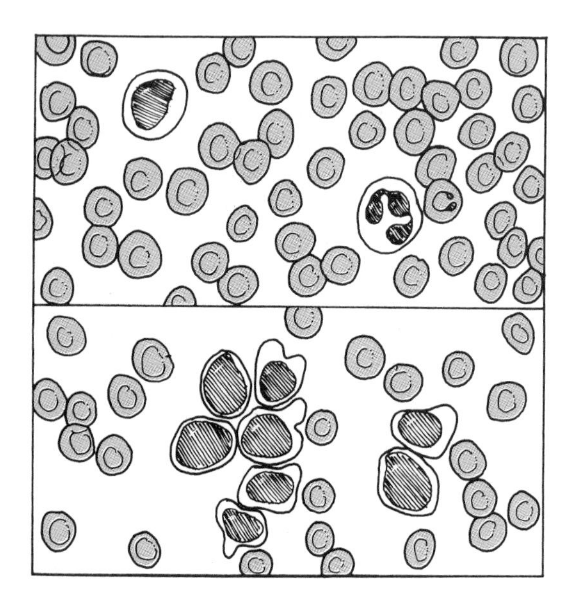

What leukemia cells look like
Normal red and white blood cells (top) have a characteristic appearance. The white blood cells are the two larger cells. The large white blood cell on the right is a neutrophil; the one on the left is a lymphocyte. Blood cells from a child with leukemia (bottom) show the typically abnormal shapes of the white blood cells. The abnormal white blood cells live longer than normal white blood cells and hinder the child's ability to fight off infection.

SIGNS AND SYMPTOMS If your child has acute leukemia, he or she will usually develop symptoms of anemia, including pale-looking skin, weakness, and fatigue, because the number of red blood cells supplying oxygen to his or her body are too low. Your child may also bruise and bleed easily. Flulike symptoms including fever and muscle aches are also common.

Your child may frequently have infections. He or she may also lose weight from a loss of appetite. There may be small, purplish-red spots on your child's skin, and he or she may have tender or swollen lymph nodes, a swollen spleen, or a swollen liver. Leukemia can also cause sores or ulcers in your child's mouth or throat and swollen or bleeding gums. If the leukemia affects your child's brain, he or she can have severe HEADACHES, confusion, seizures, or loss of muscle control. If it affects the bone, your child may have a lump or experience bone and joint pain.

DIAGNOSIS Your doctor will need to examine your child and do certain tests to diagnose leukemia, including blood tests to find out your child's blood cell count. These tests may reveal the presence of leukemia but not the specific type your child has.

To determine the type of leukemia your child may have, his or her doctor will order a bone marrow aspiration or a bone marrow *biopsy*. During both procedures, a doctor inserts a needle into one of your child's large bones, usually the pelvic bone, and withdraws a sample of bone marrow or a sample of both bone marrow and bone tissue for analysis under a microscope. Your child will receive local anesthesia (see page 292) before either procedure.

To find out how far the disease has spread, your child's doctor may order a *lumbar puncture*, in which a needle is inserted into your child's spine to take a sample of cerebrospinal fluid (the fluid surrounding your child's brain and spinal cord). Your doctor may also order chest X-rays or *computed tomography* of your child's abdomen to assess the spread of the disease.

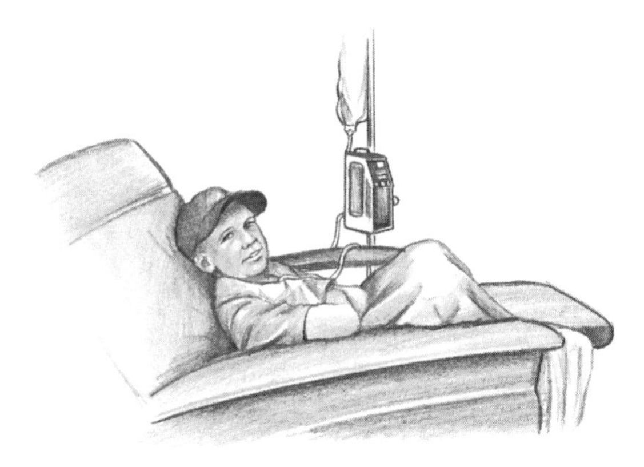

Chemotherapy for leukemia

A child typically receives chemotherapy for leukemia *intravenously*, as an *outpatient*. Doctors usually implant a stainless steel port (reservoir) under the skin of the child's chest so the tube connected to the machine that pumps the drugs can be easily and painlessly inserted before each treatment.

TREATMENT If your child has leukemia, he or she needs to go to a hospital or cancer center for *chemotherapy* with anticancer drugs to kill the leukemia cells. Your child will also receive antibiotics to treat any infections. The drugs may be given by mouth or *intravenously*. The full course of treatment lasts about 2 years and your child may be able to take the anticancer medication at home, in the doctor's office, or in the hospital as an *outpatient*.

Many of the anticancer drugs used to treat leukemia cannot cross the blood-brain barrier, which prevents many substances from passing from the bloodstream into the brain, so your child may also receive injections of anticancer drugs directly into his or her cerebrospinal fluid. He or she may also need *radiation* in addition to chemotherapy. Other treatments can include transfusions of blood or platelets.

Your doctor will monitor your child's condition closely for the disappearance of leukemia symptoms with regular blood tests and occasional bone-marrow aspirations. If your child's leukemia recurs at any time during or after treatment, he or she may need bone marrow transplantation. In this procedure, your child's bone marrow is destroyed by radiation and drugs and replaced by healthy marrow from a donor. At various times during treatment, your child may need to be isolated in the hospital because of his or her increased risk of infection. The good news is that, in most cases, treatment results in remission (see page 445) and an eventual cure for your child. A complete remission is possible in up to 95 percent of children who are treated for some forms of acute lymphocytic leukemia and in up to 80 percent of children treated for some forms of acute myelogenous leukemia.

LEUKOMALACIA

See Periventricular leukomalacia

LICE

Lice are tiny parasites that live on human hair and skin and suck blood for nourishment. Children most often get them on the head after sharing combs, brushes, hats, scarves, towels, or bedding with infected children, but they can also get lice on other parts of their bodies, such as their shoulders and buttocks, from wearing clothing that is infested with lice. The female louse attaches to the skin and then lays eggs, called nits, which cling firmly to shafts of hair on the head or body. In about a week, the nits hatch and the young lice move to the skin, where they feed. Outbreaks of lice infestation are common at school, day-care centers, or summer camps and can occur among children at any socioeconomic level. Sexually active adolescents can acquire a lice infestation in the hair and skin around their genitals by sexual contact with someone infested with lice (sometimes called crabs) living in pubic hair.

SIGNS AND SYMPTOMS Your child will experience itching on his or her scalp or any other parts of the body where infestation has occurred. If your child scratches deeply, sores may appear that scab over and can become infected. Your child may complain of dandruff (nits) that sticks to the hair or

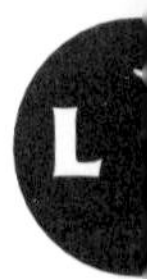

may actually see the parasites themselves. You may see red bite marks or a rash on the scalp or skin. In severe cases of head lice, your child may have swollen glands at the back of his or her neck.

DIAGNOSIS You will be able to see the nits yourself, using a magnifying glass. Head lice nits look like small grains of rice glued to the side of the hair shafts. The nits may be white, gray, or yellow. Don't confuse them with dandruff or drops of hair spray, which you can easily brush off.

TREATMENT For head lice, use an over-the-counter medicated shampoo or cream rinse that contains permethrin, which kills the lice but not the nits. A prescription shampoo containing lindane is also available. Reapply the product in a week to kill the lice that have hatched from the nits before they reproduce. Use a fine-toothed comb to remove the nits. Most doctors recommend that the entire family be treated for lice infestation, except infants. Over-the-counter products are also available for body and pubic lice. The treatment is effective in 99 percent of all cases.

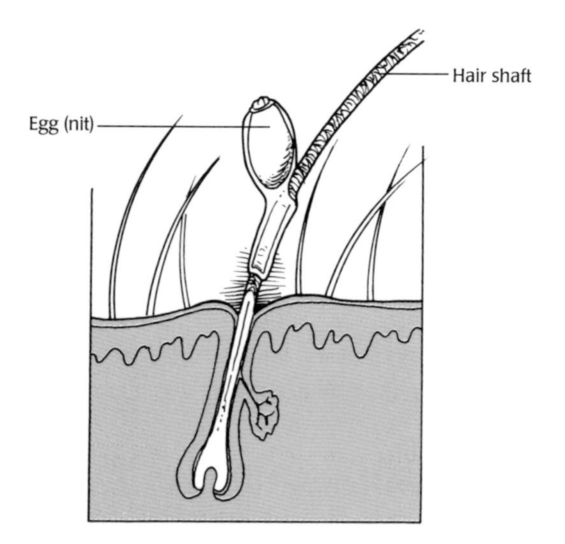

Lice eggs on a hair shaft

Female lice lay their eggs (nits) on a child's hair shaft, close to the scalp. The eggs hatch in 8 to 10 days.

Wash your child's clothing, sheets, pillowcases, blankets, toys, and towels in hot water or dry-clean your child's clothing to kill any lice. Soak your child's comb and brush in hot, soapy water for at least 15 minutes. Place any objects, such as stuffed animals, that cannot be cleaned into a plastic bag for 2 weeks to kill the lice. Furniture spray that kills lice is available for furniture that has become infested.

Keep your child out of school or day care until the lice have been eliminated, and notify the school about your child's infestation so the teachers or school nurse can check the other children for lice. Some schools have a "no nit" policy, meaning that children cannot return until all the nits are gone. If you hear that more than 20 percent of the children in your child's school are infested with lice, treat your child with a medicated shampoo to prevent him or her from getting lice.

If your child's condition does not improve after two shampooings, call your doctor.

LUPUS

Lupus is an AUTOIMMUNE DISORDER that affects the connective tissue, the tissue inside the body that holds various structures together. Lupus also affects the blood vessels in many parts of the body including the skin, heart, kidneys, brain, joints, blood cells, and lungs. There are two types of lupus: discoid lupus erythematosus (DLE), which affects only the skin, and systemic lupus erythematosus (SLE), which affects many parts of the body. In a child with lupus, the immune system—the body's natural defense against infection—attacks the child's own connective tissue and blood vessels, causing pain and swelling. Lupus tends to run in families. Viruses, ultraviolet light, female sex hormones, and drugs used to treat HIGH BLOOD PRESSURE, ARRHYTHMIAS, and SEIZURE DISORDERS are thought to play a role in triggering the abnormal immune system reaction. Among children, lupus occurs most frequently in adolescents. It is very rare for lupus to occur in children under

5 years old. Girls get the disease more often than boys. Children of Chinese, Japanese, and African descent have a higher risk of the disease.

SIGNS AND SYMPTOMS Symptoms flare up when something triggers an autoimmune response, and then the symptoms disappear. Children with DLE may have a red, raised, scaly, skin RASH on their face and scalp. The rash can leave scars. Children with SLE also develop a rash, but it is characteristically flat and red and falls over the bridge of the nose in the form of a butterfly. Neither rash is painful or itchy. Other symptoms of SLE are appetite loss, fatigue, a low fever, muscle aches, joint pain and swelling, open sores in the mouth and nose, sensitivity to sunlight, paleness, tendency to bruise, chest pain when breathing, abdominal pain, vomiting, changes in behavior and personality, seizures, and, in rare cases, PSYCHOSIS. If an affected child's kidneys are damaged, he or she may develop high blood pressure and his or her kidneys may fail (see KIDNEY FAILURE, CHRONIC). The child may also lose his or her hair (see ALOPECIA). The child's fingers and toes may be painful when exposed to cold air and they may turn blue or be colorless.

DIAGNOSIS AND TREATMENT Doctors can diagnose this disease from the signs and symptoms and from blood and urine tests. In some cases, the doctor may take a small *biopsy* of skin for analysis under a microscope. Mild cases of lupus with few or no symptoms may need no treatment at all. In other cases, the doctor may recommend or prescribe anti-inflammatory drugs. For a more serious case of lupus, the doctor may prescribe *corticosteroids* or medications that suppress the child's immune system. Blood transfusions may be needed to treat anemia (see ANEMIA, BLOOD-LOSS and ANEMIA, HEMOLYTIC) or for deficiencies in blood platelets. Significant kidney failure may require kidney dialysis (see page 545).

If your child has lupus, he or she will need lots of rest and nutritious foods, especially when flare-ups occur. He or she should avoid exposure to sunlight as much as possible and wear a sunscreen when out in the sun. Stress can trigger an attack, so try to identify possible sources of stress in your child's life and teach your child positive ways of coping with it. Most children with this disease can lead normal lives but, in a small percentage of affected children, lupus can be fatal. Flare-ups can usually be controlled with medication. Make sure your child does not abruptly stop taking the medication, otherwise his or her condition could become worse. Call your child's doctor anytime flare-ups occur.

LYME DISEASE

Lyme disease is an infection caused by a microorganism transmitted by the bite of a deer tick, a tiny insect that is the size of a pin head. To cause infection, the tick needs to remain attached to the person for 24 hours or longer. Lyme disease can occur year round, but usually occurs from May through August (tick season) when a large number of deer ticks populate outdoor areas, most frequently where woods and grasslands meet. Children can easily become infected when playing near wooded areas where deer live.

Although Lyme disease occurs in almost every state in the United States, it appears to be concentrated in the northeast coastal states, the mid-Atlantic states, northern California, Minnesota, and Wisconsin. The disease can also be found in Europe and Asia. Lyme disease is named for Lyme, Connecticut, where medical researchers first identified the illness in 1975.

SIGNS AND SYMPTOMS The most common and recognizable symptom is a slowly expanding red rash around a small red spot, which is the site of the bite. The rash spreads in a circle around the spot and then the center of the rash clears up, so that the entire circle looks like a bull's eye. A number of rashes can appear within a few weeks of the bite in different places on your child's body.

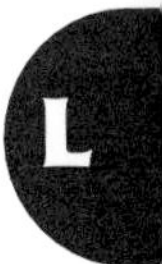

Other early signs include fever and flulike symptoms. If the illness is not promptly treated, your child may develop signs of arthritis, such as painful and swollen joints (especially in the knees), months or years after the tick bite. Untreated Lyme disease can also affect the nervous system, causing a temporary facial paralysis known as Bell's palsy, MENINGITIS, or limb numbness and weakness. Your child could also develop heart problems, such as an irregular heartbeat, along with shortness of breath and dizziness several weeks after the bite.

DIAGNOSIS Lyme disease can be very hard to diagnose because its symptoms are similar to those of other diseases. As many as one quarter of affected people don't even get the telltale rash.

How to prevent Lyme disease

Whenever your child walks or plays in the woods or near high grass, he or she needs to take certain precautions to avoid getting Lyme disease. Teach your child to follow these Lyme disease prevention guidelines:

- Wear a long-sleeved shirt with the collar buttoned, a hat, and long pants tucked into socks.
- Spray clothing and exposed skin with insect repellent that contains diethyltoluamide (DEET). Do not use any insect repellent on the skin of small children who put their fingers into their mouths. Spray clothing only.
- Don't take a pet into the woods with you during tick season. Dogs can carry deer ticks into your home.

When your child comes indoors, check his or her body for ticks. Look closely—the ticks are very small. Keep your yard clear of brush and high grass and try to keep deer off of your property. If you find a tick on your child's skin, grasp it by the head with tweezers and pull it straight out. Don't crush the tick because your child could become infected through the skin. Wash the wound with soap and water and then apply an over-the-counter antiseptic.

Your child may not remember being bitten by a deer tick because the bite is painless and the tick is hard to see with the naked eye.

If your child exhibits symptoms of Lyme disease, take him or her to the doctor. Your doctor will ask you and your child if he or she had recently been in tick-infested areas and will order a blood test for evidence of infection, but the blood test is not always accurate. If the doctor thinks your child's nervous system may have been affected, the doctor may do a test called a *lumbar puncture*, using a needle to withdraw fluid from the spine to look for evidence of infection.

TREATMENT Your child's doctor will treat an early case of Lyme disease with antibiotics taken by mouth. Later stages of the disease require antibiotics given *intravenously*. The specific antibiotics your child receives will depend on the stage of the disease and the child's symptoms. Your child should recover within a few weeks of treatment, although symptoms of the disease can linger for months or even years.

LYMPHOMA

A lymphoma is a cancer that develops in a child's lymphatic system, which is part of the body's immune system that fights infection. The lymphatic system is made up mostly of vessels—tiny tubes, much like blood vessels, that carry fluid that naturally leaks out of blood vessels and white blood cells to tissues throughout the body—and nodes or glands, which are bean-shaped organs that filter the fluid as it passes through them. Lymph nodes can be found in the head, neck, chest, abdomen, groin, and extremities. The lymphatic system also includes organs—such as the spleen, thymus, and bone marrow—that contain white blood cells.

Because the lymphatic system extends throughout the body, lymphomas can occur anywhere. Their cause remains unknown, although some types of lymphomas are thought to be

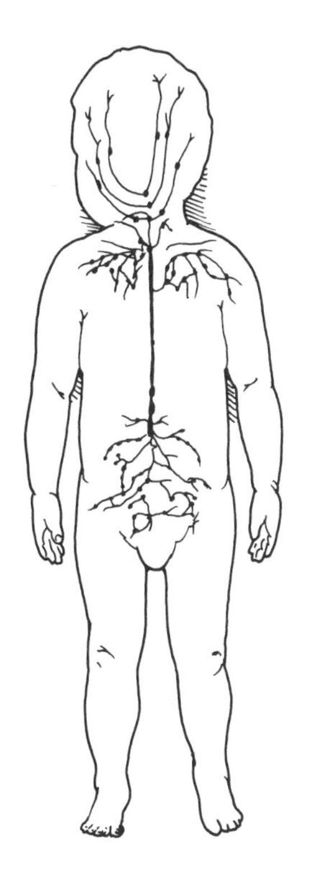

Common sites of lymphomas in children

Lymphomas develop in the network of vessels and nodes that make up the lymphatic system. The most common sites for lymphomas include the lymph nodes in the child's neck, behind the collarbone, and in the abdomen.

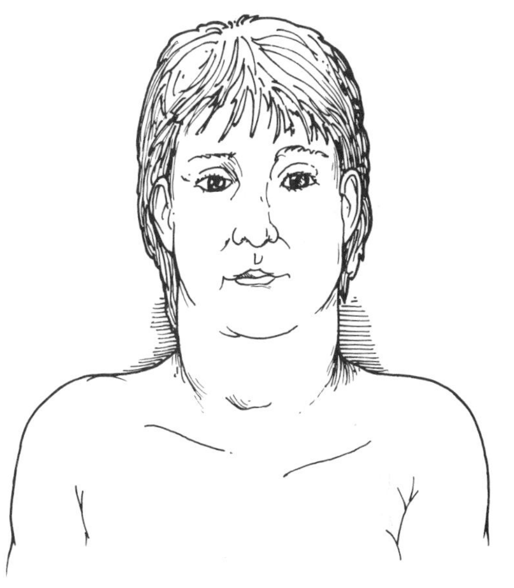

Enlarged lymph nodes in the neck

Swollen glands are usually just a sign of a common childhood infection, but they may also indicate the presence of a lymphoma. The lymph glands in the neck become enlarged but are usually painless.

linked to viral infections. Lymphomas are less common in children under 15 years of age, but become more common in young adults. There are two main types of lymphomas—Hodgkin's disease and non-Hodgkin's lymphomas. Hodgkin's disease is more common in boys than in girls.

SIGNS AND SYMPTOMS Painless swelling of the lymph glands in your child's neck, underarms, or groin that does not go away in a few weeks may be the initial sign of a lymphoma. Other symptoms can include fever, night sweats, weight loss, fatigue, itching, small purplish-red spots on the skin, or bruising. Your child may also become nauseated and vomit or have pain in his or her abdominal area. If a lymphoma develops around an airway, your child may have difficulty breathing. As the disease progresses, your child's body becomes less capable of fighting off infections than normal.

DIAGNOSIS The symptoms of a lymphoma can indicate a variety of other illnesses, so you will need to take your child to see the doctor for an evaluation. If your child's doctor suspects a lymphoma, he or she will refer your child to a cancer specialist (oncologist). The specialist will need to take a *biopsy* of the tissue in your child's lymph node to diagnosis the disease and identify the specific type of lymphoma.

The doctor may also order blood tests and *computed tomography* or *ultrasounds* of your child's chest and abdomen to determine how extensively the lymphoma has spread. Your child might also need other tests, such as bone marrow aspiration and biopsy or a gallium scan (an X-ray taken after radioactive dye is injected into your child's body to show which lymph nodes are affected), so the doctor can find out how far the disease has progressed.

TREATMENT Children with Hodgkin's disease are usually treated with *chemotherapy* combined with low doses of *radiation.* Your child may receive the drugs designed to kill the cancer cells in pill form or by injections into a vein or muscle.

Children with non-Hodgkin's lymphoma may receive only chemotherapy to treat the disease. In some cases, surgery and radiation may also be needed to kill or remove the cancer. For both types of lymphoma, treatment and outlook depend on how far the cancer has progressed, its location, and the type of lymphoma your child has.

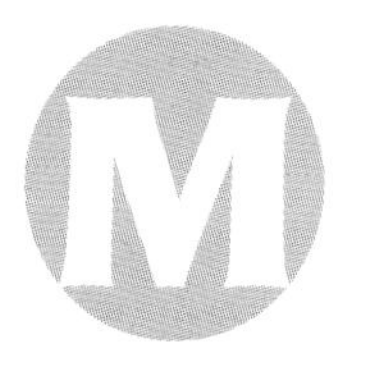

MALABSORPTION

Malabsorption is a digestive disorder in which a child's small intestine fails to absorb essential nutrients. Children may be born with the disorder, develop it following an infection, or have it because of a disease, such as CELIAC DISEASE, CYSTIC FIBROSIS, and CROHN'S DISEASE, that damages the organs that produce the enzymes needed to digest or absorb nutrients. Malabsorption may also occur after surgery that shortens the intestine and decreases the area available for absorption inside the small intestine.

One of the most common malabsorption problems in children is LACTOSE INTOLERANCE, caused by a deficiency of an enzyme called lactase that breaks down the milk sugar lactose. A child with lactose intolerance cannot drink milk without developing abdominal pain, cramps, and diarrhea.

SIGNS AND SYMPTOMS Some time after eating, a child with a malabsorption disorder belches and has gas, abdominal bloating, abdominal pain or cramping, and diarrhea. The child's stools may be loose, watery, and foul-smelling, and they sometimes float in the toilet because of their high fat content. The child may also vomit. Symptoms can last from hours to weeks, depending on the cause of the malabsorption. If the disorder is not diagnosed and treated, the child can become malnourished and lose weight. The child's growth may also be retarded. Children with malabsorption sometimes develop a prominent belly but their arms and legs may look wasted. An affected child can become weak and irritable from hunger or poor nutrition.

DIAGNOSIS If the doctor suspects that your child has malabsorption, he or she will do a thorough physical examination and ask you about his or her symptoms and their onset, diet, family history of malabsorption, and overall condition. The examination will determine the specific kinds of tests the doctor will order, but he or she will probably want to test your child's stool to look for unusual amounts of unabsorbed fat, carbohydrates, protein, or white blood cells. Blood tests will also help diagnose the condition and can show evidence of any nutritional deficiencies. Your child may also need to undergo X-ray examinations of his or her small intestine or other abdominal organs. The doctor may also order a *biopsy* of your child's liver or intestine.

TREATMENT Once the doctor has identified the specific cause of your child's malabsorption, he or she will treat the condition accordingly. In many cases, treatment includes a change in your child's diet so he or she can avoid any foods, such as milk in lactose intolerance, that are causing digestive problems. Your doctor will probably also prescribe vitamin, mineral, and enzyme supplements for your child. Medication may also be needed depending on the cause of the malabsorption. Treatment of the underlying cause should improve your child's symptoms and allow him or her to gain weight and start growing properly. But normal growth may not resume if the child has chronic (long-term) malabsorption or a disease, such as celiac disease, cystic fibrosis, or Crohn's disease, that causes malabsorption.

MALNUTRITION

Malnutrition is the inadequate intake of nutrients needed for normal growth and development. An infant, child, or adolescent may be inadequately nourished either because his or her diet does not contain enough necessary nutrients, or because the child cannot digest or absorb the nutrients because of some physical disorder. Malnutrition is a worldwide problem and one of the major causes of illness and death among children. In developing countries, malnutrition arises because of poverty, drought, famine, ignorance, and disease. In more affluent countries, malnutrition may be caused by poverty, disease, fad diets, child abuse (see page 323) or neglect, poor eating habits, or eating disorders such as ANOREXIA NERVOSA. Some of the conditions that can cause malnutrition include MALABSORPTION and related disorders—such as CYSTIC FIBROSIS, CELIAC DISEASE, and CROHN'S DISEASE in which a child is unable to digest or absorb necessary nutrients—and chronic diseases such as congenital heart disease (see HEART DISEASE, CONGENITAL) or tumors.

SIGNS AND SYMPTOMS Symptoms such as irritability, a lack of energy, and fatigue may range from mild to severe. Infants and children who have mild symptoms may grow normally in length but begin to lose a lot of weight. Eventually the child's growth is also affected and he or she may exhibit signs of DEVELOPMENTAL DELAY in intellectual, motor (movement), language, and social skills. The child's body may begin to lose fat and muscle and his or her abdomen may swell. The child may also display changes in the color and condition of his or her skin, such as abnormally dark or light patches, sores, and cracked skin on the lips or around the eyes and mouth. In severe cases, the child may develop symptoms of dehydration (see page 283) and shock, such as cold and clammy skin, dry lips, extreme thirst, quick and shallow breathing, weakness, dizziness, confusion, and fainting.

DIAGNOSIS The doctor may notice that your child has lost weight during a routine examination, or you may notice some of the symptoms of malnutrition yourself. Your child's doctor will take blood and urine tests; compare your child's weight, height, and head size against standard measurements for your child's age and sex (see page 239); and measure your child's body fat and muscle mass. The doctor will also order any additional tests that may be needed to detect an underlying disease that could be causing your child's malnutrition. Your child's doctor will question you about the growth patterns of the children in your family and about your child's diet and feeding behavior.

TREATMENT If your child has mild symptoms of malnutrition, he or she can be treated successfully with a healthy diet designed by a dietitian. Your child's doctor may also give you information about how to feed your infant or child properly and teach you about the nutrition he or she needs. The doctor may also recommend calorie or vitamin supplements. In some cases of malnutrition, the child may need to be hospitalized to be given fluids *intravenously* and to be given adequate nutrition, beginning with a liquid diet and then progressing to solid foods. With a proper diet, your infant or child should begin to gain weight in a few days. His or her strength and alertness should begin to return within a week. Most children with mild symptoms recover completely with successful treatment but, if a child's growth and development have been severely affected, he or she may be left with long-term mental and physical problems.

MANIC-DEPRESSIVE DISORDER

See Bipolar disorder

MARFAN SYNDROME

Marfan syndrome is a rare, inherited GENETIC DISORDER that affects a child's connective tissue. Children with Marfan syndrome do not produce an important component of connective tissue known as fibrillin, which acts like a glue to bind cells together. Marfan syndrome causes abnormal development of the child's bones, blood vessels, lungs, eyes, heart, and skin, giving the child's body an unnaturally slender and elongated appearance. The disorder can affect boys and girls of any racial or ethnic group.

SIGNS AND SYMPTOMS A child with Marfan syndrome begins to show the unique characteristics of the disorder at about age 10. The lack of fibrillin in the child's body causes the tissues to stretch. The child grows tall and thin and has loose joints that extend beyond the normal range or are dislocated. The bones in his or her arms, legs, and fingers become longer than usual and appear to be out of proportion to the rest of the child's body. The child's breastbone may stick out or look caved in and the spine may be curved from SCOLIOSIS. The child's face may look long and narrow, the teeth may be crowded together, and the roof of the mouth may be highly arched. These symptoms may range from mild to severe. Some affected children also have learning disabilities and require special education.

Most children with Marfan syndrome have abnormal heart valves that cause a heart murmur (unusual heart sound) or irregular heartbeat. The aorta (the main blood vessel in the body), which contains an abundance of fibrillin, can weaken and balloon out (a condition called an aneurysm) or tear, causing bleeding into the chest or abdomen and sudden death. About half of children with Marfan syndrome are nearsighted from a dislocation of the lens in the eye, lens deformities, or detachment of the retina (the light-sensitive lining at the back of the eye). They are also prone to sudden lung collapse. People with Marfan syndrome usually do not live beyond 50 years of age and often die of heart disease.

DIAGNOSIS Marfan syndrome is difficult to diagnose because there are no specific tests for the disorder. If your child's doctor suspects that your child has Marfan syndrome, he or she may order an *echocardiogram* (a picture of the heart obtained by sound waves) and an eye exam to look for the characteristic abnormalities produced by the disease.

TREATMENT Your child's doctor may prescribe beta-blocker medication to prevent the formation of an aneurysm. Heart surgery may be needed if an aneurysm occurs or to repair defective heart valves. Your child may need a brace or surgery for any spinal deformities. Both you and your child should receive genetic counseling (see page 497).

MEASLES

Measles, also called rubeola, is a highly contagious infection caused by a virus and spread by coughing and sneezing. Before the measles vaccine was developed in the early 1960s, most children got measles. Today, the disease is much less common in developed countries such as the United States. Although measles usually occurs in children, it can also occur in adults.

Doctors usually recommend two doses of the measles vaccine. Children get the first shot at 12 to 15 months of age and the second when they enter kindergarten or first grade (between the ages of 4 and 6), although the timing of the second dose varies from state to state. If an adolescent has received only one vaccination, his or her doctor will recommend getting the second immunization before age 18.

Infants under 1 year of age are usually not vaccinated unless there is a measles outbreak because the immunity may not last long enough to protect the child for life. Children whose immune system (the body's natural defense against infection) is compromised by cancer or *chemotherapy* should not receive the vaccine until their immune function returns to normal. Children infected with HIV can get the measles vaccine with their doctor's approval. If your child is allergic to eggs, remind or inform the doctor of the allergy before your child gets immunized for measles because the vaccine has an egg base and could cause a reaction. Pregnant girls or women should not get the vaccine.

SIGNS AND SYMPTOMS Initial symptoms appear 10 to 12 days after exposure to the measles virus with the development of a runny nose, hacking cough, irritability, red eyes that are sensitive to light, and a low-grade (from 101°F to 102°F) fever. These early symptoms last from 3 to 5 days.

About 2 or 3 days after the first signs occur, small, red spots with blue-white centers, known as Koplik spots, appear inside the mouth. In another day or two, the child develops a characteristic RASH that often begins on his or her forehead and spreads to the face, neck, and body (see page 24). The rash consists of large, flat, red-brown blotches that often merge and can last for 6 days. The fever can rise to 105°F and may break as the rash begins to fade.

Two or 3 days after the rash appears, complications—such as ear infections (see page 480), CROUP, BRONCHITIS, and PNEUMONIA—can occur. The child may also have muscle aches, diarrhea, abdominal pain, and vomiting. Some children develop ENCEPHALITIS 3 to 5 days after the rash appears.

DIAGNOSIS AND TREATMENT Your child's doctor can diagnose measles by asking you how the symptoms started and by examining your child for the characteristic rash. Inform your child's day-care center or school of your child's infection so that the parents of your child's playmates or classmates can be notified. Give your child plenty of fluids and acetaminophen (not aspirin) for the fever. Place a humidifier in your child's room to help keep his or her nose and mouth moist and to relieve coughing. See that your child gets plenty of rest. If your child's condition gets worse, call the doctor immediately. Your child may return to school or day care after the rash and fever have disappeared, usually in 7 to 10 days. Once your child has had measles, he or she won't get the disease again.

MECKEL'S DIVERTICULUM

Meckel's diverticulum is an abnormality, present at birth, in which a small sac protrudes from the last segment of the small intestine. The sac commonly contains tissue from other body organs, such as the stomach. Meckel's diverticulum is the most common malformation of the digestive tract. About 2 percent of all babies are born with this condition.

SIGNS AND SYMPTOMS In most children, Meckel's diverticulum causes no problems. But if the sac becomes infected, obstructs the intestine by causing it to twist or turn in on itself, or develops an ulcer (see ULCERS, PEPTIC), the affected child can become seriously ill and require emergency treatment. Signs of serious illness include sudden bleeding from the rectum or bloody stool. The child may have no pain during the bleeding, which may come and go or be continuous. If an intestinal obstruction occurs, the child develops abdominal cramping and distention, along with vomiting and sometimes bloody stool.

DIAGNOSIS If your child has rectal bleeding, a bloody bowel movement, or symptoms of an intestinal obstruction, call the doctor right away. The doctor will order a blood test to see if your child has developed anemia from blood loss. Lab tests to rule out other diseases may also be done. He or she may also order a *radionuclide scan* of your child's abdomen to locate the diverticulum in the abdomen.

TREATMENT If your child is bleeding heavily, he or she may need blood transfusions. Your child's doctor will recommend that surgery be done as soon as possible to relieve any intestinal obstruction and to take out the sac attached to it. The chances of complete recovery are very good once the sac is removed.

MENINGITIS

Meningitis is a contagious infection of the meninges, the thin tissue lining that covers the brain and spinal cord. It frequently occurs in children under 5 years of age but can affect children of any age. A variety of viruses and bacteria can cause meningitis. Bacterial meningitis is usually more serious than viral meningitis and can even be life threatening, especially when it occurs in infants younger than 6 months old.

The most common cause of bacterial meningitis in children between the ages of 3 months and 3 years is a bacterium known as Haemophilus influenzae type b. In older children, bacterial meningitis may be caused by Neisseria meningitidis and Streptococcus pneumoniae. In areas of the world where TUBERCULOSIS is common, the bacterium that causes tuberculosis can also cause meningitis. The most common cause of viral meningitis is a group of intestinal viruses known as enteroviruses.

Bacteria spread when saliva and nasal secretions are coughed or sneezed into the air. Viruses can be spread by direct contact with infected saliva and hand-to-mouth contact with the stool of an infected person.

Since the introduction of a vaccine against H influenzae type b in the mid 1980s, the incidence of H influenzae meningitis has dropped. Children as young as 2 months old are now routinely vaccinated against H influenzae type b. All children under age 5 should be vaccinated against the bacterium. If a cluster of cases occurs, public health officials may recommend that those at risk for meningitis receive both antibiotics and a vaccine against the bacterium. Vaccination against N meningitidis also exists but provides only limited protection. It is usually given only to groups, such as college students or armed forces personnel, who are at high risk because of crowded living conditions.

SIGNS AND SYMPTOMS Meningitis may follow a cold, influenza (see page 231), a throat infection, or other illnesses that lower the child's resistance to disease. Infection spreads to the meninges through the child's bloodstream or, less frequently, through a head injury. Symptoms include irritability, fever, nausea, vomiting, a severe HEADACHE, a stiff neck, back and shoulder pain, sensitivity to light, and sometimes a red or purple skin RASH. Infants may have a high-pitched cry, feed poorly, and be difficult to calm or arouse. Older children may exhibit sleepiness, disorientation, or combativeness.

Viral meningitis is usually mild and lasts less than 2 weeks, but bacterial meningitis, if left untreated, can proceed rapidly to confusion, seizures, coma (unconsciousness), and even death. A child with untreated bacterial meningitis may later develop MENTAL RETARDATION, HEARING LOSS, or BLINDNESS.

DIAGNOSIS Take your child to a hospital emergency department immediately if he or she has symptoms of meningitis. Your child's doctor or the doctor in the emergency department will confirm the diagnosis with a *lumbar puncture.* The doctor may also order blood, urine, and stool tests.

TREATMENT The doctor will begin treatment right away. Antibiotics are given *intravenously*, even before test results are available, because bacterial meningitis is so serious. If the diagnosis is confirmed, your child will stay on intravenous antibiotics for 10 days or more. If your child has viral meningitis, antibiotics won't be effective, so he or she may be discharged from the hospital. You can care for your child at home with bed rest and plenty of fluids. Your child can recover from viral meningitis completely in 2 weeks–sooner if it is mild. Most children also recover from bacterial meningitis, but recovery takes longer.

If your child has bacterial meningitis, notify the day-care center or school. Other members of your household, your child's classmates, and anyone else who has had close contact with your child may need to be treated with antibiotics to reduce their risk of getting the disease. Bacterial meningitis can cause hearing loss, even after antibiotic treatment. Affected children need follow-up to assess hearing function.

MENSTRUAL DISORDERS

Menstruation is the monthly shedding of the lining of the uterus that occurs in girls who have reached the age of menarche (the first menstrual period). The average age in the United States is 12, but menstruation can start as early as age 10 or as late as age 16.

TYPES OF MENSTRUAL DISORDERS During adolescence, the most common menstrual problems are cramping and pain (dysmenorrhea) and absent or irregular periods.

Dysmenorrhea Dysmenorrhea is cramping and pain just before or during menstruation. It is the most common menstrual problem and is caused by the release of hormones known as prostaglandins, which trigger spasms of the muscles in the uterus. Primary dysmenorrhea usually begins 6 to 18 months after a girl has had her first period and is unrelated to an underlying disorder. Secondary dysmenorrhea is not common, but is usually caused by an infection, such as PELVIC INFLAMMATORY DISEASE, or by endometriosis (a condition in which tissue from the lining of the uterus migrates to other parts of the pelvic cavity). It can also be a complication of early pregnancy.

Amenorrhea The absence of menstrual periods is known as amenorrhea. Primary amenorrhea is the delay of a girl's first period to the age of 16. In some cases, primary amenorrhea is simply related to a delay in the onset of puberty. In other cases, it can be caused by dramatic weight loss, stress, an imbalance of hormones, OVARIAN TUMORS AND CYSTS, or TURNER'S SYNDROME. Secondary amenorrhea is the cessation of menstruation for 6 months or more after menarche has occurred. The usual reason for secondary amenorrhea is pregnancy, but it can also be a sign of an eating disorder, such as ANOREXIA NERVOSA.

Irregular menstruation Irregularities can include unusual changes in the time between periods, length of the period, or amount of blood lost. For the first 2 to 3 years after menarche, it is common for adolescent girls to have irregular periods; they may even skip a period. The average time between one period and the next is 28 days, although the normal range is from 23 to 35 days. Most periods last from 3 to 5 days, but can normally vary from 2 to 7 days. Blood usually flows lightly at first, then heavily for a day or two, and then lightly again for another day or two. Irregular menstruation can be caused by an imbalance of hormones, stress, changes in contraception methods, and travel. Pregnancy, endometriosis, and ovarian tumors and cysts can also cause menstrual irregularities.

SIGNS AND SYMPTOMS A girl with dysmenorrhea experiences dull, cramping pain in the lower abdomen. The pain can be slight or very severe and can radiate down the girl's legs or to her lower back. The cramping usually starts a few hours before menstruation begins, but can begin a day or two in advance. The cramps can last a day or more during the period. The girl may also feel nauseated, vomit, and have diarrhea. The only symptom of amenorrhea is the absence of menstruation for 6 months or longer after having had menstrual periods. The symptoms of irregular menstruation are variations in the girl's normal menstrual pattern.

DIAGNOSIS Dysmenorrhea is a normal part of menstruation for many girls, but if the symptoms interfere with your daughter's ability to go to school, work, or sleep, take her to the doctor for treatment. If your daughter has or develops amenorrhea or irregular periods, the doctor will do a pelvic exam (see page 255) and may order blood and urine tests, including a test for female hormone levels. The doctor may also do a pregnancy test and order an *ultrasound* of your daughter's pelvis and abdomen and a laparoscopy (examination of the inside of the abdomen through a viewing tube). If the doctor suspects that dysfunction of the pituitary gland (see PITUITARY DISORDERS) is the cause of the problem, he or she may order *computed tomography* or *magnetic resonance imaging* of her skull.

TREATMENT If your daughter's cramps are mild, she can take over-the-counter pain relievers, such as acetaminophen or ibuprofen. A heating pad or hot water bottle placed on the abdomen might also help relieve the cramps. In severe cases, oral contraceptives (birth-control pills that contain a specific amount of hormones) can help relieve the symptoms of primary dysmenorrhea. The doctor may prescribe a drug called indomethacin to fight inflammation. Discuss treatment options and potential side effects with your daughter's doctor. Treatment for secondary dysmenorrhea depends on the underlying cause.

The treatment for amenorrhea also depends on the cause. The doctor may prescribe hormones if a hormone imbalance is causing the problem. If the doctor suspects that your daughter is losing excessive weight because of anorexia nervosa, he or she may refer her for psychological counseling.

If irregular periods are causing excessive blood loss, the doctor may prescribe iron and folic acid supplements to treat anemia (see ANEMIA, BLOOD-LOSS). The doctor may also prescribe birth-control pills to slow excessive bleeding during menstruation or to regulate your daughter's menstrual periods. In severe cases, your daughter may have to be hospitalized for further evaluation and treatment.

MENTAL RETARDATION

Mental retardation is impaired intellectual functioning as measured by an IQ (intelligence quotient) test. To fit the definition of mental retardation, a child must have an IQ score below 70 and his or her intellectual impairment must be recognized before age 18. The degree of mental retardation can range from mild to profound, according to the child's IQ score. About 80 percent of mentally retarded children fall into the mild classification. The exact causes of mild mental retardation are not known, but it tends to run in families. Doctors consider malnutrition (insufficient nutrition) to be a probable cause of mild mental retardation.

More severe degrees of mental retardation usually have a specific physical cause, such as CHROMOSOMAL ABNORMALITIES, INBORN ERRORS OF METABOLISM, or an infection of the brain (encephalitis) or meninges (meningitis), the membranes that surround the brain and spinal cord, in early childhood.

Degrees of Mental Retardation

The degree of a child's mental retardation is classified according to the child's score on a standardized intelligence quotient (IQ) test. The ranges for each category appear below.

Degree of Retardation	IQ Score
Mild	50 to 70
Moderate	35 to 49
Severe	20 to 34
Profound	Under 20

SIGNS AND SYMPTOMS About 10 percent of mentally retarded children are identified when they are infants or in early childhood because they show clear evidence of a physical disorder, such as brain damage, a BIRTH DEFECT, or a GENETIC DISORDER. The rest are usually identified when they enter school.

In infants and young children, DEVELOPMENTAL DELAY may be the first sign of mental retardation. Mildly retarded children are slow in performing mental tasks, such as reading, adding, or solving problems. Their emotional and social development may also be delayed and they may be hyperactive (see page 527) or autistic (see page 426).

Retarded infants may have difficulty sucking and forming speech sounds, while retarded children may have trouble speaking and communicating ideas. CEREBRAL PALSY, SEIZURE DISORDERS, VISION PROBLEMS, HEARING LOSS, physical deformities, behavior problems, and urinary and bowel incontinence may also occur.

DIAGNOSIS A number of screening tests can assess the mental development of infants and children. Talk to your doctor if you feel that your child is not developing normally.

TREATMENT Mentally retarded children benefit from special education and assisted living arrangements, but there is no specific treatment for intellectual impairment. Mildly retarded children can learn the skills they need to lead nearly normal lives. Moderately retarded children can be trained and may be able to live at home, but may need to live in a group home or work in a sheltered workshop. Severely and profoundly retarded children usually require continuous care either at home or in an extended care facility.

MIGRAINE

A migraine is an intense HEADACHE accompanied by disturbances of vision or nausea and vomiting, or both. Migraine headaches can occur in children of any age but most often first appear in children between the ages of 8 and 13. The condition usually lasts a lifetime. Children are at greater risk of getting migraines if they have a family history of the disorder. No one knows exactly what causes migraines, but they can be triggered by certain foods (chocolate, cheese, caffeined beverages, or alcohol), stress, fatigue, missed meals, a girl's monthly menstrual cycle, or the use of oral contraceptives.

SIGNS AND SYMPTOMS While the signs and symptoms of a migraine can vary from child to child, most children experience a warning period with symptoms before the headache begins. At first, the child may feel irritable and unusually tired. Then he or she may feel sick to the stomach, vomit, and have diarrhea. These preliminary symptoms can last from several minutes to a day or two. Some children experience visual disturbances, such as a zigzag distortion of vision, blind spots, or blurry vision, or a strong aversion to bright light. These disturbances can last from a few minutes to a few hours.

As the headache begins, the warning signs usually fade; the child is then left with throbbing, intense pain on one side of the forehead. Typically, the pain lasts for an hour or more and, during that time, the child may look pale, dizzy, and confused. He or she may also feel sick to the stomach and have bloodshot eyes. Young children often cry from the pain. Less commonly, vomiting and abdominal pain are the primary symptoms rather than intense headaches. Some children also have temporary numbness on one side of the body or in one arm and may lose consciousness or have seizures. Migraines may occur as often as two or three times a week or as infrequently as a few times a year.

DIAGNOSIS If your child has severe headaches, take him or her to the doctor for an examination. Make note of what your child eats or drinks before the attacks occur and look for signs of stress, such as a poor appetite and DEPRESSION. The doctor may need to do *computed tomography* or *magnetic resonance imaging* of your child's brain to make sure there are no other causes of the headaches.

TREATMENT The doctor may prescribe medication to control or prevent the migraines. The most typical prescribed medication for migraine is a drug called ergotamine, derived from a fungus, that narrows the blood vessels in your child's head. The doctor will probably also rec-

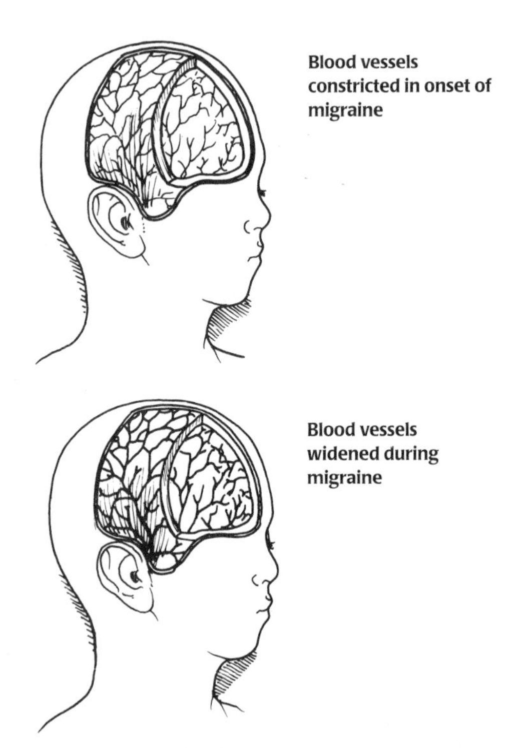

Progression of a migraine
In the first stages of a migraine headache, the blood vessels in the brain and scalp begin to narrow (top), and then widen (bottom) as it progresses. When the blood vessels narrow, the blood supply to the child's brain is reduced, probably causing the visual disturbances that often serve as a warning sign of migraine. The change in the width of the blood vessels in the scalp produces the characteristic pain of migraine.

ommend changes in your child's diet and lifestyle to avoid the foods and other factors that trigger migraine. The medication known as sumatriptan, which doctors sometimes prescribe for adults with migraine, is not recommended for children.

At the first sign of a migraine, place a cold cloth on your child's forehead and have your child lie down in a dark, quiet room so he or she can try to relax or sleep. Give your child any medication the doctor has prescribed, as directed. Notify the doctor if the headache seems to be different from those your child has had in the past.

MITRAL VALVE PROLAPSE

Mitral valve prolapse is a defect (see HEART DISEASE, CONGENITAL) in a heart valve known as the mitral valve. A healthy mitral valve has two flaps, or leaflets, that open and close, allowing blood to pass only from the atrium to the ventricle. In mitral valve prolapse, one or both flaps are larger than normal and do not close evenly when the child's heart pumps blood. Small amounts of blood can leak back over the abnormal valve from the left ventricle to the left atrium, causing a HEART MURMUR.

This condition is uncommon in young children but becomes more common in late adolescence, especially in girls. The disorder is believed to be inherited in many cases. In some children, it is linked to CARDIOMYOPATHY and other congenital heart defects, MARFAN SYNDROME, or SCOLIOSIS. Mitral valve prolapse is usually a mild condition that causes no health problems.

SIGNS AND SYMPTOMS Often, a child has no symptoms at all. Symptoms that do occur—such as fatigue, chest pains, and a sudden, brief increase in the child's heart rate—could signal a number of disorders, including arrhythmia of the heart, but are more likely to occur in adults than in children. Fainting episodes can occur. If a large amount of blood leaks back through the mitral valve, the child can develop heart failure (see HEART FAILURE, CONGESTIVE).

DIAGNOSIS If someone in your family has had mitral valve prolapse, tell your child's doctor so he or she can listen for a characteristic click or murmur in your child's heart with a stethoscope. Otherwise, your doctor may hear the murmur during a routine physical examination. If the doctor suspects mitral valve prolapse, he or she will order diagnostic exams, such as a chest X-ray, *echocardiogram* (an *ultrasound* of the heart), and *electrocardiogram* (a test that records electrical activity in the heart) to confirm the diagnosis.

TREATMENT Because mitral valve prolapse is generally a benign condition, your child usually requires no specific treatment. The doctor will listen for any changes in your child's heart sounds during routine checkups, and a cardiologist may be recommended to examine your child every 2 to 5 years. The doctor will also recommend that your child take antibiotics before any dental work or surgery to prevent a possible infection of the heart. If the prolapse gets worse and your child develops a rapid heartbeat, faints, or has other symptoms of the disease, the doctor may recommend heart medication to improve heart function and control the heart rate and rhythm. In rare cases, the doctor may recommend surgery to correct your child's heart valve defect.

MOLES

Moles are harmless flat or raised spots on the skin that are usually about the size of a pencil eraser or smaller, round or oval, and generally dark brown. Moles usually develop in childhood and last many years. They are very common among children. Most children have from 10 to 40 moles on their skin and they can appear anywhere on the body. Few children are born with moles; most develop them during childhood. While most moles are harmless, certain types can develop into a life-threatening form of skin cancer known as malignant melanoma. Moles that are present at birth and those that are larger than normal are more likely to turn into malignant melanoma.

SIGNS AND SYMPTOMS When moles first appear, they look much like a freckle. A child could have a single mole or several that are grouped together. Although they are usually brown, moles can range from pink to black. They can be flat or raised, and can range in size from a speck to 8 inches across or more.

Moles can slowly grow larger and may develop hairs. Some moles become darker with exposure to sunlight or when your child is taking certain drugs. The teen years and pregnancy are the times when moles are most active (becoming darker and larger) and when new moles may appear.

A mole that changes its size, shape, or color suddenly or one that begins to bleed, itch, or become painful, may be turning into malignant melanoma. The cancerous cells begin to grow abnormally, dividing frequently and uncontrollably. A tumor forms that can invade surrounding tissue and spread to other parts of the body. Malignant melanoma is extremely rare in childhood. In fact, under the age of 20, it is almost unheard of. It usually occurs in the late teens or in early adulthood.

DIAGNOSIS Don't worry about normal-looking moles on your child's skin. They are harmless and do not need a doctor's attention. But be on the lookout for any sudden changes in the size, color, or shape of any mole on your child's body and report these changes to your child's doctor for examination.

TREATMENT The vast majority of moles do not lead to skin cancer and do not need to be treated, unless they seriously affect your child's appearance. Moles in areas that are continually exposed to the sun or irritation, or ones that your child's doctor thinks look abnormal should be removed by the time a child has reached the middle teens to prevent them from turning into melanoma. A plastic surgeon or a dermatologist can shave off the mole with a scalpel and stitch the skin closed. Most mole removals are simple and painless and can be done in the doctor's office.

To lower your child's future risk of malignant melanoma, other types of skin cancer, or sun-damaged skin, apply sunscreen to his or her skin half an hour before he or she is exposed to the sun. Have the doctor check any abnormal-looking moles on your child's skin regularly.

MOLLUSCUM CONTAGIOSUM

Molluscum contagiosum (see page 24) is a common childhood skin infection caused by a virus from the pox virus family. The virus invades the skin and produces tiny bumps that may be mistaken for WARTS. Children get the infection from direct contact with an infected person. They can also contract it from a swimming pool or by sharing towels with an infected person. Adolescents and adults can become infected through sexual contact.

SIGNS AND SYMPTOMS Small, round, raised, pearly-white or flesh-colored bumps appear on the chest, abdomen, legs, arms, or groin, although they can emerge anywhere on the body. The firm, smooth bumps have a domed look and are filled with a cheesy material. They are covered with a thin, transparent layer of skin. If they appear on the eyelids, they can cause eye irritation. The bumps do not hurt or itch.

Symptoms can occur from 2 weeks to 6 months after infection. If the bumps are left untreated, they will increase in number in the first several weeks, and then disappear on their own from several months to 2 years later.

DIAGNOSIS Your child's doctor will be able to diagnose molluscum contagiosum by the appearance of the infection.

TREATMENT Your child's doctor will remove the bumps either by applying chemicals to kill the virus that causes the infection or by using a sharp, spoon-shaped instrument to cut open each bump and remove the center. The doctor may also freeze the bumps with liquid nitrogen and remove them surgically. During treatment, the doctor will apply an anesthetic to your child's skin to minimize pain. Your child may need treatment every 2 to 4 weeks. Otherwise, the doctor will recommend that you or your child wash his or her skin with an abrasive skin scrubber at home to open the bumps.

Encourage your child not to scratch the bumps because scratching will spread the infection to other parts of the body. Have your child's clothes dry-cleaned or wash them in hot water to kill the virus and prevent further spread. Keep the bumps dry after treatment and cover them with small bandages if the bumps are in areas that might rub against clothing.

MONONUCLEOSIS, INFECTIOUS

Infectious mononucleosis is an infection caused by the Epstein-Barr virus, a member of the herpes virus family. Most people are exposed to the Epstein-Barr virus at some time in their lives, but not all will get infectious mononucleosis. Young children tend to get very mild cases of mononucleosis, while adolescents get more seriously ill. Mononucleosis is sometimes called the "kissing disease" because the virus can be spread in saliva through kissing. It can also be spread by any other direct contact with infected saliva and by breathing infected droplets that are sneezed or coughed into the air.

SIGNS AND SYMPTOMS Symptoms appear a week or two after exposure to the virus. The first signs include an overall feeling of fatigue, loss of appetite, cold symptoms, and chills. These symptoms last 1 to 3 days. Then the child or adolescent may develop more serious symptoms, such as a sore throat, fever of up to 104°F, and swollen glands in the neck and armpits. The tonsils may enlarge and develop a white coating. The liver and spleen can swell. Some children also develop a splotchy red RASH. Many affected children become too weak to get out of bed.

DIAGNOSIS AND TREATMENT Your child's doctor will examine your child for the signs or symptoms of infectious mononucleosis. He or she will order blood tests to confirm the diagnosis.

If your child has only a mild case, he or she will generally feel better in about a week with no treatment. Children with more severe mononucleosis will improve within 2 to 4 weeks but may still feel tired for 1 or 2 months. The doctor will recommend that you give your child acetaminophen (not aspirin) for the fever, sore throat, and swollen glands. Occasionally, a child may need *corticosteroids* to reduce throat swelling if it interferes with breathing, eating, or drinking. Gargling with salt water several times a day relieves sore throat pain. Your child should drink plenty of liquids, such as plain broth, sports drinks, and juices.

Your child should not engage in contact sports for at least 4 weeks to avoid the life-threatening risk of rupture of the spleen. He or she should also avoid strenuous exercise for 3 or 4 months if the fatigue lingers. A child with a fever should remain in bed. Your child can resume normal activities gradually as his or her strength and feeling of well-being return.

MOTION SICKNESS

Motion sickness is a physical reaction to constant movement. Motion, such as from the rocking of a boat, upsets fluids in the inner ear that control a child's sense of balance. Traveling in a car, bus, boat, plane, or train can cause motion sickness. Amusement park rides are another common source of motion sickness. Motion sickness affects more children than adults, although infants do not seem to get it. Symptoms lessen with age.

SIGNS AND SYMPTOMS The first signs of motion sickness are fatigue, yawning, cold sweats, HEADACHE, salivating, and abnormally deep or rapid breathing. These early signs are followed by nausea and vomiting if the movement continues. Certain circumstances can bring on motion sickness more readily, such as ANXIETY about getting sick, focusing on nearby objects (for example, reading in a moving car), a full stomach, inadequate ventilation, and the sight or smell of food.

DIAGNOSIS AND TREATMENT If your child seems to be getting motion sickness, try to get him or her on steady ground–pull over and stop if you are in a car or remove the child from the boat or ride as soon as possible. Let your child rest. Give him or her something noncarbonated to drink, and light food such as crackers to help settle his or her stomach. If your child gets motion sickness frequently, you can buy over-the-counter antihistamines designed to prevent motion sickness. Follow the package directions carefully; some medications need to be taken just before a journey and others the day before. Be sure your child has fresh air while traveling and teach him or her to look at the horizon or into the distance instead of reading or concentrating on objects that are nearby.

MOVEMENT DISORDERS

A movement disorder is the constant repetition of an involuntary, purposeless movement. In children, movement disorders can be caused by stress, a need for stimulation, MENTAL RETARDATION, AUTISM, or other diseases. Many children outgrow the problem in early childhood.

TYPES OF MOVEMENT DISORDERS Some common childhood movement disorders are tics, repetitive movements known as stereotypy, and spasms.

Tics These are the most common movement disorders in children. Tics are quick, involuntary, repetitive movements or sounds, such as head twisting, shoulder shrugging, facial grimacing, eye blinking, touching, jumping, obscene gestures, grunting, barking, snorting, throat clearing, or repeating one's own or another person's words. Tics typically come and go. They tend to get worse when a child is anxious, stressed, angry, excited, or tired. They are less apparent when the child is relaxed or focused on some activity. When a child has both motor (movement) and vocal tics, he or she has TOURETTE'S SYNDROME.

Transient cases of tics last for less than a year, while chronic cases last for a year or more.

Stereotypy These movements are repetitive and often rhythmic. Common examples include head banging, head rolling, and body rocking. Children are more likely to rock their bodies than bang their heads. The stereotyped movements typically begin just before the child goes to sleep and last only a few minutes. Children generally begin making these mechanical movements during their first year of life and stop before they become 3 years old. Boys are more likely than girls to make stereotyped movements. The movements may be a part of normal development but could also reveal an underlying disorder, such as autism or mental retardation.

Spasms Spasms are sudden, violent, involuntary muscle jerks or contractions (cramps) that typically occur in a child's face, arms, or legs. The cramps can be quite painful. Facial spasms may affect one entire side of the child's face or only the area around one eye. When a child's diaphragm goes into spasms, he or she gets hiccups. Spasms caused by nervous system disorders include myoclonus (quick, uncontrollable muscle jerks that happen while a child is active or at rest) and chorea (rapid, random, jerky movements in the child's face, arms, legs, or trunk). Myoclonus can occur during a seizure or as a result of ENCEPHALITIS. Chorea has been linked to CEREBRAL PALSY and can appear at the same time as the slow, writhing movements called athetosis. Chorea can be a side effect of certain drugs, such as neuroleptics, which are prescribed for psychiatric disorders. It can also be a complication of RHEUMATIC FEVER and Wilson's disease, a rare, inherited disorder in which copper accumulates in the child's liver.

DIAGNOSIS If your child repeats any of the movements described above, make note of them and remember when they occur so you can tell the child's doctor. Videotape your child's movements, if you can, so the doctor can see them. The doctor will try to determine whether your child's movements are just a part of normal development, are caused by stress, or signal some underlying disorder.

TREATMENT In many cases, treatment may not be necessary unless your doctor determines that a specific disease is causing the movement disorder. If stress or lack of stimulation is the cause, your doctor may recommend ways to relieve your child's stress or increase the stimulation in his or her environment. If your child is old enough, the doctor may recommend that he or she see a mental health professional to help cope with the stressful circumstances.

If an underlying disease causes your child to move in abnormal ways, the doctor will treat the disease, if possible, and refer your child to a physical therapist for help in controlling his or her movements.

MUMPS

Mumps is a contagious infection caused by a virus that affects the salivary glands in the back of the cheeks along the jaw line. Mumps can also affect other organs, including the brain, testicles, and pancreas. It occurs most frequently in children between the ages of 2 and 12 years. The virus spreads in infected saliva that is coughed or sneezed into the air or by direct contact with infected saliva. It can also be transmitted through contact with the urine of an infected child.

Most children are vaccinated against mumps, along with MEASLES and GERMAN MEASLES, at 12 to 15 months and 4 to 6 years of age. The vaccine is effective in about 95 percent of the children who receive it. Infants under 1 year old and children whose immune system (the body's natural defense against infection) is weakened by another illness (such as cancer) should not receive the vaccine until their immune function returns to normal. If your child has an allergy to eggs, ask the doctor if your child should get the mumps vaccine because it is egg-based and your child could have an allergic reaction. The vaccine should be avoided during pregnancy.

SIGNS AND SYMPTOMS Some children have no symptoms or the symptoms are very mild. When symptoms do occur, they include swollen, painful salivary glands, a fever up to 103°F, appetite loss, and HEADACHE. Symptoms do not usually develop until 12 to 25 days after the child becomes infected. The symptoms last 10 to 12 days and then the child usually recovers fully. An infected child may be contagious from 2 days before his or her glands swell up to 10 days afterward.

Initially, only one salivary gland may swell. The others then swell 4 or 5 days later. Occasionally, glands under the child's tongue or jaw and on the sides of the face are affected. Some teenage boys who get mumps experience painful swelling of the testicles and a high fever for 3 to 7 days. In some cases, the infection spreads to the brain and pancreas and, in girls, the ovaries. Long-term complications of mumps can include infertility in the male and HEARING LOSS. Mumps may trigger the development of type I diabetes (see DIABETES MELLITUS, TYPE I) in children with an inherited predisposition to the disease.

DIAGNOSIS AND TREATMENT Your child's doctor can diagnose mumps during a physical examination and may also order blood tests. No treatment is currently available for mumps. At home, you can apply heat or an ice pack—whatever feels best—to your child's swollen glands. Give your child acetaminophen (but not aspirin) to relieve the pain. You don't need to keep your child in bed or away from other members of the family because, by the time your child has the symptoms, the virus has already had a chance to spread. Give your child plenty of liquids, but avoid orange and grapefruit juices, which could irritate the already inflamed glands. Keep your child home from school or day care until the symptoms completely disappear. Once your child gets mumps, he or she cannot be infected again.

MUSCLE DISORDERS

Children can develop a number of disorders affecting the muscle tissue during physical activity or illness.

TYPES OF MUSCLE DISORDERS Common muscle problems include cramps, tears, and inflammation.

Muscle cramps Muscle cramps are involuntary contractions (shortenings) of muscles in a child's arms or legs, usually following strenuous exercise or long periods of standing, sitting, or lying down in an uncomfortable position. They occur most often in children between the ages of 6 and 12 years and most commonly affect the foot, calf, and thigh muscles. Muscle cramps can also happen at night and awaken the child from sleep.

Muscle tears An injury can cause partial or complete tearing of the muscle. When muscles tear, blood oozes into muscle tissue. In children, muscles can tear during sports or play. The muscles in the back of the thigh (hamstring muscles) are the most vulnerable to tearing.

Myositis Myositis is inflammation of muscle tissue from accidental injury, a viral infection, or an AUTOIMMUNE DISORDER, in which the body's natural defense mechanisms against disease begin to attack the child's own tissue (see DERMATOMYOSITIS). It often accompanies colds and the flu (see page 231).

SIGNS AND SYMPTOMS Muscle cramps produce sudden, persistent pain in the affected muscle. The pain usually occurs following exercise or after being in an uncomfortable position for a long time. Muscle tears also cause sudden pain, along with swelling and tenderness. The pain increases if the muscle is stretched. Myositis can cause a dull ache in the arm, shoulder, neck, or back muscles. The muscles can become swollen and tender and the child may have a mild fever. The muscle may feel warm to the touch. The child may feel tired, have restricted motion in the affected muscle, experience muscle weakness, and generally feel ill.

DIAGNOSIS AND TREATMENT Muscle cramps can be treated right away at home by slightly warming the muscle with a heating pad or warm towel, gently stretching the muscle, and massaging it until the pain subsides. You can help prevent your child from getting muscle cramps by encouraging him or her to do stretching exercises and drink plenty of fluids before and after exercise or sports.

Muscle tears need to be seen by a doctor to assess the severity of the injury. In many cases, all that is required is the simple first-aid treatment known as RICE–rest, ice, compression, and elevation. Place an ice pack or ice wrapped in a towel on the torn muscle for 30 minutes every hour until the swelling subsides. Never massage or apply heat to a torn muscle. Elevate the injured limb to slow the flow of blood to the area and wrap the muscle in an elastic bandage. The doctor may recommend complete bed rest for your child. After a day or two, your child can begin to move the injured muscle gradually. Muscle tears can take 3 to 6 weeks to heal completely.

Myositis may require blood and urine tests, an electromyograph test, or a nerve conduction velocity test for a proper diagnosis. The two latter tests measure electrical activity in your child's muscles and nerves. Ice, elevation, and rest help reduce the swelling caused by myositis. Your child's doctor may also prescribe drugs to fight inflammation. Your child can gradually begin to use the muscle again after the pain subsides. Healing can take from 1 to 6 weeks or more, depending on what caused the child's muscle to become inflamed.

MUSCULAR DYSTROPHY

Muscular dystrophy is a rare, inherited GENETIC DISORDER producing muscle weakness that gets worse as a child grows older. The child's muscles waste away as muscle cells die and are replaced by fat and connective tissue.

Nine different types of muscular dystrophy can occur, but the two most common types that affect children are Duchenne's muscular dystrophy and Becker's muscular dystrophy. These two forms are actually the same disease, except that Duchenne's muscular dystrophy develops at an earlier age and progresses more rapidly. Both usually affect only boys, although girls can be carriers of the disease.

SIGNS AND SYMPTOMS Some signs may appear in infants as DEVELOPMENTAL DELAY or muscle weakness, but the disease does not become apparent until about age 3. A boy with Duchenne's muscular dystrophy begins to lose strength in his legs and hips from the gradual wasting away of muscle. He may walk with his feet wide apart to keep his balance and have trouble climbing stairs. He may also fall frequently and have difficulty getting up or standing up straight. His calf muscles may look larger than normal because fat and connective tissue have replaced the calf muscle. By

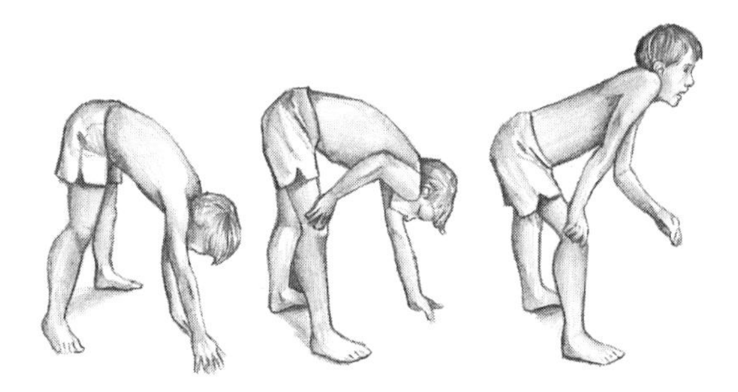

Leg muscle weakness in muscular dystrophy
When sitting on the floor, boys who have muscular dystrophy need to stand up by pushing their body up with their arms and hands because the muscles in their legs are weak. This characteristic position is called Gower's maneuver.

the time the boy turns 10, he may need braces to help him walk. By age 12, he may require a wheelchair.

The disease progresses to the muscles in the boy's arms, neck, and the upper half of his body. His growing bones develop abnormally and he may have a deformed chest or SCOLIOSIS. These bone deformities and muscle weakness may make it hard for him to breathe properly and interfere with the functioning of his heart. Some boys with this disease become mentally impaired or have MENTAL RETARDATION. Boys with Duchenne's muscular dystrophy usually die of PNEUMONIA or other lung problems by late adolescence.

Becker's muscular dystrophy produces similar symptoms, but they develop over a longer period of time. Initial symptoms appear at about age 7 and progress slowly, but affected males usually die before age 40.

DIAGNOSIS See your doctor right away if your son has any of the symptoms of muscular dystrophy. To diagnose muscular dystrophy, your son's doctor will order a blood test that can detect levels of certain proteins in your son's blood. He or she will also order a test called electromyography, which analyzes the electrical activity in a muscle and can show what is causing the muscle weakness. Your doctor may also order a *biopsy* of your son's muscle tissue to confirm the diagnosis.

TREATMENT No specific treatment for this disease is currently available, but the doctor will probably treat your son's symptoms with braces, a wheelchair, and other devices that can help your son manage in the activities of daily living and make his life as comfortable as possible. Physical therapy may help increase your son's muscle strength and can help prevent his joints from contracting. Be sure your son remains active; staying in bed for long periods will make his symptoms worse. Your son's doctor will probably recommend genetic counseling (see page 497) for your entire family.

NECK INJURIES

See Head, neck, or spine injuries

NECROTIZING ENTEROCOLITIS

Necrotizing enterocolitis is a life-threatening disease of infancy in which the lining of a child's intestine dies and sloughs off. In severe cases, an entire segment of the intestine could die, causing scarring, narrowing, or even rupture. No one knows for sure what causes necrotizing enterocolitis, but it is thought to be caused by either a decrease in blood flow to the intestine or a bacterial infection. It has also been linked to feeding overly concentrated formulas to an infant, overly rapid feeding, and stress. Outbreaks of the disease in hospital nurseries suggest that the disease might be contagious. Small, premature infants are especially vulnerable to this disease.

SIGNS AND SYMPTOMS In the first few weeks of life, the infant develops a swollen abdomen and has gas in the intestines. Some infants may have blood that is visible in the stool, vomiting, a lack of energy, an unstable temperature, and diarrhea. In very low birthweight infants, these symptoms may take as long as 2 months to develop. If scarring occurs, signs of INTESTINAL OBSTRUCTION develop. If the enterocolitis causes a hole in the intestine, the infant may quickly develop a painful infection known as peritonitis in the abdominal cavity, go into shock, and even die. The symptoms of shock include rapid and shallow breathing, weakness, cold and clammy skin, and unresponsiveness.

DIAGNOSIS If you have already taken your baby home from the hospital and he or she has symptoms of necrotizing enterocolitis, get him or her to a hospital emergency department immediately. If your baby is still in the hospital, your child's doctor will diagnose this disease from its symptoms and will confirm it with an X-ray of the abdomen. He or she will also take blood and stool tests and may use *ultrasound* or X-rays to detect gas in your baby's abdomen.

TREATMENT If your child's doctor even suspects that your infant has necrotizing enterocolitis, he or she will stop all formula or breast-milk feedings and order feeding and fluids to be given *intravenously*. The doctor will also insert a small tube through your baby's nose and into his or her stomach to relieve trapped intestinal gas. Your baby will need antibiotics to fight infection. If part of the bowel has died, surgery may be needed to remove it. The child may temporarily need help breathing with a machine called a ventilator and may need medication and fluids given intravenously if shock develops. Later on, if narrowing of the intestines occurs, the child may need surgery to prevent or relieve intestinal obstruction. Nutrition given intravenously or additional surgery may be needed depending on how much bowel was removed.

NEPHRITIS

Nephritis is a kidney disease in which the kidneys become inflamed and fail to filter waste products from the child's bloodstream. Over time, continual inflammation of the tiny filters, called the glomeruli, inside the kidneys can cause serious kidney damage, including kidney failure (see KIDNEY FAILURE, ACUTE and KIDNEY FAILURE, CHRONIC). This disorder is most common in children between the ages of 2 and 12. It can follow an infection by streptococcal bacteria, especially of the throat or skin. When the child's body produces antibodies (infection-fighting substances) to destroy the bacteria, the antibodies also damage the glomeruli.

Other causes of nephritis include a rare disease known as HEMOLYTIC-UREMIC SYNDROME, which causes blood clots to form throughout the body and destroys red blood cells, and some AUTOIMMUNE DISORDERS, which cause the child's immune (disease-fighting) system to attack the body's own cells.

SIGNS AND SYMPTOMS Children with mild cases of nephritis may experience no symptoms. Those with severe cases caused by a bacterial infection begin having symptoms of nephritis 2 or 3 weeks after signs of a sore throat or skin infection appear. Symptoms of severe nephritis include nausea, appetite loss, decreased urination, and a general feeling of ill health. The urine may become smoky or slightly red from blood in the urine. Excess water and other fluids begin to build up in the child's body and can cause swelling around the eyes, the face, or the entire body. A child with nephritis may also have headaches, fever, vomiting, shortness of breath, and high blood pressure. The child may develop anemia and acute kidney failure.

DIAGNOSIS If your child has a mild case of nephritis that produces no symptoms, the only way your doctor will be able to detect it is through a urine test done for another reason. Symptoms of severe nephritis, especially after a sore throat or skin infection, need to be checked by a doctor right away. The doctor will order blood and urine tests and check your child's blood pressure. He or she may also recommend a *biopsy* of your child's kidney to confirm the diagnosis. The doctor will continue to test your child's urine, monitor his or her kidney function with blood tests, and check his or her blood pressure during the course of the illness.

TREATMENT About 90 percent of children who develop either mild or severe cases of nephritis recover spontaneously or with treatment in 6 to 8 weeks without further complications. While your child is recovering, he or she should rest in bed until the symptoms disappear. Lying down helps blood flow to the child's kidneys, which helps speed recovery. Your child may also need a special diet to reduce fluid, salt, and protein intake. If your child still has signs of infection, the doctor may prescribe antibiotics or other medication to increase your child's output of urine. If your child's condition worsens, the doctor will probably hospitalize him or her to treat potential kidney failure and high blood pressure.

NEPHROSIS

Nephrosis, or nephrotic syndrome, is a rare kidney disorder in which the tiny filters (glomeruli) in a child's kidneys are damaged, causing protein to leak out of the child's blood into the urine. Fluid in the blood vessels leaks into the child's body tissues, giving the child a puffy appearance. This condition occurs most often in children between the ages of 1 and 6, especially those between 2 and 3 years of age. It affects boys more often than girls.

SIGNS AND SYMPTOMS At first, the child's eyes become puffy as fluid fills the tissues; then the child's ankles and legs swell up. In time, the skin over the child's entire body starts to look puffy. The child's abdomen swells as fluid accumulates. A boy's scrotum can also become swollen. The child urinates less than normal and may also look sick, feel tired, and become irritable.

DIAGNOSIS AND TREATMENT If your child begins retaining fluid, take him or her to the doctor. The doctor will order urine and blood tests to diagnose nephrosis and may recommend a *biopsy* of your child's kidneys to find out the cause. Your child will probably be placed in the hospital for treatment with medication and a special diet. The usual medications prescribed are *corticosteroids* to treat the damage to the glomeruli and diuretics to help your child eliminate excess fluids through urination. Your child may have to stay in the hospital for about 2 weeks until the symptoms clear up.

When your child comes home, make sure he or she continues to take the prescribed medication and follows his or her special diet. With treatment, many children recover completely while others have recurrent episodes over several weeks or months. In rare cases, the episodes continue. Each new episode requires treatment. If your child develops a fever (a sign of infection), notify the doctor, because children with active nephrosis are at risk of serious infection.

NEURAL TUBE DEFECTS

A neural tube defect is a BIRTH DEFECT in which a baby is born with a malformation of the brain, spinal cord, or spinal column. Neural tube defects range from ANENCEPHALY, in which the child is born with incomplete development or absence of a brain, to SPINA BIFIDA, in which part of the child's spinal cord and meninges (thin membranes that surround the brain and spinal cord) are exposed or visible under a thin layer of skin. Neural tube defects have been linked to a deficiency of folic acid in the mother before and during pregnancy; excessive body heat, as from a high fever, in the mother during pregnancy; and a family history of the disorder.

SIGNS AND SYMPTOMS Infants born without a fully developed brain have malformed faces and skulls at birth and cannot function. Protrusion of the spinal cord and meninges commonly causes nerve damage at the site of the defect and below. Walking and bladder and bowel control are usually affected. The infant may show poor reflexes and not respond to touch or pain.

DIAGNOSIS Elevated levels of a protein called alpha-fetoprotein in the mother's blood or amniotic fluid (the fluid that surrounds a fetus in the uterus) should alert the doctor to the possibility of a neural tube defect. An *ultrasound* of the fetus

Folic acid helps prevent birth defects

Women who are planning to get pregnant need to consume 400 micrograms (0.4 milligrams) of the B vitamin folic acid (also known as folate) every day. Folic acid prevents neural tube birth defects, such as anencephaly and spina bifida, that can occur during the first months of pregnancy—so early that a woman may not even know she is pregnant. Folic acid is found in spinach and other dark green leafy vegetables, orange juice, fruits, dried beans and peas, and liver. To ensure that you get enough folic acid every day, you can also take a supplement of 400 micrograms of this important vitamin. Most doctors agree that all women of childbearing age should double their current intake of folic acid—even if they are not planning a pregnancy—to reduce the risk of birth defects in case an unplanned pregnancy occurs.

may detect the type of defect and its severity. After your baby is born, the doctor will be able to see the defect during a physical examination.

TREATMENT Treatment for a neural tube defect depends on the type of defect and its severity. You should seek genetic counseling (see page 497) to understand your risks of having another child with this birth defect and to find out how to prevent it in future pregnancies.

NEUROBLASTOMA

Neuroblastoma is a cancer found in the nerve cells that make up the autonomic nervous system, which regulates involuntary body functions, such as digestion, and in the adrenal glands, located just above the kidneys. In this form of cancer, immature nerve cells known as neuroblasts multiply uncontrollably and form a tumor.

Most neuroblastoma tumors occur in children under the age of 10, and especially in very young children under 2. The disease is slightly more common in boys than in girls. Neuroblastoma most often begins in the adrenal glands and then may spread quickly to the child's lymph nodes, lungs, liver, brain, bones, and bone marrow.

Doctors do not know what causes this cancer. When it occurs in newborns and infants, it sometimes disappears spontaneously without treatment.

SIGNS AND SYMPTOMS The most common initial sign of neuroblastoma is swelling in your child's abdomen, where the adrenal glands are located. You or your doctor may be able to feel a lump or mass in your child's abdomen. Your child may become extremely tired and cranky, have no appetite, lose weight, and look pale. His or her eyes may look swollen and dark circles can develop under the eyes. Your child may also have a fever, diarrhea, and, in some cases, high blood pressure and flushed skin. As the disease progresses, your child may develop masses in his or her neck. A tumor in your child's spine may cause loss of movement in his or her arms and legs and loss of bladder control.

DIAGNOSIS Call the doctor right away if your child shows any of the symptoms of neuroblastoma. The chances that your child will survive this disease are better with early treatment, especially if your child is a newborn or infant.

Your child's doctor will examine your child and, if he or she suspects neuroblastoma, will refer your child to a doctor who specializes in cancer treatment (oncologist). The specialist will order *computed tomography*, *ultrasounds*, and *radionuclide scans* to find out the extent of the cancer. The doctor will probably do blood and urine tests and a *biopsy* of your child's bone marrow or of the tumor to confirm the diagnosis.

TREATMENT If your child's tumor is in the early stages of development, it may be possible to remove it surgically. Your child may also receive radiation after surgery to kill any remaining cancer cells. Additional surgery may be needed later if the cancer surgeon was not able to remove the entire tumor.

In some cases, your child may be given *chemotherapy* before surgery to shrink the tumor. He or she might also receive chemotherapy in combination with surgery and radiation.

Your child's outlook depends on how far the disease has progressed and how severe it was before he or she received treatment. Children under 1 year of age have a better chance of long-term survival than older children with more widespread disease.

NEUROFIBROMATOSIS

Neurofibromatosis is a GENETIC DISORDER that causes tumors (abnormal masses) to grow along the nerves, including the nerves in the brain. Tumors can also appear beneath the skin and in a child's bones. The disorder is the result of a single defective gene that may be inherited or may become abnormal through a gene mutation (a sudden change in the gene). Most of the tumors that grow throughout a child's body are not cancerous, but occasionally a cancerous tumor of the brain or spinal cord does develop.

There are two types of neurofibromatosis, type 1 and type 2. Neurofibromatosis type 1 (NF-1) is one of the most common genetic disorders in children, affecting one in 4,000 babies in the United States. From 50 to 70 percent of new cases of NF-1 are inherited from a parent, and the rest are caused by a gene mutation. Neurofibromatosis type 2 (NF-2) is much more rare than NF-1 and causes tumors to grow around the nerves for hearing on both sides of the brain. In some cases, these tumors can cause brain damage and threaten the child's life. Tumors can also occur elsewhere in the brain.

SIGNS AND SYMPTOMS Most children with NF-1 have only mild symptoms of the disease and live normal lives, but others may have very serious symptoms. The most common sign of NF-1 is the appearance of flat, light-brown spots on the child's skin, called café au lait (French for "coffee with milk") spots. These spots can appear at birth or in early infancy. Children with NF-1 typically have six or more of these spots on their bodies, each measuring more than ⅕ of an inch. By puberty, the skin spots begin to grow to about ½ inch in diameter. Tumors begin to grow around the nerves in the child's body during adolescence and can be seen as small lumps or bumps under the skin.

A child with NF-1 may also have freckles in his or her armpits and groin area, abnormal tissue in the iris (the colored part of the eye), poor vision because of tumors growing on the nerves around the eyes, and deformed spinal or leg bones. Some children with NF-1 also have learning disabilities or develop a SEIZURE DISORDER.

A child with NF-2 experiences progressive HEARING LOSS beginning in adolescence because tumors grow around the nerves for hearing. He or she may also have tinnitus (a ringing in the ears) and problems with balance. Skin growths and thickening of the lens in the eyes can also occur, causing VISION PROBLEMS. Tumors in the child's head can cause HEADACHES, numbness, and pain in the face. In extreme cases, an affected child may die of BRAIN TUMORS.

DIAGNOSIS If the doctor knows that either parent or another family member has neurofibromatosis, he or she can screen for the disorder in the fetus before birth through genetic testing (see page 498). To diagnose the disorder in a child who develops the symptoms of either type of neurofibromatosis after birth, the doctor will probably order X-rays, an eye examination, vision and hearing studies, *magnetic resonance imaging,* or *computed tomography* of the brain. The results of these tests, combined with laboratory tests and a knowledge of the child's family history, will confirm the diagnosis of neurofibromatosis.

TREATMENT Your child should get regular checkups after the first signs of neurofibromatosis so his or her doctor can monitor its progression and treat any new symptoms. If your child has disfiguring or painful tumors under the skin, he or she may need surgery to remove them, although the tumors may grow back. Tumors that affect your child's hearing or eyesight may also require surgery to preserve hearing and vision.

Your child's doctor can treat bone deformities, such as SCOLIOSIS, with surgery, a brace, or both. If your child's brain or spinal cord tumors are cancerous, he or she may need *radiation* and *chemotherapy* in addition to surgery. You and your child should receive genetic counseling (see page 497) to learn the risk of passing the disorder on to future children.

Newborn infections

See Infections in newborns

Nosebleed

Nosebleeds–bleeding from one or both nostrils–are common in childhood, especially among children between the ages of 2 and 10 years, because the lining of a child's nose contains a rich supply of tiny blood vessels that are easily injured. The most likely causes of nosebleeds in children are dryness in the nose from dry indoor heat in the winter and nose picking. Children tend to pick their noses more often when they feel dry, crusty matter inside. Other causes of nosebleeds include a blow or injury to the nose, colds, ALLERGIES, irritation from an object stuck inside the nose, or the use of cocaine by an adolescent. In rare cases, frequent nosebleeds may signal a BLEEDING DISORDER, tumor in the nose, or LEUKEMIA.

Signs and symptoms A nosebleed is usually a minor problem that clears up in a few minutes. The child's nose starts bleeding, often from one nostril only. The bleeding usually comes from the front of the nostril and lasts 5 or 10 minutes. If the blood goes down your child's throat, he or she may vomit and feel sick to the stomach.

Diagnosis and treatment If your child has a minor nosebleed, you can treat it at home with a little first aid. Have your child sit straight up, bend his or her head forward (not back) to keep the blood from going down the throat, pinch the sides of his or her nose together, and breathe through the mouth. Your child will need to keep his or her nostrils pinched shut for about 15 minutes. Then you can apply an ice pack to the nose. If your child feels blood running down his or her throat, have him or her spit it out. Tell your child not to blow his or her nose for about 24 hours to avoid irritating the lining of the nose.

If the bleeding does not stop when your child lets go of his or her nostrils, call the doctor for further advice. Always take your child to the doctor if the bleeding was caused by an injury, or if your child gets dizzy while having a nosebleed or has frequent nosebleeds. The doctor may have to place gauze inside your child's nostrils to stop the bleeding or may cauterize (burn) the injured blood vessels in your child's nose with a special chemical or device to stop the bleeding.

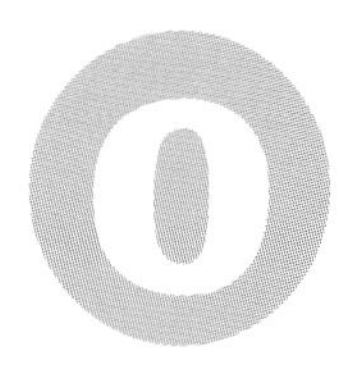

Obesity

Obesity is a condition in which a child has an excessive amount of body fat and weighs 20 percent or more over the ideal body weight for his or her height and sex. About 5 to 10 percent of children in the United States under age 12 are obese. Another 15 percent of American adolescents are obese. Fully 80 percent of obese teenagers are likely to become obese adults. Obese children and teens are at greater risk than other children of having HIGH BLOOD PRESSURE and high blood cholesterol levels (see CHOLESTEROL

ABNORMALITIES). If they continue to be obese into adulthood, they are at greater risk of developing certain diseases—such as heart disease, high blood pressure, diabetes, gallbladder disease, kidney disease, arthritis, and some types of cancer (see page 444)—at a younger age than other adults.

There are a variety of possible causes for obesity in children. Some underlying disorders can cause obesity, including HYPOTHYROIDISM and CUSHING'S SYNDROME. But in most instances, children simply eat too much and do not get enough exercise. Their bodies don't need all of the calories they take in, and they do not burn off the excess calories with physical activity. Many children inherit a predisposition to obesity. If a child has one obese parent, he or she has a 40 percent chance of being obese. If the child has two obese parents, he or she has a 70 to 80 percent chance of being obese.

Social and psychological disorders or problems, such as DEPRESSION, low self-esteem, child abuse (see page 323), and family or relationship trouble can cause a child to overeat and become obese. Obese children who are teased by others about their weight may eat for comfort, causing them to overeat even more.

DIAGNOSIS Your child's doctor or a trained nutritionist can measure excess body fat. He or she may measure the thickness of the folds of skin of the triceps area (the back portion of the upper arm). If the skin fold is in the top 15 percent of standard measurements for the child's age and sex, he or she is considered obese. The doctor will also take your child's weight and compare it to standard weight charts and assess your child's height and growth rate (see page 238).

The doctor will take blood and urine samples to determine your child's nutritional status and possible causes of your child's obesity. He or she may also order X-rays of your child's bones to rule out hormonal or GENETIC DISORDERS. You should tell the doctor about your child's eating habits, levels of physical activity, and emotional state and about any family history of obesity or eating disorders.

TREATMENT Doctors don't usually give children drugs to treat their obesity and you should not give your child over-the-counter diet pills to help decrease his or her appetite. The best treatment methods emphasize changes in your child's diet and physical activity. Your child's doctor may refer you to a dietitian or nutritionist who will develop a healthful eating plan that will reduce your child's total calorie intake and the amount of fat he or she consumes. At the same time, the diet will provide the right balance of calories, fat, protein, vitamins, and minerals for proper growth.

Your child's doctor will also recommend that your child exercise regularly to burn off excess calories. You can help by encouraging activities that he or she really enjoys and by involving the whole family in healthy physical activities—such as walking, bike riding, or swimming. Give your child healthy foods and snacks, keep a record of your child's food intake, make sure he or she avoids eating high-fat snacks, and reward your child for sticking to his or her diet. Set realistic goals for your child's weight loss. Try to deter-

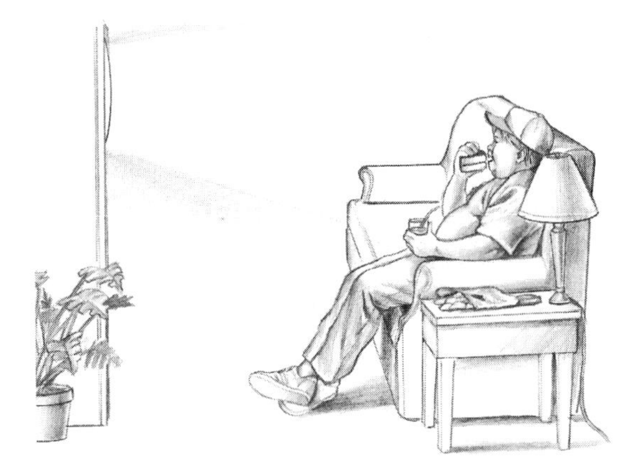

Unhealthy eating habits
Children are naturally attracted to sweet, high-fat foods, but it's important to provide healthful snacks, such as cut-up vegetables or pretzels with low-fat dip, especially if your child is overweight. Encourage physical activity—not TV watching—during your child's leisure time.

mine what stresses cause your child to overeat and teach your child to cope with stress in ways other than eating. Your child will need to change his or her behavior for life; otherwise, his or her chances of successfully losing excess fat and weight, and keeping them off, are low.

Obsessive-compulsive disorder

Obsessive-compulsive disorder is an emotional disorder in which a child has persistent or recurrent thoughts that lead to repeated behavior that the child cannot resist. The obsessive thoughts and compulsive behavior can be so severe they interfere with normal activities. At one time or another, most children display some obsessive-compulsive behaviors such as bedtime rituals or wanting things done in a certain way as a normal part of growing up. You don't need to be concerned unless these behaviors interfere with normal living, consume excessive time, and cause anxiety in your child. Obsessive-compulsive disorder is linked to some other disorders, such as the eating disorder ANOREXIA NERVOSA, the nervous system disorder TOURETTE'S SYNDROME, and epilepsy (see SEIZURE DISORDERS). Obsessive-compulsive disorder most commonly begins in adolescence.

Signs and symptoms Some children have obsessive thoughts only and others have compulsive behaviors only, but most often the two are linked. The obsessive thoughts, ideas, or images enter a child's mind involuntarily and become intrusive. The child may be aware that the thoughts do not make much sense, but he or she is unable to ignore them. Some common obsessive thoughts have to do with cleanliness, fear that something terrible will happen, sex, and religion. Along with the obsessive thoughts, the child may also feel disgust, doubt, fear, and DEPRESSION.

In response to these thoughts, the child begins to perform specific repetitive behaviors. For example, if a child is obsessed about germs and cleanliness, he or she will wash his or her hands ritualistically—many more times than they need to be. The hand washing itself may relieve the child's anxiety temporarily, but the obsessive thoughts and anxiety return and the child feels he or she has to perform the behavior again.

Many children with obsessive-compulsive disorder exhibit checking behavior, a response to obsessive thoughts about something terrible happening. The child may repeatedly check locks at bedtime to make sure he or she is safe.

Children may display more than one obsessive thought or compulsive behavior at a time. Other common compulsive behaviors include repeated touching, counting, arranging things in an orderly fashion, hoarding, and praying.

Diagnosis and treatment If you see symptoms of obsessive-compulsive disorder in your child or he or she tells you about these symptoms, take him or her to the doctor for an evaluation. The doctor will give your child a full physical

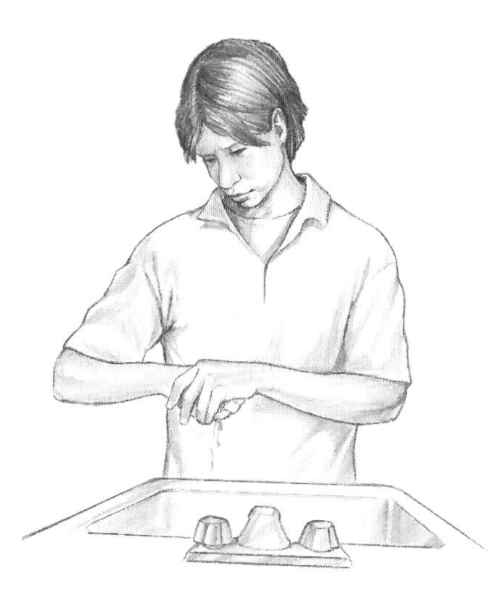

Compulsive hand washing

One of the most common obsessive-compulsive behaviors that children exhibit is repeated hand washing. The child can't stop thinking about germs or about the need for cleanliness. The hand washing makes the child feel better for a while, but then the obsessive fear returns and he or she feels compelled to repeat the hand washing.

examination to rule out other disorders. He or she may also refer your child to a psychiatrist or psychologist for a complete evaluation. Your child may need psychotherapy to change his or her behavior. Your child's doctor or psychiatrist may also prescribe drugs to relieve your child's anxiety or depression. Most children respond well to behavioral therapy with or without drugs. Your child may have relapses after the initial treatment, but the condition can be brought under control again so that your child can lead a normal life.

ORCHITIS

Orchitis is the inflammation of one or both testicles. It usually follows inflammation of one of the tubes that carries sperm from the testicles and can occur after a child has had mumps, TUBERCULOSIS, or SYPHILIS. From 25 to 30 percent of boys who get mumps after puberty develop orchitis.

SIGNS AND SYMPTOMS One or both of the boy's testicles becomes enlarged and painful. The skin of the scrotum (the pouch that holds the testicles) may look red and the scrotum may be swollen. The tube that carries sperm from the testicles may be tender and swollen as well. The boy may have a fever as high as 104°F. If orchitis is caused by mumps, symptoms appear about 3 or 4 days after the child's salivary glands in the neck become swollen (a sign of mumps). In severe cases when the orchitis follows mumps, a boy may lose his ability to generate sperm in the affected testicle. If both testicles are affected, the boy can become permanently infertile. An affected testicle sometimes becomes smaller than normal after infection.

DIAGNOSIS The doctor will order blood and urine tests to confirm a diagnosis based on the physical signs. He or she may also order an *ultrasound* or a *radionuclide scan* of the boy's testicles to rule out twisting of the testicle (see page 644).

TREATMENT The doctor will prescribe antibiotics to treat infections caused by bacteria and painkillers to relieve the boy's discomfort. He or she may also prescribe *corticosteroids.* Keep your child in bed until the symptoms begin to subside in 3 to 7 days. Your son should support his scrotum with an athletic supporter or place a towel underneath his scrotum until he feels better. An ice pack may help reduce the swelling and pain.

OSGOOD-SCHLATTER DISEASE

Osgood-Schlatter disease is an inflammation in the bone called the tibia in a child's shin, just below the knee, in a place known as the tibial tuberosity. It occurs most often in physically active boys between the ages of 9 and 14 years; girls sometimes also develop the disorder. The disorder arises from repeated stress or pulling on the thigh muscle and tendon (strong, fibrous tissue) that are attached to the tuberosity.

SIGNS AND SYMPTOMS The condition causes pain, swelling, and tenderness in the bone below the child's knee. The tibial tuberosity becomes more prominent in the affected leg. The child may also have pain above the knee. The pain becomes worse when the child is physically active.

DIAGNOSIS AND TREATMENT The doctor will diagnose this disorder from your description of the symptoms and from a physical examination. He or she may also order X-rays to rule out other possible causes of your child's symptoms. The pain, swelling, and tenderness will usually subside with rest and restricted activity. The doctor may prescribe a pain reliever that also fights inflammation, such as ibuprofen. He or she may also put a temporary brace on your child's knee to support and immobilize it. Your child might need to do special exercises to strengthen the muscles around the knee. He or she will outgrow the condition by late adolescence.

Osteogenic sarcoma

Osteogenic sarcoma, osteosarcoma, or bone cancer is a rare form of cancer that begins in bone. Cancers that spread to bone from other areas in the body are not considered bone cancer. Osteogenic sarcoma occurs most frequently in children over 10 years old, especially in teenagers during the peak years of growth. Boys get the disease more often that girls. In children, it most commonly occurs around the knee, at the ends of the long bones of the legs, where new bone is formed as the child grows. It can also occur in the upper arms or in any other bones in a child's body.

Cancer cells from the tumor that initially formed in a bone can enter the child's bloodstream through bone marrow and spread to other parts of the child's body, especially to the child's lungs.

Signs and symptoms Children with bone cancer have pain in the affected bone, often accompanied by swelling around the bone. Your child may have a slightly tender lump on the bone that you can feel through the skin. If your child develops a lump, along with pain and swelling in one of his or her bones, he or she needs to be seen by a doctor. Some children have trouble using the affected limb. Your child's bone may become weakened and break. Some children also have fever and weight loss.

Diagnosis To make a proper diagnosis, your child's doctor will order X-rays of the bone to show the size, location, and shape of the tumor. He or she will probably refer your child to a surgeon for a *biopsy*. Your child's doctor will probably also order a *radionuclide scan* of the bone (see illustration), *computed tomography*, or *magnetic resonance imaging* to find out how far the cancer has spread.

Treatment Initially, your child will receive *chemotherapy* for several months to destroy the cancer cells in the affected bone. Then a cancer surgeon will perform surgery to determine how much of the tumor has been destroyed by the chemotherapy and to remove the remaining cancer. The surgeon will try to keep your child's limb intact but, if the tumor is large and has spread, he or she may have to amputate the limb. Otherwise, the surgeon may replace the bone removed during surgery with a metal device that lengthens the bone as it heals.

If your child loses his or her arm or leg during surgery, he or she will be fitted with an artificial

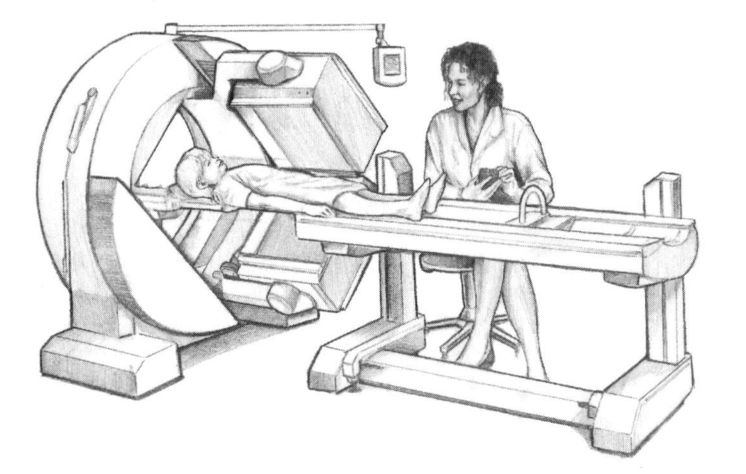

How a radionuclide bone scan works

One of the tests that a cancer specialist uses to determine the extent of osteogenic sarcoma is a radionuclide bone scan. Before the scan, the child receives an injection of a radioactive chemical, which is absorbed by the child's bones. A special device called a gamma camera detects the amount of radiation emitted by the bone. Cancer cells show up as hot spots on the scans. The radiation levels of the chemicals used in the injection are low and are harmless to the child.

limb known as a prosthesis. A physical therapist will teach your child how to use the artificial limb and a nurse will educate you and your child about the care and function of your child's stump and prosthesis.

Several months of chemotherapy will follow the surgery to destroy any cells that have spread to other parts of your child's body. Cancer specialists sometimes also use *radiation* therapy to treat this form of cancer. If treated early, your child's bone cancer may go into remission (see page 445). It is important for you to take your child in for periodic checkups after treatment, even if the cancer has gone into remission, because the cancer could recur. If the cancer has spread to other parts of your child's body, it will require additional surgery or other cancer treatment.

OSTEOMYELITIS

Osteomyelitis is an infection of the bones and bone marrow, the soft, fatty tissue inside bone cavities that is responsible for blood cell formation. The infection occurs most commonly in children 5 to 14 years old and usually affects the arm or leg bones. The infection is usually caused by bacteria, although in rare cases it can be caused by a fungus. The bacteria can enter the bone directly through a wound or burn, or from a bacterial infection of the skin called cellulitis. The infection can also spread to the bone through the bloodstream. In infants and young toddlers who have septic arthritis (see ARTHRITIS, SEPTIC), it can spread to the bone from the infected joints.

SIGNS AND SYMPTOMS The child develops pain, swelling, and tenderness around the infected bone. The skin covering the bone may be red and warm. Nearby joints, such as a knee or elbow, may also become red, swollen, and painful. An infant or child often does not want to move the affected limb or may scream in pain when moving the limb. The child may limp or refuse to walk. He or she may also have a fever and a general feeling of ill health. If the infection is not treated promptly or does not respond to treatment, osteomyelitis can last for years. In chronic osteomyelitis, pus sometimes drains through the skin around the infected bone.

DIAGNOSIS AND TREATMENT Your child's doctor will order blood tests to identify the bacteria and X-rays or a bone scan to confirm the diagnosis. He or she may also take a sample of bone–using a needle or through a surgical procedure–to identify the bacteria. The doctor will treat the infection with high doses of antibiotics. Your child may need to be hospitalized so he or she can initially receive the antibiotics *intravenously*. After treatment in the hospital, your child will be treated as an *outpatient*, getting the antibiotics either orally, intravenously, or by injection into a muscle, for 3 to 6 weeks, depending on the severity and location of the infection.

If your child develops chronic osteomyelitis, he or she may need surgery to remove dead bone tissue and to receive a bone graft that would fill in the area where the tissue was removed. Doctors give antibiotics for 3 weeks or more after surgery. In very rare cases, amputation of the infected limb is necessary if surgery has not been effective.

With successful early treatment, your child's chances of recovery are good, but if treatment is delayed or the osteomyelitis becomes chronic, the outlook is not as promising.

OVARIAN TUMORS AND CYSTS

Ovarian tumors are abnormal growths of new tissue in an ovary. Ovarian tumors can be malignant (growing uncontrollably, invading surrounding tissue and organs; see CANCER) or benign (growing slowly without spreading to other organs). Ovarian cysts are abnormal growths filled with fluid or semisolid material in an ovary. Most ovarian cysts are benign and usually disappear on their own without treatment in a month or two.

Ovarian tumors are relatively rare in children and adolescents, while ovarian cysts are somewhat common. About two thirds of growths diagnosed in adolescent girls as ovarian tumors may actually be ovarian cysts. Doctors do not know what causes ovarian tumors, but they think that ovarian cysts develop as a normal part of the menstrual cycle in response to changes in hormone levels.

SIGNS AND SYMPTOMS Ovarian tumors and cysts often cause no symptoms. When symptoms do occur, they may begin with discomfort in the lower abdomen, along with a bloated feeling and vague discomfort in the digestive tract. A tumor can cause a noticeable lump in the abdomen that may be tender to the touch. Other symptoms include pain during intercourse, cramping during menstruation or other MENSTRUAL DISORDERS, and breast tenderness. The girl may be nauseated, vomit, and either retain urine or urinate frequently. Some girls experience sharp pain in the abdomen, which can indicate that the tumor or cyst has twisted. Abnormal bleeding from the vagina may signal that a cyst has ruptured. In girls who have not yet gone through puberty or had their first period, an ovarian tumor or cyst can cause signs of precocious puberty (puberty before age 8), such as enlargement of the breasts, growth of pubic hair, and a white, sticky discharge from the vagina or vaginal bleeding.

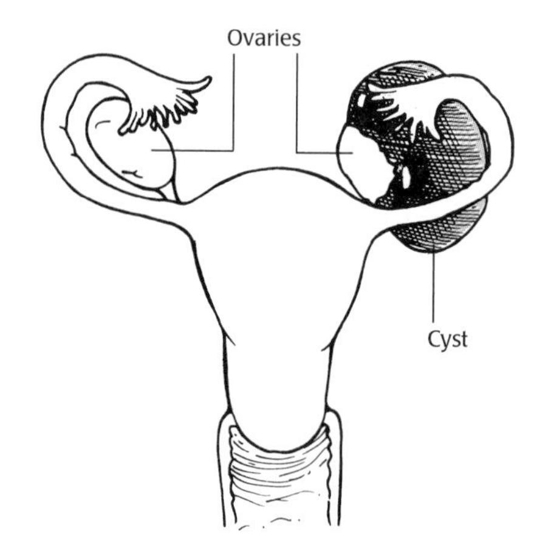

Ovarian cyst

One common type of ovarian cyst is known as a functional ovarian cyst, a sac filled with blood and fluid. A functional cyst does not indicate the presence of disease and usually disappears on its own without treatment. About 95 percent of ovarian cysts are functional.

DIAGNOSIS Your daughter's doctor may detect an ovarian tumor or cyst during a routine physical examination. If your daughter experiences sharp pain in her lower abdomen or any abnormal vaginal bleeding, notify the doctor immediately. Sharp pain in the abdomen could indicate that an ovarian cyst has twisted. Bleeding from the vagina could be caused by a ruptured cyst, which is a medical emergency.

Your child's doctor or a gynecologist (a doctor who specializes in disorders of the reproductive system of women) will do a pelvic exam (see page 255) and order blood tests and hormone-level tests. He or she may also do an *ultrasound* to look for the presence of a cyst. Laparoscopy (examination of the inside of the abdomen through a flexible viewing tube inserted into the abdomen) may be necessary to detect either tumors or cysts. The doctor may perform a laparotomy (exploratory abdominal surgery) to determine the size and type of tumor. Your daughter's doctor or gynecologist might also use other diagnostic tools, such as X-rays or *computed tomography*.

TREATMENT If the doctor suspects that your daughter has an ovarian cyst, he or she may not treat her because cysts often clear up on their own within about 2 months. The doctor may prescribe birth-control pills that contain a specific amount of hormones to establish a normal menstrual cycle and promote the natural disappearance of the cyst. If the cyst causes sharp pain or bleeding, or if it is unusually large, your daughter may need surgery to remove it. In extreme cases, a surgeon may also need to remove one or both ovaries and fallopian tubes.

If your daughter has an ovarian tumor, she will need surgery to remove the tumor and, most likely, the ovary. If the tumor is cancerous, she will probably also require *radiation* or *chemotherapy*, or both. Discuss the impact of treatment on your daughter's future reproductive ability with your daughter's doctor.

OVEREATING

Overeating is a disorder in which a child consistently consumes excessive amounts of food for psychological and emotional reasons. Such children equate food with comfort and emotional support. The disorder may begin in infancy if parents always feed their baby when the infant cries or is irritable instead of providing physical and emotional comfort. The child learns to want food at times of stress or when he or she is upset. Parents may reinforce this pattern throughout the child's life.

SIGNS AND SYMPTOMS Children who overeat are frequently overweight or obese (see OBESITY). They routinely overeat when they are depressed (see DEPRESSION), frustrated, having problems at home or at school, or upset with friends. In some cases, overeating may be the first sign of BULIMIA. Friends and peers may taunt these children because they are overweight, and the child may then overeat for comfort. Children may also overeat to please their parents if parents equate food with love and affection.

DIAGNOSIS AND TREATMENT Your child's doctor can determine if your child is overweight by comparing your child's weight with standard weight charts for age and sex (see page 239). To diagnose overeating, the doctor will ask about your child's eating habits, physical activity, emotional state, and any family history of eating disorders. He or she may refer your child to a mental health professional to identify the problems underlying your child's overeating. Behavior modification therapy has been very successful in treating overeating. Your child will be taught the right foods to eat and the right quantities. He or she will also need to exercise to lose weight. Provide a low-fat, low-calorie diet and keep high-fat snacks out of the house. Reward your child for sticking to his or her diet and exercise program with plenty of praise and affection—not with food. Try to involve the whole family in healthy activities, such as walking, bike riding, or swimming.

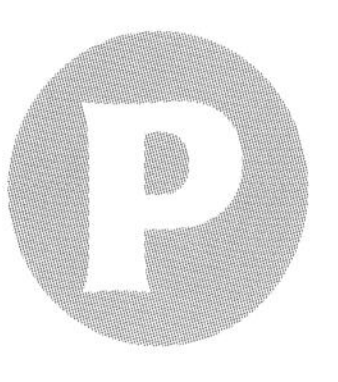

PATENT DUCTUS ARTERIOSUS

Patent ductus arteriosus is a heart defect (see HEART DISEASE, CONGENITAL) in which the blood vessel connecting the pulmonary artery (the artery that transports blood from the heart to the lungs) and the aorta (the main artery that transports blood from the heart to the body) remains open after birth. Because this vessel is open, or patent, some of the blood pumped from the left side of the newborn's heart goes to his or her lungs instead of to the rest of the body.

This vessel, known as the ductus arteriosus, is normally present in every fetus before birth. It permits blood to bypass the fetus's lungs while the fetus receives oxygen from the mother's placenta and umbilical cord. Shortly after birth, the channel normally closes so blood can go to the baby's lungs for oxygen and then return to the left side of the heart to be pumped to the rest of the body. If the channel fails to close, the newborn's heart pumps too much blood to the lungs, causing symptoms of congestive heart failure (see HEART FAILURE, CONGESTIVE). Patent ductus arteriosus occurs most often in babies born prematurely or in those who have breathing difficulties such as RESPIRATORY DISTRESS SYNDROME.

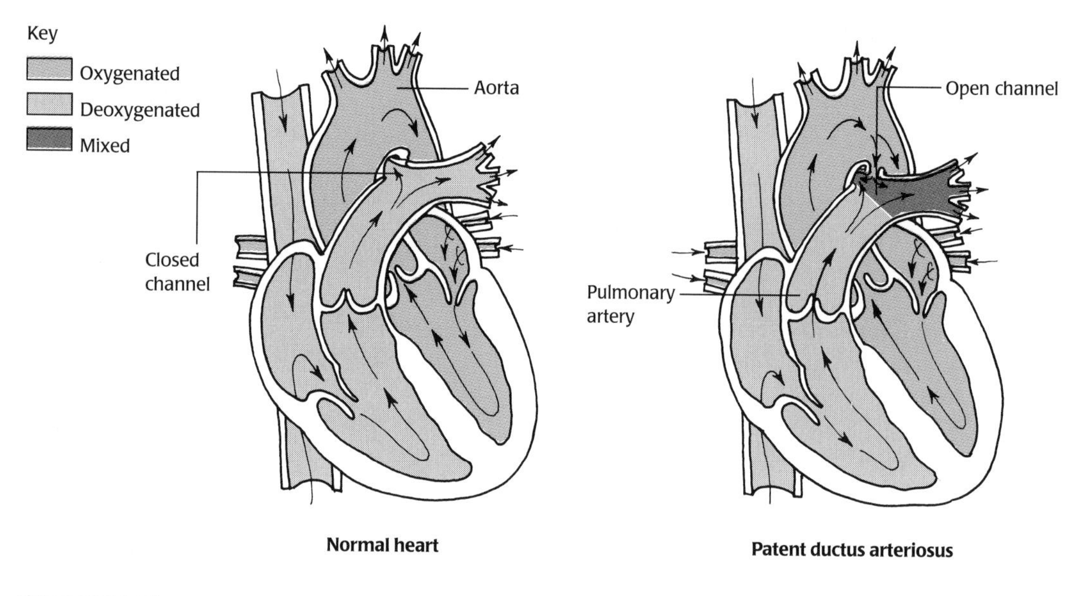

Open channel
Before birth, the heart has a special channel, known as the ductus arteriosus, that connects the pulmonary artery and the aorta. The channel allows blood to bypass the lungs because the fetus receives oxygen from the mother's placenta and umbilical cord. In a baby born with a normal heart (left), the channel closes shortly after birth so that the newborn's blood can travel to the lungs for oxygen. In a baby with patent (open) ductus arteriosus (right), the channel remains open. Oxygenated blood flows back to the baby's lungs and accumulates there, making it difficult for the lungs to function properly.

SIGNS AND SYMPTOMS Patent ductus arteriosus often causes only mild symptoms or none at all. In more severe cases, infants may have rapid breathing, shortness of breath, a HEART MURMUR, a very strong pulse, difficulty feeding, poor weight gain, frequent chest infections, and irritability. The symptoms get worse without treatment. Eventually, the child develops congestive heart failure.

DIAGNOSIS If your baby is born with patent ductus arteriosus, the doctor may be able to diagnosis this defect by listening for a heart murmur through a stethoscope. To confirm the diagnosis, the doctor will order additional tests, such as a chest X-ray, an *echocardiogram* (an *ultrasound* of the heart), or an *electrocardiogram* (an external monitor that records electrical activity in the heart). These tests are painless.

TREATMENT If your infant is born prematurely and has patent ductus arteriosus, the doctor will first try a medication known as indomethacin to try to close the channel. He or she will also administer drugs called diuretics to reduce the fluids in your child's body through increased urination and will place restrictions on the amount of fluids your baby gets so that excessive fluids do not build up.

If the treatment fails, if the infant is born at full term, or if symptoms occur in an older infant, the doctor will recommend surgery to correct the problem. A cardiac surgeon will perform the operation. He or she will tie off the open channel so the baby's blood begins circulating normally. The operation is usually quite effective and carries a low risk of complications. After surgery, your child should grow and develop normally.

PELVIC INFLAMMATORY DISEASE

Pelvic inflammatory disease (PID) is a bacterial infection affecting the internal organs of the female reproductive tract–the endometrium (lining of the uterus), the fallopian tubes (the tubes that transport eggs from the ovaries to the uterus), and the ovaries. PID most often results from infection with a sexually transmitted disease (STD), such as CHLAMYDIA or GONORRHEA, that spreads to the inner reproductive organs. Sexually active adolescent girls between the ages of 15 and 19 years are at high risk of developing PID because they often have multiple sexual partners and engage in sex without using a barrier contraceptive, such as a condom.

The cervix (the opening to the uterus) prevents most bacteria from spreading into the internal reproductive organs. But after sexual contact with an infected partner, the bacteria can easily spread beyond the cervix and into the internal organs. Sometimes the bacteria that are normally present in the vagina can spread to the internal organs, causing PID. The disease can also be caused by infections that occur after childbirth, a miscarriage, or an abortion, or by an intrauterine contraceptive device.

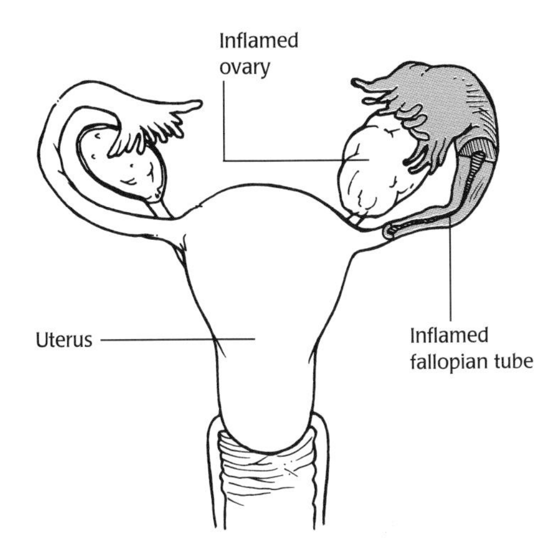

PID: A serious threat

When bacteria pass through the cervix (the narrow opening to the uterus) and into a girl's internal reproductive organs, they can cause pelvic inflammatory disease. The infection inflames the lining of the uterus, fallopian tubes, and ovaries, causing redness, pain, and swelling. The infection can permanently block the fallopian tubes, preventing fertilization (making it difficult or impossible for the girl to have children), or preventing a fertilized egg from reaching the uterus, which results in an ectopic pregnancy, in which the egg implants in the fallopian tube.

SIGNS AND SYMPTOMS Adolescent girls with PID often have tenderness or pain in the lower abdomen; a yellow or greenish, foul-smelling discharge from the vagina; and MENSTRUAL DISORDERS, such as periods that last an unusually long time or abdominal cramps in between periods. Other symptoms include chills, a high fever, vomiting, diarrhea, and a general feeling of ill health. Pain may occur during intercourse or immediately after menstruation. Some girls with PID have no symptoms.

If the infection is not treated right away, it can cause infertility (the inability to bear children), ectopic pregnancy (growth of a fertilized egg outside the uterus), an abscess (collection of pus) in the fallopian tubes or ovaries, and chronic pelvic pain.

DIAGNOSIS If your daughter has symptoms of PID, she needs to have the infection diagnosed and treated as quickly as possible. Your child's doctor or a gynecologist (a doctor who specializes in treating disorders of the female reproductive system) will do a thorough pelvic exam (see page 255) and order urine and blood tests, a pregnancy test, and *cultures* for gonorrhea and chlamydia. The doctor may also need to do a laparoscopy (examination of the inside of the abdomen through a viewing tube inserted into the abdomen) to look for abscesses in your daughter's internal reproductive organs. The doctor might also test your daughter for other STDs, such as SYPHILIS, HEPATITIS B, and the human immunodeficiency virus.

TREATMENT If your daughter has a mild infection, she may be treated as an *outpatient* with antibiotics that she must take by mouth or by injection for about 2 weeks. After the first examination, the doctor will want to see your daughter again in a few days to check her progress. She needs to take all of the antibiotics or the infection will not be cured and could get worse. You can expect to see a significant improvement in your daughter's health in a couple of days. In more complicated cases, she may need to be hospitalized for 2 to 4 days and given antibiotics *intravenously*, followed by antibiotics taken by mouth and close follow-up care. Recovery can take 3 to 5 days.

An abscess in the fallopian tubes or ovaries may require emergency surgery to remove the pus and possibly even to remove any damaged reproductive organs. Surgery may also be needed if drug therapy does not work. If the infection was caused by the use of an IUD, the doctor will remove it.

How to prevent pelvic inflammatory disease

Pelvic inflammatory disease (PID) can cause serious complications and can make it difficult for your daughter to have children of her own. You can help your daughter avoid getting this infection by making sure she knows how to prevent it. Stress these important preventive measures when you talk to your daughter about her sexuality:

- Abstain from having sex; this is the only complete protection. Sexual intercourse increases your risk for PID.
- Know the risks; it takes only one sexual encounter to get infected. The more partners you have, the greater your chances of getting PID and other sexually transmitted diseases (STDs).
- If you do have sex, always use a condom. Condoms help prevent the transmission of bacteria that can cause PID and STDs.
- Make sure your partner gets treated for infection. If you have been treated for PID, your sexual partner or partners should also be treated so that you do not become infected again.

If your daughter has PID, her sexual partner also needs to be notified and treated, or he could infect your daughter again. Talk to your daughter about her sexual activity and teach her how to prevent infection from STDs.

Penis disorders

See Balanitis; Hypospadias; Phimosis

Periventricular hemorrhage

See Intraventricular and periventricular hemorrhage

Periventricular leukomalacia

Periventricular leukomalacia is a brain disease, usually found in premature infants, in which the brain tissue lining the fluid-filled spaces, called the ventricles, is damaged. It occurs when fluid treatment, given *intravenously* for a life-threatening condition, causes the vessels around the ventricles to leak or rupture, causing brain injury. Periventricular leukomalacia has been linked to INTRAVENTRICULAR AND PERIVENTRICULAR HEMORRHAGE.

Signs and symptoms There are usually no signs or symptoms of periventricular leukomalacia in the newborn, but affected babies are vulnerable to developing SEIZURE DISORDERS and intellectual and motor (movement) problems (see CEREBRAL PALSY AND DEVELOPMENTAL DELAY). The child may be slow to or unable to sit, crawl, stand, or walk. He or she develops tight or stiff leg muscles and holds the legs straight most of the time. At 3 or 4 months of age, the infant may still not respond to a voice. At 8 or 9 months, he or she may not yet be making a variety of sounds. At the age of 1 year, the child may not speak or be able to understand speech. The child may also have HEARING LOSS and VISION PROBLEMS. LEARNING DISABILITIES, a short attention span, behavior problems, and poor hand-eye coordination often appear when the child enters school.

DIAGNOSIS AND TREATMENT Because there are usually no symptoms at birth, a premature infant needs to have an *ultrasound* of the head to detect this disease. If something looks suspicious on the first ultrasound, the doctor will do a series of ultrasounds. *Computed tomography* or *magnetic resonance imaging* of the head may be done to determine the severity of the disease. If the child develops a seizure, an electroencephalogram will be done to measure electrical activity in the brain. There is no treatment for periventricular leukomalacia. If your infant has the disease, he or she will need frequent checkups as he or she develops. The doctor will treat your child's symptoms as they occur. Your child may need therapy for physical, mental, and behavioral problems; special education; and medication to control seizures.

PERTUSSIS

See Whooping cough

PHENYLKETONURIA

See PKU

PHIMOSIS

Phimosis is a disorder in which the foreskin of the penis is so tight that it cannot be drawn back over the head of the penis comfortably. Phimosis usually occurs in uncircumcised boys, but it can also affect circumcised boys if an excessive amount of skin is left after circumcision.

SIGNS AND SYMPTOMS Some phimosis is normal in uncircumcised boys under 3 years of age, but it usually goes away on its own as the child grows older. If the problem persists, the boy may have difficulty urinating and the foreskin may balloon out during urination. The foreskin can also become swollen, red, and tender. Adolescent boys can experience extreme pain during an erection or may not be able to get an erection. Phimosis makes it difficult for a boy to clean the head of his penis, setting the stage for an infection called BALANITIS. In some cases, the child's foreskin can be drawn back over the head of the penis but then cannot be returned to its normal position. A tight, painful ring of skin then forms under the head.

DIAGNOSIS AND TREATMENT If your son is more than 3 years old and still has a tight foreskin, he may be able to stretch the skin gradually by pulling it gently, using soap and water, in the shower or bath. He should be careful not to force the skin or he could injure it. The stretching process can take several weeks. If this treatment at home does not work, take your son to the doctor. The doctor might recommend circumcision (see page 32) to remove the foreskin. This procedure is relatively minor and your son could return home the same day.

PICA

Pica is an eating disorder in which a child eats nonfood substances, such as dirt, wood, clay, paint chips, string, plaster, charcoal, animal feces, or hair. The abnormal eating behavior may go on for a month or more. About 10 to 20 percent of children, especially hyperactive children, under 6 years old exhibit pica. Pica is most common—and completely normal—in children under 2 years old. Most children outgrow the habit, but a small number continue the behavior into adulthood.

Pica is more common among children living in poverty and those deprived of emotional support and intellectual stimulation. It has been linked to MENTAL RETARDATION and infantile AUTISM, and it occurs more frequently in children who have behavior disorders, such as ATTENTION DISORDERS or sensory impairment such as BLINDNESS. Iron-deficiency anemia (see ANEMIA, IRON-DEFICIENCY) and lead poisoning commonly accompany pica.

SIGNS AND SYMPTOMS Most children put things into their mouths, but children who have pica routinely eat nonfood items. These substances–especially those containing lead, which can be ingested in chips of lead-based paint or soil–can endanger a child's health. If your child has LEAD POISONING, he or she may have severe stomach pain, diarrhea, vomiting, weakness or paralysis in his or her arms and legs, and possibly seizures. Other nonfood substances can cause a child to develop abdominal pain and vomit. INTESTINAL OBSTRUCTION can also result from pica.

DIAGNOSIS AND TREATMENT If your child starts eating nonnutritious substances, take the child to the doctor. He or she will test your child for lead poisoning and iron-deficiency anemia. The doctor may give you information about using syrup of ipecac in case you need to induce vomiting and the telephone number of a hotline in case of poisoning. The doctor will ask about your child's home environment, emotional state, and intellectual development. He or she will try to assess not only your child's needs but the changes your family may need to make to prevent your child from ingesting nonfood substances. The doctor may involve a social worker and mental health specialist in the care of your child and the assessment of your family's needs. Counseling can help your child change his or her behavior. You can help your child by making sure his or her home environment is free of dangerous substances (see page 76). Be sure to keep unsafe substances, especially medications, in childproof containers and out of reach (see page 302). Praise and reward your child for changing his or her behavior.

PIGEON TOE

Pigeon toe is a minor foot deformity in which a child's feet and toes point inward. The problem can be caused by an abnormal rotation or turning in of the bones in the child's legs, ankles, or feet. Pigeon toe is extremely common among infants and toddlers. A fetus's feet or legs can be forced into an abnormal position for a long period before birth. Toddlers often develop pigeon toe as a normal part of the development of their thighbones. A child's feet and toes usually straighten out without treatment by the time the child reaches the age of 5 or 6 years.

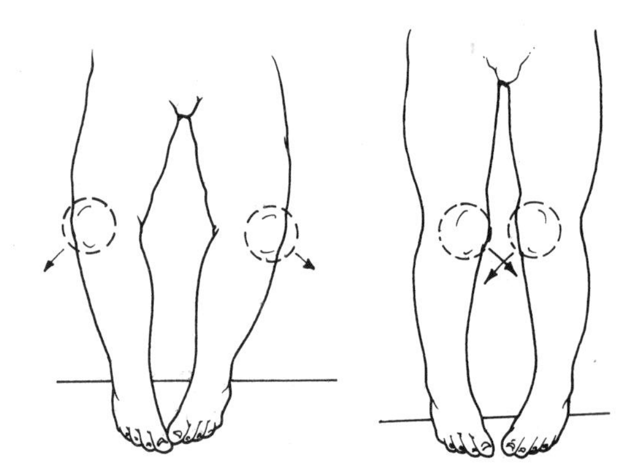

Two types of pigeon toe

Pigeon toe is caused by the rotation of bones in a child's legs. Two common types are known as internal tibial torsion and femoral anteversion. Internal tibial torsion (left) refers to the twisting out of a child's shinbone (tibia). The twisting causes the child's toes to turn in. Parents often notice this condition about the time a child begins to walk. It usually straightens out in the baby's first year of life. Femoral anteversion (right) is the twisting inward of a child's thighbone (femur). This condition usually occurs in children between the ages of 2 and 4 years. The child's toes usually straighten out by the time he or she is 8 years old.

DIAGNOSIS AND TREATMENT If your child has pigeon toe, you will be able to recognize the problem on your own. The doctor will determine the cause of your child's pigeon toe by watching him or her stand and walk. The doctor may also need to take X-rays to check for other possible bone problems. If your child has only a mild turning in of the toes, he or she may not need any treatment at all, although the doctor may recommend exercises to help strengthen the leg muscles and straighten your child's feet. For a more severe case of pigeon toe, the doctor will probably prescribe special shoes that your child will need to wear at night. In some cases, putting the limb in a cast is required, beginning at about 6 months of age and lasting until your child starts to walk. In rare cases, the doctor may recommend surgery to reposition the affected bones, but surgery is usually not necessary unless other bone problems exist.

PINWORMS

Pinworms are tiny worms that live in a child's intestines. Pinworm eggs spread from child to child on contaminated fingers, shared toys, toilet seats, or through other means of direct contact. The eggs can also be inhaled from the air. They enter the body through the nose or mouth and migrate to the upper part of the intestine to hatch. Once hatched, the worms move to the child's anus to lay eggs. When the child scratches his or her anus, the eggs lodge under the child's fingernails and spread to the child's mouth, reinfecting the child, or spread to other children or family members. Pinworms are annoying but they are not a serious health problem.

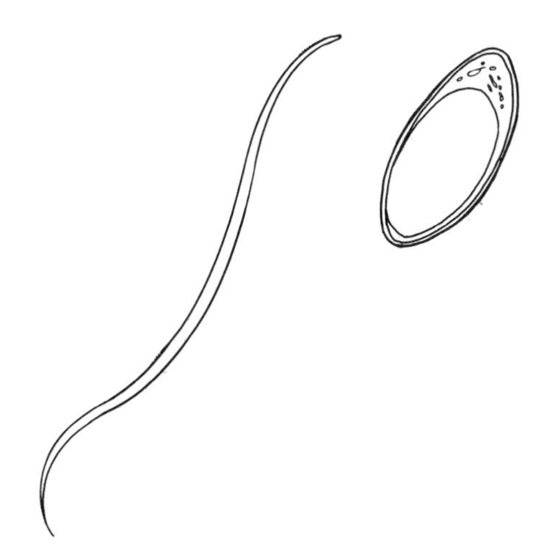

Pinworm infestation
Adult pinworms (left), which are ¼ to ½ inch long, live in a child's intestine and lay their tiny eggs (right) around the anus. Children can scratch the anal area, then transfer the eggs to their mouth and start a new life cycle.

SIGNS AND SYMPTOMS The skin around the child's anus becomes red and irritated and the child may scratch his or her anus or buttocks, especially during sleep. The child sleeps restlessly and, if the itching is intense, he or she may frequently wake up at night. In girls, the pinworms may crawl into the vagina or urethra (the opening to the bladder), causing a vaginal discharge, itching, irritation, and sometimes pain while urinating.

DIAGNOSIS AND TREATMENT Your child's doctor will take samples of the eggs for examination under a microscope to confirm the diagnosis. He or she will press a strip of cellophane tape against the skin near your child's anus to obtain the samples. The test is most accurate if the child has not bathed the night before and if you have not applied any medication. Pinworms last only for 2 or 3 weeks if you can break the reinfection cycle. Try to prevent your child from putting his or her hands in his or her mouth. Make sure that all contaminated bedding, towels, and dirty clothing have been laundered in hot, soapy water. Cut and clean your child's fingernails and wash all toys with hot water. Most children reinfect themselves and eventually need to be medically treated. The doctor will prescribe medication for your child; it probably will have to be taken by all members of your family to prevent the worms from infecting them. The medication is taken in two doses about 2 weeks apart. You can ease your child's rectal irritation with a warm bath or soothing creams.

PITUITARY DISORDERS

Pituitary disorders affect the pea-sized pituitary gland, which is located at the base of the brain. The pituitary gland is made up of two parts: the anterior (front) and the posterior (back) parts. The back portion controls water balance in the body and the release of breast milk in women. The front portion controls growth, metabolism (the rate at which nutrients and chemicals break down or build up in the body), and sexual development through the release of hormones into the bloodstream. The pituitary gland is sometimes called the master gland because it regulates the activities of other glands in the body. The pituitary gland produces many hormones that have specific functions. Too little or too much of these hormones can affect the functions they control. The two main pituitary disorders are hypopituitarism and hyperpituitarism. Both affect functions controlled by the anterior portion of the pituitary gland.

Signs and symptoms Hypopituitarism causes a decrease in one or more pituitary hormones. It can be caused by a tumor on the pituitary gland, a defective pituitary gland, injury to the pituitary or hypothalamus (the area of the brain that controls the pituitary gland), or a disease, such as MENINGITIS. Surgery and *radiation* can harm the gland and cause hypopituitarism. The signs of hypopituitarism include retarded growth, short stature (see HEIGHT PROBLEMS), delayed sexual development, weight gain or loss, weakness, fatigue, HEADACHE, VISION PROBLEMS, and low blood pressure. Symptoms develop slowly and often begin in the first few years of the child's life.

Hyperpituitarism results in an increase in one or more of the pituitary hormones. This disorder is usually caused by a tumor on the pituitary gland or hypothalamus. It can also be caused by an injury or disease. The signs of hyperpituitarism include rapid growth, tall stature, delayed sexual development or loss of sexual function, excess weight gain or loss, and muscle weakness.

Diagnosis To diagnose pituitary disorders, the doctor needs to order blood tests to measure hormone levels in your child's blood. The doctor also needs to do tests to rule out diseases in the organ affected by the increase or decrease of pituitary hormones. He or she may also order X-rays, a *computed tomography* scan, or *magnetic resonance imaging* of your child's head to look for a possible tumor or to see if the pituitary gland is missing or damaged.

Treatment If your child has a tumor in his or her pituitary gland or hypothalamus, he or she will need surgery, radiation, or both to remove or destroy the growth. After treatment, your child will need to take hormone replacement therapy to treat delayed growth and development. If your child's pituitary disorder is caused by something other than a tumor, he or she will also need to take hormone replacement therapy. If something other than a tumor has caused your child's pituitary disorder, the doctor will offer appropriate treatment, depending on the cause.

Pityriasis rosea

Pityriasis rosea is a common skin RASH that can occur in infants as young as 3 months but usually appears in children 10 years and older. This mild condition affects children more often in the winter, fall, and spring, but the cause of pityriasis rosea is not known. The rash does not leave permanent marks, although dark-skinned children might have flat brown spots that disappear in a few months.

Signs and symptoms The symptoms usually begin with one large, flat, pale pink or light brown, slightly scaly patch that is round or oval in shape. This large patch is called the herald or mother patch. In a week or two, several smaller, faint pink areas appear, most commonly on the chest, abdomen, and arms, although they can occur anywhere on the child's body. In children under age 10, the rash may appear more frequently on the face, scalp, and legs.

The rash usually lasts from 6 to 12 weeks. Some affected children feel slightly ill, with mild fatigue, slight fever, and a headache. The rash can also begin to itch, particularly when the child becomes overheated. The rash can get worse or reappear after fading when the child engages in vigorous activities, such as running, or bathes in hot water. The disease usually occurs only once, but in rare cases can recur within weeks of the first episode and last for months.

DIAGNOSIS Your child's doctor will be able to diagnose the condition from its appearance.

TREATMENT There is no treatment available for pityriasis rosea. The disease will usually run its course in about 6 weeks. For a child who experiences severe itching, a doctor may recommend antihistamines or a 1 percent hydrocortisone cream and warm (not hot) baths.

PKU

PKU (phenylketonuria) is an inherited INBORN ERROR OF METABOLISM in which a child's body cannot process an amino acid (a building block of protein) called phenylalanine, which is present in many common protein-containing foods, such as milk, eggs, cheese, meat, and fish. If a baby born with PKU does not receive treatment soon after birth, phenylalanine and its by-products build up in the child's bloodstream and cause MENTAL RETARDATION.

SIGNS AND SYMPTOMS Newborns with PKU may appear normal for the first several weeks of life, but then gradually lose interest in their surroundings and eventually begin to show signs of mental impairment. By the time they reach 1 year old, they may show signs of delayed mental skills. Children with PKU may have jerky arm or leg movements, are restless and destructive, and give off a musty odor from the accumulation of phenylalanine. Some have a skin RASH; others have seizures. Affected children characteristically have light complexions, blond hair, and blue eyes.

DIAGNOSIS Every state requires newborn testing for PKU (see page 223). During the test, a doctor or nurse pricks your baby's heel and takes a few drops of blood that are analyzed for phenylalanine levels. If your baby has a high level of the amino acid, he or she will receive more sensitive tests to confirm the diagnosis.

TREATMENT If your child is found to have PKU, he or she will have to follow a strict diet that eliminates foods containing phenylalanine. You will not be able to breast-feed your child or give him or her regular formula. Your child will need regular follow-up care so the doctor can check the levels of phenylalanine in his or her blood and adjust the diet as he or she grows. Your child may have to stay on the special diet for life, but will otherwise be able to lead a normal life.

If you are thinking about having more children, and either have PKU yourself or are a carrier of the disorder, you should seek genetic counseling (see page 497). You will have to follow a strict PKU diet throughout your pregnancy to avoid the possibility of brain damage to your fetus.

PNEUMONIA

Pneumonia is a lung infection caused by bacteria, viruses, or fungi. Children catch pneumonia by breathing in the microorganisms in small droplets sneezed or coughed into the air. They can also develop pneumonia when bacteria or viruses normally present in their nose or throat enter their lungs. There are two types of pneumonia. One type affects the lobes of one or both lungs. The other type first affects the air passages leading to the lungs and then spreads to the lungs. Infants and children are especially vulnerable to developing life-threatening cases of pneumonia. It often appears as a complication of other diseases.

SIGNS AND SYMPTOMS The initial symptoms may resemble those of a cold, including fatigue and a stuffy nose. Then the child suddenly develops a high fever up to 105°F, shaking chills, and a cough. A child 10 years old or older may cough up yellow-green sputum (phlegm), sometimes with blood in it. He or she may also develop shortness of breath, rapid breathing, chest pain on one or both sides of the body, or blue lips or nails. The child could also have a HEADACHE, diarrhea, vomiting, and abdominal pain.

Severe cases of pneumonia can cause serious complications, including a collection of fluid around the lung called pleural effusion that makes breathing difficult, and an accumulation of pus around the lung known as empyema that produces severe chest pain. Without treatment, an affected child could die of respiratory failure.

DIAGNOSIS AND TREATMENT If the doctor suspects that your child has pneumonia, he or she will listen to your child's chest through a stethoscope, will order a chest X-ray and blood tests, and may also take a sample of your child's sputum for laboratory analysis. The doctor will prescribe antibiotics if bacteria or fungi have caused your child's pneumonia. Antibiotics are not effective against viruses and your child's immune system (the body's natural defense against infection) will fight off viral pneumonia over time. Your child will probably not have to be hospitalized. He or she should rest in bed, drink plenty of fluids, and stay home from school or day care until the fever is gone. You can give your child acetaminophen (but not aspirin) to relieve the fever and pain. With treatment, your child should recover completely within about 2 weeks.

PNEUMOTHORAX

A pneumothorax is an abnormal pocket of air in the chest cavity from a ruptured lung or injury to the chest wall. When the lung leaks air, the air becomes trapped in the spaces between the lungs, rib cage, and diaphragm. The air then pushes the lung inward and eventually causes it to partially or totally collapse. The pneumothorax can occur as a consequence of ASTHMA, BRONCHOPULMONARY DYSPLASIA in premature infants, or emphysema (damaged air sacs in the lungs). It can also occur spontaneously during such activities as scuba diving or flying at high altitudes. A penetrating wound to the chest or lungs or broken ribs that puncture the lungs can also produce pneumothorax.

SIGNS AND SYMPTOMS The symptoms vary according to the size of the pneumothorax and the overall health of the child's lungs. The child can experience sharp chest pain that extends to the shoulders and abdomen, shortness of breath, and a dry, hacking cough. The lips or fingers can become blue from inadequate oxygen intake.

DIAGNOSIS AND TREATMENT The doctor will order chest X-rays to determine the size of the pneumothorax and to detect any other lung diseases. If the pneumothorax is small and your child is otherwise healthy, no treatment may be necessary because the condition will heal on its own in a few days. But, if your child has an underlying lung disease or if the pneumothorax is large, your child may need to be hospitalized to remove the trapped air from the chest cavity. To remove the air, the doctor will insert a suction tube or needle through your child's chest wall. The tube may need to remain in place for several days. If your child's lung does not return to normal size or continues to leak, surgery may be needed.

POISON IVY

Poison ivy (see page 597) is a plant with three shiny leaves that grows throughout the United States and causes a severe skin reaction. Upon contact with the skin, a yellowish oil found in the plant's sap produces an itchy, burning, blistering RASH. Also present in the sap of poison oak and poison sumac, the oil can even cause a rash when a child touches something that has come into contact with the sap, such as the fur of a

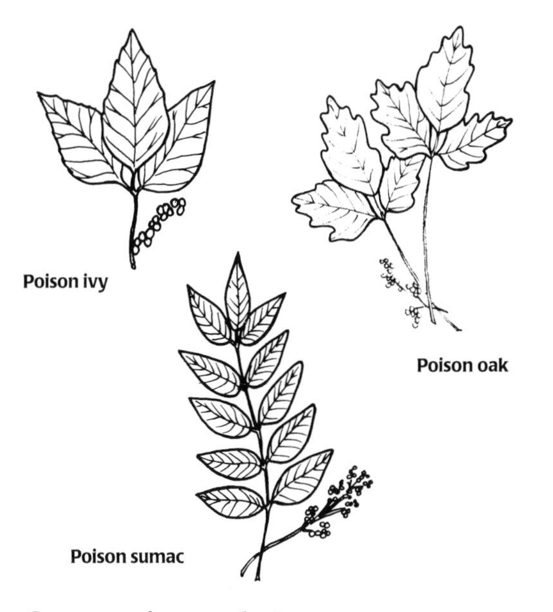

Common poisonous plants
Learn to identify common poisonous plants, such as poison ivy, poison oak, and poison sumac, so you can teach your child to identify them. Poison ivy has three shiny leaflets on its stem. It may grow as a vine, bush, or plant. Like poison ivy, poison oak has three leaflets on its stem, but the leaflets look like oak leaves. Poison sumac has two parallel rows of leaflets on its stem, with a single leaflet at the top. It grows as a bush or tree.

dog. Poison ivy usually grows as a shrub or vine east of the Rocky Mountains. Poison oak is a shrub that grows in the West and Southwest. Poison sumac is a shrub or tree found east of the Mississippi River.

SIGNS AND SYMPTOMS Within 24 to 72 hours after exposure to the oil in poison ivy, your child will develop a rash that is made up of lines or patches of red, swollen spots and BLISTERS. The rash is extremely itchy. The blisters break, crust over, and become scaly in a few days. The fluid from the blisters does not spread the rash. The rash erupts wherever the skin has been exposed to the oil. Areas where the skin is thick, such as the soles of the feet or the palms of the hands, are less susceptible. The rash usually heals on its own in 1 to 3 weeks.

DIAGNOSIS Your child's doctor will be able to diagnose poison ivy from its appearance. You may be able to recognize it on your own.

TREATMENT If you or your child can wash the exposed skin with water from a stream or lake within 5 minutes of exposure to the oil, you can stop the rash from developing. Otherwise, wash your child's skin and anything else that has come into contact with the oil, such as his or her clothing, with water and a strong soap as soon as you can.

Your child can take cool showers or oatmeal baths to relieve the itching. Over-the-counter medications such as antihistamines, calamine lotion, Burow's solution, or a cortisone cream can help reduce itching and soothe the rash. Call your doctor if the rash spreads to your child's face, eyes, or lips; lasts more than 2 weeks; or becomes infected (has pus or soft, yellow scabs on it) from too much scratching.

POLIO

Polio is a contagious infection caused by three different strains of viruses that attack a child's brain and spinal cord. Until the 1950s, when the polio vaccine was developed, the disease was fairly common and widely feared. Today, polio is very rare in the United States. The polio virus lives in the nose, throat, and intestines of infected people and spreads through contact with the stool of an infected person, by direct contact with another person, or indirectly through food. Poor sanitation promotes the spread of polio.

Most children are first immunized against polio when they are 2 months old by an oral polio vaccine given as drops in the mouth or by an injectable vaccine. Children then receive additional doses of the vaccine at 4 months, at 6 to 18 months, and at 4 to 6 years of age—when they start school. If a child will be traveling to a foreign country where polio is common, the doctor may recommend that the child have an additional dose of the vaccine.

SIGNS AND SYMPTOMS Most cases of polio are mild and do not affect the nervous system, so an affected child may have no symptoms. When symptoms do occur, they include a low-grade fever, sore throat, stomach ache, and HEADACHE. The symptoms may begin suddenly and last only a few days. But in about 3 percent of all cases, polio can also be a very serious infection that initially causes muscle aches and twitching, and pain and stiffness in the neck, legs, and back. Within a week, these symptoms progress to muscle paralysis, especially in the legs and lower part of the body. In very severe cases, the child may have difficulty breathing and swallowing and the condition could be fatal.

DIAGNOSIS AND TREATMENT To confirm a diagnosis of polio, the doctor may take a stool sample and order a *lumbar puncture* to identify the virus. There is no effective treatment for polio. Some children experience permanent paralysis, some have only temporary paralysis, and others endure muscle weakness for the rest of their lives. Some have no long-term effects. A child who is paralyzed may be hospitalized and will need physical therapy. He or she may also need assisted breathing with the help of a ventilator.

POLYMYOSITIS

Polymyositis is a persistent inflammation of the muscles that frequently begins when a child is in his or her teens. It is characterized by periodic flare-ups. The cause remains unknown. Some children may have a predisposition to getting polymyositis if either of their parents has the disorder. The most severe form of the disease, known as inclusion body myositis, may be triggered by a viral infection. Polymyositis sometimes occurs along with other diseases, such as LUPUS and JUVENILE RHEUMATOID ARTHRITIS.

SIGNS AND SYMPTOMS Children with polymyositis have weakness in the muscles in or near the trunk. They may have difficulty climbing stairs or lifting their arms above their shoulders. Their muscles ache and feel tender. Affected children feel very fatigued and lose weight. They may have a low-grade fever; a poor appetite; a red, swollen RASH on the face, elbows, or knees; and an overall feeling of discomfort.

DIAGNOSIS AND TREATMENT If your child has symptoms of polymyositis, the doctor will test his or her muscular strength and order blood and urine tests. He or she may also order tests such as electromyography and nerve conduction velocity tests that measure muscle and nerve activities. Your child's doctor may take a muscle *biopsy* to confirm the diagnosis.

To treat polymyositis, the doctor will prescribe *corticosteroids*, which your child may have to take for years. If the corticosteroids are not effective, the doctor may prescribe medications that suppress the immune system to reduce the inflammation. Your child will also need physical therapy to strengthen his or her muscles and improve movement. With successful early treatment, your child should be able to maintain his or her normal activities. Even after treatment, polymyositis continues to be a chronic condition in some children. For a small percentage of children, the disease is fatal.

POLYPS, INTESTINAL

Intestinal polyps are small growths of abnormal tissue in the lining of a child's intestines. They can be found throughout the intestines, but occur most often in the colon (the large intestine). Most intestinal polyps that occur in children are harmless and disappear as the child gets older. But in rare cases, some types of polyps can become cancerous.

TYPES OF INTESTINAL POLYPS Most common in children are polyps caused by Peutz-Jeghers syndrome, juvenile polyps, and familial polyps.

Polyps caused by Peutz-Jeghers syndrome This inherited condition produces polyps in the small intestine of infants and young children and causes small brown spots to appear on their lips and in their mouth. This type of polyp bleeds easily. The polyps are harmless in most cases, but in rare instances can become cancerous.

Juvenile polyps This type rarely occurs in children under 1 year of age but is the most common type of polyp in children, especially in those between the ages of 2 and 5 years. Most occur in the colon and rectum and are harmless. They usually disappear without treatment by the time a child reaches age 15.

Familial polyposis This rare inherited disorder causes a large number of polyps to develop in the colon and rectum. These polyps should be treated in childhood because they have a high risk of becoming cancerous by the time the child reaches age 40. This type can develop in children between the ages of 4 months and 10 years, but is most commonly discovered in early adolescence.

SIGNS AND SYMPTOMS The most common sign of intestinal polyps is the appearance of a small amount of bright red blood in the stool. The blood may appear every time the child passes a stool or only occasionally. Peutz-Jeghers syndrome usually causes no symptoms, other than the brown spots on the child's lips and mouth, but it sometimes causes bleeding, abdominal pain after meals, INTUSSUSCEPTION, anemia (see ANEMIA, BLOOD-LOSS), or vomiting. Juvenile polyps cause bleeding upon defecation and, in rare cases, abdominal pain, diarrhea, and blood-loss anemia. Familial polyposis can cause rectal bleeding and diarrhea or produce no symptoms at all until cancer develops in adulthood.

DIAGNOSIS Even though many intestinal polyps are harmless, your child should see the doctor for a diagnosis if he or she has bloody stools or any other symptoms of polyps. The doctor will want to know if your family has a history of intestinal polyps, colon cancer, or blood in the stool. The doctor will perform a thorough physical examination that includes a rectal examination. He or she will probably refer your child to a gastroenterologist (a doctor who specializes in disorders of the stomach and intestinal tract) who will examine your child's colon and rectum through an endoscope inserted into your child's anus. An endoscope is a flexible viewing tube containing a light that allows your doctor to see the intestinal polyps and take a *biopsy* of them. The doctor may also order a *barium X-ray* study to aid in the diagnosis, although this procedure is becoming less common because of the use of endoscopes. Blood tests may be needed to detect complications of the polyps, such as anemia.

TREATMENT The doctor may choose not to treat your child's polyps if they are harmless and cause no symptoms. If they are causing bleeding or INTESTINAL OBSTRUCTION, he or she will probably treat them with electrocoagulation (see below). The endoscope the doctor uses to diagnose your

What is electrocoagulation?

Destroying diseased tissue or stopping bleeding by burning the tissue is an ancient technique. Early physicians used a piece of iron heated in a fire. Modern physicians have used caustic chemicals, heat, and, more recently, electricity. Electrocoagulation is the use of a high-frequency electrical current to burn tissue. Surgeons use it to treat intestinal polyps by passing an instrument known as an electrocautery snare through an endoscope (a probe with a viewing instrument) to burn away the polyps with electricity. Electrocoagulation is more efficient and easier to use than chemicals or heat. Your child will need general anesthesia (see page 292) before the operation, but the procedure itself is simple and relatively painless. The surgeon may need to do more than one electrocoagulation treatment to remove all of your child's polyps.

child's polyps can also be used to treat the polyps with electrocoagulation.

Polyps caused by familial polyposis require more aggressive treatment because of the danger of cancer in adulthood. The polyps must be surgically removed. The doctor may even recommend surgical removal of your child's entire colon to prevent cancer from occurring in the future. If your child's colon is removed, the surgeon will either connect your child's small intestine directly to his or her rectum or create a permanent artificial opening, called an ileostomy, on the outside of your child's abdomen and connect the small intestine to the opening. Your child will then have to pass feces into a bag attached to the outside of his or her abdomen. After surgery, your child should continue to be checked often for the appearance of additional polyps, which should be treated promptly.

POLYPS, LARYNGEAL

Laryngeal polyps are small outgrowths of abnormal tissue on a child's voice box (larynx). They are usually caused by overuse or straining of the child's voice.

SIGNS AND SYMPTOMS The major symptoms of laryngeal polyps are a hoarse voice and LARYNGITIS, an inflammation of the child's voice box. Most laryngeal polyps are harmless, but, in rare cases, they can develop into cancer of the larynx. Polyps that progress to cancer usually occur in children who have inherited a genetic predisposition to laryngeal cancer (see GENETIC DISORDERS).

DIAGNOSIS Most laryngeal polyps are harmless and disappear on their own without treatment. A visit to the doctor is warranted if your child's hoarseness does not clear up in a week or two.

TREATMENT The doctor may refer your child to an otolaryngologist (ear, nose, and throat specialist) who will diagnose the polyps in your child's larynx with a special viewing instrument inserted into the child's throat. The doctor will want to examine your child periodically afterward to see whether the polyps grow or disappear. If the polyps get bigger or if there is any chance they might become cancerous, the doctor will recommend surgical removal.

POLYPS, NASAL

Nasal polyps are small outgrowths of abnormal tissue inside a child's nose. CYSTIC FIBROSIS is the most common cause of nasal polyps in children, but they can also be caused by ASTHMA or HAY FEVER or an allergy to aspirin. A child may have only one polyp or many, usually in both sides of the nose. The polyps appear most frequently in children over 10 years of age.

SIGNS AND SYMPTOMS A child with nasal polyps sometimes has a stuffy nose because the polyps obstruct the flow of air. He or she may also have a watery discharge from the nose and an impaired sense of smell. The child's voice may sound the way it does when he or she has a cold. The child may breathe through his or her mouth because breathing through the nose becomes difficult. Sometimes the polyps grow so large and numerous that they cause the child's nose to look large and deformed.

DIAGNOSIS AND TREATMENT The doctor can detect polyps in your child's nose by looking through a special viewing instrument. If the polyps are small and not causing problems, your child's doctor may take a wait-and-see attitude toward treatment. If the polyps completely obstruct your child's nose or cause the nose to look deformed, the doctor will recommend minor surgery to remove the polyps using a local anesthetic. The polyps often return, even after surgery. The doctor will want to treat any underlying diseases, such as cystic fibrosis or allergies, that are causing the polyps. Never give a child with polyps aspirin because he or she could have a severe allergic reaction to the drug.

PREMATURITY

See page 35

PRETERM INFANTS

See page 35

PRICKLY HEAT

Prickly heat, or miliaria rubra, is an itchy skin RASH caused by clogged sweat-gland ducts. The condition is brought on by excessive sweating. It can occur in people of all ages, but is most common in infants.

SIGNS AND SYMPTOMS Prickly heat is characterized by tiny red spots that cover the skin in areas where sweat glands are clustered, such as the waist, armpits, upper torso, and the inside of the elbows. In infants, the rash can also appear on the face. The affected skin itches and becomes irritated. If your infant or child has prickly heat, he or she may be uncomfortable because of irritation from the rash.

DIAGNOSIS You will probably be able to recognize prickly heat on your own. Your doctor will be able to diagnose it during a physical examination.

TREATMENT Give your infant or child cool sponge baths or showers to relieve the discomfort. Use mild soap; harsh soaps will irritate the rash further. For older children, use calamine lotion or dusting powder to relieve the irritation. Dress your child in cool, lightweight clothing. Keep your infant or child in a cool, dry environment as much as possible to avoid excessive sweating.

Call your doctor if your child's skin does not clear up after 10 days of care at home. Your doctor may recommend a *corticosteroid* cream to reduce inflammation.

PROCTITIS

Proctitis is an inflammation of the rectum and the area around the anus. In children, it is most common in adolescents. The inflammation can be caused by diseases such as CROHN'S DISEASE or ULCERATIVE COLITIS, by infection with streptococcal bacteria, by sexually transmitted diseases such as GONORRHEA spread through anal intercourse, or (in rare cases) by *radiation* therapy, drugs used in the rectum, food allergies, tuberculosis, injury to the rectum, or chronic constipation.

SIGNS AND SYMPTOMS Proctitis can cause bleeding or discharge of mucus from the rectum, soreness and pain in the rectum and anus, cramping on the left side of the abdomen, rectal itching, and a persistent urge to move the bowels even when there is no stool.

DIAGNOSIS If your child has signs of proctitis, the doctor may recommend examination of the child's rectum with a proctoscope (a viewing tube) and a *biopsy* of rectal tissue to determine the cause of inflammation. A *culture* of the tissue around and inside your child's rectum will help the doctor diagnose proctitis caused by streptococcal bacteria.

TREATMENT Treatment depends on the underlying cause of the inflammation. The doctor may prescribe suppositories or enemas containing *corticosteroids* to treat Crohn's disease or ulcerative colitis. Sexually transmitted diseases are treated with antibiotics. Proctitis caused by streptococcal bacteria is also treated with antibiotics. The doctor will advise a sexually active teenager to avoid anal intercourse and to practice safe sex by using a latex condom. At home, your child can take baths in hot water to relieve pain. He or she should keep the anal area clean by taking frequent showers or baths.

Psoriasis

Psoriasis is a persistent skin condition marked by areas of dry, scaly skin. It usually begins in childhood and can come and go throughout life. The condition varies in intensity, ranging from mild cases with small patches of scaly skin that get better on their own to severe cases that can cover large areas and require intensive treatment. There are different types of psoriasis, defined by the shape and pattern of the scales and the severity of the condition. The most common type among children is guttate psoriasis, which is generally a mild form. A child often develops guttate psoriasis after a sore throat. The condition clears up on its own in a few weeks or a few months.

The exact cause of psoriasis is not known. In children, certain infections, such as strep throat, can trigger the condition. Psoriasis also runs in families. Flare-ups can occur in winter from the combination of dry weather and little sunlight, or at other times when the skin has been cut, scratched, or severely sunburned.

Signs and symptoms Psoriasis usually begins with little red bumps on the skin of the elbows, knees, lower back, or scalp. The red areas gradually grow larger. Then silvery scales begin to form on top. The top layer of scales flakes off easily, while the lower layer sticks together and thickens. The skin cracks, becomes painful, and sometimes itches. When the scales are removed, the exposed skin bleeds.

The scaly areas of skin often appear on both sides of the body in the same places. The child's nails are frequently affected, developing tiny pits, and can become loose or thick or even fall off. Some types of psoriasis appear in the armpits; on the buttocks, groin, or genitals; or under the breasts. Some children also experience pain and swelling in their joints.

Diagnosis Your child's doctor will probably take a scraping of the scaly skin and examine it under a microscope to confirm the diagnosis.

Treatment There is no cure for psoriasis, but your child's doctor can prescribe medications and treatments that will control the symptoms. The doctor may refer your child to a dermatologist (doctor who specializes in disorders of the skin). Treatment will depend on the seriousness of the disease and its location.

For mild cases, the doctor may prescribe creams or ointments that contain *corticosteroids*, tar, or a compound known as anthralin. If your child has a severe case of psoriasis, he or she may receive etretinate or methotrexate pills along with the creams or ointments. Severe cases may also require treatment in the doctor's office with ultraviolet light, sometimes in combination with tar baths given at home or a medication called psoralen given in tablet form. The doctor will discontinue treatment once the psoriasis has cleared up but treatment will have to resume if the condition returns.

Psychosis

Psychosis is a serious mental disorder in which a child loses touch with reality and lives in a fantasy world. Psychosis is not common among children; it occurs more often in adolescents. Not much is known about psychosis in infants and preschool children because they do not yet have the sophisticated language skills necessary to express their symptoms. Psychosis can result from other illnesses, such as a high fever, HYPERTHYROIDISM, ENCEPHALITIS, or MENINGITIS; from the use or abuse of prescription or illegal drugs and alcohol (see DRUG AND ALCOHOL ABUSE); from extreme stress; or from a brain injury or disorder. Researchers do not know if it can be inherited or not. Psychosis has been linked to other mental disorders, including SCHIZOPHRENIA, BIPOLAR DISORDER, and DEPRESSION. Psychotic episodes may occur temporarily during an illness or stressful situation or they may be long-lasting.

SIGNS AND SYMPTOMS There are three major symptoms of psychosis: hallucinations, delusions, and illogical thinking. Hallucinations are perceptions of objects or sounds that do not exist. A delusion is an irrational idea that has no basis in reality, such as a false belief by the child that someone is trying to harm him or her. Illogical thinking means not thinking clearly or rationally. Children with psychosis may have mood swings from extreme excitement to deep depression. They can also not show emotion and have irrational fears and ANXIETY. Psychosis can impair a child's normal development and social interaction.

DIAGNOSIS If your child has symptoms of psychosis, he or she will need a thorough physical examination to detect any illnesses that might be causing the symptoms. Psychological evaluation and testing from a mental health specialist may be necessary to determine a specific diagnosis. Your child's doctor may order blood and urine tests and a *computed tomography* scan, *magnetic resonance imaging* scan, or *positron emission tomography* scan of your child's brain. He or she may also refer your child to other specialists—such as a speech and language specialist or a specialist in child development—for an evaluation.

TREATMENT Even if your child's psychosis is temporary and his or her symptoms disappear after treatment for an underlying illness, he or she should receive psychotherapy, if only for a short period, to help the child understand what happened. For longer-lasting episodes, your child may need to take antipsychotic drugs and undergo psychotherapy for a longer time. The combination of drugs and therapy is usually quite effective in relieving symptoms. In some cases, your child may need to be hospitalized for a short time until he or she gets over the worst symptoms. The entire family may be included in all or part of the therapy.

PYLORIC STENOSIS

Pyloric stenosis is the abnormal overgrowth and narrowing of the pylorus, a muscular ring surrounding the lower outlet of the stomach that blocks the passage of food from the stomach into the small intestine. The condition develops most often in infants 2 to 6 weeks old, but can occur as late as 4 months after birth. Boys, especially firstborn boys, are far more likely to have pyloric stenosis than girls. If the condition is not diagnosed and treated quickly, it can cause severe dehydration (see page 283) and shock.

SIGNS AND SYMPTOMS After a feeding, the baby's stomach fills up but the narrowed pylorus blocks the partially digested milk or formula from passing into the small intestine. Within minutes after eating, the infant begins to vomit forcefully, ejecting food from his or her stomach several feet away (projectile vomiting). The baby may vomit with increasing intensity as the disease progresses. An affected infant may not be in pain and may even seem happy, although hungry, after vomiting. He or she may produce less stool because food cannot pass through the intestine. Eventually, the infant becomes irritable and weak, begins to lose weight, becomes dehydrated, and fails to gain weight.

DIAGNOSIS If your baby vomits after most feedings or develops projectile vomiting, take him or her to the doctor for an evaluation right away. If your child has pyloric stenosis, the doctor may be able to feel a lump in your baby's abdomen where the pyloric muscle is located. Blood tests will help the doctor diagnose the condition. The doctor may want to watch your child eat and then observe how he or she vomits in the office. To confirm the diagnosis, the doctor may order a *barium X-ray* study or an *ultrasound* examination of your child's abdomen.

TREATMENT Your infant will need surgery to correct the narrowing in his or her pylorus. Your baby will be given general anesthesia (see page 292) and then a surgeon will make an incision in the thickened muscle of the pylorus to split it, relieving the obstruction and allowing food to pass into the small intestine. Doctors sometimes try to correct the condition with drugs, but surgery is quicker and much more effective in most cases. Your baby will recover quickly and will be able to eat within hours of the surgery, but will have to remain in the hospital for about 3 to 5 days.

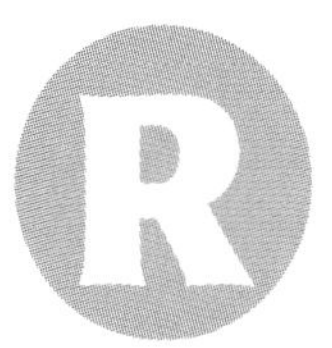

RABIES

Rabies is an infectious disease of the nervous system caused by a rhabdovirus. The virus is spread through the saliva in the bites of infected animals. Occasionally, infected saliva that accidentally contaminates a scratch or open sore can also cause rabies. Animals commonly infected with rabies include bats, ferrets, raccoons, and skunks. Squirrels, rodents, and domestic cats and dogs can become infected if bitten by an infected animal, although the incidence is infrequent. The disease can occur 5 days to 1 year after exposure to the virus. Rabies can be prevented by vaccinating all household pets and by avoiding contact with animals that carry a high risk of infection.

SIGNS AND SYMPTOMS After becoming infected, a child will have a fever that lasts 2 to 10 days. The disease then affects the child's nervous system, producing high excitability, delirium, agitation, and fear of drinking liquids (hydrophobia). Convulsions and paralysis follow. Human rabies is usually fatal.

DIAGNOSIS Doctors diagnose rabies by looking for either antibodies to the virus or the virus itself in the child's saliva or spinal fluid.

TREATMENT A human bite can also transmit rabies, so the infected child will be hospitalized in isolation. If an animal that could have rabies has bitten your child, a veterinarian will either observe the animal for signs of rabies for 10 days or destroy it so its brain can be autopsied for evidence of the rabies virus. Bites from a bat or ferret, or from any animal known to have rabies, warrant immediate preventive treatment, before any symptoms appear. Treatment consists of a shot of human rabies immune globulin and a shot of rabies vaccine, given at the same time. The child then receives shots of the rabies vaccine again 3, 7, 14, and 28 days after the initial dose. If the disease develops, doctors treat the child with sedatives and painkillers, but survival is rare.

RASH

A rash is a cluster of red or purple spots, bumps, or BLISTERS on the skin. Rashes can appear anywhere on a child's body and occur in children of all ages. They can affect only one small area of skin or the child's entire body and may or may not be accompanied by fever and itching. Rashes are usually only temporary. They may be caused by an infection, by something that irritates the skin, by allergic reactions to food, medications, or plants, or by insect bites. (See the color photographs on pages 23 and 24 to help you identify common childhood rashes.)

TYPES OF RASHES Rashes can be caused by infections, allergies, and insect bites. Certain rashes are common mainly in newborns and infants.

Rashes in newborns and infants Up to half of all newborns develop a harmless rash known as erythema toxicum (see page 23) in the first few days of life, characterized by flat, red spots or pimples that usually disappear in a week or two. The cause is not known. Many babies between the ages of 4 and 15 months develop diaper rash around the stomach, genitals, and the folds of the skin on the buttocks and thighs. Other rashes that are common among infants include CRADLE CAP and PRICKLY HEAT.

Infection-related rashes Rashes can indicate an underlying infection caused by a virus, bacterium, or fungus. Viral infections that can cause a rash in children include CHICKENPOX, GERMAN MEASLES, FIFTH DISEASE, MEASLES, and HAND-FOOT-AND-MOUTH DISEASE. Common bacterial infections that produce a rash are MENINGITIS, SCARLET FEVER, and IMPETIGO. Among the fungal infections that cause a rash are RINGWORM and THRUSH.

Allergy-related rashes Rashes can also signal an allergic reaction to food, medication, or plants. Examples of allergy-related rashes include HIVES, ATOPIC DERMATITIS, CONTACT DERMATITIS, and POISON IVY. Drugs, such as antibiotics and barbiturates, can also cause an allergic reaction that produces a rash.

Rashes caused by insect bites Insect bites and infestations, such as LICE and SCABIES, can also cause a rash. Bites from bees, wasps, mosquitoes, and fleas may also trigger a rash.

SIGNS AND SYMPTOMS The symptoms of specific rashes vary. Some rashes produce blisters; others consist of flat, discolored spots or small bumps. Still others have both flat and raised spots. Rashes may also consist of swollen red or pink patches of skin, as in hives, have small, solid spots, or have blue or purple bruises. Some change into open sores.

DIAGNOSIS Doctors look for characteristic symptoms of a rash that offer clues to diagnosis. Your child's doctor will diagnose a rash based on its appearance; location on the body; or whether or not it spreads, changes, or itches.

How to prevent and care for diaper rash

Your baby can easily get diaper rash (see page 59) from wet, dirty diapers that chafe or rub against his or her delicate skin. A yeast infection, a bacterial infection, or an allergic reaction to the diaper can also trigger diaper rash. Mild cases usually clear up in 3 or 4 days. To prevent diaper rash, change your baby's diapers frequently and keep the diaper loose so it doesn't irritate his or her skin. Wipe your baby's skin with a warm wet cloth after every diaper change and pat the area dry—don't rub the skin. If diaper rash does occur, let your baby's skin air-dry thoroughly after you have wiped it after each diaper change. Apply an ointment or cream containing zinc oxide to protect the skin. Don't use baby powder because your baby can inhale the powder, which can irritate his or her airways. You usually won't have to call your baby's doctor for a simple case of diaper rash, unless:

- Your baby's diaper rash does not clear up within 3 days.
- The rash contains blisters or sores filled with pus.
- The rash gets worse.
- The rash extends beyond the area covered by a diaper.
- Your baby has a fever or other symptoms of illness.
- Your infant is under 3 months old.

TREATMENT Once a diagnosis is made, your child's doctor will treat the cause of the rash—for example, an underlying infection. Common drugs given to relieve the symptoms of a rash include antihistamine drugs to relieve itching and soothing creams or lotions for itching and discomfort.

REACTIVE AIRWAY DISEASE

Reactive airway disease is a group of disorders characterized by a high-pitched whistling sound known as wheezing. The child wheezes when the airways inside his or her lungs become irritated and inflamed. The airways swell up, become clogged with mucus, and constrict, making breathing difficult. Causes of reactive airway disease include ASTHMA, BRONCHITIS, PNEUMONIA, CYSTIC FIBROSIS, BRONCHIOLITIS, colds, congenital lung defects, inhalation of a foreign object, or a tumor.

SIGNS AND SYMPTOMS The wheezing that the child produces each time he or she takes a breath is the most characteristic symptom. The doctor can hear the wheezing through a stethoscope, but if the wheezing is severe, you may be able to hear it easily without one. Other symptoms include rapid breathing, straining of the chest muscles while breathing, chest pain, or a change in skin color.

DIAGNOSIS AND TREATMENT Your child's doctor may order blood tests, chest X-rays, sputum (phlegm) *cultures*, and lung-function tests to confirm the diagnosis of reactive airway disease. The doctor will monitor your child's lung function with a peak flow meter (see page 421) and may prescribe bronchodilators, drugs that relax the muscles in the air passages and open up the bronchial tubes. These medications can either be taken by mouth or inhaled. Your child's doctor may also prescribe *corticosteroids* to reduce the swelling and inflammation in the airways. If your child has asthma caused by ALLERGIES, the doctor may prescribe allergy medication and recommend allergy testing to determine whether your child needs allergy shots. The doctor will also treat the underlying cause of the wheezing. If your child has a severe breathing problem, he or she may need to be hospitalized for oxygen therapy or fluids given *intravenously,* or to get more aggressive airway treatment. If the wheezing is caused by an inhaled object—such as a coin—that is obstructing an airway, an ear, nose, and throat specialist will remove the object with a viewing instrument called a bronchoscope. Surgery may be needed to treat a congenital lung defect or a tumor.

RECTAL PROLAPSE

Rectal prolapse is the protrusion of the inside of a child's rectum out of his or her anus. The condition usually occurs when a child strains to defecate. Causes include long-term malnutrition from such diseases as CYSTIC FIBROSIS or CELIAC DISEASE, or from intestinal infection, polyps, or chronic constipation.

SIGNS AND SYMPTOMS Prolapse is most common in infants and children under 3 years of age. It develops gradually and causes rectal bleeding, discomfort during defecation, and mucus in the stool. The reddened, protruding tissue is readily visible and may be painful.

DIAGNOSIS The doctor can diagnose rectal prolapse during a physical examination, based on your child's medical history. The doctor may order blood and other laboratory tests to determine the underlying cause.

TREATMENT Rectal prolapse is usually only temporary in children and disappears as the child grows. Reversal of the child's malnutrition alleviates the problem. A change in diet may be the only treatment your child needs to prevent constipation. Your child's diet should include foods rich in fiber, such as cereals, bran, whole-grain breads, fruits, and vegetables.

If a digestive tract disorder causes rectal prolapse, the doctor will treat the underlying disease. If your child does not respond to medical treatment, he or she may need corrective surgery.

RESPIRATORY DISTRESS SYNDROME

Respiratory distress syndrome is a life-threatening lung disease found in premature infants caused by incomplete development of the lungs. It is the most common lung disease in premature babies and is a common cause of death. About 20 percent of all infants born prematurely have respiratory distress syndrome. The more premature the baby is, the greater the risk of having the disease. Respiratory distress syndrome stems from a deficiency of a chemical fluid called surfactant that is produced naturally in the lungs. Surfactant coats and protects the tiny air sacs, known as alveoli, in the lungs, and allows these sacs to stay open so they can deliver oxygen to the bloodstream and exchange it for carbon dioxide. Premature infants with respiratory distress syndrome are born before their lungs are able to produce adequate amounts of surfactant. The alveoli collapse and cannot sustain normal breathing.

SIGNS AND SYMPTOMS At delivery or soon after, the infant's breathing becomes labored and very rapid, the nostrils flare when the infant inhales, and he or she makes grunting noises and draws in his or her chest while struggling to breathe out. The infant's condition gets progressively worse as he or she becomes tired from the effort needed to breathe. Irregular breathing patterns or long pauses in breathing begin to occur. Because the infant is not getting enough oxygen, his or her skin begins to turn blue. Without treatment, the baby can die within a few hours or days.

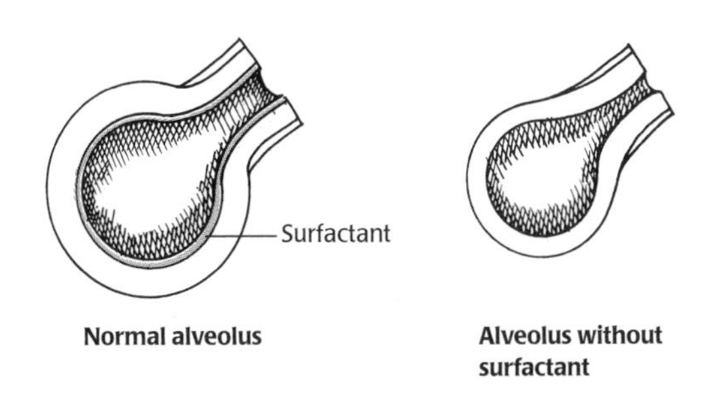

The role of surfactant

The tiny air sacs in the lungs called alveoli produce surfactant, which normally coats and protects the alveoli and allows them to stay open (left) so they can absorb oxygen from inhaled air. An alveolus without surfactant (right) collapses, causing the labored breathing characteristic of respiratory distress syndrome.

DIAGNOSIS AND TREATMENT If the doctor suspects that your newborn has respiratory distress syndrome, he or she will listen to your baby's lungs with a stethoscope and will order a chest X-ray and an analysis of the oxygen and carbon dioxide levels in the child's blood to confirm the diagnosis. Your infant will need immediate treatment in a hospital intensive care unit. Mild symptoms need only oxygen treatment given through a mask or plastic hood. If your infant's condition is initially severe or worsens, he or she will be connected by a tube placed in the windpipe to a machine called a ventilator that assists with breathing. The ventilator provides the baby with oxygen and keeps the air sacs open by applying a sufficient amount of pressure to expand the lungs. Oxygen pumped into the ventilator is filtered through a humidifier that produces water vapor so the infant's lungs won't dry out. The ventilator and the oxygen can both cause unwanted side effects, such as a chronic lung disease called BRONCHOPULMONARY DYSPLASIA.

Your baby may also be given a commercial surfactant replacement administered through a tube inserted into your child's trachea (windpipe). The surfactant replacement reduces your baby's risk of death by as much as 50 percent. In some cases, doctors give the surfactant replacement as a preventive measure to premature infants who are at risk of developing respiratory distress syndrome. Treatment may also be started before a premature birth. Doctors may be able to stop or slow premature labor with medication and then give the mother *corticosteroids* to stimulate surfactant production in the fetus.

Respiratory distress syndrome usually resolves in a week. Eventually, your infant's lungs will mature and will be able to produce their own surfactant. As soon as the baby is able to breath normally without help, he or she will be taken off the ventilator. With treatment, most infants have a good chance of recovering completely in 1 or 2 weeks.

RETINOBLASTOMA

Retinoblastoma is a rare cancer of the eye that develops in a child's retina, the light-sensitive layer of tissue at the back of the eyeball. It occurs most frequently in children under the age of 5. Cancer cells from the initial tumor in the retina can quickly spread to other parts of the child's body, especially the brain.

Most children get this type of cancer in only one eye, but about a quarter of affected children have the disease in both eyes. Retinoblastoma is an inherited disorder in some children, especially those who are affected in both eyes. If one child in the family has the disease, other children in the family may also develop it, so they should be checked by a doctor for retinoblastoma.

SIGNS AND SYMPTOMS If your child has retinoblastoma, he or she will experience a gradual loss of vision and may eventually go blind in the eye affected by cancer. An ophthalmologist (doctor who specializes in diseases of the eye) can usually see a white reflection in the pupil (colored part) of the child's eye in the early stages of the disease. Some children develop strabismus (VISION PROBLEMS, see page 659) or bulging eyes. Your child may feel pain in his or her eye. You may actually be able to see the tumor in your child's eye through the pupil.

DIAGNOSIS If either parent has a family history of retinoblastoma, your newborn should have regular eye exams to screen for the disease. If your child develops symptoms of retinoblastoma, he or she should be seen by an ophthalmologist who will conduct a thorough examination of your child's eyes. The ophthalmologist will order a *computed tomography* scan or *magnetic resonance imaging* examination of your child's skull to see the site of the tumor and assess whether it has spread.

If your child is diagnosed with retinoblastoma, the doctor may also draw samples of your child's bone marrow and cerebrospinal fluid (the fluid in and around your child's brain and spinal cord) through a needle and send them to a laboratory for testing to determine if the cancer has spread.

TREATMENT If the disease is detected before it becomes large and spreads, the ophthalmologist will probably treat it with *radiation* therapy and *chemotherapy* to kill the tumor cells and preserve your child's vision. Otherwise, some form of surgery will be necessary. Treatment for a large tumor is removal of the entire eye and replacement with an artificial eye. In another type of surgery called cryosurgery, the surgeon attempts to kill the cancer cells by freezing them. A third type of surgery, known as photocoagulation, uses a narrow beam of light to destroy the blood vessels that feed the tumor.

Tumors sometimes recur after treatment. If the treatment is successful, your child may still be at risk of developing another type of cancer, OSTEOGENIC SARCOMA. People who survive retinoblastoma and anyone with a family history of the disease should receive genetic counseling (see page 497) before having children.

RETINOPATHY OF PREMATURITY

Retinopathy of prematurity is an eye disorder found in preterm infants in which the developing blood vessels of the retina (the light-sensitive lining at the back of the eyeball) become damaged before or shortly after birth. Extreme prematurity, exposure to excessive oxygen given to manage a premature infant's respiratory problems, and vitamin deficiencies can all contribute to retinopathy of prematurity. The condition is more likely to occur in extremely low birthweight babies (those weighing about 2 pounds or less).

SIGNS AND SYMPTOMS Retinopathy of prematurity develops in the first weeks after the premature birth of a baby. Soon after birth, the damaged blood vessels in the baby's retina begin to repair themselves. But the regrowth of the vessels can be so excessive that blood vessels begin to grow into other parts of the baby's eye, causing blood to seep into the eyeball, scarring of the retina, and retinal detachment (the pulling away of the retina from the back of the eye). If the excessive blood vessel growth stops in time, the baby's eye may heal completely. But, if the abnormal growth continues and causes retinal detachment, the infant can have VISION PROBLEMS ranging from mild nearsightedness to partial or complete BLINDNESS.

DIAGNOSIS Only an ophthalmologist (a doctor who specializes in disorders of the eye) can detect the abnormal growth of blood vessels in a baby's eye. The ophthalmologist will dilate your baby's pupils and examine his or her eyes with an ophthalmoscope (an instrument used to examine the interior of the eye). The examination is not painful. If your baby was born prematurely, he or she should be examined by an ophthalmologist frequently during the first year of life.

TREATMENT If your baby's retinopathy does not heal on its own, the doctor may recommend surgery using cryotherapy (freezing) or laser therapy to treat the part of the retina that contains damaged blood vessels. The doctor will want to monitor your child's vision closely after surgery. Your child may need eyeglasses or therapy for the visually impaired if the surgery only partially corrects the problem.

REYE'S SYNDROME

Reye's syndrome is a rare, life-threatening disorder that causes a child's brain and liver to swell following a viral infection (especially influenza, see page 231), CHICKENPOX, or an upper respiratory tract (nose and throat) infection. The swelling causes various degrees of liver and brain injury. It most often affects children between the ages of 4 and 16, but it can occur in children of all ages. Children get Reye's syndrome most frequently in the winter months when viral infections are most common. At least a third of the cases of Reye's syndrome occur in children who have had chickenpox. Research has shown an association between Reye's syndrome and the use of aspirin and other salicylate-containing medications, such as some cold remedies, to treat viral infections. Don't give aspirin or aspirin-containing products to children under 18 years old; give them acetaminophen or ibuprofen instead.

SIGNS AND SYMPTOMS Symptoms may range from mild to life threatening. About 3 to 7 days after a child gets sick with influenza (see page 231), chickenpox, or another type of viral infection, the child begins to vomit forcefully. The vomiting may continue and get worse over the next 3 hours to 3 days. The child may also have a headache. As the syndrome progresses, the child can develop signs of encephalopathy (abnormal brain function), which include staring spells, confusion, memory loss, disorientation, slurred speech, listlessness, drowsiness, hallucinations, or sudden outbursts of aggressive behavior. The child may also have a rapid heartbeat (see ARRHYTHMIAS) and take quick, deep breaths. In later stages of the disorder, the child can develop seizures or a coma, or stop breathing because of excessive brain swelling and injury.

DIAGNOSIS If your child has symptoms of Reye's syndrome, get him or her to a hospital emergency department immediately. A doctor will order blood tests to monitor your child's blood sugar level and to look for high concentrations of certain liver enzymes in his or her blood. The doctor will examine your child to see if his or her liver is enlarged. The doctor may do a biopsy to check for liver damage and order an electroencephalogram to detect unusual brain-wave activity; he or she may also do a *lumbar puncture* to rule out other disorders. A *computed tomography* scan or *magnetic resonance imaging* scan will be performed to determine the extent of the brain swelling.

TREATMENT Even if your child has a mild case of Reye's syndrome, he or she will need to be hospitalized so the doctor can *intravenously* replace fluids lost through vomiting. There is no cure for Reye's syndrome, but surgery to implant brain pressure monitors and medication may be used to monitor and control brain swelling. Your child may need blood transfusions or kidney dialysis. He or she may be placed on a mechanical breathing device called a ventilator that helps control pressure in the brain by increasing the breathing rate. The outlook for recovery depends on the seriousness of the illness. In some cases, the symptoms of the syndrome stop progressing and the child may recover fully in 5 to 10 days. In other cases, the child may survive a serious attack, but is left with brain damage. The death rate was once high for children with Reye's syndrome, but has dropped dramatically with earlier treatment and better treatment methods.

RHABDOMYOSARCOMA

Rhabdomyosarcoma is the most common type of soft tissue cancer in children, primarily affecting a child's muscles, tendons (fibrous bands that connect muscles to bone), and the connective tissue around joints, nerves, and fat. It can occur in a child's head, neck, abdomen, bladder, vagina, testicles, or limbs. Rhabdomyosarcoma grows rapidly in muscle and spreads to other tissue in the child's body. Most tumors occur in children under 10 years old.

SIGNS AND SYMPTOMS The signs of rhabdomyosarcoma vary depending on where the disease strikes. If your child has a tumor in his or her throat or nose, he or she may have NOSEBLEEDS, congestion, changes in his or her voice, or difficulty swallowing. A tumor around the eye causes bulging of the eye and difficulty moving the eye. A tumor in a girl's vagina or on the bladder may make it difficult for her to urinate or have a bowel movement. Rhabdomyosarcoma may also appear as a swelling or lump in your child's muscle or testicle. The lump may or may not be painful.

DIAGNOSIS Call your doctor if your child has any of the symptoms of rhabdomyosarcoma. If your doctor suspects your child has a tumor, he or she will order a *biopsy* of the tumor to confirm the diagnosis. Your doctor will refer your child to a cancer specialist who will conduct further testing to assess the extent of the cancer's spread. The tests will vary depending on the site of the cancer.

TREATMENT The most common form of treatment for rhabdomyosarcoma is surgery to remove the tumor. After surgery, your child will receive *chemotherapy* and *radiation* therapy to kill any cancer cells that may remain. The specific treatment and long-term outlook for your child depend on how much the tumor has spread.

RH AND ABO INCOMPATIBILITY

Rh and ABO incompatibility refer to a mismatch between the blood of a fetus and the mother's blood. Rh is a protein found on red blood cells. In Rh incompatibility, the mother's blood is Rh negative (lacks the Rh protein) while the fetus's blood is Rh positive (has the Rh protein). In ABO incompatibility, the blood types—A, B, AB, or O—differ between fetus and mother. The most common type of ABO incompatibility occurs when the mother's blood type is O and the fetus's blood type is not O. ABO incompatibility and Rh incompatibility both cause red blood cell destruction, but ABO incompatibility is a milder condition.

In Rh incompatibility, the mother's blood develops antibodies (proteins that help fight foreign substances in the blood) against the fetus's blood. When the mother's antibodies pass through the placenta (a tissue formed in the uterus during pregnancy that links the blood supplies of mother and fetus), the antibodies attack and destroy the fetus's blood cells. As a result, the fetus or newborn can develop anemia (see ANEMIA, HEMOLYTIC), JAUNDICE, brain damage, or heart failure. In severe cases, the fetus or newborn may die. In ABO incompatibility, the antibodies in the mother's blood cause less severe symptoms.

SIGNS AND SYMPTOMS Rh-incompatible fetuses often grow and move more slowly than normal. An affected newborn is usually pale and shows signs of jaundice (yellowing of the skin and eyes) from high levels of bilirubin (a yellow pigment in bile, a fluid produced by the liver). The child may also have unexplained BRUISES or spots of blood under the skin, generalized swelling, breathing difficulties, seizures, poor reflexes, and heart failure. ABO-incompatible newborns develop high levels of bilirubin, producing jaundice within 24 hours of birth. They rarely have anemia or severe complications.

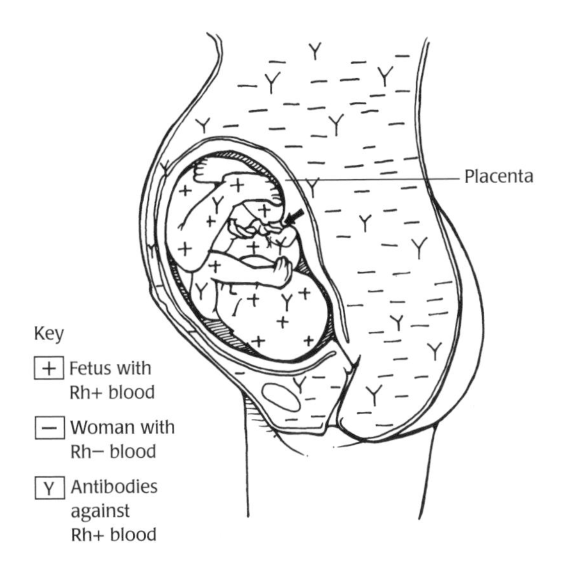

Rh incompatibility

A pregnant woman with Rh-negative blood develops antibodies against the fetus's Rh-positive blood. The antibodies pass into the fetus's bloodstream through the placenta and begin to destroy the fetus's blood cells.

DIAGNOSIS Doctors test the blood from both the mother and child to detect Rh or ABO incompatibility. High bilirubin levels and signs of anemia in the fetus and antibodies in the mother's blood are indicators of the disorders.

TREATMENT If you are a pregnant woman who has Rh-negative blood, you need to seek prenatal care early so your doctor can closely watch your condition. You will receive an injection of a blood product known as Rh immunoglobulin at the 28th week of your pregnancy and again within 72 hours after your child is born or if the pregnancy is terminated for any reason. Rh immunoglobulin destroys the fetal blood cells before the mother can form antibodies against them.

Fetuses with severe cases of Rh incompatibility often receive blood transfusions at the 18th week of gestation or later. Alternatively, the newborn may receive blood transfusions after birth, or exchange transfusions in which the baby's blood is withdrawn and replaced with blood from a donor. Blood transfusions require hospitalization for the pregnant mother or newborn infant.

Phototherapy (light therapy, see page 39) sometimes corrects mild jaundice in newborns produced by ABO incompatibility. Phototherapy may cause side effects such as diarrhea, a RASH, or dehydration, which can be treated in a hospital with rehydration fluids (see page 283) given by mouth or *intravenously.*

RHEUMATIC FEVER

Rheumatic fever is a rare complication of untreated strep throat infection (see STREP INFECTION) marked by pain and swelling of tissues in various parts of the body, such as the joints and the heart. Rheumatic fever most likely occurs when the immune system (the body's natural defense mechanism against infection) attacks the body's own tissues in response to an invasion of streptococcus bacteria (see AUTOIMMUNE DISORDERS). Unlike strep throat, rheumatic fever is not contagious. The disease most often affects children between the ages of 5 and 15.

SIGNS AND SYMPTOMS Most of the symptoms of rheumatic fever occur about 2 to 4 weeks after the onset of strep throat. Children with rheumatic fever have joint pain, swelling, and redness, especially in their wrists, ankles, elbows, and knees. The inflammation moves from joint to joint and the pain can be quite severe.

The child may also develop a red RASH on the chest, back, and stomach; tiny lumps under his or her skin, especially on the forearms; a low-grade fever; and fatigue. Occasionally, he or she may display involuntary jerky movements known as chorea months later. Chorea may occur without other symptoms. Rheumatic fever can damage a child's heart and heart valves, causing HEART MURMURS, chest pain, shortness of breath, inflammation of the heart, and congestive heart failure (see HEART FAILURE, CONGESTIVE).

DIAGNOSIS AND TREATMENT If your child has symptoms of rheumatic fever after he or she has had a strep throat infection, call the doctor. He or she may order blood tests, a throat *culture*, an *electrocardiogram*, an *echocardiogram*, and X-rays of your child's chest to check for any damage to the heart. To treat rheumatic fever, the doctor will prescribe anti-inflammatory drugs (which may include aspirin) to relieve the swelling and inflammation. He or she will also prescribe antibiotics to treat strep throat. Your child may also need heart drugs and, if the disease has damaged the heart valves, he or she may need surgery later in life to repair or replace the valves.

Your child will need to rest for 2 to 12 weeks, depending on the seriousness of his or her condition. Rheumatic fever can recur if your child gets another strep throat infection. The doctor may recommend that your child take antibiotics daily until he or she is an adult to prevent streptococcus infections and a recurrence of rheumatic fever.

RINGWORM

Ringworm (see page 24) is an infection of the scalp or skin that occurs in children of all ages but most commonly affects those between the ages of 2 and 10. A child can pick it up easily through direct contact with another infected child or a pet, or by sharing hats, brushes, combs, barrettes, pillows, or towels used by infected children. The infection is caused by a fungus known as tinea, not by a worm.

SIGNS AND SYMPTOMS The fungus infects the roots of the hair on your child's head and body, causing the hair to fall out and leaving small, round, red patches that slowly enlarge. The skin in the infected areas sometimes becomes scaly and itchy. Some children get ringworm on the face in the form of a round, pink RASH with a red, ringlike, raised border and clear center. Others develop small, tender, pus-filled swellings on the scalp called kerions, which may drain. The child's nails sometimes become pitted, thick, and discolored.

Untreated, ringworm can spread over your child's scalp and body. Your child can spread the infection to other people until he or she gets treatment.

DIAGNOSIS To diagnose ringworm, your child's doctor will examine a scraping of infected skin under a microscope, but will probably be able to recognize ringworm by its appearance.

TREATMENT For scalp infections, your child's doctor will probably prescribe an antifungal medicine known as griseofulvin, which your child will have to take by mouth in liquid or capsule form for 6 to 8 weeks. Give your child the medication with fatty foods, such as whole milk, cottage cheese, ice cream, or yogurt, which will help your child absorb the medicine. Wash your child's hair with an over-the-counter shampoo that contains the antifungal ingredient selenium sulfide twice a week for 8 weeks. Schools and day-care centers encourage parents to keep a child with ringworm home until the child has started taking the medication and using the antifungal shampoo.

For skin infections on other areas of your child's body, the doctor will prescribe an antifungal lotion that you can apply to your child's affected skin at home until the rash completely disappears in 2 to 4 weeks.

ROCKY MOUNTAIN SPOTTED FEVER

Rocky Mountain spotted fever is an infection transmitted by tick bites. People can get the infection at any age, but it is most common in children. Although the infection was first discovered in the Rocky Mountains, it most often occurs on the eastern seaboard from Massachusetts to Florida and in southern states from Alabama to Texas. The infectious organism, a bacterium known as rickettsia, lives in certain wood and dog ticks. The infection can also be spread when secretions from a crushed tick enter a child's body through a cut or wound, but the infection cannot be spread from person to person.

SIGNS AND SYMPTOMS It may take 1 or 2 weeks after a tick bite before symptoms occur. The symptoms usually begin suddenly and include a high fever up to 105°F, chills, muscle aches, muscle weakness, and a severe HEADACHE. One to 5 days later, a RASH begins on the child's hands and feet and spreads to the rest of the body (except the face). Initially the rash is made up of small red spots, but may change to look like BRUISES. The child may also have a stiff back, red eyes, mental confusion, seizures, nausea, and vomiting. If the infection is left untreated, it can damage the child's lungs, liver, and kidneys. In severe cases, it can even cause death.

DIAGNOSIS AND TREATMENT To confirm a diagnosis of Rocky Mountain spotted fever, the doctor will order blood tests but may start treatment before the test results are back. He or she may also do a *lumbar puncture* to test your child's spinal fluid for the rickettsia bacteria. Mild symptoms can be treated at home with oral antibiotics. Give your child plenty of liquids and acetaminophen (not aspirin) to relieve the pain. Your child should stay home from school or day care until the fever disappears. Keep the doctor informed of your child's progress while he or she is at home. If your child has moderate to severe symptoms, he or she will need to be hospitalized and receive the antibiotics *intravenously*.

ROSEOLA

Roseola is a common viral infection characterized by a red RASH that usually occurs in about a third of all infants and toddlers between the ages of 6 months and 3 years. Not much is known about how the infection spreads or how long it takes for an infant to show signs of the illness after exposure to the virus.

SIGNS AND SYMPTOMS The infant develops a rapidly rising fever that lasts for 4 or 5 days, with temperatures ranging from 101°F to 104°F or higher. Your child's fever may go up and down, but there may be no other signs of illness. He or she may be fussy or irritable, but not all the time. Then your child's temperature will return to normal, but he or she will develop a skin rash consisting of small red blotches that break out all over his or her body. The rash (see page 24) appears within 1 to 2 days after the fever ends. Your child may become slightly irritable. Many children get mild cases of roseola and show no symptoms at all. Even a mild case confers lifelong immunity against new roseola infection.

DIAGNOSIS Your child's doctor will be able to diagnose your child's condition based on your description of the characteristic rash after a fever.

R

Treatment You can treat your child at home with a fever-reducing over-the-counter medication containing acetaminophen or ibuprofen. Make sure to give your child plenty of fluids. Lukewarm baths will help to reduce the fever. Let your child get plenty of rest. Your child should recover fully in about a week. If he or she does not, call your doctor again.

Roundworms

Roundworms, also called nematodes, are parasites that reside in the intestines and, sometimes, the lungs and liver. There are many different types. Worm eggs enter a child's mouth when he or she ingests water, food, or soil contaminated by the feces of infected animals or other children. The roundworms may also enter a child's body through the skin or an insect bite.

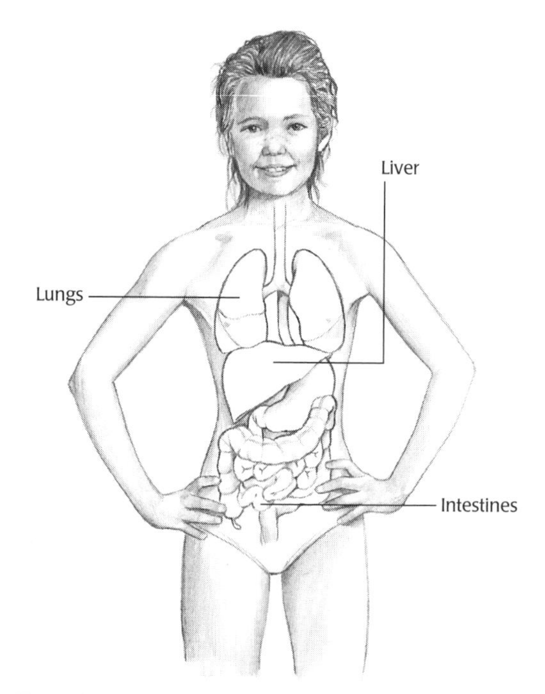

Roundworms migrate throughout the body
Roundworm eggs hatch in the intestine and the worms can migrate to such organs as the liver and lungs.

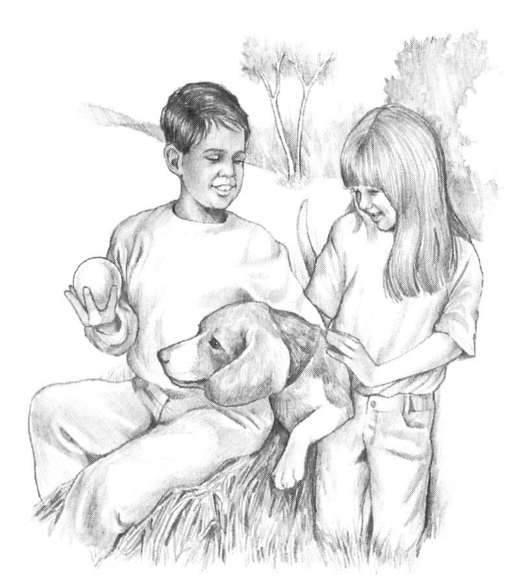

Roundworms from infected animals
A child can ingest roundworms by touching soil containing the feces of an infected animal and then transferring the worms to his or her mouth. Make sure your child washes his or her hands thoroughly after playing with an animal or after playing outdoors. Have your dog dewormed regularly.

Signs and symptoms The worms look like earthworms and can sometimes be seen in a child's stool or bed. Some children have no symptoms; others lose weight and become restless at night, irritable, and fatigued. An affected child may also have hives, a fever, diarrhea, bloody stools, and abdominal discomfort. If roundworms infect the lungs, the child will cough up blood and have symptoms of REACTIVE AIRWAY DISEASE.

Diagnosis and treatment If you can provide a sample of some of the worms, put them in a jar for your child's doctor to examine. The doctor will take a stool sample and may also order an X-ray of your child's lungs. The doctor will prescribe an antiworm medication and your child should recover in about a week. In the meantime, launder your child's soiled bedding, underwear, towels, washcloths, and nightclothes in hot water or soak them in ammonia and water to kill all the worms. Keep your child's fingernails short and remind your child to keep his or her hands away from his or her mouth to avoid reinfection. Be sure your child washes his or her hands thoroughly and often, especially before meals, after using the toilet, and after he or she has been playing outdoors.

Rubella

See German measles

Rubeola

See Measles

Rumination

Rumination is a rare eating disorder in which a child repeatedly throws up partially digested food and then chews and swallows it again. It most often occurs in infants from 3 to 12 months old, although it can also occur in children and adolescents. No one knows for sure what causes rumination. It has been linked to intestinal disorders and GASTROESOPHAGEAL REFLUX AND HIATAL HERNIA. Adolescents with BULIMIA may also experience rumination. It is also sometimes found in children with MENTAL RETARDATION. Rumination is also linked to stressful interactions between an infant and a parent at feeding times and poor bonding between parent and child. The parent may need to interact more closely and lovingly with the baby to create a close bond. Rumination is a controlling behavior in these infants; they use it to gain attention.

Signs and symptoms The child may begin to suck in air or make chewing motions, arch the back, and repeatedly move his or her head. The child's abdominal muscles stiffen. The infant may stick a finger in his or her mouth both before and during regurgitation or gag on his or her tongue to make the food come up. The child then chews and swallows the food repeatedly. Any food that spills out of the child's mouth may be small, but it can contribute to lowered resistance to disease, MALNUTRITION, and FAILURE TO THRIVE.

Diagnosis and treatment The doctor will order *barium X-ray* studies to detect any physical causes of rumination. The usual treatment is behavior modification therapy or psychotherapy to change your child's behavior and improve the parent-child bond. The therapist may want to observe your interaction with your child while you are feeding him or her to suggest ways of improving the feeding process. If your child has gastroesophageal reflux, the doctor will probably prescribe medication. If medication fails, surgery may be necessary to prevent reflux or to repair a hiatal hernia.

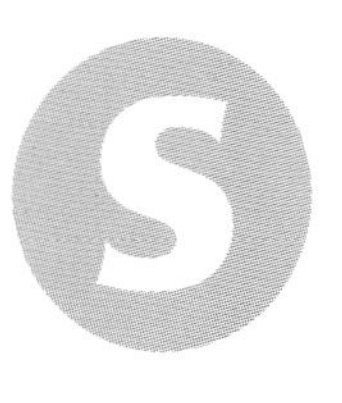

Scabies

Scabies is an extremely itchy skin condition caused by a mite that burrows under the skin and lays eggs. A child can contract scabies from direct contact with an infected person or by sharing clothing, bedding, and towels that have been used by an infected person. Children often become infected at day-care centers and at school. Once infected, your child can infect your whole family. Infants and young children tend to get worse cases than teens and adults because their skin is more sensitive.

Signs and symptoms You will see your child scratching areas of his or her body where the mites have burrowed under the skin. The itching may be most intense at night, robbing your child of sleep, so he or she may be tired and irritable during the day. The mite is attracted to warm, moist areas of the body, such as the skin between the fingers, the wrists, the armpits, the waist, the buttocks, and the genitals, but it can infest any area of the body. The mites cause small, red bumps and a noticeable RASH. You may be able to see red streaks on your child's skin caused by the mites burrowing under the skin. The rash itches and the child's scratching can produce sores and scabs. Intense scratching can lead to a bacterial infection, such as IMPETIGO. Bacterial infections produce crusty sores that sometimes have pus draining from them.

Diagnosis Call your child's doctor at the first signs of scabies because the infection is very contagious and should be diagnosed and treated right away. The doctor may diagnose your child through physical examination alone or might take a scraping of infected skin and examine it under a microscope.

Treatment Your child's doctor will prescribe a lotion or cream to kill the mites. Give your child a bath before applying the insecticide. The doctor may or may not tell you to apply the lotion to your child's scalp and head, but the medication should always be applied in a thin layer all over your child's body from the neck down. Young infants may need different treatment because the insecticide may be too strong for them. The doctor may also prescribe *corticosteroid* creams or antihistamines to relieve the itching. If your child has also developed a bacterial infection, he or she will probably need to take antibiotic ointments or pills.

The mites can live in clothing and bedding for up to a week, so you will have to wash your child's clothing, bedding, washcloths, and towels in hot, soapy water and dry them in a dryer to kill the mites. Dry-clean any clothing that cannot be washed.

Apply a moisturizing lotion to your child's skin after treatment to relieve dryness and itching. Your child can return to day care or school the day after treatment with the lotion or cream. All evidence of scabies should be gone within 2 to 4 weeks. If new areas of rash develop, you may need to apply the insecticide lotion or cream again. All of the members of your family will need to be treated for scabies infestation to prevent recurrence.

Scarlet fever

Scarlet fever is a contagious infection caused by a streptococcus bacteria. It most often occurs in children between the ages of 2 and 10. Scarlet fever usually follows a throat infection by streptococcus (see STREP INFECTION) but occasionally occurs following a skin or blood infection with the bacteria. The streptococcus bacteria produce a scarlet-fever *toxin* that causes the symptoms. The bacteria are spread when an infected person coughs, sneezes, or breathes the germs into the air. Scarlet fever most often occurs in the winter and spring.

Signs and symptoms Scarlet fever causes a bright red RASH that begins on the neck, armpits, and groin and then spreads to the chest, back, and extremities. The rash is made up of red bumps that look like sunburn and have a sandpapery texture. The child's tongue also becomes bright red. Other possible symptoms include a fever up to 104°F, a sore throat, swollen glands in the neck, coughing, and vomiting. The child may have swollen tonsils and develop red lines in the creases at the elbows and in the groin area. The child's rash may last up to 7 to 10 days and then fade. The skin on the fingers may peel as the rash goes away.

Diagnosis and treatment Your child's doctor can diagnose this disease from its characteristic rash. He or she may order a throat *culture* and blood tests to confirm the diagnosis. The doctor will prescribe antibiotics that your child should take by mouth. Follow the doctor's instructions and make sure your child takes all of the medication. In some cases, your child's doctor may recommend an injectable antibiotic instead of an oral medication. With treatment, your child should recover in about 10 days. Your child will need to rest and drink plenty of liquids until the symptoms are gone. Give your child acetaminophen or ibuprofen (not aspirin) for the fever.

SCHIZOPHRENIA

Schizophrenia is a type of PSYCHOSIS, a serious mental disorder that causes bizarre behavior, disturbed thinking, and abnormal emotional reactions. It is rare in children and difficult to recognize before a child reaches 4 or 5 years old. Boys are affected more often than girls. Schizophrenia tends to run in families. Children with parents or siblings who have schizophrenia have a 10 percent chance of developing the disorder, and a 50 percent chance if an identical twin is schizophrenic. Doctors do not know for sure what causes schizophrenia, but studies have shown that it may be related to brain damage before or after birth, stress in a child's life, or the use of drugs such as amphetamines. Schizophrenia is a lifelong illness.

SIGNS AND SYMPTOMS Children with schizophrenia have a variety of symptoms that affect their behavior, thinking, and emotions. They may have hallucinations (perceiving objects or hearing voices that are not real) or have trouble distinguishing dreams from reality. Delusions, false but persistent thoughts or beliefs, are usually present. They may speak extremely loudly or softly without reason. Children with schizophrenia often make up words and string words together in sentences that make no sense, a phenomenon known as a "word salad." They have difficulty keeping their minds on one thing and may illogically jump from one topic to another in a conversation. They usually have learning problems because they cannot concentrate. An affected child's emotional responses may be flat, or he or she may have extreme high and low mood swings. Withdrawal, angry outbursts, ANXIETY, and the expression of incongruous emotions, such as laughing at something sad, also occur. Schizophrenic adolescents are at risk of violent behavior and suicide. The symptoms can vary in intensity from severe to mild at various times in the child's life. A child may have episodes of severe symptoms followed by periods of mild symptoms or no symptoms at all.

DIAGNOSIS If your child displays any symptoms of schizophrenia, the doctor will thoroughly examine your child and may order a *computed tomography* scan, *magnetic resonance imaging* exam, or *positron emission tomography* scan of your child's brain. The doctor will also refer your child to a psychiatrist for a complete evaluation and testing. Other specialists may be called on to evaluate your child's speech, language, or behavior.

TREATMENT Your child will need psychotherapy and your family may need group therapy to cope with the demands of caring for a schizophrenic child. Your child's doctor may recommend medication to control symptoms such as hallucinations and delusions. Your child may need to be hospitalized if he or she has severe symptoms or is suicidal or violent. Adolescent schizophrenics may require treatment in a residential treatment center. At school, your child will need special education to meet his or her specialized needs. At home, you will need to have great patience in teaching your child the difference between fantasy and reality, nonsense and reason, and inappropriate and acceptable behavior. Some children respond well to treatment but many do not. Ask your child's doctor or a social worker at your local hospital about support groups in your community for families of children with schizophrenia so you can share your concerns with similarly affected families

SCOLIOSIS

Scoliosis is an abnormal curvature of a child's spine. The most common type of scoliosis, known as idiopathic scoliosis, develops in adolescents during the period of rapid growth beginning at about age 10 or 12 years. Girls are more commonly affected than boys. Other types of scoliosis can be present at birth or develop at any time during childhood. For most cases of scoliosis, the cause is unknown. But the deformity is sometimes inherited and can be caused by an underlying condition, such as uneven leg length, or by a disease, such as MUSCULAR DYSTROPHY, CEREBRAL PALSY, SPINA BIFIDA, NEUROFIBROMATOSIS, or MARFAN SYNDROME.

SIGNS AND SYMPTOMS The most obvious sign of scoliosis is a curvature of the child's spine. The curve may cause one of the child's shoulders to be higher than the other or one hip to be out of line with the other. The child's legs may also appear to be unequal in length, and his or her ribs may stick out on one side more than on the other. In many children, the curvature is so slight that it causes no noticeable physical problems. However, if the curve becomes severe, it can affect the child's heart and lungs and hamper the ability of these organs to work properly. A significant curvature can also affect the child's height.

DIAGNOSIS You may be able to detect scoliosis in your child. Have him or her bend over and then look for a curve in the spine or a hump on one side of his or her back (see page 233). Many schools screen for scoliosis in the fifth or sixth grade. Your doctor will check for scoliosis as part of your child's routine physical examination. If your child has any sign of scoliosis, the doctor may refer your child to an orthopedic (bone) specialist for evaluation and treatment. The orthopedist will examine your child's back, shoulders, and hips and order X-rays to confirm the diagnosis. Your child's doctor or a specialist will measure the degree of spinal curvature to see how much it deviates from the norm.

TREATMENT Your child's treatment will depend on the degree of the curvature of his or her spine. If the curvature is less than 10 degrees, your child may need no treatment at all, but the doctor will want to examine your child again in 1 year to see if the curvature has gotten any worse. If the curvature is between 10 and 20 degrees, the doctor will examine your child every 4 to 6 months to see if the scoliosis has progressed. Scoliosis of more than 20 degrees requires treatment.

The initial treatment is usually a lightweight brace that your child can wear under his or her clothing to stop the curvature from getting worse. The child needs to wear the brace almost 24 hours a day until he or she stops growing. He or she may also need physical therapy to help strengthen the muscles in his or her back.

If the brace does not work or the curvature of your child's spine is more than 40 degrees, the doctor or specialist may recommend surgical correction. An orthopedic surgeon will fuse the bones in your child's spine together to strengthen it and may also need to place one or more metal rods inside your child's back to straighten the spine. Your child will have to be in the hospital for about a week for the surgery and then will need about 6 months of recuperation. During this time, the doctor might place a brace around your child's torso to protect his or her spine. Your child should be able to resume normal activities in 6 months to a year after surgery.

SEBORRHEIC DERMATITIS

Seborrheic dermatitis is a common skin condition characterized by red, inflamed patches of skin covered by white scales. It can occur in children and adults, but commonly affects infants in the first year of life. If seborrheic dermatitis affects an infant's scalp, it is known as CRADLE CAP. The cause of seborrheic dermatitis is not known, but it has been linked to a variety of conditions, including oily skin, ACNE, PSORIASIS, and obesity.

Hot or cold weather conditions and infrequent shampooing can also bring on the condition.

SIGNS AND SYMPTOMS The red, scaly areas of skin (see page 23) commonly occur where sebaceous (oil) glands are located in the skin–on the scalp, eyebrows, sides of the nose, eyelids, behind the ears, in the middle of the chest, and in skin folds. The white scales can be greasy or dry, and may itch. Scratching the scales can break the skin and promote infection. When infection occurs, the skin crusts over and can drain pus.

Cradle cap usually clears up on its own by the time the infant reaches 8 to 12 months of age. Children who get seborrheic dermatitis may have it off and on for life. It could also disappear in childhood and then reappear in middle age or old age.

DIAGNOSIS Your child's doctor will be able to diagnose the condition based on its appearance.

TREATMENT If you detect cradle cap on your child's scalp, apply baby oil and leave it on overnight. Then shampoo your child's hair once a day, scrubbing his or her scalp with your fingertips to loosen the scales. Comb the scales out with a fine-tooth baby comb. On other areas of your child's body, apply a low-strength, over-the-counter, cortisone or hydrocortisone (anti-inflammatory) cream. Keep the affected areas clean and dry. Call your doctor if you see that the condition does not clear up after treatment at home. He or she may prescribe a medicated shampoo or a stronger cortisone cream.

SEIZURE DISORDERS

The human brain normally sends out electrical signals along nerve pathways to control activities, such as moving, thinking, and feeling. Seizure disorders are conditions in which an abnormal electrical discharge occurs in the brain causing a sudden change in behavior and involuntary convulsive body movements that are commonly called seizures.

Seizures happen more frequently in children than in adults, especially in newborns. They can manifest as mild inattention or frightening convulsions of the body with loss of consciousness. The child's developing brain is most susceptible to some of the common causes of seizures–fever (see FEBRILE SEIZURES), abnormal body chemistry (see PKU), infections (see MENINGITIS), injury to the brain, or a BRAIN TUMOR.

If the underlying cause of the seizure is temporary, such as a fever, the seizure may be an isolated incident. Recurrent seizures are defined as epilepsy. Most seizures that occur in children have no known causes and do not signal abnormal development.

TYPES OF SEIZURES Seizures result from an underlying disorder in the electrical system of the child's brain. There are generalized seizures (grand mal seizure, status epilepticus seizure, absence seizure) and partial seizures (focal seizure, infantile spasm). A partial seizure affects only a small area of the child's brain, while a generalized seizure begins in one or more parts of the brain and spreads throughout the entire brain.

Grand mal seizure This type of seizure, often called a tonic-clonic seizure, occurs in all age groups. The classic features of grand mal seizures are loss of consciousness and convulsions (sudden, uncontrolled body movements). The child first loses consciousness, may cry out involuntarily, and falls to the floor. His or her eyes roll back and the child has convulsions that affect both sides of the body and that can last for several minutes. Some children turn blue around the mouth or face and have difficulty breathing. A child can bite his or her tongue while convulsing. The child's eyes may turn to one side and he or she may lose control of his or her urinary or bowel functions. He or she may perform automatic, repetitive movements, such as lip smacking. After the seizure stops, the child returns to consciousness but is extremely tired and usually wants to sleep.

Status epilepticus seizure This type of seizure lasts for at least 30 minutes. Status epilepticus may appear as one, continuous seizure or as a series of seizures within at least 30 minutes. Status epilepticus seizures can be life threatening or cause permanent brain damage. Call 911 or your local emergency number and get your child to a hospital emergency department immediately if he or she has breathing difficulty or the seizure lasts longer than a few minutes.

Absence seizure Often called petit mal seizures, these seizures are much less severe but may occur many times in a day. They last for only 5 to 10 seconds. During an absence seizure, the child appears to be merely daydreaming, staring straight ahead with a blank expression. The child's hands, lips, mouth, or eyelids may flutter. The child returns to normal quickly and may not be aware that anything happened. These seizures most commonly occur in children age 4 to 15 years.

Focal seizure These seizures vary according to the part of the brain involved. The child may smell a bad odor, feel dizzy, or turn his or her head or eyes to one side involuntarily for a minute or so. Other possible symptoms include speaking nonsense, walking aimlessly, or engaging in other senseless activity, and repetitive movements of the lips, hands, head, or limbs. After the seizure, the child may be confused and sleepy but usually does not remember what happened.

Infantile spasm These seizures first appear in infants. The baby tenses or shakes his or her body suddenly and briefly several times a day. The infant may also lose consciousness and have difficulty breathing. Infantile spasms can occur until the baby is about 18 months old and then may disappear. The infant may develop other types of seizures as he or she gets older and usually has delayed development (see DEVELOPMENTAL DELAY).

SIGNS AND SYMPTOMS Just before having a seizure, the child may smell an unusual odor or feel an unusual sensation in his or her body.

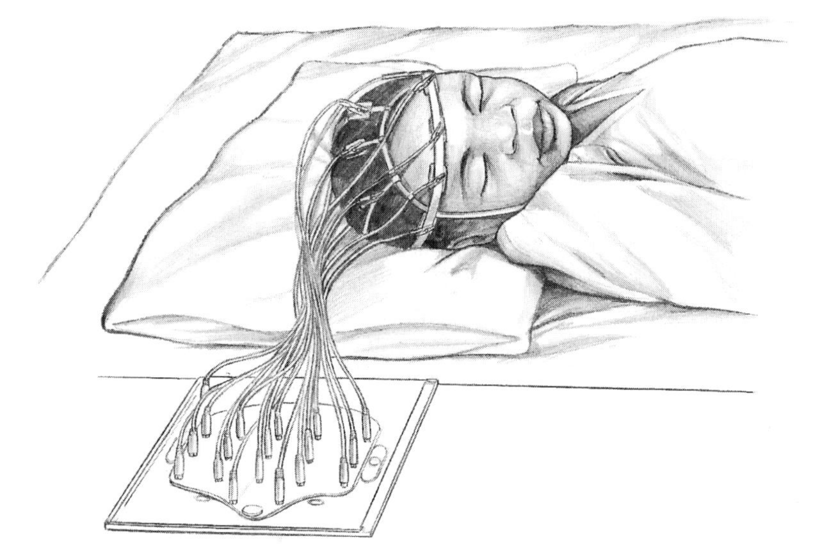

Having an EEG
When a child has an electroencephalogram (EEG), electrodes are attached to his or her head to monitor brain-wave activity. The test can take from half an hour to half a day, depending on the age of the child, and causes no pain or discomfort. The doctor takes readings when the child is both asleep and awake.

These preliminary, warning signs are known as an aura. An infant's or child's body response during a seizure will vary according to the type of seizure he or she has.

DIAGNOSIS If your child has a seizure, take him or her to the doctor immediately for an evaluation. Your child will probably need an electroencephalogram (EEG), a painless test that measures the electrical activity in the child's brain. The doctor may also test your child's blood and urine, and take a sample of his or her spinal fluid to test for meningitis. A *computed tomography* scan or *magnetic resonance imaging* scan of your child's brain will also help the doctor find out the cause of the seizure.

TREATMENT If your child loses consciousness and falls to the floor, try to ease his or her fall and clear away any furniture or other objects that could cause injury. Lay your child on his or her side, if possible, with his or her head turned to the side. Don't put anything in your child's mouth or you could push his or her tongue back and block the airway. Don't try to restrain your child in any way.

S

Living with recurrent seizures

A child with recurrent seizures needs to live as normal and active a life as possible: playing with friends, participating in sports, and, when the time comes, learning to drive a car. But you need to modify or avoid certain activities for the sake of your child's safety. Avoid contact sports, such as football, because of the risk of a head injury that could trigger a seizure. Your child should swim only when a lifeguard is on duty or when he or she is with a responsible person, such as a parent or sitter– never alone. Diving from a high board is not recommended. Your child should avoid high-risk activities, such as hang gliding or scuba diving, because he or she could lose control should a seizure occur.

A parent or responsible sitter should always stay with your young child when he or she is taking a bath. Periodically check on older children who want privacy in the bath or shower to make sure they are all right. Certain anticonvulsant medications cause inflammation of the gums, so your child should floss and brush his or her teeth and see a dentist regularly.

Ask your child's doctor about the possible side effects, such as a rash or JAUNDICE, of any prescribed medication and be alert to any signs of overdose reactions. Inform your child's teachers about his or her condition in case a seizure occurs in school, or if the school nurse needs to give a dose of medication to your child.

Check your state's regulations before your teenager is old enough to get a driver's permit or license. Most states require that the teenager be under a doctor's care and free of seizures for at least 2 years before getting a driver's license. Sexually active adolescent girls should protect against pregnancy because anticonvulsant medications can cause physical deformities, such as CLEFT LIP AND CLEFT PALATE, in a baby. Teens must not drink alcohol or take drugs while taking anticonvulsant medication because taking the two together could cause respiratory (breathing) failure or trigger a seizure.

As a parent, you need to know what to do to protect your child from physical harm. But you also need to give your child the emotional support he or she needs to cope with having a physical disorder that he or she can't control. The loss of consciousness and lack of control over body movements during a seizure can be very frightening and embarrassing to a child, who may fear having a seizure in front of friends. Boost your child's confidence by assuring him or her that taking seizure medication on schedule will help to control the seizures. Teach an older child how to take the medicine him- or herself so your child can feel that he or she has some control over the disorder. Most important of all, emphasize your child's many abilities and remind him or her that you will be there to give needed emotional support.

The doctor will treat the specific causes of the seizures, such as fever or infections. If your child has epilepsy, the doctor will probably prescribe anticonvulsant drugs, taken by mouth, that are usually effective in controlling or eliminating recurrent seizures. Make sure your child takes his or her medication as prescribed. If your child does not take the medicine on schedule or stops taking it abruptly, more seizures could result.

The doctor will want your child to return for regular checkups and to monitor the levels of the anticonvulsant drug in his or her bloodstream. Your child should wear a medical identification tag to warn emergency medical workers of his or her condition. As your child gets older, the seizures may disappear and your doctor may recommend that your child gradually stop taking the medication.

SEPTAL DEFECTS

A septal defect is a heart defect (see HEART DISEASE, CONGENITAL) in which a baby is born with a hole in the wall, or septum, that separates the left and right sides of the baby's heart. There are two types of septal defects. The most common type is a ventricular septal defect, or a hole in the septum between the two lower chambers (the ventricles) of the baby's heart. Less than 1 percent of all babies are born with this defect, but it is one of the most common congenital heart diseases. The other type is an atrial septal defect, or a hole in the septum between the two upper chambers (the atria) of the infant's heart.

Septal defects allow blood from the left side of the infant's heart to flow into the right side. If the hole is large enough, it can make the baby's heart work harder, resulting in congestive heart failure (see HEART FAILURE, CONGESTIVE) and putting excessive strain on the heart muscle.

SIGNS AND SYMPTOMS Ventricular septal defects are often small and close up on their own in the baby's first year of life without producing any symptoms other than a HEART MURMUR. Atrial septal defect causes few problems in childhood, but, if untreated, can cause ARRHYTHMIAS and serious heart dysfunction in middle age.

If the baby has a large defect–either atrial or ventricular–he or she may develop signs of congestive heart failure, such as rapid, labored breathing, shortness of breath, excessive sweating while feeding, a heart murmur, poor weight gain, and delayed growth. He or she is also at risk of developing ENDOCARDITIS, an infection of the heart.

DIAGNOSIS If your child has a septal defect, the doctor may detect a heart murmur during a physical examination while listening to your child's heart through a stethoscope. To confirm the diagnosis, the doctor will order additional tests, such as a chest X-ray, *echocardiogram* (an *ultrasound* of the heart), or *electrocardiogram* (an external monitor that records electrical activity in the heart). The doctor may refer your child to a cardiologist, a doctor who specializes in treating disorders of the heart.

TREATMENT If your baby has a small septal defect and no signs of heart disease are present, the doctor will probably not treat the problem but only observe your baby's progress. Over 80 percent of ventricular septal defects close on their own. The doctor may recommend giving your child antibiotics before having any dental work or surgery; this precaution will help prevent endocarditis.

If your baby has signs of congestive heart failure, the doctor will prescribe heart medications and a high-calorie diet. If your child's condition does not improve, the doctor will probably recommend surgery to repair the defect. Most atrial septal defects require surgical correction during childhood. Surgery is extremely effective in correcting the problem. After surgery, your child will grow and develop normally and can expect to lead a normal life.

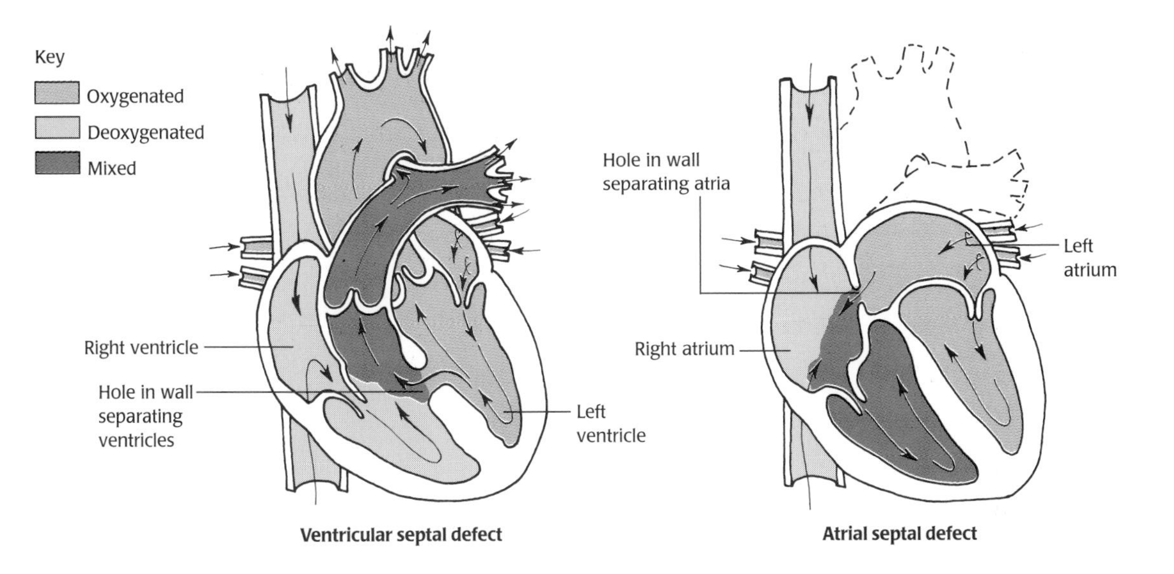

Two types of septal defects

A baby born with a ventricular septal defect (left) has a hole in the septum (wall) that separates the right and left ventricles (the lower chambers of the heart). Some oxygenated blood flows through this hole, mixes with deoxygenated blood, and recirculates through the lungs. An infant born with an atrial septal defect (right) has a hole in the septum separating the right atrium from the left atrium (the upper chambers of the heart). This defect causes the same kind of abnormal blood flow as a ventricular septal defect. If the hole is large enough, too much blood flows through the child's lungs.

SEPTIC ARTHRITIS

See Arthritis, septic

SEPTICEMIA

Septicemia, a more severe form of BACTEREMIA, is a life-threatening bacterial infection that spreads throughout a child's body through the bloodstream. The source of the infection can be a surgical or other type of wound, an abscess (collection of pus), or a major burn. Certain illnesses (such as diabetes, cancer, or sickle cell anemia) that lower resistance to infection can increase a child's risk of getting septicemia. Newborns, low-birthweight babies, and infants under 18 months of age are at higher risk because their immune systems are not yet fully developed. If treatment is delayed, the child can go into shock and even die. Other potential complications of septicemia include infection of the child's heart valves and multiple organ failure.

SIGNS AND SYMPTOMS A child with septicemia becomes seriously ill very suddenly. Symptoms include shaking chills, a rapidly rising temperature, a fast heartbeat, flushed skin that is warm to the touch, low blood pressure, headaches, irritability, lethargy, and confusion. The child may also have a skin rash or jaundice (yellowing of the skin and whites of the eyes). Shock and convulsions can develop. A child in shock (see page 678) becomes dizzy or faint, breathes rapidly, and has a quick, weak pulse. The child also has pale, clammy, cool skin and experiences thirst.

DIAGNOSIS If your child develops the symptoms of septicemia, take him or her to the hospital immediately. The doctor will test your child's blood to see if an infection is present and identify the bacteria. Blood culture results may take from 1 to 3 days to obtain. Your doctor may also test your child's urine, spinal fluid, or fluid from identifiable sites of infection.

TREATMENT Your child will be hospitalized–in severe cases, in an intensive care unit–and will receive antibiotic drugs given *intravenously*. Your doctor will also treat the source of the infection. Your child should recover fully as long as the source of infection is found and treated promptly.

SERUM SICKNESS

Serum sickness is an adverse physical reaction to a foreign substance. It was originally described as a reaction to a medication known as antiserum used to treat children and adults who are exposed to dangerous infections, such as those caused by rabies or snake bites (see page 604). The antiserum was made from the clear, fluid part of blood–the serum–taken from animals that are immune to the infection. The body's immune system can react adversely to the foreign protein in the antiserum. Presently, drugs–especially penicillin–are the leading cause of serum sickness, although insect stings can cause serum sickness as well.

SIGNS AND SYMPTOMS Symptoms develop 1 to 2 weeks after exposure to the foreign substance. The child develops HIVES, fever, swollen glands, and pain in his or her joints. Some children have nausea, vomiting, and abdominal pain. In severe cases, the child may develop heart, kidney, or neurologic (nervous system) disease.

DIAGNOSIS AND TREATMENT Your child's doctor will determine if your child has serum sickness from his or her signs and symptoms. Tell your child's doctor what substance or insect your child may have come into contact with. If a medication caused your child's symptoms, he or she must stop using the medication immediately and avoid it for life. You can apply anti-itch creams or lotions to relieve your child's itching. Your child's doctor may prescribe anti-inflammatory drugs including aspirin for joint pain and antihistamines to relieve symptoms more quickly. In severe cases, your child's doctor may prescribe *corticosteroids*.

SEXUALLY TRANSMITTED DISEASES

See Chlamydia; Genital herpes; Genital warts; Gonorrhea; Syphilis

SHOCK

See page 678

SICKLE CELL ANEMIA

Sickle cell anemia is a potentially life-threatening inherited blood disease in which red blood cells contain abnormal hemoglobin (the protein in red blood cells that carries oxygen to body tissue). The abnormal hemoglobin causes the red blood cells to change their shape from round to curved, like a sickle. The sickle-shaped blood cells can stick together and block the flow of blood through small blood vessels.

In the United States, the disease occurs most frequently among African Americans and Hispanics of Caribbean ancestry. About 1 in 10 African Americans carries the gene for sickle cell anemia. Carriers of the sickle cell trait are usually healthy and have no signs of the disease but, if two carriers have children together, they have a 25 percent chance of having a child with the disease and a 50 percent chance that the child will be a carrier. There is no possibility that the child of only one parent who is a carrier will have the disorder.

SIGNS AND SYMPTOMS Symptoms usually begin to appear in infants at about 6 months of age and can last for life. A child with sickle cell anemia often becomes anemic (has a reduced level of

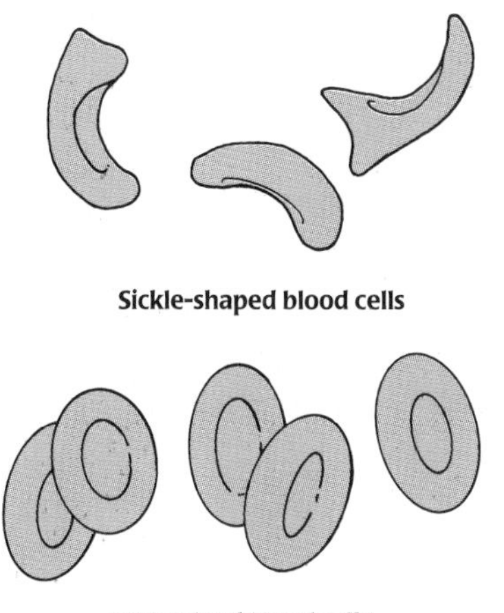

Abnormally shaped red blood cells

Sickle cell anemia produces abnormal, crescent-shaped red blood cells (top) that contrast strongly with the round, "doughnut" shape of normal red blood cells (bottom). Normal red blood cells pass easily through your child's blood vessels, but sickle cells clump together and can block the vessels, producing anemia (a reduced level of oxygen-carrying hemoglobin in the blood).

oxygen-carrying hemoglobin in the blood) because the misshapen red blood cells become trapped in the spleen, liver, or other organs and are destroyed. But because the anemia is chronic (long-term), the child may not feel any worse than usual unless the anemia suddenly gets worse. Then the child becomes easily tired, short of breath, and pale. He or she may also have a rapid heartbeat and JAUNDICE.

A child with sickle cell anemia is at high risk of bacterial infections, especially PNEUMONIA and MENINGITIS, because the sickle cells damage the spleen, which helps fight infection. Infections are the leading cause of death in infants and children with sickle cell anemia.

When the sickle cells block small blood vessels, they cut off the blood flow and prevent oxygen from reaching the surrounding tissue, causing extreme pain in affected areas. A painful episode such as this is called a sickle cell crisis and can occur frequently and last for several hours or even days. Sickle cell crises can be triggered by infection, dehydration (see page 283), fever, emotional or physical stress, cold temperatures, and high altitudes (because of decreased oxygen). Infants and toddlers usually experience pain in their hands and feet during a sickle cell crisis, while older children most often have arm and leg pain.

Other complications of sickle cell disease include FAILURE TO THRIVE and stroke. Blockage of the blood vessels in the brain causes brain damage, producing weakness, speech problems, seizures, or coma. The blood vessels in the child's intestines and lungs can also become blocked.

DIAGNOSIS Doctors use a blood test known as hemoglobin electrophoresis to identify children who have sickle cell anemia and those who are carriers of the disease. Many states now require that all newborns be given a screening test for this and other inherited diseases (see page 223).

TREATMENT No cure for sickle cell anemia exists, but you can work together with your child's doctor to minimize the occurrence of painful sickle cell crises. Beginning at 2 months of age, your child will need to take the antibiotic penicillin by mouth every day. Penicillin substantially reduces the risk that your child will develop a serious infection. Your child's doctor will also give your infant and toddler a series of vaccinations to protect against Haemophilus influenzae type b, a type of bacteria to which children with sickle cell disease are susceptible, and another shot to protect your baby against HEPATITIS B, which is caused by a virus that can be transmitted through blood transfusions. In infancy, your child will probably receive a vaccine against pneumonia and meningitis. Of course, your child should also get the other routine childhood vaccines as well as yearly flu shots (see page 231).

Episodes of mild pain can be treated with acetaminophen with or without the narcotic painkiller codeine, or with other nonsteroidal anti-inflammatory medications as prescribed by your child's doctor. A child with severe pain caused by blocked blood vessels may need to be treated in a hospital. If your child develops a fever of 101°F or higher, call your doctor immediately because a fever can signal a serious infection that requires hospitalization and treatment with antibiotics. Stroke, rapid spleen enlargement, or difficulty breathing also warrant hospitalization. Treatment depends on the child's specific symptoms, but could include fluids given *intravenously*, oxygen, blood transfusions, antibiotics, and pain relievers.

At home, make sure your child drinks plenty of liquids, especially during hot weather, to help prevent his or her red blood cells from blocking the blood vessels and bringing on a sickle cell episode. Don't let your infant or child become chilled because cold temperatures can also trigger a sickle cell crisis. Encourage your child to avoid stressful circumstances and extremely strenuous exercise as much as possible. Teach your child to brush and floss his or her teeth every day and take him or her to the dentist for regular checkups to avoid infections in the mouth. Feed your child a balanced diet to promote healthy growth. Your child should wear a medical identification tag or bracelet to warn emergency medical personnel of his or her condition. With antibiotic treatment and good care at home, your child will be able to live into adulthood.

You and your child should seek genetic counseling (see page 497) to find out your chances of passing the disease on to future children.

SIDS

SIDS (sudden infant death syndrome) is the sudden, unexpected, and unexplained death of an infant under 1 year old. Typically, the infant appears to be healthy and then is found dead after a nap or a night's sleep with no evidence of a struggle to breathe, no bodily trauma, and no crying having been heard. Previously called crib death, SIDS is the leading cause of death among infants between the ages of 1 month and 1 year, affects slightly more boys than girls, and occurs most frequently in the winter. Most deaths occur in babies who are between 1 and 4 months old. In the United States, about 6,000 infants die of SIDS every year.

Doctors believe there are a variety of causes, including the abnormal regulation of heart and breathing rates, poor airway control, and an immature sleep arousal capability. There is no way to predict SIDS, but parents can take certain measures to help reduce the risk (see page 56). A number of factors place an infant at risk for developing SIDS, including premature birth; low birthweight; insufficient prenatal care; laying the baby on his or her stomach during sleep; and a mother who abused narcotics or alcohol (see DRUG AND ALCOHOL ABUSE), was very young, or smoked during pregnancy. All other causes of death must be ruled out through an autopsy and on-sight investigation of the child's death before a diagnosis of SIDS can be established.

Sinusitis

Sinusitis is an inflammation of the lining of the sinuses (air passages in the bones) surrounding a child's nose. The inflammation is usually caused by an infection such as a cold that spreads from the child's nose, but it can also be caused by ALLERGIES, HAY FEVER, nasal polyps (see POLYPS, NASAL), a DEVIATED NASAL SEPTUM, an injury to the nose, an abscess in one of the child's teeth, or an irritant, such as dry or polluted air or tobacco smoke. The sinuses that lie between a child's eyes and in his or her cheekbones are most often affected. Children can get sinusitis at any age. Children under 2 years old usually get milder cases than older children. Single or infrequent episodes last about a week to 10 days. Chronic, persistent sinusitis can last 3 months or more.

Signs and symptoms A child with sinusitis feels pressure inside his or her head around the nose.

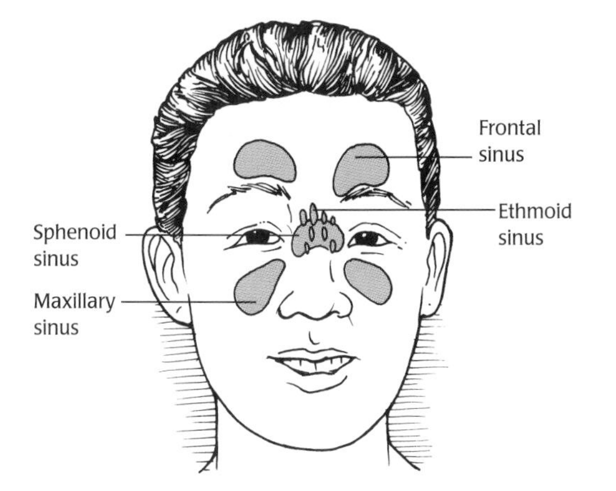

Where the sinuses are located
Sinuses are air-filled cavities in various bones of a child's face. The sinus cavities are located behind the forehead, over the nose, and under the eyes. Inflammation most often affects the ethmoid sinuses, which are located between the eyes, and the maxillary sinuses, which are located in the cheekbones.

He or she may have a throbbing headache that is at its worst in the morning, a runny nose, nasal congestion, postnasal drip (fluid running down the throat from the nose), a fever, bad breath, pain in the cheekbones, swelling around the eyes, and a chronic cough. A child with sinusitis may also look tired, lack energy, and have trouble sleeping.

DIAGNOSIS AND TREATMENT The doctor will examine the inside of your child's nose with a viewing instrument or a strong light and palpate (push on) the sinus areas for tenderness. He or she may order X-rays or a *computed tomography* scan of your child's sinuses to look for evidence of infection. The doctor may also take a sample of your child's nasal discharge for laboratory analysis or do skin tests to check for allergies (see page 406). The doctor will prescribe antibiotics for a bacterial infection, along with salt water nose drops, *corticosteroid* nasal sprays, or decongestant pills to clear the congestion. He or she may also prescribe antihistamines if your child has allergies.

Don't give your child nonprescription nasal sprays or nose drops. Overuse of these decongestants can make your child's symptoms worse. Warm, moist air from a vaporizer might make your child feel better. You can give your child pain relievers, such as ibuprofen or acetaminophen, but do not give aspirin. Place a humidifier in your child's room in the winter when indoor air is dry.

SLEEP DISTURBANCES

A sleep disturbance is an abnormal sleep pattern or an interruption of sleep. A variety of problems can disturb a child's sleep, including nightmares, night terrors, sleepwalking, sleeptalking, sleep apnea, insomnia, and excessive sleepiness.

NIGHTMARES Nightmares are frightening dreams that cause a child to wake up completely. They usually occur late at night when dreaming is most intense. When the child wakes up, he or she may be frightened, breathe rapidly, or cry. Children of all ages have nightmares, but they most commonly affect children younger than 6 years old. If your child has a nightmare, encourage him or her to tell you about it, reassure your child that nothing will harm him or her, and try to get your child to go back to sleep when he or she is calm again. Leaving a night-light on may help.

NIGHT TERRORS Night terrors differ from nightmares and are far less common. They occur as a child is in transition from deep sleep to light sleep or partial wakening; they often happen about an hour or more after the child starts to go to sleep. Night terrors are most common in young children between 2 and 5 years old. When a child is having a night terror, he or she may sit up, look confused or anxious, and let out a loud scream while still partially asleep. He or she may begin kicking, screaming, thrashing, and showing physical signs of terror, such as sweating, shaking, and heavy breathing. The child may stare,

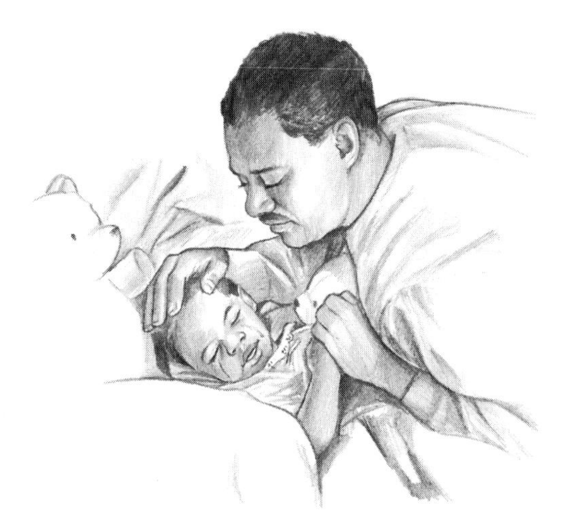

Comforting a child with nightmares
Children younger than 6 years old commonly have nightmares that wake them up and leave them frightened and crying. If your child has had a nightmare, comfort and reassure him or her. Stay with your child until he or she is ready to go back to sleep.

won't recognize you, may try to escape the room, and may push you away if you try to offer comfort. A night terror can last from a few minutes to up to 45 minutes. The child will probably fall back into a complete sleep again and will not remember what happened. If your child has a night terror, try to remain calm and do not wake the child. Gently hold the child if he or she tries to leave the bed. In time, your child will calm down and return to sleep. Be sure to let your baby-sitters know what to do if your child has night terrors. Talk to the doctor if your child has frequent night terrors.

SLEEPWALKING A sleepwalker may sit up, get out of bed, and walk around. Some even get dressed or play with toys. Sleepwalking tends to run in families. It usually occurs when a child is coming out of a deep sleep. The child is fully asleep, is often difficult to wake, and has a blank expression, but is able to see objects in his or her path. The child may return to bed and not remember what happened. He or she may not respond to being spoken to or may answer with only one or two words. If your child sleepwalks, clear a path so he or she does not fall. Don't try to wake your child; instead, lead him or her back to bed. Your child will eventually fall back asleep. You may have to put a gate in your child's doorway to prevent injury.

SLEEPTALKING Some children talk during sleep. They may just make sounds, speak in single words, or talk in understandable sentences. The sleeptalking may occur with or without night terrors. In some instances, sleeptalking arises during periods of stress or illness. If you hear your child talking in his or her sleep, do not wake the child. Sleeptalking is harmless and your child will probably not remember doing it the next morning.

SLEEP APNEA Sleep apnea means the cessation of breathing during sleep for 20 seconds or longer. In many cases, enlarged tonsils or small masses of tissue at the back of the nose called adenoids cause the apnea. Sleep apnea can also be caused by the excessive weight and narrowing of the upper airways that accompanies OBESITY. The child may snore loudly (see SNORING), have labored breathing, sleep excessively during the day, be irritable, have a poor appetite, wet the bed at night (see BED-WETTING), and have a headache in the morning. Premature infants often have apnea because the area of the brain that controls breathing is not yet fully developed. The apnea usually goes away as the child matures. Rarely, a child's brain regulates breathing improperly, causing apnea. If your child has episodes of sleep apnea, see the doctor. Treatment will depend on the cause. Your child may need surgery to remove enlarged tonsils and adenoids, a monitor to assess breathing function, or a ventilator to assist his or her breathing.

INSOMNIA Children with insomnia have repeated difficulty falling asleep or sleeping through the night. The most common cause is stress or worry. Other possible causes include sleep apnea, too much noise or light in the bedroom, sleeping excessively during the day, too many liquids before bedtime that prompt the urge to urinate, a change in the sleep schedule or location, or an illness. To help your child fall asleep and sleep through the night, establish a consistent sleep schedule and bedtime routine. Make sure he or she does not get too much sleep during the day. Reassure and comfort your child if he or she seems anxious or fearful. Read a bedtime story. Calm your child and let him or her know you will be near during the night. Leave a night-light on or play the radio or children's tapes softly. If your child has severe insomnia that interferes with normal activities, talk to your child's doctor.

EXCESSIVE SLEEPINESS Some children sleep too much. They may sleep late in the morning or fall back asleep during the day. Sometimes, excessive sleepiness is related to insomnia. The child has not had enough sleep at night and naps excessively during the day. Excessive sleeping may also be caused by sleep apnea. Make sure your child is on a regular sleep schedule to avoid excessive sleepiness during the day. In some cases, sleeping excessively may be a symptom of DEPRESSION. If your child seems to be sleeping too much, talk to the doctor.

SNORING

Snoring is noisy breathing through the nose or mouth during sleep. In children, snoring can be a sign of TONSILLITIS, a cold, HAY FEVER, sleep APNEA, enlargement of the adenoids (small masses of tissue behind the nose), or other conditions that partially obstruct the child's breathing passages. The noise is caused by vibrations of the child's soft palate, the soft tissue at the back of the roof of the mouth. Snoring occurs more often when the child is sleeping on his or her back. Adenoids are part of the body's infection-fighting system. It is normal for them to enlarge in early childhood, but they usually shrink after the child reaches age 5 and then disappear at puberty. In some children they grow larger in response to infection or irritation, causing partial obstruction of the passage of air from the nose to the throat; this obstruction is what results in snoring.

SIGNS AND SYMPTOMS Aside from noisy breathing during sleep, snoring can produce a dry mouth, bad breath in the morning, cracked lips, and restlessness during sleep. Some children also have sleep apnea (cessation of breathing during sleep for 20 seconds or longer, see page 416), which can cause sleepiness during the day because the child awakens frequently during the night to catch his or her breath.

DIAGNOSIS AND TREATMENT The doctor will do a thorough examination of your child's nose, mouth, and throat to look for signs of an underlying disease or obstruction that could be causing your child's snoring. The doctor might also want to X-ray your child's adenoids. To pinpoint a diagnosis of apnea, the doctor will order a sleep study.

Mild cases of snoring may improve if your child sleeps on his or her side or if the head of the bed is raised up. If your child is a heavy snorer or shows signs of apnea, the doctor may recommend surgery to remove the tonsils, adenoids, or other obstructions in your child's nose or throat. The doctor will treat any underlying infections or ALLERGIES that are causing the snoring.

SORE THROAT

Sore throat–a raw, painful feeling in the back of the throat that causes discomfort when swallowing–is very common in children. A sore throat may be caused by a variety of viral or bacterial infections, including colds, influenza (see page 231), a STREP INFECTION, LARYNGITIS, TONSILLITIS, mononucleosis (see MONONUCLEOSIS, INFECTIOUS), MEASLES, and MUMPS. A sore throat can also accompany HAY FEVER and other ALLERGIES and be caused by irritants, such as air pollution, smoking or inhaling secondhand smoke, and drinking excessive amounts of alcohol.

SIGNS AND SYMPTOMS In addition to throat pain, the child may have difficulty swallowing, a tickle or lump in his or her throat, and a fever. The throat may look red and the neck glands may be swollen. The pain can last a day or two. A child with a sore throat may show signs of an underlying infection, such as a cold or flu. Infants are often irritable, cry a lot, refuse to eat, and have trouble sleeping.

DIAGNOSIS AND TREATMENT You can treat a mild sore throat at home by mixing 1 teaspoon of salt in an 8-ounce glass of warm water and having your child gargle with the solution several times a day. Place a humidifier in your child's room to moisten the air, especially in the winter. Give your child plenty of liquids to drink. Older children can have cough drops or lozenges. You can give your child over-the-counter pain relievers, but never give a child under 18 years of age aspirin unless your doctor recommends it. Studies have linked aspirin with REYE'S SYNDROME in children.

If your child's sore throat does not go away in a few days or if he or she has a high fever, a rash, and other symptoms of a serious infection, take the child to the doctor for evaluation. The doctor may prescribe antibiotics if your child has a bacterial infection, such as strep throat, but antibiotics do not work against viral infections such as a cold.

SPEECH PROBLEMS

Children can have a number of different problems related to speech, such as stuttering, articulation problems, and voice problems.

STUTTERING Stuttering means that the flow of speech is interrupted by stopping, repeating sounds or syllables (as in "sp-sp-speaking"), or prolonging sounds or syllables ("sssssspeaking"). Most children go through a stage when they appear to be stuttering, especially between the ages of 2 and 4, as they develop complex language skills. Almost all of them outgrow the problem by the time they go to school. Children who continue to stutter need your understanding and encouragement. Do not draw attention to the problem by constantly asking your child to talk slower or start again. Instead, listen to your child carefully and patiently. Show approval and love. Making your child feel self-conscious could make the stuttering worse. Talk to the doctor about your child's stuttering. Your child's doctor will refer you to a speech and language pathologist for an evaluation and possible treatment (see box on next page). An assessment of your child's hearing may also be necessary if the stuttering persists or if other language problems are apparent.

ARTICULATION PROBLEMS Children with articulation problems pronounce sounds, syllables, or words incorrectly. They may omit sounds (say "at" for "cat"), substitute one sound or syllable for another ("wabbit" for "rabbit"), or distort a sound or syllable. Articulation problems can result from learning sounds incorrectly, imitating poor speech, or physical disorders such as CEREBRAL PALSY, a cleft palate (see CLEFT LIP AND CLEFT PALATE), or a HEARING LOSS. Children master sounds in stages and should be able to make all the correct English sounds by about the age of 8 but speech therapy is more effective if begun around age 3. If your child has trouble pronouncing words, see the doctor. Your child may need speech therapy and a hearing evaluation.

VOICE PROBLEMS Examples of voice problems include hoarseness, unusual pitch or loudness, harshness, shrillness, abnormal resonance (such as a nasal-sounding voice), or breathiness. Some of these problems may be temporary, caused by straining or overuse of the voice or by a cold. Others may be caused by an underlying physical problem, such as damage to the child's voice box (larynx), damage to the soft tissue at the back of the roof of the mouth, dental problems, or polyps

Speech therapy

Many speech problems can be corrected or at least helped by speech therapy, which should be administered by a trained speech and language pathologist—someone who has a master's or doctorate degree with special training in the evaluation and treatment of speech and language problems. He or she may either be certified by the American Speech-Language-Hearing Association or licensed by your state.

The therapist will listen to your child's speech patterns and examine his or her mouth, nose, and throat. He or she may also give your child a hearing test. Once a specific problem has been identified, the therapist will teach your child speech exercises to improve your child's speech. The therapist may also work with your family and your child's teachers to explain the speech problem and suggest ways to help.

on the larynx or in the nose (see POLYPS, LARYNGEAL and POLYPS, NASAL). Talk to the doctor if your child has a voice problem that lasts for more than 4 weeks. The doctor will refer your child to an ear, nose, and throat doctor (otolaryngologist), who can detect any underlying physical problems. If polyps cause your child's voice problem, he or she may have to undergo surgery to remove them. The doctor may refer your child to a speech and language pathologist for speech therapy (see box).

SPHEROCYTOSIS, HEREDITARY

Hereditary spherocytosis is an inherited blood disorder characterized by a large number of abnormally shaped red blood cells. These unusually small, round blood cells, called spherocytes, have a fragile outer membrane that makes them vulnerable to destruction when they pass through the spleen (an organ in the upper left abdomen that is part of the body's immune system). At times, these red blood cells are destroyed faster than new red blood cells can be produced by the bone marrow (the tissue at the core of bone). When this happens, an affected child develops anemia (see ANEMIA, HEMOLYTIC). Hereditary spherocytosis is the most common cause of hemolytic anemia among people of northern European descent, but is much less common among people of other racial groups. Half of all children born to someone who has hereditary spherocytosis have a chance of inheriting the disorder. Spontaneous mutation (change) of a gene can also result in spherocytosis

SIGNS AND SYMPTOMS The most common symptoms of hereditary spherocytosis are fatigue, weakness, and shortness of breath upon exertion. Your child may also become pale or develop JAUNDICE (yellowing of the skin and eyes) and an enlarged spleen. Affected newborns sometimes have severe and prolonged jaundice. An infection can cause the symptoms to become worse. Gallstones (tiny stones in the gallbladder) are a common complication of hereditary spherocytosis.

DIAGNOSIS Your child's doctor will diagnose this condition by taking some samples of your child's blood and looking at it under a microscope for evidence of the abnormally shaped red blood cells. Special tests are also done to assess how fragile the red blood cell membranes are.

TREATMENT If your child has hereditary spherocytosis, the doctor will watch him or her closely for signs of anemia. Later in life, your child may need to have his or her spleen removed should the anemia become severe. This procedure produces a significant drop in the destruction of the child's red blood cells and a marked improvement in health.

SPINA BIFIDA

Spina bifida is a group of NEURAL TUBE DEFECTS in which a child is born with malformed or underdeveloped vertebrae (the bones surrounding the spine). The vertebrae do not close completely, causing part of the baby's spinal cord and the membranes covering the spinal cord, known as the meninges, to protrude from the baby's back. Spina bifida has been linked to a deficiency of the B vitamin folic acid (see page 578) in the mother before and during the first months of pregnancy.

SIGNS AND SYMPTOMS The most common type of spina bifida, known as spina bifida occulta, is a mild form of the condition in which the vertebrae are malformed, but the spinal cord and meninges remain inside the spinal column. A dimple, birthmark, or wisp of hair along the spine may be the only external sign of this disorder. A small proportion of affected children have a physical impairment. In the most severe form of spina bifida, meningomyelocele, the meninges and spinal cord are exposed on the baby's back. In another form of the disorder, known as meningocele, a bulging sac containing the meninges appears on the baby's back. This sac may or may not be covered by skin.

DIAGNOSIS Spina bifida can be detected before birth. Doctors look for high levels of a protein known as alpha-fetoprotein in the mother's blood early in pregnancy. If the protein is present, the doctor will order *amniocentesis* and fetal *ultrasound* to confirm and identify the defect. After a baby is born, mild spina bifida is often detected as an incidental finding on an X-ray of the spine and more severe forms can be found by a doctor during a physical examination.

TREATMENT If your baby has spina bifida, he or she will need surgery shortly after birth to cover the spinal cord and close the opening in the bones of the spine. A *computed tomography* scan or *magnetic resonance imaging* of the brain may be needed to look for any related brain malformation or hydrocephalus. If the child has hydrocephalus, he or she may need additional surgery to place a shunt (a small plastic tube) in his or her brain to drain excess fluid.

To counteract the bladder control problems that sometime occur with a spinal defect, the doctor will show you how to place a *catheter* through your child's urethra and into his or her bladder to drain urine. Catheterization needs to be done four or five times a day. For a child with bowel problems, the doctor will recommend a high-fiber diet and may prescribe enemas or laxatives to keep the child on a regular bowel-movement

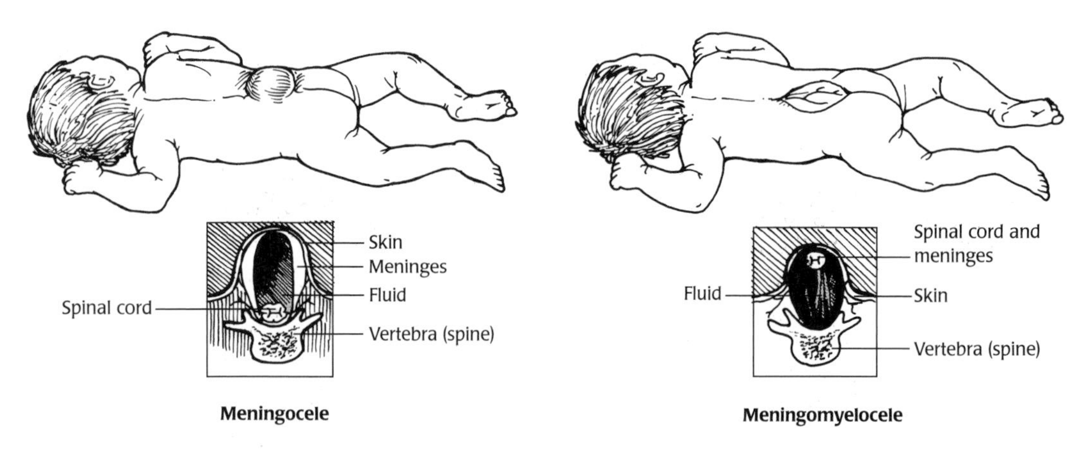

Two types of spina bifida

The two most common types of spina bifida are meningocele, the less severe form, and meningomyelocele. In a baby with meningocele (left), the protruding meninges are covered by skin. In the most severe form of spina bifida, meningomyelocele (right), the baby's malformed spinal cord protrudes from the child's back, covered by meninges but not skin.

schedule. Because the nerve damage is permanent, your child will have to remain on the catheter and bowel-movement schedule indefinitely. You should seek genetic counseling (see page 497) to understand your risk of having another child with this condition and to find out how to prevent it in future pregnancies.

SPINAL INJURIES

See Head, neck, or spine injuries

SPRAINS

A sprain is a stretching or tearing of a ligament, the fibrous tissue that holds the bones of a joint together. Ligaments can be stretched or torn during a sudden twist, pull, or blow to the joint, often during sports. Sprains most commonly occur in a child's ankles, but they can also occur in the knee or wrist. Doctors grade sprains I, II, or III, depending on how serious they are and whether the ligament is partially or completely torn.

SIGNS AND SYMPTOMS When a child sprains a joint, he or she immediately feels severe pain and may also feel as if something has popped in the joint. The joint begins to swell and the pain gets worse if the child tries to move it. If the ligament in the joint is partially torn, the joint will remain stable. However, if the ligament is completely torn, it will no longer be able to hold the bones in place.

DIAGNOSIS AND TREATMENT To determine the extent of the injury, the doctor will examine the joint and order X-rays. The initial treatment for any sprain is RICE–rest, ice, compression, and elevation (see page 677). Put an ice pack or ice wrapped in a towel on the injured joint to reduce the swelling. The doctor will wrap the joint with an elastic bandage for compression and will advise your child to elevate it above the level of the heart so that less blood flows to the joint. Tell your child not to put pressure on the joint to avoid further injury.

The doctor will probably prescribe pain relievers and your child may need crutches and a cast or splint to protect the joint against further injury. The sprain should heal in 6 to 8 weeks. If the ligament has been seriously damaged, your child may need corrective surgery.

STENOSIS, AORTIC AND PULMONARY

Aortic stenosis is a narrowing of the heart valve that normally permits blood to flow from the child's heart into his or her aorta or in the part of the aorta that surrounds the valve. Pulmonary stenosis is a narrowing of the heart valve (or the area around it) that normally allows blood to flow from the heart to the child's lungs. Both types of stenoses impede the flow of blood from the child's heart to the lungs or body. Children can be born with either type of stenosis, or they can develop a stenosis as a complication of another disease, such as RHEUMATIC FEVER, ENDOCARDITIS, or NEUROFIBROMATOSIS.

SIGNS AND SYMPTOMS Many children have mild stenosis and may not experience any symptoms, or may develop them when they get older. Shortness of breath, especially during activity, is a sign of both aortic and pulmonary stenosis. Other common symptoms include fatigue, weakness, and chest pains. Both types of stenosis can cause fainting, but it is more common in aortic stenosis. The severity of the symptoms does not always match the severity of the stenosis.

An infant born with severe pulmonary stenosis can have an enlarged heart, difficulty feeding, poor weight gain, FAILURE TO THRIVE, and congestive heart failure (see HEART FAILURE, CONGESTIVE). In some cases, the baby's skin may also turn bluish. Such symptoms require emergency medical treatment. An older child with severe aortic stenosis can also develop heart failure. His or her shortness of breath may occur initially only during activity, but eventually becomes continuous.

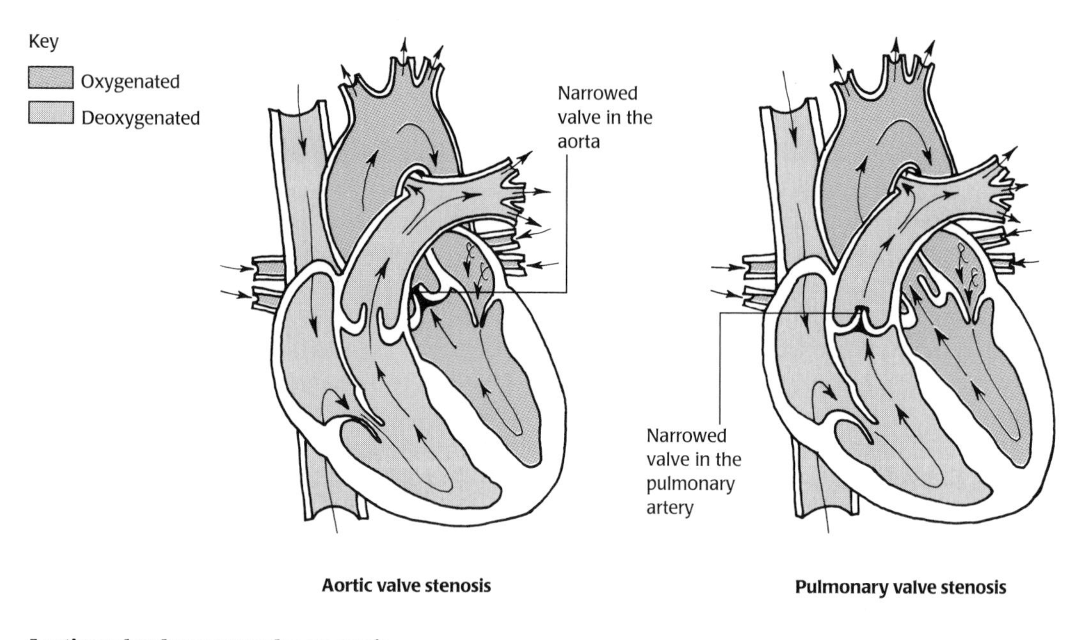

Aortic and pulmonary valve stenosis

A heart with aortic valve stenosis (left) has a narrowed valve in the aorta (the main artery in the body). The narrowing obstructs the flow of blood to the child's body, causes the heart to work harder, and thickens the wall of the lower chamber of the heart. A heart with pulmonary valve stenosis (right) has a narrowed valve in the pulmonary artery (the large blood vessel that leads to the lungs). The narrowing obstructs the flow of blood into the lungs and makes the child's heart work harder.

DIAGNOSIS If your child has stenosis, with or without symptoms, the doctor will detect it during a physical examination by listening for a HEART MURMUR with a stethoscope. To confirm a diagnosis, the doctor will consult a cardiologist and will probably order a chest X-ray, *echocardiogram* (an *ultrasound* of the heart), *electrocardiogram* (an external monitor that records electrical activity in the heart), or *cardiac catheterization* examination.

TREATMENT If your child has mild stenosis, the doctor will probably not treat the disease but only monitor your child's progress. If symptoms become more severe or the stenosis is found to be serious, your child may need to be hospitalized and given heart medications, especially if he or she has developed congestive heart failure.

In severe cases of pulmonary stenosis, the doctor may recommend a procedure known as a balloon valvuloplasty. In this procedure, the doctor threads a small plastic tube with an attached balloon into your child's heart valve through a blood vessel. The balloon is then inflated to open up the narrowed valve. To treat severe aortic stenosis, the doctor may recommend heart-valve surgery to correct the narrowing or to replace the child's heart valve with a mechanical valve. Children with both aortic and pulmonary stenosis need to take antibiotics before any future dental work or surgery to prevent possible bacterial infection of the heart.

STRAWBERRY MARK

See Hemangioma

STREP INFECTION

Strep infection is a contagious infection caused by a streptococcus bacteria. It can occur at any age but is most common in school-age children. Strep throat, the most common form of strep infection, is spread when an infected person sneezes or coughs the bacteria into the air. Strep infection of the skin or blood can also occur, usually following a wound or cut. Most strep infections are caused by a specific type of streptococcus bacteria called group A.

SIGNS AND SYMPTOMS Children with strep throat get a sore throat, a fever (see page 279), and swollen, tender glands in the neck 1 to 3 days after exposure. Left untreated, a strep throat infection can cause RHEUMATIC FEVER. Strep infection of the throat or skin can also cause NEPHRITIS, a serious infection of the kidneys, even if the child receives early treatment. Strep infection of the skin produces red, swollen, tender areas that can drain pus or form red streaks if left untreated. If the infection spreads to the bloodstream, it can cause serious consequences.

DIAGNOSIS AND TREATMENT To diagnose strep throat, the doctor will need to do a throat *culture* (see below). He or she may also order blood tests.

What is a throat culture?

A throat culture is a medical examination in which the doctor takes a sample of the bacteria growing in your child's throat for laboratory analysis. To take a throat culture, the doctor will use a soft cotton swab to gather bacteria from your child's throat and tonsils. The sample bacteria are smeared on a small dish and sent to a laboratory. Within 24 to 48 hours, the bacteria are cultured, or grown, in the dish and can easily be identified by trained medical technicians. Many doctors now use a rapid strep test that screens children for strep throat. The presence of infection is confirmed by a throat culture.

Antibiotics taken by mouth will be prescribed to treat the infection. Give your child plenty of fluids and acetaminophen (not aspirin) for aches and fever. Ice pops and tea with honey will help soothe a sore throat. Try to get your child to gargle with salt water to relieve the throat pain. Your child will begin to feel better 2 or 3 days after starting antibiotic treatment, but needs to continue the medication for 10 to 12 days. Your child is still contagious for 24 hours after starting the antibiotics.

The doctor will diagnose a strep infection of the skin by a *culture* of the wound site to identify the organism causing the infection. He or she will treat a skin infection by cleaning the affected site, draining any pus, and prescribing antibiotics that the child might have to take by mouth, through an injection, or *intravenously.*

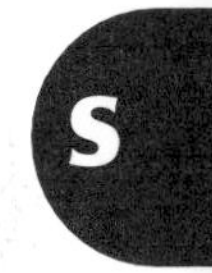

STUTTERING

See Speech problems

STYES

A stye is an inflamed, pus-filled sac on the edge of a child's eyelid caused by a bacterial infection. The infection usually appears in a gland near the root of an eyelash. It can spread to other glands in the child's eyelid.

SIGNS AND SYMPTOMS A painful, red swelling or lump, similar to a BOIL, develops on the child's eyelid near the eyelashes, and then a small whitehead filled with pus appears. The head of the stye is visible on the outside of the eyelid. Within a few days, the head breaks open and pus oozes out, relieving the pain. In about a week, the stye disappears on it own, but new ones may develop if the bacteria have spread to other areas on the edge of the eyelid.

DIAGNOSIS Because the head of a stye can be seen on the eyelid, you will probably be able to recognize a stye on your own.

TREATMENT You can treat a stye yourself at home. Place a warm, moist washcloth on the stye for about 10 or 15 minutes. The moist cloth will hasten the drainage of pus from the stye. Apply the warm cloth at least four times a day until the head disappears. Call your child's doctor, who will prescribe an antibiotic ointment to kill the bacteria. If the stye does not disappear in a month, call the doctor again. He or she may recommend surgical drainage of the stye.

SUBDURAL HEMATOMA

A subdural hematoma is a blood clot that lies inside the skull between the brain and the outer layer (dura mater) of the meninges (thin membranes that cover the brain). The blood clot develops from bleeding usually caused by a severe head injury that damages the blood vessels in the dura mater.

SIGNS AND SYMPTOMS Some time after a head injury—anywhere from minutes to weeks and especially if he or she lost consciousness—the child may get recurring headaches that get worse every day. The child also feels tired, irritable, confused, drowsy, or dizzy. He or she may experience weakness or paralysis on one side of his or her body. The child may also vomit without feeling sick to the stomach and have blurry or disturbed vision. In children, subdural hematomas that appear suddenly most often occur within several hours to a day after a head injury from a fall or motor vehicle collision and produce seizures and difficulty speaking. Chronic subdural hematomas arise from a slow, gradual bleeding and can develop several weeks after a head injury, causing more subtle symptoms that affect the child's ability to think or concentrate.

DIAGNOSIS If your child develops symptoms of a subdural hematoma after a head injury, call the

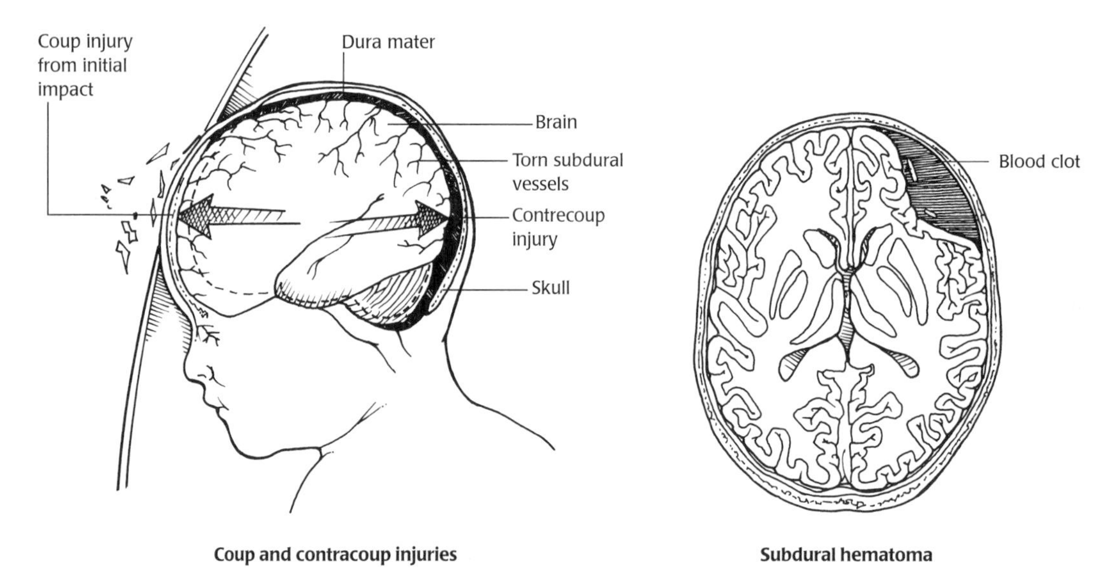

Coup and contracoup injuries

Subdural hematoma

The effects of a head injury

A head injury can occur from the direct impact of a severe blow to the head as the brain moves in the skull (coup injury) or from its opposite reaction (contrecoup injury) as the impact propels the brain in the opposite direction. The movement of the brain can tear vessels in the dura mater (the outermost membrane that covers the brain) or bruise the brain itself. The torn vessels in the dura mater bleed and create a blood clot or subdural (under the dura mater) hematoma between the brain and dura mater.

doctor right away and get your child to a hospital for emergency medical care. The doctor will order a *computed tomography* scan or a *magnetic resonance imaging* scan of your child's head to locate the subdural hematoma. If diagnosed and treated in time, your child can recover fully. If not treated, the child can sustain permanent brain damage, paralysis, or speech impairment. Subdural hematoma can be fatal.

TREATMENT Your child will need surgery to remove the hematoma. During surgery, the surgeon drills into the child's skull and drains the blood clot. The child remains in the hospital after surgery for about a week and may be fed *intravenously* or through a tube at first. He or she may also receive drugs to reduce the swelling inside his or her skull or to prevent seizures. Once home, the child can be as active as his or her strength permits during recovery. Moderate exercise and activity are recommended, although the child needs to rest when he or she is tired and needs to avoid activities that increase the risk of further head injury. The child may also need speech or physical therapy.

SUDDEN INFANT DEATH SYNDROME

See SIDS

SUNBURN

Sunburn is a painful skin condition caused by overexposure to the ultraviolet rays from the sun or artificial tanning lights. Overexposure to the sun in childhood can lead to skin cancer in adulthood. Sunburns bad enough to cause blistering in children or teens double the child's risk of malignant melanoma, the most serious form of skin cancer, later in life. Sun exposure can also cause premature aging of the skin in adults.

SIGNS AND SYMPTOMS Sunburn causes redness, pain, and swelling of the skin 2 to 4 hours after exposure to the sun or a sunlamp. The peak reaction occurs about 24 hours after exposure. Your child's skin will turn pink or red after a minor sunburn and will develop BLISTERS after a more severe one. Your child might develop a fever and become dehydrated (lose body fluids) as well. Swelling is common in the badly sunburned legs. Pain and a feeling of heat on the skin can last for 2 days. The damaged skin begins to peel away 3 to 8 days after exposure.

DIAGNOSIS You will be able to recognize a sunburn in your child on your own.

TREATMENT A baby's skin is thinner and burns more easily than an adult's, so keep your baby out of direct sunlight until he or she is at least 6 months old. If you take your baby outside, dress him or her in clothing that covers his or her entire body and shade the baby's face with a hat. Use a sunscreen to protect children older than 6 months from the sun whenever they go outside. (Don't use sunscreen on an infant 6 months old or less.) The sunscreen should have a sun protection factor (SPF) of at least 15 (meaning that it provides protection from the sun 15 times longer than without it). Children with fair skin should use a sunscreen with an SPF of 30. Apply the sunscreen half an hour before your child is exposed to the sun and reapply it often, especially if he or she is sweating or swimming. Make sure that, whenever your child is outside on a sunny day, he or she wears sunglasses that are labeled "UV (ultraviolet) absorption up to 400mm," "maximum or 99 percent UV protection," or "meets ANSI (American National Standards Institute) UV requirements" to protect his or her eyes from sunlight.

To treat the pain and heat of a sunburn, give your child the pain reliever acetaminophen or ibuprofen (not aspirin). Over-the-counter antihistamines can help relieve the swelling and itching. You can also apply an over-the-counter moisturizing cream on peeling skin, but don't pull off the papery dead skin before the skin underneath has healed. If you see that the sunburn has blistered, trim off the dead skin when the blisters break and apply an antibiotic ointment. Make sure your child drinks plenty of water to replace lost fluids. Give your child cool baths to help relieve the pain.

Swimmer's ear

Swimmer's ear is an inflammation in the outer ear canal that leads to the eardrum. The inflammation is usually caused by a bacterial or fungal infection picked up while swimming in lakes, pools, or the ocean. Children are most likely to get swimmer's ear from swimming in lake water in the hot summer months when bacteria levels build up in lakes or from poorly chlorinated swimming pools. Swimmer's ear can also arise from other types of ear infections (see page 480) and from colds. Children can introduce bacteria into their ear when they insert a dirty finger, cotton swab, or small object into the ear canal when trying to clear out earwax. Irritation of the skin in the canal by hair sprays, shampoos, and hair dyes can also set the stage for infection. Swimmer's ear frequently recurs.

Signs and symptoms The ear canal becomes itchy, red, swollen, and painful. The pain gets worse when the child pulls his or her earlobe up and down or against the ear canal. A discharge of fluid often drains from the child's ear and can turn yellow if the condition is not treated. The skin in the ear canal may be scaly, and the child may feel as if the ear is plugged up.

Diagnosis and treatment The doctor will examine your child's ear with a special viewing instrument and may take a sample of any fluid that is draining from your child's ear for analysis in a laboratory. If the condition is caused by an infection, the doctor may prescribe antibiotic or antifungal ear drops that also fight inflammation. Your child's symptoms should improve in 3 days. For a mild case of swimmer's ear, the doctor may simply clean and dry your child's ear canal thoroughly. Your child should avoid swimming until the inflammation is gone. If your child is on a swim team and needs to keep swimming or if the condition keeps recurring, you can rinse your child's ear canal after a swim with a mixture made of half rubbing alcohol and half white vinegar to dry the ear out and kill germs.

How to prevent swimmer's ear

To prevent your child from getting swimmer's ear, it's important to keep his or her ears as dry as possible. Take these precautions:

- After your child has been swimming, get water out of his or her ears quickly by having the child tilt his or her head and gently drying the ears with a soft towel.
- Tell your child not to stick his or her finger or put any object "smaller than your elbow" into the ears.
- Ask your doctor to recommend an over-the-counter drying agent for the ears or use the remedy described above.
- If your child swims a lot, have him or her wear a swim cap.
- Take extra precautions in a hot, humid climate, when bacteria levels are high in lakes.

Synovitis, toxic

Toxic synovitis is a hip disorder that causes inflammation inside the hip joint. The disease most commonly occurs in children between the ages of 3 and 6 years, but it can also affect infants and children in early adolescence. Boys are more likely to get the condition than girls. Toxic synovitis disappears on its own without treatment in 1 to 4 weeks. The cause is unknown, but may be related to infection by a virus.

Signs and symptoms Children with toxic synovitis develop hip pain, usually on one side of the body only, and a painful limp. They may also have pain in the thigh or knee of their affected leg and a low-grade fever of less than 101°F. The child may have a viral illness, such as a cold or the flu (see page 231). In about 70 percent of cases, the symptoms disappear in a week. In 90 percent of cases, the symptoms disappear within 4 weeks.

DIAGNOSIS AND TREATMENT The doctor will check for pain or a decreased range of motion of the child's hip joint and check for a limp when the child walks. If the doctor suspects that your child has toxic synovitis, he or she will order an *ultrasound* examination to differentiate the disease from other possible illnesses. The doctor might also order a *radionuclide scan, magnetic resonance imaging,* or X-rays. A sample of the fluid in your child's hip joint may also be taken for laboratory analysis. To obtain a sample of the fluid, the doctor will have to insert a needle into your child's hip joint and draw the fluid out.

To treat the disease, the doctor will recommend that your child rest in bed at home. Only in very serious cases will he or she need to be hospitalized and placed in traction (see page 491). Your child will have to avoid bearing weight on his or her hip until the pain subsides and the hip joint has regained its full range of motion. The doctor may also prescribe nonsteroidal drugs that fight inflammation.

SYPHILIS

Syphilis is a contagious infection caused by a bacterium known as Treponema pallidum. Among children, syphilis occurs most often in sexually active adolescents during sexual contact with an infected person, but it can also occur in infants born to mothers who have syphilis during pregnancy. The bacterium crosses the placenta in the mother's blood or contaminates the fetus as it passes through the birth canal.

SIGNS AND SYMPTOMS The symptoms of syphilis occur in three stages. The main symptom of the first stage is a painless open sore, known as a chancre, that appears at the point of infection, usually the penis, vulva, vagina, mouth, or rectum. The sore develops 3 to 21 days after infection. It can last from 1 to 6 weeks with or without treatment. The child may have swollen glands near the site of infection. Untreated, syphilis enters its second stage, marked by a RASH that may appear on any part of the body, but usually appears on the palms, soles, penis, vagina, or mouth. The rash occurs about 2 to 10 weeks after the chancre heals. The child may also have a fever (see page 279), sore throat, a hoarse voice, HEADACHE, loss of appetite, and swollen glands that last 2 to 6 weeks. The child's hair may fall out in patches. The final stage of syphilis occurs years later. Symptoms can include insanity, BLINDNESS, sexual impotence, bone and tissue loss, heart failure, and eventually death.

Infants born with syphilis may have discolored spots or bumps on their skin, peeling skin, fever, and a runny nose. They may also fail to gain weight (see FAILURE TO THRIVE). Commonly, the liver or spleen are enlarged. If the disease is left untreated, the infant may experience liver failure, PNEUMONIA, bleeding sores, and damage to his or her teeth, bones, and brain.

DIAGNOSIS AND TREATMENT If your infant or adolescent has symptoms of syphilis, see your child's doctor immediately. He or she will order blood tests or an examination of the discharge from the chancre. In some cases, especially in newborns, your child's doctor may need to take a sample of cerebrospinal fluid to see if the brain or the membranes that protect the brain and spinal cord called the meninges are affected. Pregnant adolescents are routinely tested for syphilis during prenatal care. Newborns may also be tested at the time of delivery.

Syphilis is usually treated with penicillin by injection. If your child is allergic to penicillin, other antibiotics will be given. During the first stage, syphilis can be cured within 3 months with antibiotics. If it is not properly treated, reinfection can occur. Your adolescent should avoid intercourse for about 2 months after treatment and should be evaluated for the presence of any other sexually transmitted diseases. The child's sexual partner or partners need to be notified so they can also be treated.

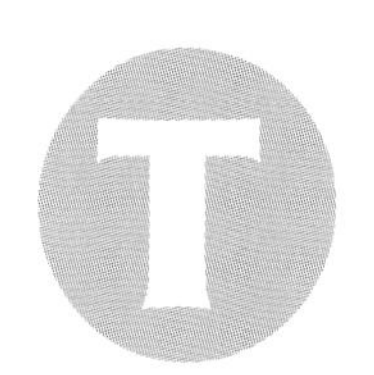

TAY-SACHS DISEASE

Tay-Sachs disease is a rare and devastating inherited INBORN ERROR OF METABOLISM that affects the central nervous system (the brain and spinal cord) of infants and causes paralysis and early death. Babies with Tay-Sachs disease lack a protein known as hexosaminidase A, which helps break down certain fats in brain and nerve cells. Without hexosaminidase A, the fats build up and destroy the baby's central nervous system. The disease occurs most frequently in Jewish children of Central and Eastern European descent (Ashkenazi Jews). It can also occur in French Canadians and Louisiana Cajuns.

Carriers of the disease have no symptoms of illness, but, if two carriers have children, each child has a 25 percent chance of getting the disease and a 50 percent chance of becoming a carrier. If only one parent is a carrier, each child has a 50 percent chance of becoming a carrier but no chance of getting the disease.

SIGNS AND SYMPTOMS In most cases, a newborn with Tay-Sachs disease appears normal at birth but begins losing muscle strength at around 3 to 6 months of age. The child has difficulty turning over or sitting up, stops smiling, loses interest in his or her surroundings, and shows delayed development of mental and physical skills. During an eye examination, the doctor can see a cherry red spot on the child's retina (the light-sensitive membrane at the back of the eye). The child gradually becomes blind, deaf, and paralyzed and may also have seizures and severe constipation. Most affected children die by age 4 or 5.

In a rare form of the disease, symptoms appear between the ages of 2 and 5 and progress more slowly, but the child gradually deteriorates until death occurs at around age 15. Infrequently, children can develop somewhat milder symptoms, such as slurred speech, an unsteady walk, muscle weakness, and mental illness, but do not become deaf or blind.

DIAGNOSIS Tay-Sachs disease can be diagnosed using *amniocentesis* before birth or by a blood test that measures levels of hexosaminidase A after birth.

TREATMENT Unfortunately, no treatment exists for Tay-Sachs disease. The most you and your child's doctor can do is make your child as comfortable as possible. If you care for your child at home, ask your doctor the best way to meet your child's special needs. If you cannot care for your child at home, you will probably need to place him or her in an extended-care center. You and your other children may need psychological counseling to manage the stress of having a child or sibling with this disease. You and your other children should also seek genetic counseling (see page 497) to find out how likely you are to pass on the disorder to future children.

TEAR-DUCT OBSTRUCTION

Tear-duct obstruction is a blockage or narrowing of the tiny tubes that drain tears from a child's eyes. Many infants are born with the condition. In up to 95 percent of them, the obstruction clears up on its own in the first year of life. A child can also develop blocked tear ducts from an eye infection, such as CONJUNCTIVITIS.

SIGNS AND SYMPTOMS The eyes of an infant who is born with blocked tear ducts will overflow with tears and may discharge some mucus when the child is about 3 to 12 weeks of age. The mucous discharge can cause your child's eyes to become red and infected. A child with tear-duct obstruction caused by an infection will have redness, pain, and swelling in his or her eyes; frequent tearing; and a discharge of mucus or pus from the eyes.

DIAGNOSIS AND TREATMENT If your child has an obstructed tear duct from a bacterial infection, the doctor will prescribe an antibiotic to kill the bacteria. If your infant's tear ducts are obstructed but not infected, you can treat the problem at home by massaging your child's tear ducts (located at the inner corner of the eyes, near the nose) with your fingertips or a warm, moist towel to release the contents. Massage the tear ducts with each diaper change until your child's symptoms clear up. Don't forget to wash your hands before touching your baby's face.

If these treatments do not work, your child may need to have his or her ducts opened surgically. Before the surgery, your child will be given general anesthesia (see page 292). The surgeon will insert a tiny probe into the opening of the tear duct and drain the contents.

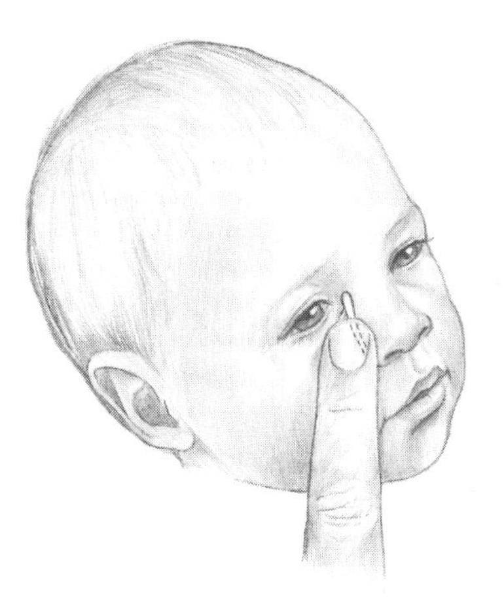

Unblocking a tear duct

If your baby has a blocked tear duct, you can drain the duct by massaging your baby's lower eyelid near his or her nose several times a day. Use a gentle, circular motion to open the clogged duct. Wipe away any discharge with a cottonball or soft washcloth.

TEETH DEVELOPMENT PROBLEMS

Children can have a number of developmental problems that affect their teeth, such as malocclusion (an overbite or underbite), overcrowding of the teeth, defects in the tooth enamel, and early or late tooth development.

MALOCCLUSION Malocclusion means an abnormal alignment of the top and bottom teeth when the child's jaw is closed. The most common malocclusion in children is an overbite. The upper front teeth should overlap the lower teeth slightly but, if the child has poorly spaced or tilted front teeth, the overlap may become exaggerated. The child's lower jaw may also lie too far back, causing an overbite. If the child's lower jaw juts out too far forward, he or she has a malocclusion known as an underbite. Malocclusions usually develop in childhood and are often inherited. They can also result from thumb-sucking, unusually large teeth, or overcrowding of teeth in the mouth. To correct a malocclusion, your child may need braces or a retainer (see page 265) to reposition his or her teeth. Some of your child's teeth may also need to be pulled out. In severe cases, your child may need surgery on his or her jaw to reposition the bones by either removing some bone in the jaw or adding a bone graft from another part of the body to make the jaws line up properly.

OVERCROWDING Overcrowding of the teeth means that the teeth are bunched too close together. Teeth can become overcrowded when they move out of their normal position or are too large, or if there are too many teeth for the size of the child's jaw. Overcrowding can cause tooth decay and gum disease because the child's teeth are hard to clean. It can also produce malocclusion. To relieve overcrowding, your dentist or orthodontist may need to remove some of your child's teeth and fit him or her for braces or a retainer. Braces can straighten crooked teeth, move teeth into their correct position, and guide erupting teeth into position. As your child's permanent teeth come in and the bones of the jaw develop, your child's orthodontist may prescribe a retainer to alter the shape of the palate (the roof of the mouth) to allow for better tooth alignment.

ENAMEL DEFECTS Defects in the enamel (the hard, white substance that covers the teeth) can include pitting, discoloration, an irregular shape, and abnormal thinness. These defects can arise because of an injury or serious illness before or after birth, as a complication of premature birth, or because the child is taking certain medications, such as the antibiotic tetracycline. A family history of enamel defects can also predispose a child to the condition. If your child has defects in the tooth enamel, he or she may need to have caps fitted onto the defective teeth. Other potential treatments include internal bleaching with a hydrogen peroxide solution, or bonding with a white resin.

EARLY OR LATE DEVELOPMENT A child's teeth can come in sooner or later than usual. The primary teeth of newborns and infants sometimes develop too early, but a child's permanent teeth usually do not develop before the normal time. Permanent teeth can develop later than normal if a child loses his or her primary teeth prematurely or keeps the primary teeth for an unusually long time. Tooth development can also be delayed by certain disorders, such as DOWN SYNDROME or HYPOTHYROIDISM. A child's teeth may also fail to erupt because of overcrowding, an existing tooth that is blocking a new tooth's entry, or a dense bone that impedes the erupting tooth.

Your child's dentist may remove teeth that develop early if they are loose. To treat teeth that fail to erupt, the dentist may need to remove extra teeth from your child's mouth or cut away surrounding gum tissue and bone to allow the impacted tooth to grow in. Your child may also need braces to align the teeth, permitting an impacted tooth to erupt.

TERATOMA

Teratomas are tumors made up of many different types of cells, such as bone, hair, and teeth cells, which are unlike the cells normally found in the part of the body in which they occur. A teratoma may be benign or malignant. Most teratomas are benign, meaning they do not spread into surrounding tissue and are not a threat to the child's life. They are rare in children and most often occur in a girl's ovaries or a boy's testicles. They can also appear in the space in the chest between the lungs, called the mediastinum, and in the pineal gland (a small gland deep inside the brain that secretes the hormone melatonin). When a teratoma occurs in newborns, it is most often found near the bones of the lower back.

SIGNS AND SYMPTOMS The most obvious symptom of a teratoma is a noticeable lump on a boy's testicles or in a girl's abdomen, but sometimes there are no signs at all. A teratoma in an ovary may develop a cyst (a sac filled with fluid). Girls with ovarian teratomas often urinate frequently or have difficulty urinating if the growth affects the urinary tract. They may also have pain in the abdomen. A lump may be present anywhere in the body where a teratoma can occur, such as the lower back in a newborn. Teratomas located in a child's chest may produce chest pain, a cough, or difficulty breathing.

DIAGNOSIS Teratomas are often found during a routine physical examination. Your child's doctor may also notice one incidentally on an X-ray taken for another purpose. He or she may order *computed tomography* scans, *magnetic resonance* *imaging*, or an *ultrasound* examination to determine the size, location, and nature of the growth.

TREATMENT In most cases, the tumor is removed by surgery. Microscopic examination of the tissue after surgery will determine whether the tumor is benign (unable to spread to other parts of the body) or malignant (able to spread and invade other body tissue). If your child has a tumor that is malignant, he or she may need *radiation* therapy and *chemotherapy* to destroy any remaining cancer cells after surgery. The results of treatment will depend on how far the cancer has progressed and if it has spread to other parts of the body. Surgery can cure your child completely if his or her tumor is benign.

TESTICLE AND SCROTUM DISORDERS

A variety of disorders can affect a boy's testicles (the organs that produce sperm and the male hormone testosterone) and scrotum (the pouch that contains the testicles) at any time from birth to late adolescence. Some of these disorders require immediate treatment, while others may resolve on their own. Some of the most common testicle and scrotum disorders in boys include the following problems.

UNDESCENDED TESTICLES The testicles of a newborn boy may not have descended from his pelvis or abdomen into his scrotum at birth. Undescended testicles occur in about 2 percent of full-term and up to 10 percent of premature baby boys. In most cases, only one testicle fails to descend. The doctor usually detects the disorder in the hospital when the baby is examined immediately after birth. The undescended testicle often descends on its own within the first year of life. If it does not descend, the doctor will recommend surgery when the boy is about 1 year of age to move the testicle into the scrotum.

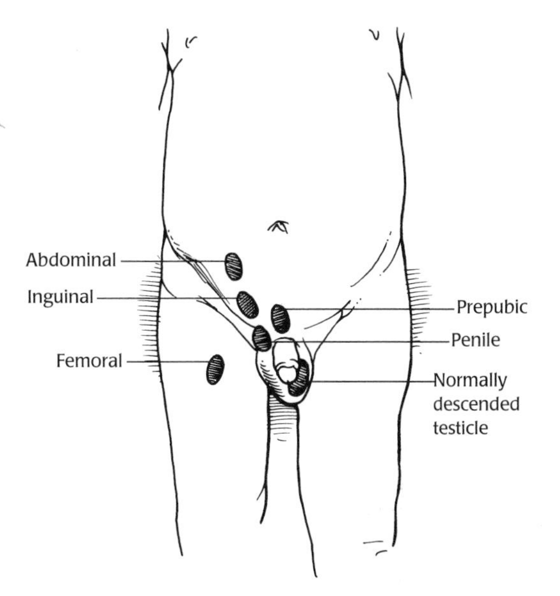

Common types of undescended testicles
The testicles of a male fetus normally descend into his scrotum during the last 3 months of fetal development. But sometimes a testicle has not descended by the time the baby is born. It may descend within the first year of life, but surgery is sometimes needed to bring the testicle down into the scrotum. An undescended testicle can be located in the boy's abdominal cavity (abdominal) or groin (inguinal), above the penis (penile), just above the pubic bone in the lower pelvis (prepubic), or in the upper thigh (femoral).

Without treatment, the child could become infertile and both testicles could become cancerous later in life.

EPIDIDYMITIS An infection that spreads from the urinary tract (see URINARY TRACT INFECTIONS) can infect a boy's epididymis (the tube that carries sperm away from each testicle), causing it to become extremely painful and swollen. The boy's scrotum can also become inflamed and swollen. The doctor gives antibiotics to fight the infection and recommends plenty of bed rest. In some cases, the doctor may order an *ultrasound* or *radionuclide scan* of the testicle to rule out a more serious disorder. Occasionally, surgery may be needed to ensure that the testicle is not twisted.

TESTICLE TORSION (TWISTING) The spermatic cord contains nerves and blood vessels that run from a boy's abdomen to his testicle. Movement of the testicle inside the scrotum can cause the spermatic cord to become twisted, cutting off the blood supply to the testicle and severely damaging it, sometimes irreversibly. This type of twisting occurs most often in adolescent boys. The symptoms include sudden, intense pain, swelling, and tenderness in one testicle; swelling and redness in the scrotum; nausea; and vomiting. Take your son to the emergency department of a hospital immediately if he experiences any of these symptoms because a testicle can be irreversibly damaged in as little as 12 hours. Your son will need surgery to correct the twisted cord. Another type of twisting of the testicle can occur—torsion of the testicular appendix. Attached to each testicle is a small structure known as the testicular appendix, which can become twisted and cause some of the same symptoms as a testicular torsion. Usually, however, the only symptom is a tiny, hard lump in the scrotum. The testicular appendix has no known function and, when it becomes twisted, no treatment is necessary. But, because the symptoms can mimic those of testicular torsion, your child may need an ultrasound, radionuclide scan, or exploratory surgery so the doctor can rule out that disorder.

HYDROCELE Sometimes fluid accumulates in the scrotum in the space around a boy's testicle. This disorder is called a hydrocele. It most commonly occurs at birth or in early infancy. The scrotum swells, but the condition is usually painless. The hydrocele usually disappears without treatment during the first few months of life, but it may signal the presence of a hernia, so the doctor will want to examine your son's scrotum. Surgical correction of the hydrocele is sometimes necessary, especially if it occurs later in life.

VARICOCELE A defect in the veins surrounding the testicles can cause the veins to enlarge, producing swelling and aching discomfort in the scrotum. This disorder, called varicocele, most often occurs in the left testicle. Frequently, varicocele requires no treatment, but, if it interferes with sperm production or growth of the testicle, or if it causes a lot of discomfort, the doctor will recommend surgical correction.

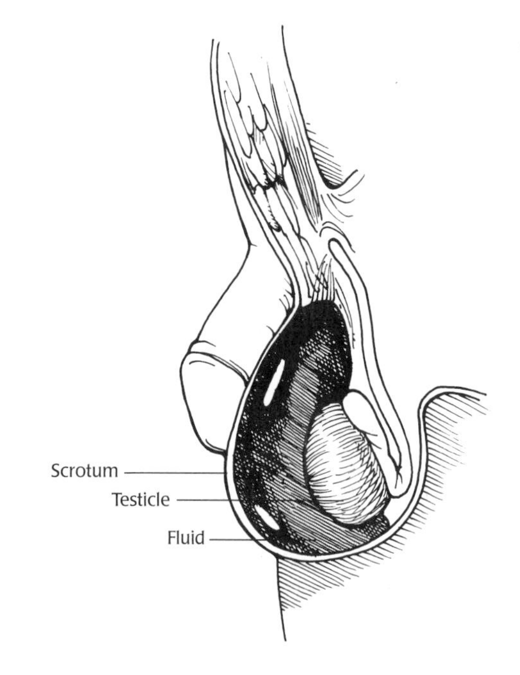

Fluid accumulation in a hydrocele

A hydrocele causes one or both sides of a boy's scrotum to swell up from an accumulation of fluid. The problem can occur at birth or later in life.

INJURY Various kinds of injuries to the testicles, such as a sports injury or falling onto the crossbar of a bicycle, can cause excruciating pain, nausea, and sometimes vomiting. The pain usually goes away within minutes after most injuries, but the testicles can feel sore for several days after a severe blow. Such injuries usually cause no permanent damage, but more serious injuries—for example, one sustained in a motor vehicle collision—can require surgical repair or removal of the testicle.

TESTICULAR CANCER

See Cancer

TETANUS

Tetanus is a life-threatening bacterial infection that affects the central nervous system. The disease is rare in the United States and other developed countries because most children are immunized against it beginning at 2 months of age. The tetanus bacteria enter the body through a wound. The bacteria reside in many places, especially in soil, dust, and animal feces. Once in the body, the bacteria produce a *toxin* that affects the nerves that control the muscles. The tetanus vaccine is usually given in combination with vaccines for DIPHTHERIA and WHOOPING COUGH to infants and children at 2, 4, 6, and 15 to 18 months and 4 to 6 years old. Supplementary doses of the vaccine known as booster shots are recommended 10 years after the last dose and every 10 years after that for life.

SIGNS AND SYMPTOMS The muscles of the jaw and neck are usually affected first. The muscles stiffen, which is why tetanus is commonly known as lockjaw. The stiffness spreads to other muscles, such as those in the child's arms and legs. The child may also have muscle pain and severe muscle contractions. Difficulty swallowing, breathing problems from stiffened chest muscles, fever (see page 279), a rapid pulse, profuse sweating, and seizures also occur. From 30 to 50 percent of those who get tetanus die of the disease.

DIAGNOSIS AND TREATMENT If your child has symptoms of tetanus, see your child's doctor immediately. He or she can confirm the diagnosis from the symptoms and from blood tests and lab *cultures* of tissue from your child's wound. Usually your child will need to be hospitalized for treatment. The wound will be cleaned and the doctor will give your child injections of human tetanus immunoglobulin or tetanus *antitoxin*, penicillin, and a tetanus vaccine booster. Your child may also need help breathing with a machine called a ventilator or respirator and have a breathing tube inserted into his or her windpipe. He or she will be given fluids *intravenously*. With early diagnosis and treatment, your child should recover completely in about 4 weeks.

If your child gets a serious burn or wound, see your child's doctor immediately to avoid infection with the bacteria that cause tetanus. If your child's last tetanus shot was more than 5 years before the injury, he or she will need another dose of tetanus vaccine. If your child has not been adequately immunized in the past, he or she will get both a tetanus vaccine and tetanus immunoglobulin. You will still need to observe your child for symptoms of tetanus after treatment.

TETRALOGY OF FALLOT

Tetralogy of Fallot is a congenital heart disease (see HEART DISEASE, CONGENITAL) in which a baby is born with four different defects in his or her heart. The four defects include:

- A hole in the wall separating the two lower chambers of the heart (see SEPTAL DEFECTS).
- A narrowing of the valve in the pulmonary artery (the blood vessel that sends blood from the heart to the lungs) (see STENOSIS, AORTIC AND PULMONARY).
- A displaced aorta (the main blood vessel carrying blood from the heart to the rest of the body).
- A thickened wall in the lower right chamber (ventricle) of the heart.

These four defects prevent some of the child's blood from reaching his or her lungs, allowing blood that is not carrying oxygen to be pumped to the body and causing the child's tissues to be deficient in oxygen. No one knows what causes these defects to develop, but certain factors affecting the mother during pregnancy have been linked with a higher-than-normal occurrence of the disease in newborns. Such factors

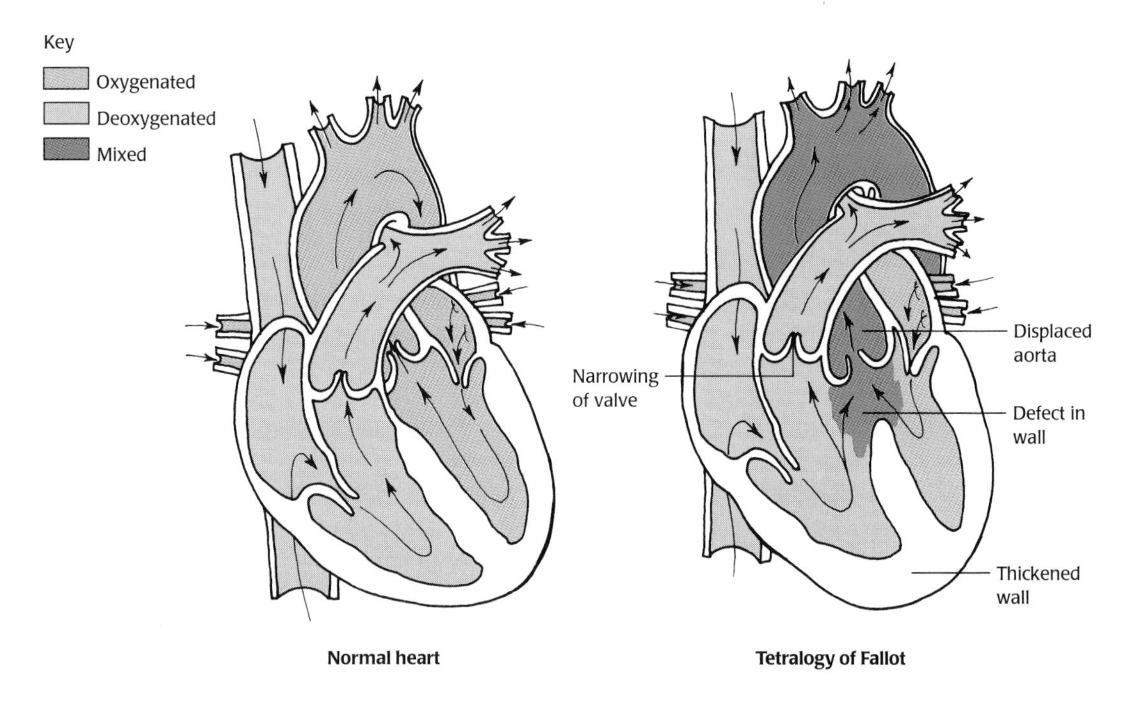

Four characteristic defects

Tetralogy of Fallot is a birth defect comprised of four distinct heart defects: a defect in the wall separating the lower chambers (ventricles) of the heart, a narrowing of the valve in the pulmonary artery, displacement of the aorta, and a thickening of the wall of the right ventricle. Together, the defects cause insufficient amounts of oxygen in the blood.

include GERMAN MEASLES, infection by a virus, poor nutrition, drinking alcohol, being over 40, and diabetes (see DIABETES MELLITUS, TYPE I).

SIGNS AND SYMPTOMS At birth, the baby may appear normal, but gradually the deoxygenated blood begins to turn the infant's skin bluish, especially when he or she is crying or feeding. Signs of the disorder include shortness of breath, rapid breathing, a HEART MURMUR, difficulty in feeding, failure to gain weight, an inability to tolerate exercise, and slowed growth.

If the child does not receive treatment in infancy, he or she may develop thickened, clubbed fingers. The child may also need to squat down after strenuous exercise to catch his or her breath.

DIAGNOSIS Doctors often diagnose this disease shortly after birth, when they see a bluish skin color in the newborn after detecting a heart murmur during a physical examination. A chest X-ray will reveal an abnormally shaped heart. The doctor will also order an *echocardiogram* (an *ultrasound* of the heart) and *electrocardiogram* (a test that records the flow of electricity through the heart) to determine the defects of tetralogy of Fallot and to differentiate the condition from other heart diseases. The child will be referred to a pediatric cardiologist (a doctor who specializes in disorders of the heart in children) for further evaluation and treatment. The cardiologist may order a *cardiac catheterization* with a series of *angiograms* to determine the severity of the defects.

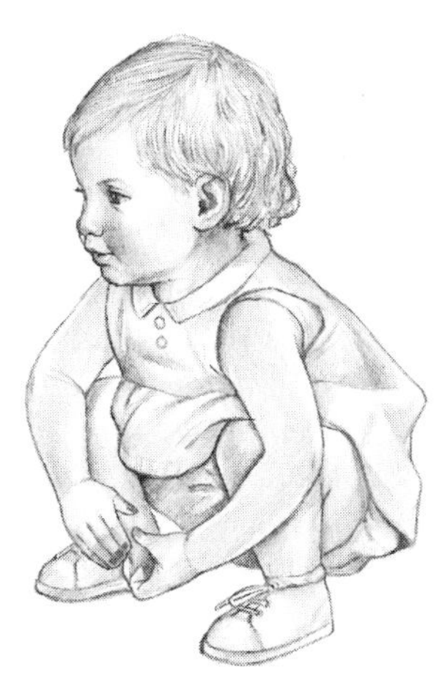

Relieving shortness of breath

A child with uncorrected tetralogy of Fallot assumes a characteristic squatting position to recover from shortness of breath after strenuous activity. The child's lips and fingernails may also appear bluish.

TREATMENT Your child will need surgery to correct this BIRTH DEFECT, preferably before he or she starts school. Before corrective surgery, the doctor may recommend a temporary operation, known as a Blalock-Taussig operation, to relieve your child's immediate symptoms. As new advances in cardiac surgery emerge, more and more children with tetralogy of Fallot are having their defects repaired in early infancy, without the initial, temporary surgery.

The doctor will prescribe antibiotics that your child should take before any dental work or surgery to prevent ENDOCARDITIS, a bacterial infection of the heart. Following surgery, the chances are excellent that your child will grow and develop normally.

THALASSEMIA

Thalassemia is the name for a group of inherited blood disorders characterized by a lower-than-normal production of hemoglobin, the oxygen-carrying protein in red blood cells. This deficiency in hemoglobin produces anemia that can be mild or severe. There are two major types of thalassemia: alpha-thalassemia, which occurs in children of Southeast Asian, Chinese, and Filipino ancestry, and beta-thalassemia, which occurs in children of Italian, Greek, Middle Eastern, and African descent. Beta-thalassemia is further divided into beta-thalassemia minor, intermedia, and major. Beta-thalassemia major (also called Cooley's anemia) is more severe than beta-thalassemia intermedia or minor.

SIGNS AND SYMPTOMS Most children with alpha-thalassemia have anemia to varying degrees and, in severe cases, a fetus or newborn with alpha-thalassemia may die.

A child with beta-thalassemia minor may have no symptoms at all. Children who have beta-thalassemia major look healthy at birth but grow slowly; become pale, tired, and fussy; and eat poorly in the first year or two of life. They are often out of breath, sometimes produce bloody or dark urine, and develop JAUNDICE. Untreated, beta-thalassemia major can cause an enlarged spleen, liver, and heart and enlarged facial bones. Ultimately, the child can die of heart failure. Beta-thalassemia intermedia causes similar symptoms, but the anemia is less severe.

DIAGNOSIS If your child's doctor suspects that your child has thalassemia, he or she will order blood tests and an examination of the bone marrow, where blood cells are produced, to diagnose the disorder. Because the disease is inherited, the doctor will probably also test your blood to confirm the diagnosis and offer genetic counseling (see page 497) if you plan to have any more children.

TREATMENT If your child is found to have thalassemia major, he or she may need to go to the hospital for blood transfusions every 3 or 4 weeks to promote healthy growth. He or she may also need daily doses of a drug that removes the excess iron that accumulates in the blood from multiple blood transfusions. Excessive iron stores can damage your child's liver. The drug is dispensed through a mechanical pump while your child sleeps. In severe cases, your doctor may recommend a bone marrow transplantation (see page 410) if an appropriate marrow donor becomes available. Milder forms of the disorder require treatment of the symptoms, but no blood transfusions.

With blood transfusions and drug therapy, a child with thalassemia major can expect to live another 20 or 30 years or more. People with the milder forms of thalassemia usually live a normal life span.

THRUSH

Thrush is an infection by a fungus known as Candida albicans that most often occurs in the mouth of both breast- and bottle-fed newborns. It can also occur in children whose resistance to infection is low because of some other illness such as cancer, or in those who take certain antibiotics. Newborns can get thrush when they pass through the birth canal if their mother has a vaginal yeast infection at the time of birth. Infants can get it from infected baby bottle nipples or from their mother's infected breast. Thrush is an infection by a fungus that is normally present in the mouth but is kept in check by bacteria in the mouth. When children are given broad-spectrum antibiotics, the antibiotics kill the bacteria and allow the fungus to grow out of control.

SIGNS AND SYMPTOMS White or creamy-yellow spots appear in the child's mouth, on the tongue, on the roof of the mouth, on the gums, inside the cheeks and lips, and in the throat. The spots look like tiny milk curds that do not wipe off easily. They are not painful unless rubbed. If the spots are rubbed off, open sores appear underneath.

DIAGNOSIS AND TREATMENT The doctor can usually diagnose the infection by simply examining your child, but he or she may want to take a sample of the spots for examination under a microscope. The doctor will prescribe antifungal drugs to treat this infection. With treatment, the infection should clear up in a few days, but can recur. If you bottle-feed your infant, boil the nipples for 20 minutes before using them. Always wash your breasts after breast-feeding.

THYROID DISEASES

See Hyperthyroidism; Hypothyroidism

THYROIDITIS

Thyroiditis is the inflammation of a child's thyroid gland. The thyroid gland is located just below a child's Adam's apple. It wraps around the trachea (windpipe) and is shaped like a butterfly. Thyroiditis takes a number of different forms. The most common type is a chronic (long-lasting) form known as Hashimoto's disease. Hashimoto's disease is an AUTOIMMUNE DISORDER in which the child's own immune system (the body's natural defense system against infections) attacks his or her thyroid gland. It commonly affects children in their teens–girls more often than boys. Acute and subacute thyroiditis are two other forms of the disease. Acute thyroiditis is a rare disease usually caused by a bacterial infection that spreads to the child's thyroid gland from some other part of the body. Subacute thyroiditis is a more common form thought to be caused by a viral infection.

SIGNS AND SYMPTOMS Hashimoto's disease causes a goiter (an enlarged thyroid gland), which may result in a noticeable swelling in the child's neck below the Adam's apple. It also causes progressive degrees of HYPOTHYROIDISM, which may be marked by slow growth, changes in behavior, low energy levels, weight gain, muscle weakness, muscle cramps, a general feeling of fatigue, flaky or coarse skin, a husky voice, and hair loss. Acute thyroiditis can cause severe pain and extreme tenderness in the child's neck and redness in the skin over the thyroid gland. It can also cause signs of bacterial infection, such as chills, fever, and shivering. Subacute thyroiditis usually starts with a low-grade fever and sore throat and progresses to pain in the back of the neck and tenderness in the area of the thyroid gland.

DIAGNOSIS The doctor can diagnose thyroiditis from your child's symptoms and from blood tests that measure the levels of thyroid hormones in your child's blood. The doctor will also test your child's blood for any autoimmune disorder.

TREATMENT If your child has mild symptoms or no symptoms at all, the doctor may simply observe your child's progress without treatment. Subacute thyroiditis can disappear on its own. But, if your child has a thyroid-hormone deficiency, he or she will need to take drugs that replace the missing thyroid hormones for life. Many children who have signs or symptoms of thyroiditis need to take thyroid replacement medication even if they have normal blood hormone levels. Taking the medication prevents hypothyroidism from developing in the future and alleviates symptoms. Your child should return to normal health within several months after treatment begins.

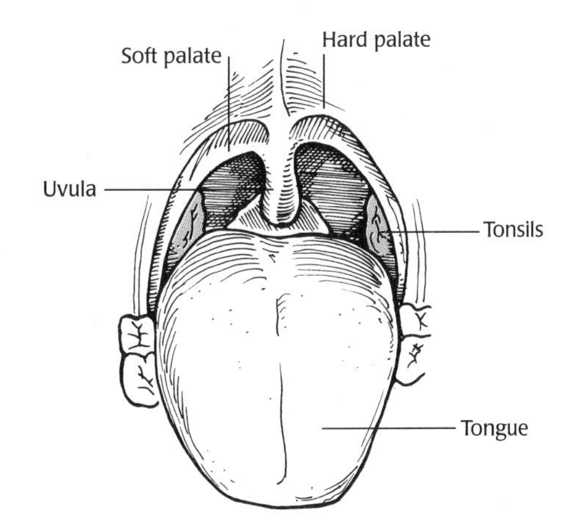

Checking your child's tonsils

If you ask your child to open his or her mouth and stick out his or her tongue, you will be able to see the tonsils. The roof of the mouth is made up of the hard palate in the front and the soft palate in the back. The uvula is a tiny appendage that hangs from the soft palate. You will see the tonsils on either side of the uvula, attached to the back of the throat.

TONSILLITIS

Tonsillitis is an inflammation of the tonsils, caused by infection. The tonsils are two small masses of tissue at the back of the mouth, on both sides of the throat. Their job is to filter out and fight bacteria and viruses that enter the body through the mouth and nose. Sometimes, however, the tonsils can become so overwhelmed by infectious organisms that they become inflamed. Tonsillitis is most common in children between the ages of 5 and 10 years. Most children have at least one episode of tonsillitis.

SIGNS AND SYMPTOMS A child's tonsils become red, swollen, and sore, and the child has difficulty swallowing. Babies may be irritable and refuse feedings. A child may also have chills and fever, swollen and tender glands in the neck, a HEADACHE, foul-smelling breath, and sometimes a cough. The child's voice or the baby's cry may sound throaty. A child with tonsillitis may snore during sleep (see SNORING). Several days after infection, the tonsils may develop a white or yellow coating. If the tonsillitis is severe, the child may experience some ear pain or have difficulty breathing.

DIAGNOSIS AND TREATMENT If the doctor suspects that your child has tonsillitis, he or she will *culture* your child's throat to identify the infectious agent causing the tonsillitis. The doctor will prescribe antibiotics for a bacterial infection. Your child should take the medication for the full course prescribed, even if he or she feels better after a day or two. Antibiotics are not effective against viruses, so don't insist on a prescription for antibiotics if the doctor does not think they are necessary (see page 278). With treatment, your child should feel better in 2 or 3 days.

Your child will need to rest in bed until his or her health improves, drink plenty of liquids, and take nonprescription pain relievers, such as aceta-

What you should know about tonsillectomy

The tonsils are two small masses of tissue visible in the back of the throat. The adenoids are tiny clusters of tissue on top of the soft palate, behind the nose. The adenoids look like clusters of little grapes and they are not visible without a mirror or viewing instrument.

Until the 1960s, surgeons routinely removed children's tonsils and adenoids as a preventive measure, but doctors now know that the tonsils and adenoids help the body fight infection. Operations to remove them, known as tonsillectomy and adenoidectomy, are now done only under certain circumstances. If your child has severe or frequent bouts of tonsillitis, the doctor might recommend a tonsillectomy. The adenoids are very close to the tonsils and can also become inflamed, so the surgeon may want to take out your child's adenoids at the same time. The operation is usually done when a child is 6 or 7 years old.

The surgery can be done on an *outpatient* basis, meaning that your child will usually not have to stay overnight in the hospital; he or she may be able to go home after 8 to 10 hours of observation. Make sure that your child understands what will happen before, during, and after the surgery. You should be there at the hospital to comfort your child before and after the operation and then bring him or her home. Like any operation, a tonsillectomy or adenoidectomy carries some risk. The main potential complication is bleeding after surgery. If your child starts to bleed, make sure he or she lies on his or her side so he or she does not choke on the blood. Your child's throat will be sore for up to 2 weeks. You can give your child pain relievers such as acetaminophen or ibuprofen, plenty of liquids, and soft foods to ease the discomfort.

minophen (but not aspirin). If your child develops an abscess (a collection of pus) on his or her tonsils, if tonsillitis frequently recurs, if your child has difficulty breathing or swallowing, or if he or she has ear infections frequently, the doctor may recommend relatively simple surgery to remove the tonsils (see box).

TORCH syndrome

See Infections in newborns

Tourette's syndrome

Tourette's syndrome is a nervous system disorder marked by sudden, involuntary body movements and uncontrollable vocal sounds, known as tics. These muscular and vocal tics begin in childhood, generally between the ages of 2 and 16, but most frequently occur around age 6 or 7. Boys are at higher risk of this disorder than girls.

Signs and symptoms The first signs of Tourette's syndrome usually appear in a child's face. The child may begin to blink excessively or twitch the nose and head. The MOVEMENT DISORDER progresses to a point at which the child may contort the face, jump up and down, stamp the feet, stretch the neck, twist or bend the body, or constantly touch other people. Vocal tics include grunting, barking, clearing the throat, coughing, sniffing, and shouting sounds or phrases. In rare cases, a child may shout obscene words or constantly repeat his or her own words or those spoken by other people.

Some children with Tourette's syndrome also have other conditions, such as OBSESSIVE-COMPULSIVE DISORDER, ATTENTION DISORDERS, LEARNING DISABILITIES, ANXIETY, DEPRESSION, and a tendency to injure themselves by biting their hands or banging their head.

Diagnosis and treatment If a child displays the symptoms of Tourette's syndrome, the doctor may prescribe a medication, such as haloperidol or clonidine, that relieves tics, but these medications have unwanted side effects, such as drowsiness, depression, and weight gain. At home, try to minimize any emotional stress your child may be under because stress can make the condition worse. Be careful not to scold your child for his or her uncontrollable behavior because scolding will only increase your child's distress. Make sure your child's teachers understand the condition. In some cases, the tics disappear on their own or the child learns to control them. The doctor may refer the child to a neurologist (a doctor who specializes in treating disorders of the nervous system) or psychiatrist for further evaluation.

TRANSPOSITION OF THE GREAT ARTERIES

Transposition of the great arteries is a heart defect (see HEART DISEASE, CONGENITAL) in which the two major blood vessels that transport blood from the heart—the aorta and the pulmonary artery—are transposed. The result of this BIRTH DEFECT is that the infant's blood receives insufficient amounts of oxygen from the lungs and carries too little oxygen to the child's body. Without treatment, the baby is likely to die within the first weeks or months of life.

SIGNS AND SYMPTOMS Because of a lack of oxygen, the baby's skin turns bluish within the first few hours or days of life. He or she may have difficulty feeding, rapid breathing, or shortness of breath. The infant is sometimes larger than normal at birth. A doctor can hear a HEART MURMUR through a stethoscope.

DIAGNOSIS If your baby turns blue after birth, the doctor will order a chest X-ray, *electrocardiogram, echocardiogram,* and blood tests to determine the exact cause.

TREATMENT Once the defect is diagnosed, your child will need *cardiac catheterization* right away to create a large hole in the wall between the right and left atrium (upper chambers of his or her heart). The hole will allow blood that has traveled to the lungs to pick up oxygen to pass to the right side of your baby's heart and into his or her aorta to be circulated throughout the body.

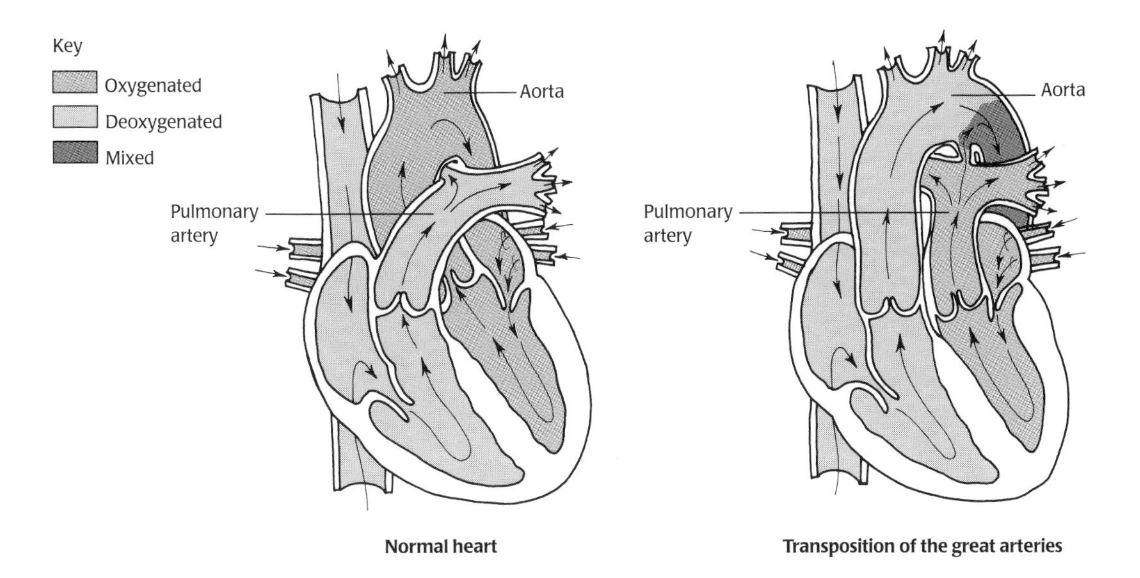

Major vessels switched

Transposition of the great arteries describes a heart defect in which the major vessels that carry blood away from an infant's heart are transposed, or switched. The pulmonary artery, which carries blood from the heart to the lungs, is where the aorta (the main artery in the body) should be and vice versa. This defect causes blood that has already passed through the baby's lungs to flow back to the lungs instead of out to the rest of the body.

Your baby will also need an operation within the first 3 or 4 months of life to switch the aorta and pulmonary artery so they are in the correct places. After having surgery, the chances are excellent that your baby will live a full and healthy life.

TUBERCULOSIS

Tuberculosis, commonly called TB, is a contagious, life-threatening infection caused by a bacterium known as Mycobacterium tuberculosis. It usually affects the lungs, but it can also enter the child's bloodstream and affect his or her brain, kidneys, intestines, liver, and spine. The bacterium is spread by coughing or sneezing tiny droplets containing the TB bacterium into the air so, to become infected, a child needs to be in close contact with someone who has tuberculosis. The body's immune system (the natural defense mechanism against infection) can "wall off" the bacteria and prevent the infection from progressing. Although tuberculosis is a major cause of death in many developing countries, it was relatively rare in the United States until 1985, when the incidence of tuberculosis began to rise in this country.

SIGNS AND SYMPTOMS Some people infected with the TB bacterium have no symptoms or have only influenzalike symptoms such as fever and muscle aches, but they are still able to spread the disease. If the immune system fails to stop the disease from progressing, an infected child develops a fever, weight loss, night sweats, tiredness, and an overall feeling of ill health. When the lungs are infected, he or she also has chest pain, shortness of breath, and a cough that may or may not produce sputum (phlegm) with blood in it. Tuberculosis can also produce symptoms that mimic those of digestive diseases such as CROHN'S DISEASE or ULCERATIVE COLITIS. MALABSORPTION, FAILURE TO THRIVE, and MENINGITIS can all be caused by tuberculosis.

DIAGNOSIS If the doctor suspects tuberculosis, he or she will prick the skin on your child's forearm and inject a protein derived from the TB bacterium under the skin that causes a reaction in people exposed to the disease (see page 234). The reaction occurs 2 days after the skin test. A positive reaction causes redness, swelling, and firmness of the skin at the site of injection but these signs may mean that your child has only been exposed to the bacteria that causes tuberculosis, not that he or she actually has the active disease. If you see such a reaction on your child's skin, call the doctor. He or she will order chest X-rays to determine if your child has an active infection. Analysis of your child's sputum, stomach contents, or spinal fluid are not necessary to confirm a diagnosis unless other signs of tuberculosis exist.

TREATMENT The doctor will prescribe an antibiotic to treat your child, even if he or she does not have an active case of tuberculosis but only has a positive skin test and no signs of active disease. Your child will need to take the antibiotic for 6 to 9 months. With treatment, he or she will recover from tuberculosis completely. Once your child has had a positive skin test, he or she will not need to be tested again because future tests would always be positive.

TURNER'S SYNDROME

Turner's syndrome is an inherited CHROMOSOMAL ABNORMALITY in which a female infant is born with a missing X *chromosome* (females normally have two X chromosomes). The missing chromosome affects the child's physical and sexual development. This abnormality occurs when one X chromosome becomes lost or defective when the mother's egg is fertilized by the father's sperm.

SIGNS AND SYMPTOMS A girl with Turner's syndrome is usually a low-birthweight infant. She may have loose skin and a low hairline at the base of the neck, drooping eyelids, swollen hands and feet, a broad chest, and a heart condition known as COARCTATION OF THE AORTA. As the child gets older, she may have short stature (see HEIGHT PROBLEMS), and will not mature sexually without treatment. She will not be able to have children because of improper formation and function of the ovaries, resulting from the missing X chromosome.

DIAGNOSIS AND TREATMENT The doctor can diagnose this syndrome in your child by ordering a chromosomal analysis and blood tests to detect levels of female sex hormones. Your daughter will be given female sex hormone medication every day for 6 months to a year beginning at about age 12 or 13 to stimulate sexual development. She will then take sex hormones to stimulate her menstrual cycles. She must continue taking these hormones until menopause (until she is about 50 years of age). Hormones will not give her the ability to bear children. If your daughter has coarctation of the aorta, she will need surgery to correct the defect in her heart.

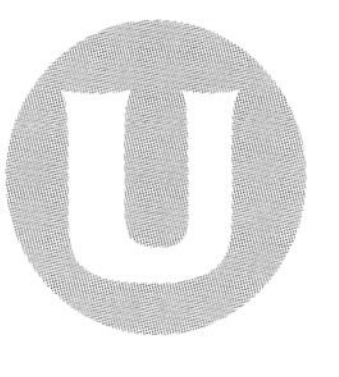

ULCERATIVE COLITIS

Ulcerative colitis is a chronic (long-term) inflammation in the lining of a child's colon (large intestine). It affects children over the age of 9 years and its symptoms often come and go throughout the child's life. The inflammation usually begins in the child's rectum and can spread throughout the child's colon. As the condition progresses, the affected cells in the lining of the colon begin to die and slough off, causing ulcers (open sores) to form. Doctors do not know what causes ulcerative colitis, but it seems to run in families and is most common in young white adults in the United States and northern Europe.

SIGNS AND SYMPTOMS Ulcerative colitis flares up without warning, causing a frequent and urgent need to have a bowel movement, abdominal cramps, and pain before having a bowel movement. The stools sometimes contain pus, mucus, and blood. The child may also have diarrhea.

If ulcerative colitis affects only the rectum, rectal bleeding may be the only sign of the disease. When a larger part of the colon is affected, the child has extensive bloody diarrhea, sharp abdominal pain, weight loss, fever, and a general feeling of ill health. Months may go by without symptoms between flare-ups, although a small number of children have continuous symptoms. Untreated, ulcerative colitis can cause anemia (see ANEMIA, BLOOD-LOSS), a life-threatening condition called toxic megacolon (an enlargement and swelling of the colon), a skin RASH, arthritis, poor weight gain, and growth retardation. Ulcerative colitis that affects the entire colon for 10 years or more increases a child's risk of colon cancer later in life.

DIAGNOSIS If your doctor suspects that your child has ulcerative colitis, he or she will refer your child to a gastroenterologist (a doctor who specializes in disorders of the stomach and intestines). The specialist will examine your child's rectum and colon through an endoscope (a flexible viewing instrument) inserted into your child's anus. He or she may also do a *biopsy* of the tissue to confirm the diagnosis. A *barium X-ray* study of the colon is another alternative, but is less accurate than use of the endoscope. The doctor may have a sample of your child's stool analyzed to rule out other causes of his or her symptoms. The doctor will also order blood tests to check for signs of inflammation in the colon and for complications, such as arthritis.

TREATMENT Drugs work well to reduce the severity and frequency of flare-ups in a child with

U

ulcerative colitis. Salicylate drugs, which are anti-inflammatory drugs in the aspirin family, are commonly used to treat mild to moderate cases of the disorder. Other drugs that the doctor may prescribe are sulfa drugs and *corticosteroids.* If drug therapy does not work, or complications, such as toxic megacolon, develop, your child may need surgery to remove the entire colon. In that case, the surgeon will create an artificial opening in your child's abdomen and connect the final part of the child's small intestine, called the ileum, to the opening to create an ileostomy. Your child will then pass stool into a bag attached to the outside of his or her body. The ileostomy may or may not be permanent. If it is only temporary, the surgeon will later connect your child's ileum directly to his or her rectum during a second operation.

Ulcers, duodenal

See Ulcers, peptic

Ulcers, peptic

Peptic ulcers are raw areas or open sores that occur in the lining of a child's stomach (gastric ulcers) or duodenum, the first part of the small intestine (duodenal ulcers). Duodenal ulcers are primarily caused by excessive stomach acid exposure, while gastric ulcers can be caused by several factors, including stress. Infection with a bacterium known as Helicobacter pylori is a known cause of peptic ulcers. Children get mainly duodenal ulcers, although they can develop duodenal or gastric ulcers as complications of another disorder. The ulcers can be temporary or chronic (long-lasting).

Duodenal ulcers tend to run in families. They have been linked to the use of aspirin, ibuprofen, and *corticosteroids*; cigarette smoking; overuse of alcohol; stress; severe infections; and chronic liver disease. Gastric ulcers can be caused by excess production of stomach acid or slow emptying of the stomach, so that acid sits in the stomach for long periods. Smoking and the use of aspirin and other inflammation-fighting drugs can also contribute to the development of gastric ulcers. How these factors affect ulcer formation is not clearly understood.

Signs and symptoms The primary symptom of peptic ulcers is a burning or gnawing pain in the stomach a few hours after eating. The pain is relieved by eating, drinking milk, or taking antacids and can be so bad it wakes the child at night. Nausea, vomiting, abdominal bloating, gas, and heartburn can also occur. Infants and toddlers are more likely to vomit, have bloody stools, and eat poorly than older children. Some children with duodenal ulcers actually gain weight because they eat more to relieve the pain. If the child loses a lot of blood from the ulcer, he or she can develop anemia (see ANEMIA, BLOOD-LOSS). In rare cases, the ulcer can erode through the wall of the stomach or intestine, causing infection or bleeding into the abdomen, both of which are life threatening.

Diagnosis If your child has symptoms of a peptic ulcer, the doctor will order blood and stool tests and confirm the diagnosis with a *barium X-ray* study. He or she may also insert an endoscope (a flexible viewing instrument) inside your child's mouth and down his or her esophagus (the muscular tube that connects the mouth and the stomach) to look at the inside of your child's stomach or duodenum.

Treatment Antacids are the usual treatment for ulcers. The antacids neutralize excess stomach acid and help heal the ulcers. If your child's symptoms continue after taking antacids, the doctor may prescribe special ulcer medications that reduce the secretion of acid from the cells in the lining of the stomach, or medication that coats the ulcer, protecting it from further erosion. The doctor may also prescribe an antibiotic if the bacterium H pylori has been found in your child's digestive tract. Most ulcers clear up within 6 to 8 weeks with treatment. If your child has lost a lot of blood from a bleeding ulcer, he or she may need a blood transfusion. An ulcer that has eroded through the wall of the stomach or intestine also needs to be treated in the hospital.

UNDESCENDED TESTICLES

See Testicle and scrotum disorders

UREA-CYCLE DISORDERS

Urea-cycle disorders are a group of inherited illnesses that cause excessive amounts of ammonia to build up in a child's blood. The disorders arise from a deficiency in one of the enzymes (proteins that regulate chemical reactions) needed to produce urea, one of the main components of urine. Urea is produced in the liver in a five-step process known as the urea cycle. Each step of the cycle requires a specific enzyme. The individual disorders are named for the missing enzyme. Normally, the child's liver converts ammonia (a by-product of the breakdown of proteins) to urea during the cycle. When an enzyme is missing, excessive amounts of ammonia build up in the child's bloodstream. Ammonia is extremely poisonous and can damage the brain, causing mental retardation, seizures, and even death.

SIGNS AND SYMPTOMS Newborns with a urea-cycle disorder begin to show signs of the disorder in the second or third day of life. They become irritable, start vomiting, feed poorly, and become weak. These initial symptoms are followed quickly by seizures, breathing difficulty (see RESPIRATORY DISTRESS SYNDROME), and coma. Without treatment, the infant will die. In milder cases of these disorders, symptoms may not appear until later in infancy or early childhood. Mental retardation and seizures are common even in less severe cases. Symptoms can flare up when the child eats protein or gets an infection.

DIAGNOSIS A newborn is often diagnosed with a urea-cycle defect in the hospital on the basis of his or her condition and blood and urine tests.

TREATMENT The specific treatment depends on the enzyme the child lacks, but in most cases the doctor will prescribe a low-protein diet and give medication that helps correct the chemical imbalances in the child's blood. In some cases, the child may need dialysis treatments (see KIDNEY FAILURE, CHRONIC) to filter out waste products from his or her blood. In extreme cases, the child may need a liver transplant (an operation that replaces a diseased liver with a healthy, donated liver) to survive.

URINARY TRACT DEFECTS AND OBSTRUCTION

A variety of structural defects in a child's urinary tract–including the kidneys, ureters (the tubes that carry urine from the kidneys to the bladder), bladder, and urethra (the tube that carries urine out from the bladder)–can interfere with the normal flow of urine. A child's urinary tract can also become obstructed by kidney stones, tumors, or blood clots that develop in or near the urinary tract. Damage to the nerves that serve the bladder can obstruct urine flow because they prevent the child from releasing urine from his or her bladder.

KIDNEY STONES Small, solid crystals can form in a child's kidneys and migrate to the ureters or bladder to obstruct the flow of urine. Kidney stones can range in size from a grain of sand to a golf ball. If your child has kidney stones that do not pass easily through the urinary tract, he or she will have sharp pains in the back, just below the ribs, that move to the groin as the stones move down to the bladder. He or she may also have painful urination, blood in the urine, nausea, and vomiting. The stones sometimes pass out on their own in a few days, but, if they become lodged, they need to be removed either by surgery or using high-frequency sound waves that break up the stones.

EPISPADIAS In rare cases, a baby boy can be born with the opening of his urethra on the upper surface of his penis instead of at the tip. The penis of a boy with this condition, called epispadias, may also curve upward. The boy's urethra must be surgically reconstructed, using tissue from the foreskin, to create an opening at the tip of the penis. The infant may need more than one operation to correct this problem.

HYDRONEPHROSIS A malformation at the junction of the ureters and kidneys that is present at birth, or a kidney stone, tumor, blood clot in or around the ureters, or nerve damage can block the flow of urine, causing urine to build up in the kidneys, a condition known as hydronephrosis. One or both kidneys can become enlarged or severely damaged, and possibly fail (see KIDNEY FAILURE, ACUTE and KIDNEY FAILURE, CHRONIC). A child with acute hydronephrosis has sharp, sudden pain in the lower back. If the blockage develops slowly and on both sides, signs of chronic kidney failure—weakness, nausea, and appetite loss—appear. If only one kidney is affected, the child may develop high blood pressure. A URINARY TRACT INFECTION can develop as a complication of hydronephrosis. A doctor can sometimes feel an abdominal mass in an infant during a physical examination. In older children, X-rays or *ultrasound* scans aid in the diagnosis. Surgery is needed to correct the blockage. If one kidney is so severely damaged it can no longer function, it may need to be surgically removed. If both kidneys fail to work, the child may need a kidney transplant.

URETEROPELVIC JUNCTION OBSTRUCTION During the first 3 months of fetal development, a defect at the junction of the kidneys and ureters can cause an obstruction, producing hydronephrosis (see above). A baby born with this defect may have a noticeable lump in his or her abdomen, along with vomiting, blood in the urine, a urinary tract infection, and high blood pressure. Older children may also develop a urinary tract infection and high blood pressure. A doctor can diagnose this defect with an ultrasound, X-rays, and other tests. Surgery—sometimes done on an emergency basis—is needed to repair the defect.

VESICOURETERAL REFLUX A valve normally regulates the flow of urine from the ureter to the bladder. Some children are born with a faulty valve, causing urine to flow back from the bladder toward the kidneys when the bladder contracts. This condition, called vesicoureteral reflux, can cause kidney damage. Common symptoms include pain upon urination, blood in the urine, and fever. Most children are diagnosed after they develop a urinary tract infection and are evaluated by an X-ray examination of the bladder called a *cystogram*. The doctor will prescribe antibiotics to treat the urinary tract infection. Many cases clear up on their own. In severe cases, surgery may be needed to repair the defective valve.

POSTERIOR URETHRAL VALVES The valves that control the flow of urine in a boy's urethra can develop abnormally before birth, obstructing the flow of urine. An infant born with this defect often has symptoms similar to those of ureteropelvic junction obstruction (below left), along with an enlarged bladder and constipation. Older children experience an urge to urinate frequently, have poor bladder control, and may get a urinary tract infection or have blood in the urine. Left untreated, the condition can eventually lead to chronic kidney failure. This defect can be diagnosed by a radiographic cystogram. Surgical correction of the defect is the usual treatment.

DYSPLASTIC KIDNEY The cells and structures of the kidneys can develop abnormally before birth, creating a small, poorly functioning kidney that produces little urine. Usually, only one kidney is abnormal. During the physical examination immediately after birth, the doctor will detect a noticeable mass in the baby's abdomen. The infant may develop a urinary tract infection, blood in the urine, and high blood pressure. If both kidneys are affected, the infant could die.

Doctors sometimes detect this defect during an ultrasound scan before birth. In older children, doctors often discover the condition during an evaluation for high blood pressure. Ultrasound and *radionuclide scans* can also help in diagnosis after birth. The child's doctor may recommend removing the affected kidney surgically, but if the condition causes no health problems, he or she may recommend no treatment because a child can survive with only one functioning kidney.

HORSESHOE KIDNEY Some babies are born with their kidneys joined together at the base, in the shape of a horseshoe. In most cases, the kidneys function normally and cause no symptoms, but in some children the flow of urine becomes obstructed and can damage the kidneys.

URETERAL DUPLICATION An infant can be born with two sets of ureters attached to his or her kidneys. In many cases, the defect causes no symptoms and the infant's kidneys function normally, but sometimes ureteral duplication can cause obstruction or reversal of the flow of urine, infections, or loss of bladder control. In such cases, the child may need surgery to correct the defect.

URINARY TRACT INFECTIONS

Urinary tract infections, usually caused by bacteria, affect one or more organs of the urinary tract, comprised of the kidneys, ureters (the tubes that carry urine from the kidneys to the bladder), bladder, and urethra (the tube that carries urine out from the bladder). Bacteria, viruses, and fungi can enter the urinary tract through the urethra and migrate into the bladder. In infants, infectious organisms can also spread through the bloodstream from other parts of the body. Normally, urine is sterile (free from infectious organisms) and frequent urination keeps it sterile, but abnormalities in the structure of the urinary tract can cause a child to retain urine, increasing the chances of infection. The most common urinary tract infection is cystitis, or infection of the bladder. An infection in the urethra is known as urethritis, and an infection in the kidneys is called pyelonephritis. After 1 year of age, girls get urinary tract infections more often than boys, primarily because their urethra is shorter.

SIGNS AND SYMPTOMS Cystitis causes an urge to urinate frequently. Sometimes the urine has an offensive odor and contains blood. Other symptoms include a burning sensation while urinating, difficulty urinating, and sometimes a fever. Urethritis causes pain while urinating and frequent, sometimes bloody, urination. Pyelonephritis causes similar symptoms—although an affected child has a higher fever, generally looks more ill, and may have pain in the lower back, just above the waist, where the kidneys are located. The pain may spread into the child's groin. Sometimes a child has no symptoms. Infants often are irritable, feed poorly, vomit, and have a fever and diarrhea.

DIAGNOSIS If your infant or child has symptoms of a urinary tract infection, take him or her to the doctor for an evaluation. The doctor will order a urine *culture* and might also order X-rays, *ultrasound* scans, or *radionuclide scans* to assess the location of the infection and to check the urinary tract for any abnormality that may be causing the infection.

TREATMENT Urinary tract infections, urethritis, and cystitis can usually be treated effectively with antibiotics taken by mouth. Pyelonephritis requires treatment with antibiotics taken *intravenously* or given as an injection into the muscle. Your child should drink plenty of liquids to help him or her urinate frequently. Children who get a urinary tract infection before age 4, boys of any age with a urinary tract infection, or a child with recurrent infections need to be evaluated with a radionuclide scan or ultrasound of the kidney and a *cystogram* to detect any abnormalities in their anatomy. If the doctor finds an abnormality in your child's urinary tract, he or she will refer the child to a urologist (a doctor who specializes in disorders of the urinary tract).

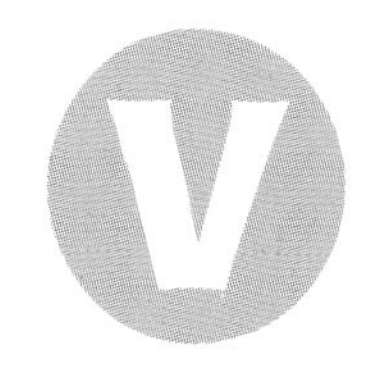

VAGINITIS

Vaginitis is an inflammation of the vagina (the muscular passage that connects the cervix with the external genitals) caused by an infection, a chemical or physical irritant, or poor hygiene. Girls of all ages can develop vaginitis, although most cases occur for the first time in adolescence. The most common infections that cause vaginitis are vaginal candidiasis (yeast infections caused by a fungus), bacterial vaginosis (infection with the bacteria known as Gardnerella vaginalis), and trichomoniasis (infection with the microorganism known as Trichomonas vaginalis). Common irritants that can cause vaginitis include the chemicals in douches, creams used with condoms to kill sperm, feminine hygiene sprays, and some soaps or bath oils. Tampons and sanitary pads with deodorant can also irritate the vagina and cause vaginitis. Infrequent bathing and wearing clothes that are too tight at the crotch, made of synthetic materials, or dirty can also cause vaginitis. Wiping from the back to the front after a bowel movement can spread bacteria from the anus to the vagina, causing vaginitis. Girls who have not yet gone through puberty lack the sexual hormones that can protect against vaginitis and may be at higher risk for infection if they are exposed to irritants or have poor hygiene.

The vagina normally contains bacteria and these germs can multiply excessively during any illness that affects a girl's natural ability to fight off disease, causing vaginitis. Vaginitis can also accompany DIABETES MELLITUS, TYPE I; herpes (see COLD SORES); PELVIC INFLAMMATORY DISEASE; pregnancy; and the use of oral contraceptives (birth-control pills).

SIGNS AND SYMPTOMS The symptoms of vaginitis include itching, swelling, pain, redness, and burning inside the vagina or on the lips that surround the vagina (labia). The girl may also have an abnormal vaginal discharge that could be thin or as thick as cottage cheese and could be white, gray, yellow, or green. The discharge may be stained with blood and have a bad odor.

DIAGNOSIS If your daughter has any of these symptoms, take her to the doctor for a thorough examination. During the examination, the doctor will take a sample of the vaginal discharge and any pus found in the vagina for laboratory analysis to look for signs of infection.

TREATMENT The treatment your daughter receives will depend on the specific cause of her vaginitis. If infection is the cause, the doctor will prescribe antibiotic or antifungal medication. If the vaginitis was caused by an irritant, the doctor will recommend removing the source of the irritation–such as a forgotten tampon or use of a feminine hygiene spray. Sitting in a warm bath (a sitz bath) can help soothe the irritation. If poor hygiene is the problem, the doctor will teach your daughter improved bathing and toilet techniques–such as daily bathing and wiping from front to back–and will tell her to avoid wearing dirty or tightly fitting clothes. He or she will probably recommend wearing underwear made of cotton instead of synthetic fabrics.

VALVE ABNORMALITIES

A valve abnormality is a defect in the valves that regulate the flow of blood through the heart. The heart contains four valves–the tricuspid, the mitral, the pulmonary, and the aortic–that connect the heart's four chambers by opening and closing to allow blood to flow from one chamber to the next without backing up. The defect is usually either a stenosis (narrowing) of the valve, causing the heart to work harder to pump blood through the valve, or a widening of the valve, allowing blood to leak backward instead of moving forward through the heart chambers.

A child can be born with a heart valve abnormality (see HEART DISEASE, CONGENITAL) or can develop it later in childhood from another heart disorder, such as RHEUMATIC FEVER that develops from strep throat (see STREP INFECTION) or ENDOCARDITIS, an infection in the heart.

SIGNS AND SYMPTOMS A child with a minor heart valve abnormality may have no symptoms. When symptoms do occur, they can include fatigue, weakness, dizzy spells, fainting, shortness of breath, and chest pains. A doctor may detect congestion in the lungs, irregular heartbeats (see ARRHYTHMIAS), HEART MURMURS, and HIGH BLOOD PRESSURE or low blood pressure during a routine physical examination. Eventually, the child may suffer heart failure (see HEART FAILURE, CONGESTIVE).

DIAGNOSIS If your child has symptoms of a valve abnormality, the doctor will listen to your child's heart with a stethoscope for a heart murmur or irregular heartbeat. To confirm the diagnosis, the doctor will order blood tests and an *electrocardiogram* and *echocardiogram*; a *cardiac catheterization* may also be necessary.

TREATMENT If your child has a heart valve abnormality, he or she will probably be referred to a cardiologist (a doctor who specializes in treating disorders of the heart). In many cases, close observation (by way of regular medical examinations) is all that is necessary. Medications to stabilize and regulate your child's heartbeat and improve the heart function may be needed. The doctor will prescribe antibiotics before any dental work or surgery to prevent endocarditis. If the valve abnormality is a complication of an infectious illness, the cardiologist will probably prescribe antibiotics to treat any infection in your child's heart. If a valve is narrowed, your child may need to have it widened through cardiac catheterization. Surgery may be required in other cases to repair a defective valve or replace it with a synthetic valve or one from a human or animal donor.

Following surgery, your child may need to take drugs that help prevent blood clots from forming around the replacement valve. After surgery, your child should grow and develop normally. He or she will need to take antibiotics before any future dental work and surgery to prevent infection of the heart. He or she will also need follow-up care with the cardiologist or cardiac (heart) surgeon to make sure the surgery has been effective.

VISION PROBLEMS

Infants and children can develop a variety of problems that affect their vision, including crossed eyes, nearsightedness, droopy eyelids, GLAUCOMA, and cataracts. Newborn babies can see but do not have fully developed vision until about 3 years of age. They may be born with vision problems or develop them later on in childhood. Children should have their eyes examined during each routine well-child examination. Regular eye examinations should begin between 3 and 5 years of age. If the vision testing reveals a problem, or if your child tells you he or she has difficulty seeing, the doctor will refer your child to an ophthalmologist (a doctor who specializes in disorders of the eye). The two most common vision problems in infants and children are strabismus and amblyopia.

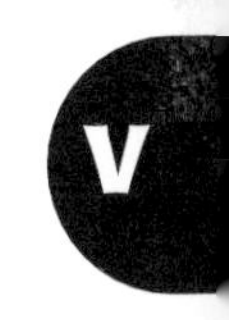

STRABISMUS A child with strabismus has eyes that are not aligned so they cannot work together to produce normal vision. The muscles of the child's eyes are not coordinated and the eyes cannot move in the same direction. One eye may look straight ahead while the other eye looks up, down, inward, or outward. The two main forms of strabismus are esotropia and exotropia.

The familiar name for esotropia is crossed eyes. One or both of the child's eyes turn inward toward his or her nose. Children can be born with esotropia or develop it later in life, especially between the ages of 2 and 7. Children who have crossed eyes usually need surgery on their eye muscles before the age of 2 years. If they develop the condition after age 2, eyeglasses can usually correct the problem.

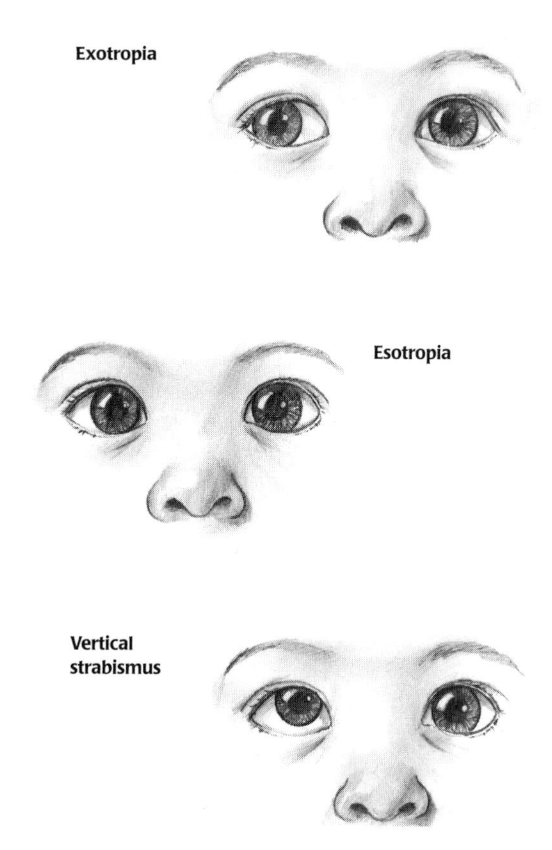

Types of strabismus

A child whose eye veers out and away from his or her nose has exotropia (top), a form of strabismus (misalignment of the eyes). When a child's eye points in and toward his or her nose, the child has esotropia (center), a form of strabismus commonly known as crossed eyes. A child whose eye veers upward or downward when the other eye looks straight ahead has vertical strabismus (bottom), a less common misalignment of the eyes.

A child with exotropia has one or both eyes turning outward away from his or her nose. Children can be born with this eye problem or develop it later in life, especially between the ages of 2 and 7. The child's eye or eyes may turn out only occasionally at first, but eventually turn out more and more often. The child may also squint in bright sunlight. Children with excessive exotropia usually need surgery on their eye muscles.

AMBLYOPIA A child with strabismus learns to "turn off" the vision in one eye so he or she can see things clearly. This loss of vision in one eye from strabismus or another eye problem is called amblyopia or lazy eye. A child can develop amblyopia anytime from infancy up to the age of 4. If the problem is not treated before 7 years of age, the child can sustain permanent loss of vision. The treatment consists of covering the eye the child uses with a patch to encourage use of the other eye, using glasses to correct the child's vision, or both. The underlying problem, such as strabismus, also needs to be treated. Other vision problems that can cause amblyopia include cataracts and ptosis.

CATARACTS A cataract is a clouding of the lens in a child's eye. The lens, which sits behind the pupil and focuses light onto the back of the eyeball, is normally clear. Over time, a cataract distorts or blocks the light coming into the child's eye, causing loss of vision. A child may have cataracts at birth or develop them later in life, sometimes as the result of injury to the eye. Surgical removal of the damaged lens is the only treatment for cataracts.

PTOSIS A child with ptosis has an eyelid that droops, usually from a weak muscle in the upper eyelid. The child may be born with this condition or develop it after an illness or injury. If the droopy eyelid covers the pupil, the child will need surgery to correct the problem and avoid amblyopia. Children with milder cases may not need surgery.

MYOPIA A child with myopia is nearsighted; he or she sees close objects clearly but faraway objects are blurred. Nearsightedness is more common among school-age children than infants. It can be corrected with glasses.

HYPEROPIA A child with hyperopia is farsighted; he or she has difficulty focusing on nearby objects initially. Eventually far away objects also become unclear. An infant may be born with the condition or develop it later in childhood. The child's eyes can adjust naturally to the condition in mild cases, but more severe cases may require corrective glasses.

ASTIGMATISM A child with astigmatism has an abnormally shaped cornea (the clear outer covering of the eyeball) that distorts light and causes blurred vision. Occasionally, the shape of the lens is abnormal. Severe cases of astigmatism require corrective glasses or contact lenses. A small degree of astigmatism is normal and does not require glasses or contact lenses.

VITILIGO

Vitiligo is a skin condition that produces white patches and small white spots on the skin. The condition is caused by a loss of the pigment that gives skin its color. For reasons that are not fully understood, the cells called melanocytes that form pigment don't function properly and destroy or fail to produce normal skin color. The risk of getting the disease increases with a family history of the condition. Patches of vitiligo can grow and spread throughout a child's lifetime and the skin rarely returns to its normal color. About half of all cases develop in children and teens under age 20, especially in children between the ages of 9 and 12.

SIGNS AND SYMPTOMS Children with vitiligo have milky-white patches of skin on their bodies that are sometimes distributed symmetrically (appearing in the same area on both sides of the body) or asymmetrically. The patches spread to form larger areas that are irregularly shaped. Hair on the affected areas sometimes turns white as well. Common sites of vitiligo include areas around the mouth, nose, and eyes; the back of the hands and fingers; and the skin on the elbows, wrists, knees, armpits, groin, genitals, legs, and nipples. Vitiligo can also appear on the skin that covers a cut or burn. Although more noticeable in dark-skinned children, vitiligo can also be seen in light-skinned children in summer when their skin becomes suntanned. Children with severe cases can lose skin pigmentation over their entire body.

DIAGNOSIS Your doctor will be able to diagnose vitiligo from the appearance of your child's skin during a physical examination.

TREATMENT If you have a child who is fair-skinned, cover the lighter patches of skin with clothing when he or she goes outside to avoid SUNBURN. Always apply sunscreen to affected areas that may be exposed to the sun, even in winter. If the vitiligo makes your child feel embarrassed about his or her appearance, disguise your child's light patches with makeup or a self-tanning lotion.

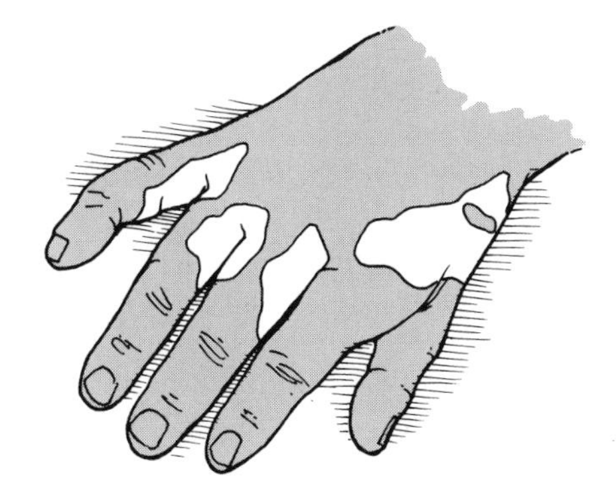

Loss of skin pigmentation
This child's hand shows the typical appearance of the skin condition known as vitiligo, which is characterized by milky-white patches or white spots on the skin.

A number of more aggressive treatments are available for vitiligo, but they are generally not recommended for children. Your child's doctor may prescribe a *corticosteroid* cream or lotion to treat your child's skin, but you and your doctor will need to monitor the treatment carefully. Your child's doctor may take a sample of your child's blood to test it for certain conditions, such as thyroid disease, that can cause vitiligo.

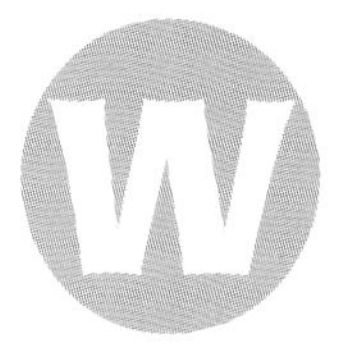

WARTS

Warts are tiny, harmless bumps on the outer layer of the skin caused by a virus known as the human papillomavirus. The virus is transmitted by direct contact between people and can also be picked up from a surface, such as a shower stall, that has been touched by an infected person. Warts are very common in children, typically appearing on the fingers, hands, soles of the feet, and face. When they appear on the genitals, they are known as GENITAL WARTS.

SIGNS AND SYMPTOMS Hand warts are elevated, flesh-colored, sometimes scaly bumps with horny projections. They start out the size of a pinhead and can grow to the size of a pea in several months. Hand warts occur around the fingernails, on the fingers, and on the back of the hand. Children who bite their nails or pick at hangnails often get hand warts around their fingernails.

Warts that occur on the foot are known as plantar warts. They have a soft, pulpy core surrounded by a hard, horny ring and tend to grow in groups that can become as big as a quarter. Plantar warts often have little black dots on them, which are blocked or clotted blood vessels. Plantar warts are more common in children who sweat or exercise a lot.

Flat warts commonly appear on a child's face. They are much smaller and smoother than hand or plantar warts and usually grow in groups of 20 to 100.

DIAGNOSIS Your child's doctor will be able to diagnose a wart based on its appearance during a physical examination.

TREATMENT In children, warts usually disappear without treatment several months to several years after they appear. But, because warts can spread to other people and to other parts of a child's body through scratching, children with warts should be seen by a doctor for treatment, especially if there is swelling around the wart that causes pain or discomfort. Check the rest of your family for warts as well.

For a very young child with a small hand wart, the doctor may recommend treatment at home with an over-the-counter lotion that contains salicylic acid. The doctor will probably treat hand warts in an older child by applying liquid nitrogen, or another chemical that freezes the warts. This treatment causes only mild discomfort. Foot warts can be removed with salicylic acid plasters or frozen with liquid nitrogen. Facial warts require daily applications of salicylic acid under the doctor's supervision.

WHOOPING COUGH

Whooping cough, also known as pertussis, is a contagious bacterial infection that affects a child's lungs. It occurs most often in children under 5 years of age, especially in infants. The bacteria usually spread when an infected person coughs or sneezes into the air. Infants are usually immunized against the disease beginning at 2 months of age. The vaccine is effective in preventing the disease in 70 to 90 percent of all children who receive it. Children usually get the vaccine five times by age 5 or 6, along with the vaccines for DIPHTHERIA and TETANUS.

SIGNS AND SYMPTOMS Symptoms can take 1 or 2 weeks to develop. Initially, the child has the symptoms of a cold, such as a runny nose, low-grade fever (see page 279), sneezing, and a mild cough. The cough gradually worsens over the next week or two, and the child has bouts of severe, continuous coughing that may last up to a minute. The child's face can turn blue during the coughing spells from a lack of oxygen. After coughing, the child gasps for breath, making the characteristic whooping sound; most infants do not whoop and some children may whoop while coughing. The child may also vomit (see page 284) from coughing so hard. If not treated right away, whooping cough can cause severe complications, such as seizures, PNEUMONIA, or even death.

DIAGNOSIS AND TREATMENT Your child's doctor will order chest X-rays, blood tests, and a *culture* of your child's sputum (phlegm) or nasal mucus to confirm the diagnosis. The doctor will then prescribe antibiotics to treat both whooping cough and its complications (such as pneumonia). Infants may need to be hospitalized. Family members will also need to take antibiotics to minimize their risk of getting the disease. Children with whooping cough are contagious from a few days before the symptoms appear to about 3 weeks after. Keep your child in bed and away from other people until the fever disappears and give him or her plenty of fluids. Most children recover without complications within 6 weeks.

WILMS' TUMOR

Wilms' tumor is a cancer of the kidney found mostly in children under the age of 4, although it can occur anytime in childhood from birth to age 15. Wilms' tumor is one of the more common childhood cancers, accounting for about 20 percent of all cases of cancer. Twice as many boys are affected as are girls.

Untreated, the tumor grows quickly and frequently spreads to other parts of the child's body, such as the liver, lungs, and brain. Usually, only one kidney is affected, but a tumor can occur in both kidneys in about 10 percent of cases.

SIGNS AND SYMPTOMS Wilms' tumor causes a child's abdomen to become swollen. Sometimes the child also has abdominal pain and blood in his or her urine. Other symptoms may include a slight fever, a general feeling of being unwell, loss of appetite, constipation, nausea, vomiting, and high blood pressure.

Wilms' tumor often appears in children who have other abnormalities that have been present from birth, including absence of the iris (colored part of the eye), abnormal enlargement of one limb or one side of the child's body, and defects in the development of the genitourinary tract. Children who have any of these abnormalities should receive routine *ultrasound* examinations of the kidney during the first few years of life to screen for Wilms' tumor because of their increased risk.

DIAGNOSIS Wilms' tumor produces abdominal swelling, and a parent sometimes finds the tumor during a child's bath. If your child's doctor suspects Wilms' tumor, he or she will do a thorough physical examination and will order an *ultrasound* examination of your child's kidneys or a *computed tomography* (CT) examination of your child's abdomen. A *biopsy* of the tumor will confirm the diagnosis. Further tests, such as a CT scan of other parts of the body, may be needed to find out if the cancer has spread.

TREATMENT Treatment of Wilms' tumor depends on its stage of development and whether it has affected only one of your child's kidneys or both. If the tumor is in its early stages and occurs in only one of your child's kidneys, a cancer surgeon may remove the entire kidney.

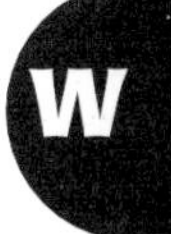

The surgeon may remove the lymph nodes that lie near your child's kidneys to make sure the disease does not spread. Your child may receive *chemotherapy* after surgery to destroy any remaining cancer cells. *Radiation* therapy may be needed, depending on the extent of the disease.

Your child can survive the loss of one kidney, but not both. If your child has a tumor in both kidneys, the cancer surgeon will try to remove part of the tumor from each kidney and then use chemotherapy to shrink the tumors. During a second operation, the cancer surgeon will try to cut away as much of the cancerous tissue as possible without removing the entire kidneys. Your child may then need chemotherapy or radiation therapy or both.

About 80 to 90 percent of children with Wilms' tumor who are treated early survive, but survival depends on how far the cancer has spread. Long-term complications can include liver problems and damage to the remaining kidney.

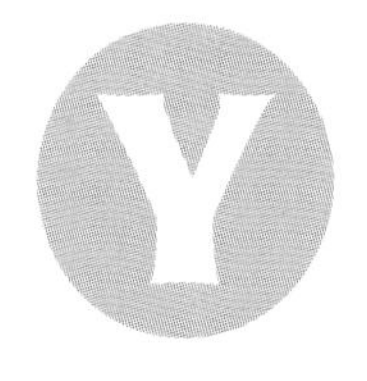

YEAST INFECTIONS

A yeast infection is caused by a type of fungus known as candida.

TYPES OF YEAST INFECTIONS Yeasts can infect infants, children, and adolescents and cause such conditions as thrush, diaper dermatitis, and vaginal yeast infections.

Thrush Thrush is a yeast infection that most commonly affects newborns and infants, but it can also occur in older children. Thrush is caused by a yeast known as Candida albicans, which is normally present in small amounts in the mouth. Sometimes the yeast grows out of control and causes infection. Newborns can develop thrush shortly after birth by being exposed to yeast in the mother's birth canal if the woman had a vaginal yeast infection. Newborns exposed to a yeast infection can develop symptoms of thrush within a day to a week of birth. Breast-feeding babies can also acquire thrush from their mother's breasts. Infants and children being treated with antibiotics can develop thrush because the antibiotics affect the natural balance of organisms in the child's mouth, allowing the yeast to multiply. Children with immune system deficiencies resulting from AIDS, cancer, transplantation, or malnutrition can also develop thrush. White or gray-white patches typically appear in the mouth and throat of a child who has thrush. These patches are not painful unless they are rubbed; they then become open sores.

Diaper dermatitis Diaper dermatitis is a candida yeast infection occurring in the diaper area that can be triggered by antibiotic treatment, especially for ear infections (see page 480). More commonly, it occurs when excess moisture created by urine and sweat become trapped in the baby's diaper. Diaper dermatitis produces small, red, pimplelike bumps around the genitals and anus.

Vaginal yeast infections Vaginal yeast infections, caused by C albicans, occur when the yeast that is normally present inside the vagina in small amounts multiplies because of menstruation, antibiotics or oral contraceptives, pregnancy, or diabetes (see DIABETES MELLITUS, TYPE I), all of which can change the vagina's environment and encourage growth of the yeast. Irritation and moisture can also encourage infection. A vaginal yeast infection produces a white discharge that resembles cottage cheese. Additional symptoms include vaginal itching and burning, swelling of the skin around the vagina, and pain during intercourse.

DIAGNOSIS AND TREATMENT If the doctor suspects that your child has a yeast infection, he or she will examine your child for signs of infection and may take a sample of the vaginal discharge, patches in the mouth, or skin rash for analysis. Doctors usually treat thrush with an antifungal medication in liquid form that is rubbed inside your child's mouth with a swab or clean finger. If your child is old enough, the medication may be given by spoon so the child can swish the liquid in his or her mouth and then spit it out. Diaper dermatitis is treated with antifungal medication in cream or lotion form applied to the affected area. Vaginal yeast infections are generally treated with an antifungal cream or a suppository placed inside the vagina. The infection should disappear in a few days with treatment but can return.

QUICK REFERENCE GUIDE

FIRST AID AND EMERGENCIES

Instructions for most common medical emergencies are in the First Aid and Emergencies section that follows. However, some minor injuries and rarer emergencies are covered in other parts of the book. The alphabetical list of emergency situations below refers you to the information you need. If you don't see the topic for which you are searching, refer to the index at the back of the book.

First aid and emergencies

To provide care to an injured child, you need to know the basics of cardiopulmonary resuscitation (CPR) and first aid. In an emergency, it's important to remain calm. But you also need to act quickly because you can make the difference in a sick child's condition until emergency medical services arrive.

Emergency phone numbers

Make sure your children know what to do in case of an emergency. Have them practice what to do by pretending to dial 911 (or your local emergency number) and describing what is wrong. They should know how to give their name, address, and phone number. Keep the following numbers near all the telephones in your home and show the list to your baby-sitter whenever you go out:

Nearest pediatric hospital emergency department
Local emergency number
Ambulance
Poison control center
Doctor or clinic
Fire department
Police department
Your own home phone
Dad's work phone
Mom's work phone
Pager or cellular phone
Nearest neighbor's phone
Nearest relatives or friends

When to call for help

In an emergency, time is of the essence. For emergencies that appear serious or life threatening, call 911 (or your local emergency number), 0 for operator, or an ambulance service and ask for immediate transportation to a hospital emergency department. The emergency squad or ambulance service will take your child to the nearest hospital. Not all hospital emergency departments have personnel trained to handle childhood emergencies or equipment designed to treat children. Call the emergency department at the hospital nearest your home and ask if it is equipped to handle pediatric emergencies. If there is a children's emergency department or a pediatric-equipped emergency department in your community, keep the number by your phone so that you can call there for help in an emergency. Keep the address of the pediatric emergency department handy in case you need to drive your child there yourself during an emergency that is not life threatening.

If your child has any of the following symptoms, he or she needs immediate medical attention and you should call your child's doctor or the hospital emergency department:

- Loss or decreased level of consciousness, drowsiness, or diminished alertness
- A seizure that continues for more than 2 minutes or produces dusky skin or bluish lips
- Bleeding that can't be stopped by direct pressure
- Difficulty breathing, especially if the child can't speak, has blue skin, or the muscles between his or her ribs are straining
- Severe choking
- Cold, clammy, pale skin
- Bloody vomit
- Bloody diarrhea
- Stiff neck
- Major injury, such as from a fall or motor vehicle collision
- Possible neck injury
- Swelling, pain, or discoloration of a testicle
- Severe abdominal pain
- Bone fracture or break

CHOKING, RESCUE BREATHING, AND CARDIOPULMONARY RESUSCITATION

Cardiopulmonary resuscitation (CPR) can help you save a life. CPR and first-aid courses may be offered by the American Red Cross or the American Heart Association, or by your local hospital, fire department, community center, school, or employer. Ask your doctor about classes in your community and sign up today. Once you learn the CPR techniques, practice them often so you will be able to remember the correct procedures in an emergency. The CPR techniques presented here are not intended as a substitute for a course.

CHOKING: FOR CHILDREN UNDER 1 YEAR

Suspect that something is obstructing an infant's airway if the baby suddenly has difficulty breathing, along with coughing, gagging, a change in color, or wheezing. If the infant can cough, cry, or make any sounds, see if the coughing reflex dislodges the object from the child's airway. Don't slap the infant on the back or give him or her anything to drink because you could make the problem worse. If coughing doesn't dislodge the object, call your child's doctor immediately and ask what to do.

If the infant is choking on a solid object and can't breathe, cough, or make a sound, his or her airway may be completely blocked. You must remove the object quickly to prevent suffocation. Ask someone to call 911 (or your local emergency number) immediately and perform the first-aid procedures described at right until help arrives.

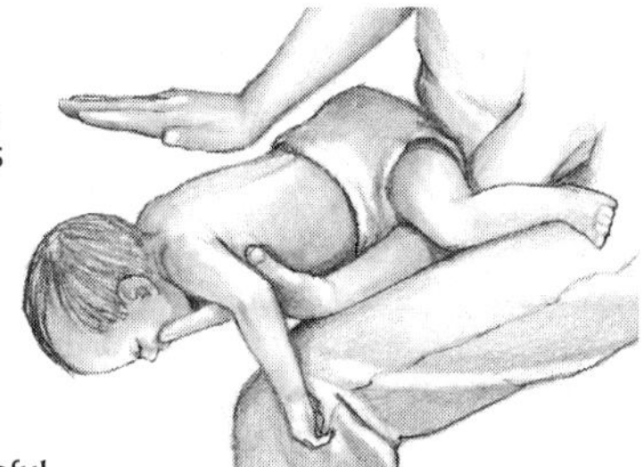

1. Position the infant facedown on your arm with the child's head lower than his or her chest. Support the infant's head at the jaw, resting your forearm on your thigh.

2. Give up to five forceful blows between the infant's shoulder blades with the heel of your hand. If the object remains lodged in the airway or the infant still can't breathe, continue to step 3.

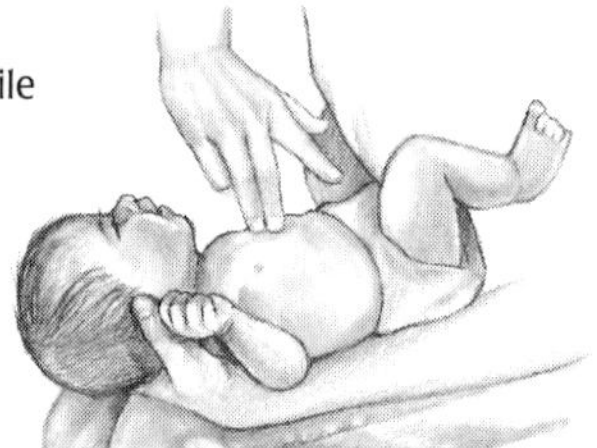

3. Turn the infant over while supporting his or her head and position the child face up on your forearm with the child's head lower than his or her chest.

4. Using two fingers, give up to five quick thrusts to the infant's chest near the center of the child's breastbone.

Repeat steps 1 through 4 until the object is coughed up, the infant starts to breathe, or medical help arrives.

If infant loses consciousness:

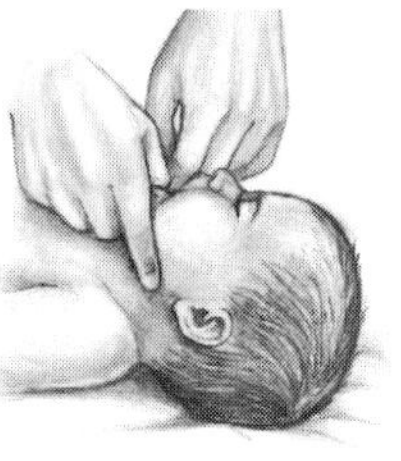

5. Lay the infant on a flat surface, open his or her mouth, and look inside. If you see an object, sweep your index finger across the back of the child's throat to remove it. Sweep with your finger only if you see an object; otherwise you could push it in farther.

6. Tilt the child's forehead back and lift his or her chin up with your fingers just until the infant's ears are level with his or her shoulders. Don't tilt the child's head back too far or you could block the airway.

7. Perform rescue breathing (below, right). Seal your lips tightly around the infant's mouth and nose and try to give two slow breaths 3 seconds apart. Look at the child's chest to see if it rises with the breaths, indicating that air is getting into the airway.

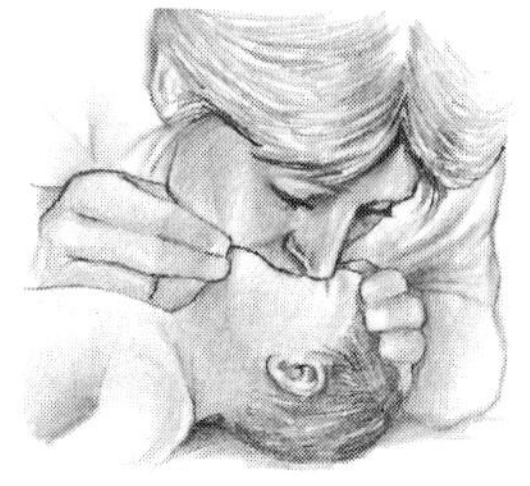

8. If air goes in, go to step 3 in the left column on the next page. If air won't go in, go to step 3 in the right column on the next page.

CPR: For children under 1 year

CPR is used when an infant is unresponsive or when his or her breathing or heartbeat has stopped. Follow these steps:

1. Try to open the infant's airway. Tilt the child's forehead back and lift his or her chin up with your fingers just until the child's ears are level with his or her shoulders. Don't tilt the head back too far or you could block the airway.

2. Perform rescue breathing. Seal your lips tightly around the infant's mouth and nose and try to give two slow breaths 3 seconds apart. Look at the child's chest to see if it rises with each breath, indicating that air is getting into the airway.

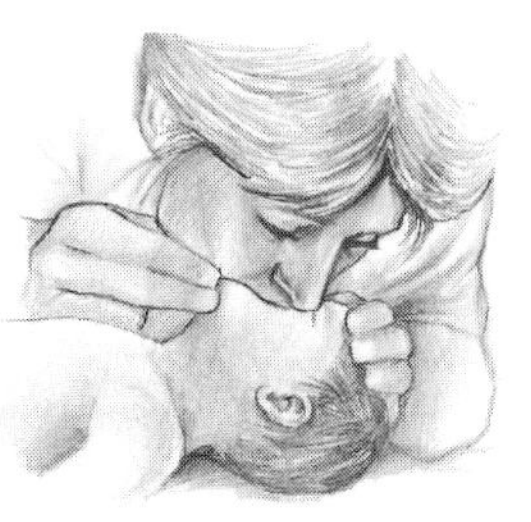

If air goes in:

3. Briefly check for a pulse by pressing gently on the artery on the inner part of the child's upper arm, just above the elbow crease.

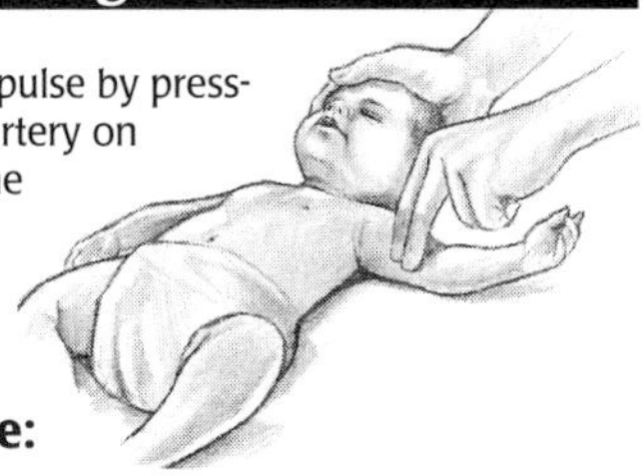

If there is a pulse:

4. Give one slow breath every 3 seconds for about 1 minute (20 breaths).

5. Check the infant's pulse once every minute.

6. Continue rescue breathing as long as the child has a pulse but is not breathing.

If there is no pulse, begin CPR:

4. Lay the infant on his or her back on a firm surface. Place two fingers on the breastbone, just below an imaginary line connecting one nipple to the other.

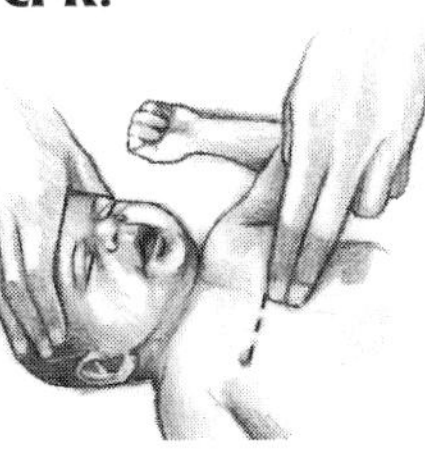

5. Compress the infant's chest five times within 3 seconds.

6. Give the child one slow breath (right).

7. Repeat cycles of five chest compressions within 3 seconds and one breath until you feel a pulse or medical help arrives.

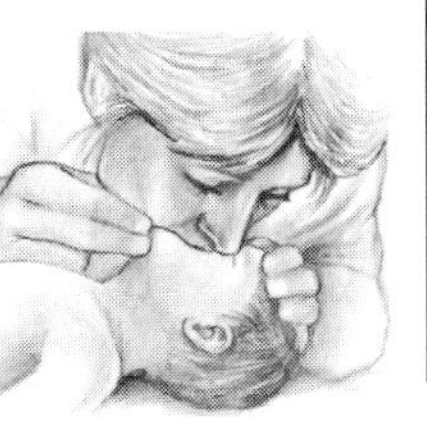

If air won't go in:

3. Try to open the airway by tilting the infant's head back again. Give two slow breaths (right).

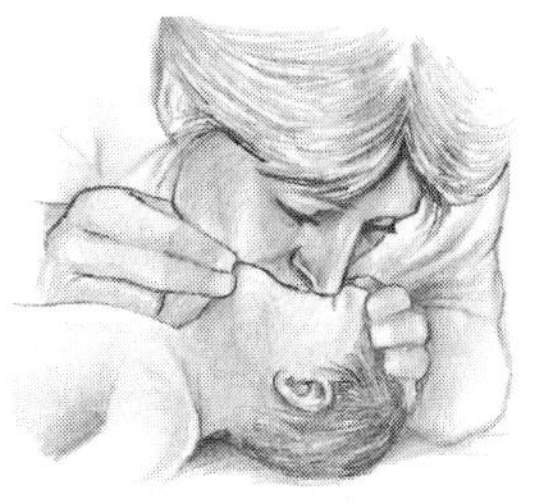

4. Try to dislodge whatever may be blocking the airway by repeating steps 2 through 4 on the facing page, giving five back blows and five chest thrusts.

5. Open the infant's mouth and look inside for an object. If you can see one, sweep your index finger across the back of the child's throat to remove it. Do the finger sweep only if you can see the object to avoid pushing it in farther.

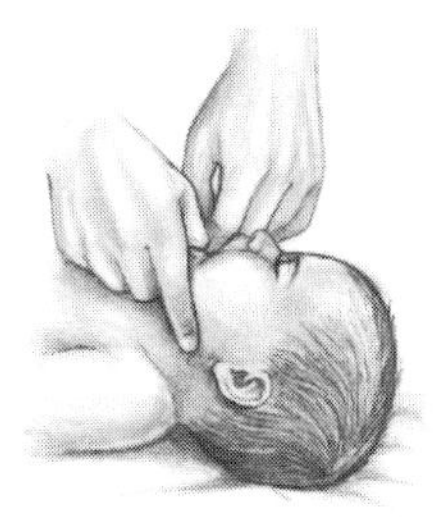

6. Repeat steps 3 through 5 until your breaths go in (you'll notice the child's chest gently rise), the child starts to breathe, or medical help arrives.

CHOKING, RESCUE BREATHING, AND CARDIOPULMONARY RESUSCITATION

CHOKING: FOR CHILDREN OVER 1 YEAR

If a child is choking on a solid object and can cough, cry, or speak, and his or her skin color is good, see if the coughing reflex dislodges the object from the child's airway. Don't slap the child on the back or give him or her anything to drink because you could make the problem worse. If coughing doesn't dislodge the object, call your child's doctor immediately and ask what to do.

If the child is choking on a solid object and can't breathe, cough, or make a sound, his or her airway may be completely blocked. You must remove the object quickly to prevent suffocation. Ask someone to call 911 (or your local emergency number) immediately and perform the first-aid procedures described at right and below until help arrives:

1. Stand behind the child and put your arms around his or her waist. Place the thumbside of your fist against the child's abdomen just above the navel and below the ribs. Grasp your fist with your other hand.

2. Give up to 10 quick, forceful, inward and upward thrusts. Use only your fist; don't squeeze the child's ribs with your arms.

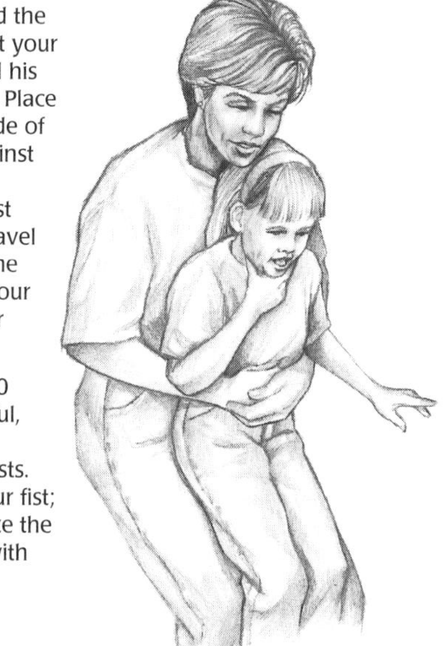

If object doesn't come out:

3. If the object doesn't come out, place the child on his or her back. Open the child's mouth and look inside for an object. If you see one, sweep your index finger across the back of the child's throat to remove it. Sweep with your finger only if you see the object to avoid pushing it in farther.

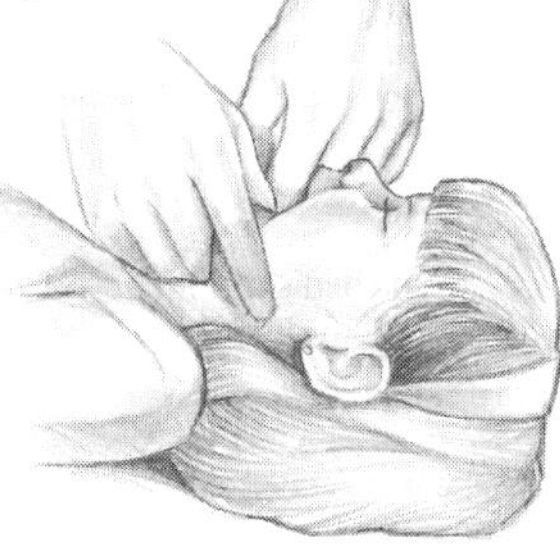

If breathing doesn't start:

4. If the child doesn't start breathing, gently push his or her forehead back and lift the chin up just until the child's ears are level with his or her shoulders. Don't tilt the child's head back too far or you could block the airway.

5. Perform rescue breathing. Seal your lips tightly around the child's mouth, pinch his or her nose shut, and give two slow breaths 3 seconds apart. Look at the child's chest to see if it gently rises, indicating that air is getting into the airway.

6. If air goes in, go to step 3 in the left column on the next page. If air won't go in, go to step 3 in the right column on the next page.

CPR: FOR CHILDREN OVER 1 YEAR

CPR is used when a child is unresponsive or when his or her breathing or heartbeat has stopped. Follow these steps:

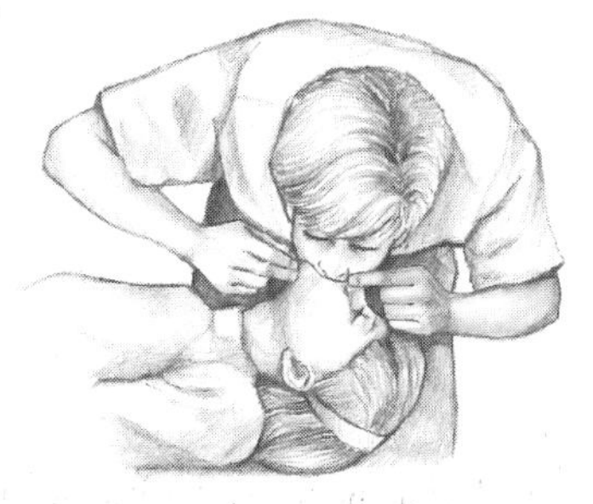

1. To open the child's airway, gently push his or her forehead back and lift the chin up just until the child's ears are level with his or her shoulders. Don't tilt the child's head back too far or you could block the airway.

2. Perform rescue breathing. Seal your lips tightly around the child's mouth, pinch his or her nose shut, and give two slow breaths over 3 seconds. Look at the child's chest to see if it gently rises, indicating that air is getting into the airway.

If air goes in:

3. Briefly check for a pulse by pressing two fingers firmly on the child's throat over the artery on either side of the Adam's apple.

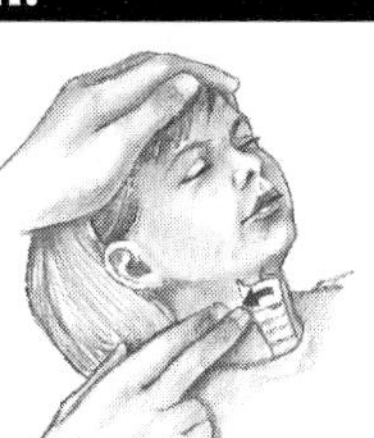

If there is a pulse:

4. Give one slow breath every 3 seconds for about 1 minute (20 breaths).

5. Check the child's pulse once every minute.

6. Continue rescue breathing (steps 4 and 5) for as long as the child has a pulse but is not breathing.

If there is no pulse, begin CPR:

4. Move your fingers up the center of the child's chest to the notch where the ribs meet the breastbone. Place the heel of your hand two finger-widths above the notch. If the child is older than 8 years, put your other hand on top of the hand on the chest, interlacing your fingers.

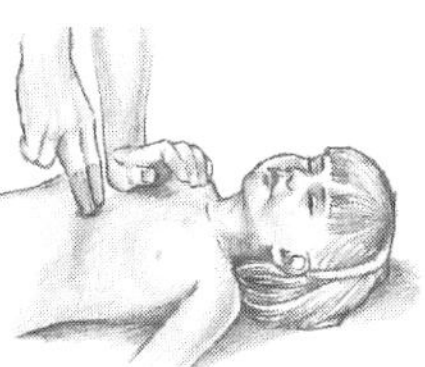

5. Position your shoulders over your hand(s).

6. Push down quickly and forcefully five times. Let the child's chest rise after each compression, but do not remove your hand(s) from the chest.

7. Give the child one slow breath.

8. Repeat cycles of five chest compressions and one breath until you feel a pulse or medical help arrives. Each cycle of chest compressions should last for 3 seconds for a child 1 to 8 years old and for 5 seconds for a child over the age of 8.

If air won't go in:

3. Try to open the airway by tilting the child's head back again. Give two slow breaths.

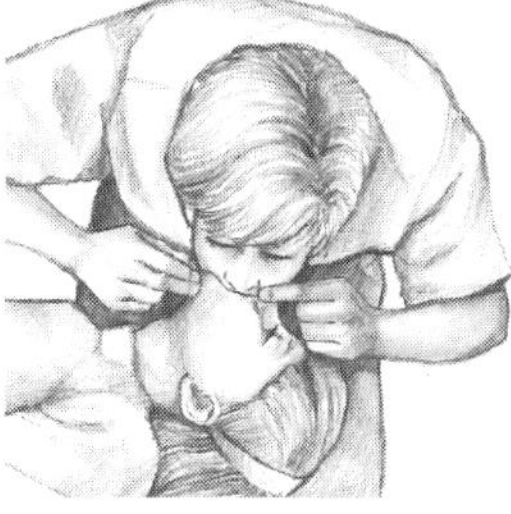

4. If air still won't go in, straddle the child's hips or kneel beside him or her. Place the heel of one hand on the center of the child's abdomen slightly above the navel and below the ribs. Place your other hand on top of it.

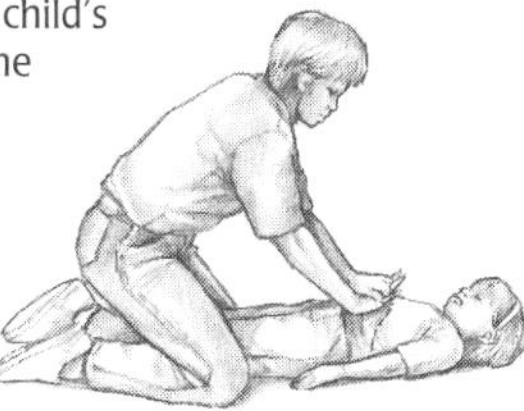

5. Keeping your elbows straight, give up to five quick, abdominal thrusts upward toward the child's head.

6. Open the child's mouth and look inside for an object. If you see one, sweep your index finger across the back of the child's throat to remove it. Sweep with your finger only if you see the object to avoid pushing it in farther.

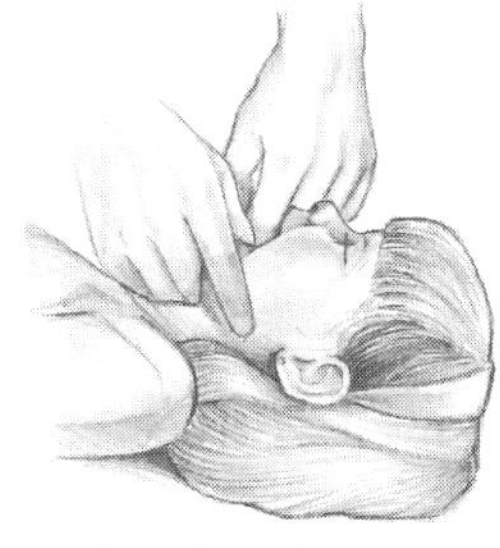

7. Repeat steps 3 through 6 until your breaths go in (you'll see the child's chest gently rise), the child starts to breathe, or medical help arrives.

BITES, HUMAN OR ANIMAL

Bites that break the skin—whether from people, pets, or wild animals—transmit organisms, especially bacteria, that can cause infection. Wild animal bites also carry the risk of infection with tetanus or rabies, two life-threatening diseases. If your child has been bitten by an animal or a person, take the following steps:

1. Clean the bite with soap and running water for at least 5 minutes. If the wound is bleeding, place a sterile bandage or clean cloth over it and apply firm, continuous pressure for 5 minutes or until the bleeding stops. Do not apply any ointment or antiseptic medication.
2. Cover the bite with another sterile bandage or clean cloth.
3. Take your child to the doctor immediately, even if the injury appears minor. The doctor can determine whether or not your child needs antibiotics to prevent a bacterial infection, shots to prevent rabies, or a tetanus booster.

BONE FRACTURES

Children are most likely to break the bones in their arms and legs. The most important thing you can do for a child with a fracture is to immobilize the broken bone because any movement can cause severe pain and further injury to the bone and surrounding tissues.

BROKEN ARM

If your child breaks a bone in his or her arm, keep the arm immobile. If the arm is bent, don't try to straighten it. Gently place the child's arm in a wide sling, adjusting it so that the injured area is at or above the level of the heart, if possible, and carefully apply ice to the area. If the bone is protruding out of the skin, cover it with a clean cloth and place firm pressure on the wound to stop the bleeding. Seek medical attention immediately by calling your doctor or 911 (or your local emergency number), or take your child to the nearest hospital emergency department.

BROKEN LEG OR FOOT

If your child has broken a bone in his or her leg or foot, carefully immobilize the injured limb, supporting it above and below the break. If the bone is protruding from the skin, apply direct pressure with a sterile cloth to stop the bleeding and then cover it with a clean dressing. Call an ambulance or, if you can transport your child without moving the injured limb too much, take him or her to the nearest hospital emergency department.

BURNS

If your child has a minor, first-degree burn on the surface of the skin and it does not blister, you can treat it at home (see page 287). Call the doctor if the burn blisters. Burns that are deep, are on the face or palms, or affect a large area of the body require treatment in the hospital emergency department. Call 911 or your local emergency number for medical help.

SECOND-DEGREE BURNS

Second-degree burns most often result from hot liquids or a serious sunburn and require immediate treatment to limit skin damage. Put the burned area in cool water, or apply cloths that have been soaked in cool water over the area for a few minutes. Cover the burn loosely with a sterile, nonfluffy bandage or clean cloth, being careful not to break any blisters, then take your child to the doctor.

If the burn occurs in the child's mouth or throat, take the child immediately to the nearest hospital emergency department. A burn in the throat can cause swelling, making breathing difficult. Give the child fre-

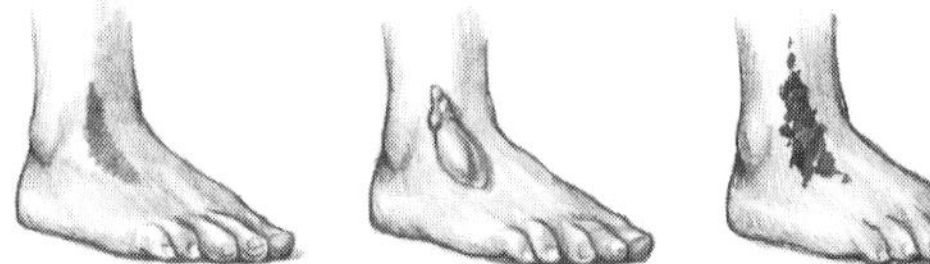

First-degree burn   Second-degree burn   Third-degree burn

Burns

First-degree burns affect only the outer layer of the skin, causing redness, pain, and, sometimes, slight swelling. Second-degree burns go deeper into the outer layer of skin and may invade the second layer, causing redness, tenderness, swelling, and blistering. Third-degree burns damage tissue and muscle underneath the skin. Third-degree burns make the skin look white or charred, tough, and leathery.

quent sips of cold water and remove any jewelry or clothing from around his or her neck.

THIRD-DEGREE BURNS

Third-degree burns are life threatening. They are usually caused by scalding or contact with fire or high-voltage electricity and extend deep into the skin and underlying muscle.

If your child has a third-degree burn, call 911 (or your local emergency number) or take him or her to the nearest hospital emergency department. Here's what to do before transporting your child or while waiting for medical help to arrive:

1. If your child's clothing is on fire, smother the flames with a blanket or jacket starting at the child's neck and working down. Check to make sure the child is breathing. If necessary, perform rescue breathing or cardiopulmonary resuscitation (see page 668). If the child is breathing, go to step 2 or 3. If the child is not breathing, perform rescue breathing.

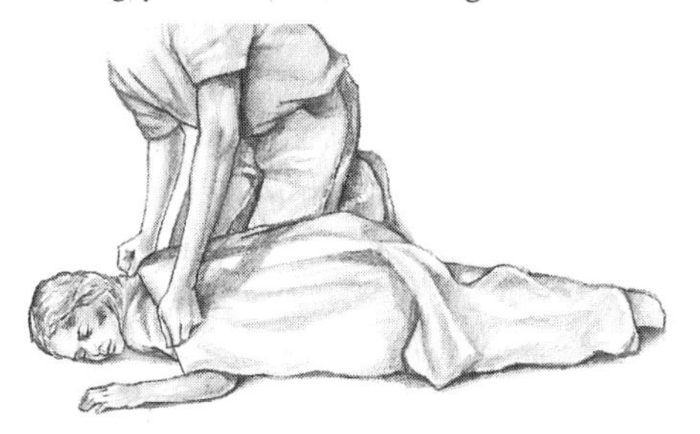

2. If the burn is extensive (for example, it covers the child's chest, an entire arm, or the face), don't put anything cold on it because you could lower the child's body temperature to a dangerous level. Instead, cover the child with a clean blanket.
3. If the burn is not extensive, place a cold, wet cloth on the area or gently pour cool or cold water (not ice) on it for a few minutes. Cover the burn with a thick, sterile, nonfluffy dressing. Do not remove any clothing or other material that is stuck to the burn.

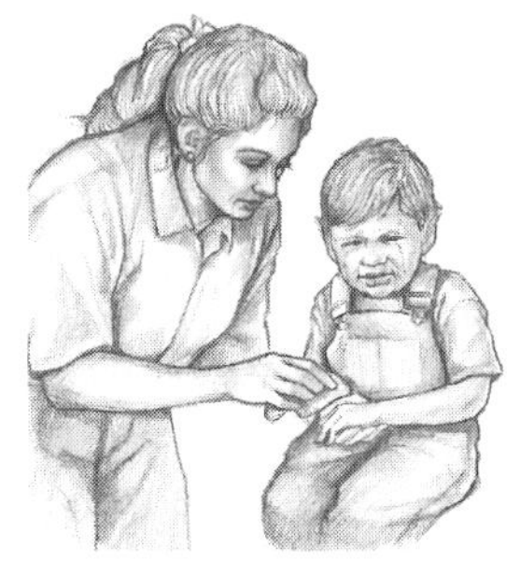

ELECTRICAL BURNS

Electrical burns are often invisible because they can affect internal tissue more than the skin. For example, a toddler who chews through an electric wire may have only a small burn at the corner of his or her mouth but could have serious internal injuries. A severe electric shock can knock a child to the ground and cause him or her to lose consciousness or stop breathing. All electrical burns need to be checked by a doctor. Here's what to do if your child gets an electric shock or burn:

1. If your child is still in contact with the source of electricity, turn off the power by pulling the plug or turning the switch off. Don't touch the child if he or she is still in contact with the electricity source; you could also get shocked. If you can't turn off the electricity, separate the child from the source with something that will not conduct electricity, such as a wooden broom handle, a rope, or a long length of cloth. (Never use anything wet or made of metal. Make sure you are standing on a dry surface.)
2. Check the child's breathing and pulse and, if necessary, perform rescue breathing or cardiopulmonary resuscitation (see page 668). If someone else is in the house, ask him or her to call 911 (or your local emergency number).
3. If you are alone, call 911 (or your local emergency number) as soon as your child starts breathing.
4. Cover all burns with a dry, loose dressing and then a bandage. Do not break any blisters, remove any loose skin, or apply any lotions or ointments.

CUTS AND WOUNDS

Most cuts that children get are minor and you can treat them easily at home (see page 286). But call your child's doctor or seek medical treatment immediately if your child has a more serious wound and any of the following circumstances apply:

- The wound is very deep or more than ½ inch long.
- The bleeding does not stop after you apply pressure for 5 minutes.
- The bleeding comes in spurts, indicating injury to a major blood vessel and risk of severe blood loss.
- The wound was caused by a dirty object.

- ◆ The wound was caused by a bite (human or animal).
- ◆ The wound has been in contact with soil or manure.
- ◆ The wound is on the child's face. (Prompt treatment can help minimize scarring.)
- ◆ Something is deeply embedded in the wound.
- ◆ You are not sure when your child last had a tetanus shot.
- ◆ The wound shows signs of infection—redness, swelling, tenderness, or pus—after a few hours or days.
- ◆ The wound is deep and on the palm side of the hand, potentially injuring a tendon.
- ◆ Your child has a bleeding disorder.

Stopping heavy bleeding

Severe loss of blood can cause shock (see page 678) and death. If your child has a deep wound with severe bleeding, call 911 (or your local emergency number) and take the following measures while waiting for medical help to arrive:

1. Place a thick, clean compress of sterile gauze or a soft, clean cloth over the entire wound and press firmly with one or both hands. Don't remove any objects, such as metal or glass, that are deeply embedded in the wound or you could worsen the bleeding. Continue to apply steady pressure until the bleeding stops or medical help arrives. If blood soaks through the compress, leave it in place, put another compress over it, and continue to apply pressure. If the wound has occurred in an arm or leg and you are sure no bones are broken, elevate the limb above the level of your child's heart. If pressure and elevation of the limb fail to stop the bleeding, tie a tourniquet around the limb above the wound.

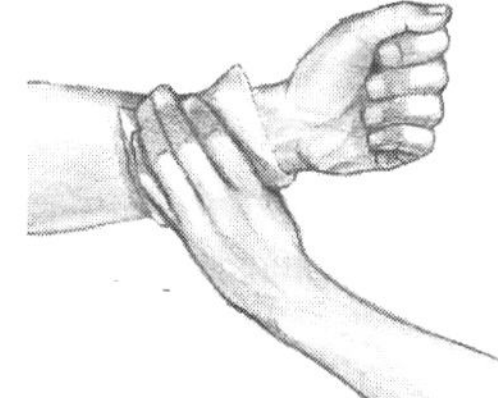

2. When the bleeding stops, apply a pressure bandage (gauze, cloth strips, or even a necktie) over the compress to hold it in place. To apply the bandage, place the center of it directly over the compress and wrap it around the wound, pulling steadily to secure. Tie a knot over the compress.

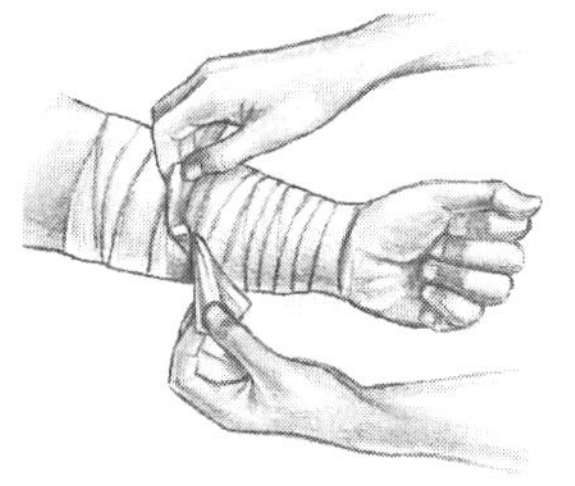

3. Check for a pulse below the level of the bandage. If you don't feel a pulse, the bandage may be cutting off the blood supply to the limb. Loosen the bandage slightly and recheck the child's pulse.

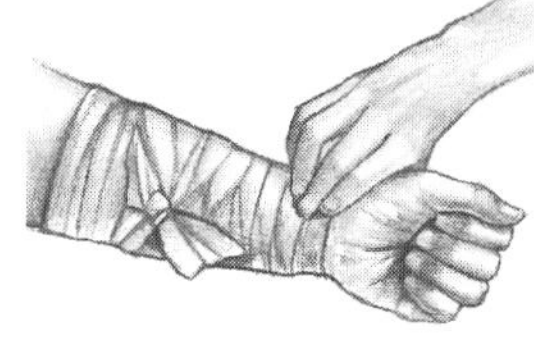

4. Keep the child warm by covering him or her with blankets or a coat, keeping the wound area in view. If the child is conscious and asks for water, moisten his or her lips and tongue. If the child is unconscious or if the injury is severe, do not give fluids. (A severe injury may require surgery and general anesthesia should only be given on an empty stomach.)

Signs of internal bleeding

Cuts or bruises on the chest, abdomen, or back should alert you to possible internal injuries that could cause internal bleeding, especially if your child has had a bad fall, been struck by a motor vehicle, been in an automobile collision, or sustained a severe blow. Call 911 (or your local emergency number) if you notice any of the following signs of internal bleeding:

- Coughing up or vomiting blood
- Pale, cold, clammy skin, which could indicate shock
- Severe pain in the chest or abdomen
- Swollen abdomen
- Difficulty breathing
- Severe swelling around the injury
- Fainting, which could indicate severe blood loss

Removing splinters

Every child gets splinters under the skin from time to time. You can usually remove them yourself at home with tweezers and a needle that you have sterilized with rubbing alcohol. If a splinter is protruding from your child's skin, grab it with a tweezers and pull it out at the same angle it entered the skin. If the splinter is not protruding from the skin but is visible beneath it, loosen the skin around the splinter with a sterilized needle until you can grasp the splinter with a tweezers and remove it. Squeeze the skin around the affected area until it bleeds to help eliminate germs and dirt. Wash the area well with soap and water and cover it with a bandage. Check the area over the next few days for redness, pus, or red streaks, which indicate infection. If the splinter breaks off underneath your child's skin or if it is deeply embedded, take your child to the doctor to have it removed.

Drowning

Recovery from a near-drowning episode depends on how long the child has been without oxygen. If you find a child who is immersed in water, get him or her out of the water and lay the child on his or her back on a flat surface. If you can't swim, don't go in the water to save the child. Instead, use a pole or throw a flotation device or rope to the child to bring him or her out of the water. Check for breathing and pulse. If he or she is not breathing, immediately begin rescue breathing; if he or she has no pulse, begin cardiopulmonary resuscitation (CPR) (see page 668). Have someone call 911 (or your local emergency number) for help. Don't stop rescue breathing or CPR until the child begins to cough or breathe on his or her own or until medical help arrives.

If the child is coughing or breathing, stay close until his or her breathing returns to normal. Remove wet clothing and wrap the child in blankets or put warm clothing on the child. Call the doctor immediately for further instructions.

Eye injuries

A number of injuries can impair vision—an object that penetrates the eyeball, chemicals that burn the eye, or a direct blow to the eye. Call your child's doctor or an ophthalmologist (a doctor who specializes in disorders of the eye) immediately after any eye injury, no matter how minor it may seem.

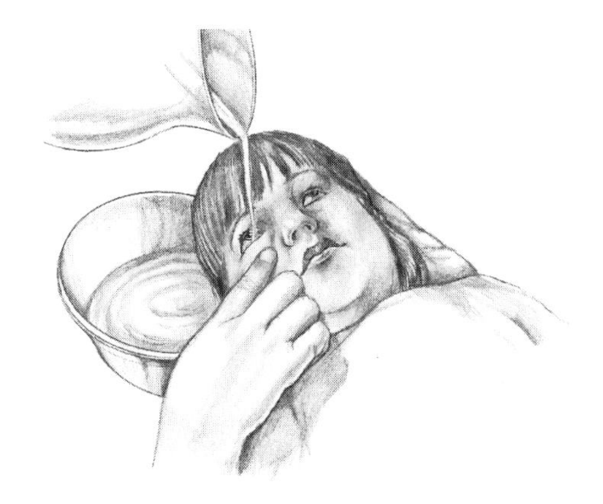

Chemical burns to the eyes

Strong chemicals, such as drain openers or bleach, can damage a child's eyes permanently. If your child's eyes become exposed to a harsh chemical, immediately flush the eyes with a gentle stream of running water for at least 15 minutes while holding the child's eyelids open. Make sure the water is not too hot and that it flushes all parts of both eyes. Then, call your doctor or the local poison control center for further instructions. Do not apply medication to the child's eyes and tell your child not to touch or rub them.

Penetrating eye injuries

If an object, such as a stick or a piece of glass, penetrates your child's eye, do not try to remove it. Ask the child to lie down or sit in a semireclining position. Gently cover both eyes with a clean cloth or pad of gauze, and tape it loosely in place. Don't put any pressure on the eye. Then, take your child to the emergency department immediately.

Removing something from the surface of the eye

If an eyelash or a speck of dirt is resting on the white part of your child's eye or inside the eyelids, you can probably remove it yourself at home by taking the following steps:

1. Wash your hands with soap and water. Gently pull your child's upper eyelid down to produce tears that

may wash out the object.

2. If the object is still there, pour water slowly from a large glass or run a gentle stream of tap water over the eyeball. Make sure the water is not too hot.
3. If step 2 fails to remove the object, pull down the child's lower eyelid. If you can see the particle, carefully remove it with a moistened, clean tissue or cloth.
4. If the object is not visible, tell your child to direct his or her eyes downward while you gently and carefully fold the upper lid back on itself and look for the object at the top of the eyeball. If the particle is visible, gently remove it with a moistened, clean tissue or cloth. If you cannot remove the object, take your child to the doctor.

Fainting

Fainting is a brief period of unconsciousness usually lasting less than 1 minute. If your child has fainted, check his or her breathing and pulse. If he or she is not breathing, call 911 (or your local emergency number) and begin rescue breathing. If he or she has no pulse, start cardiopulmonary resuscitation (see page 668).

Head injuries

Injuries to the head and neck can damage the brain and spinal cord, potentially causing paralysis, severe disability, or even death. To be on the safe side, treat any child who is unconscious as if he or she has a head, neck, or spinal injury, especially after a severe blow.

Severe injuries to the head or neck

In the event of a serious head injury, don't move the child and don't change the position of his or her head while waiting for medical help to arrive. Changing the position of the child's head or neck could make the injuries worse. Call 911 (or your local emergency number) if your child has any of the following symptoms of a severe head injury:

- Unconsciousness that lasts longer than a few seconds, drowsiness, confusion, or difficulty speaking
- Nausea or vomiting that doesn't go away
- Convulsions
- Blood or clear fluid leaking from the ears, nose, or mouth
- Extensive bleeding from head wounds
- Irregular breathing
- Dilated pupils or pupils of different size, or vision problems
- Weakness or numbness in the arms or legs, or clumsy walking
- Any symptom, including headache, nausea, irritability or sleepiness, that gets worse

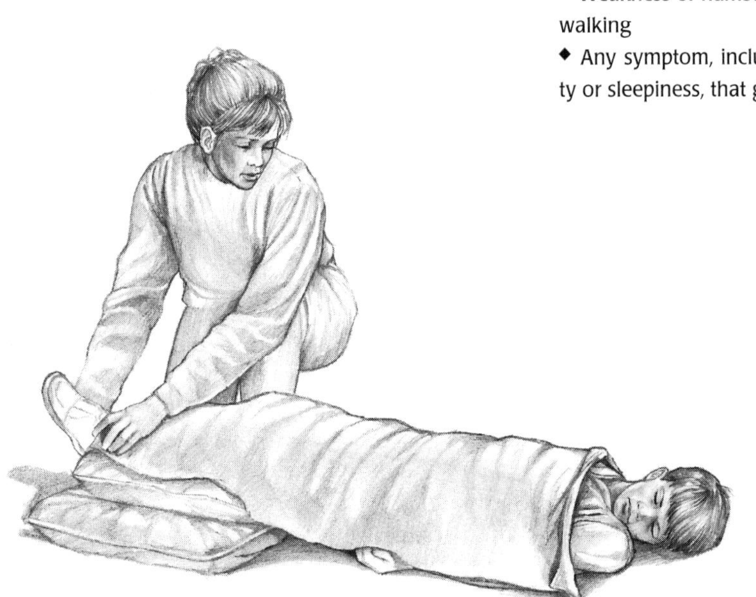

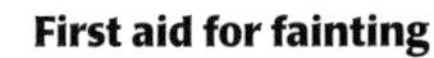

First aid for fainting

If your child has fainted but is breathing and has a pulse, lay the child down on his or her back and elevate the feet about 8 to 12 inches by resting them on folded blankets or towels. Apply a cloth soaked in cool water to his or her face and check for injuries that could have been caused by falling. Don't put anything in the child's mouth and don't offer anything to drink until he or she has fully recovered. Call the child's doctor for further instructions.

Any time that your child sustains a head injury, you should suspect injury to his or her neck, which could affect the spinal cord. Again, do not move the child or the position of his or her head. Call 911 (or your local emergency number) if your child has any of the following signs of a neck injury:

◆ Stiff neck

◆ Inability to move or loss of movement in any part of the body

◆ Tingling or change in sensation in any part of the body, especially in the arms or legs

MINOR HEAD INJURIES

A minor head injury may cause loss of consciousness for a few seconds, a headache, momentary confusion, double vision, a lump on the head, or drowsiness for an hour or two. After a minor head injury, your child should be able to move uninjured body parts and answer simple questions such as "What is your name?" Keep your child lying down and quiet while you call the doctor for advice on treatment.

◆ If the child's scalp has a small cut, clean the wound gently with soap and water. Apply gentle direct pressure to the injury to control any bleeding and cover the wound with a sterile bandage or clean cloth. Call the doctor to find out if your child needs more treatment.

◆ If the child has a lump on his or her head, apply an ice pack or chemical pack to reduce the swelling. Severe swelling that increases greatly in size over the next few hours might signal a skull fracture. Call the doctor and seek medical attention promptly.

◆ If the child's symptoms are very mild after the head injury and the child is not bleeding or in pain, watch him or her carefully for a day or two. Wake the child every 3 to 4 hours during the night of the injury and, if you notice any change in his or her mental alertness or if the child vomits, seek medical attention right away.

MUSCLE AND JOINT INJURIES

If your child sprains a joint or strains or tears a muscle, the best treatment is rest, ice, compression, and elevation (RICE). RICE helps to reduce pain and swelling during the first 24 to 48 hours after the injury.

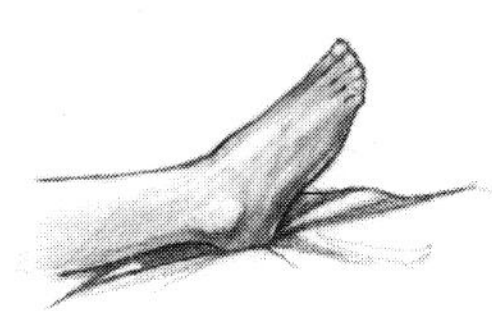

REST the injured part of the child's body. Rest helps reduce bleeding from damaged blood vessels in an injured joint or muscle, minimizes the risk of further damage, and allows time for tissues to heal.

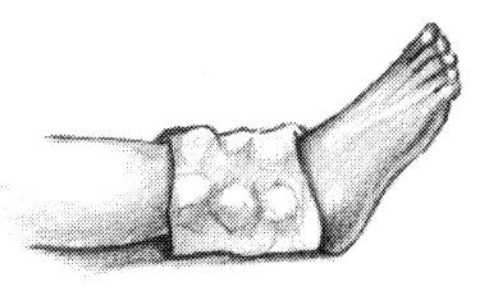

ICE, applied to the injury in an ice pack or chemical pack for 10 minutes every few hours, helps relieve pain and limits swelling.

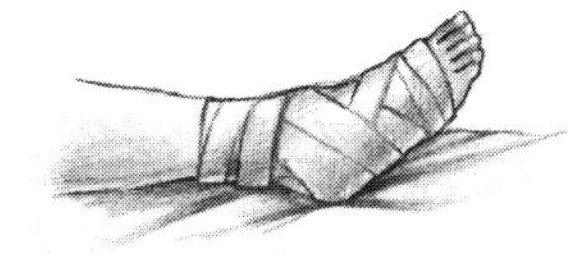

COMPRESSION limits bleeding and swelling. Wrap an elastic bandage around the injury and leave it there for at least 2 days. Be careful not to wrap it too tightly; you should be able to slip your finger under the bandage.

ELEVATION of the injured limb above the level of the child's heart reduces swelling by preventing blood and other fluids from collecting at the site of injury.

NOSEBLEEDS

Nosebleeds are common during childhood and some children get them frequently, especially if they have allergies that affect the nasal passages. Although blood streaming from a child's nose looks frightening, it rarely signals a serious condition. Nosebleeds usually happen when the nasal lining becomes dry or irritated, when children rub and pick their noses, or when they blow their nose too vigorously. Take the following steps if your child gets a nosebleed:

1. Ask your child to sit up or stand and tilt his or her head forward slightly to keep from swallowing the blood. Hold a container in front of his or her mouth to collect any blood that drains into the throat. If the child is old enough, ask him or her to blow his or her nose gently.
2. Pinch the soft part of your child's nostrils closed between your thumb and forefinger. Hold firmly for

10 minutes. If your child is old enough to pinch his or her own nostrils together, ask the child to do it. Tell your child to breathe through his or her mouth. Don't release the grip during the 10 minutes, even to see if the nose is still bleeding.

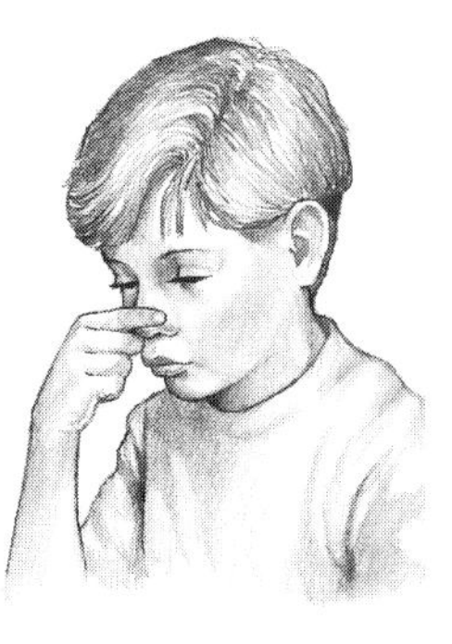

3. When the 10 minutes are up, release the pressure and wait, keeping your child quiet, to see if the bleeding has stopped.
4. If the bleeding has stopped, ask your child to remain quiet and to avoid laughing or blowing his or her nose for 1 or 2 hours. If the nose is still bleeding after 10 minutes, repeat steps 2 and 3.
5. If the bleeding continues after applying pressure for two 10-minute periods, call the doctor or take the child to the nearest hospital emergency department. You should also call the doctor if you think your child may have lost an excessive amount of blood, if the blood is coming only from his or her mouth, or if your child is coughing up or vomiting blood or brown material that looks like coffee grounds from discolored, clotted blood that has been in the stomach for a long period.

Poisoning

If you suspect that your child has been poisoned, call the local poison control center immediately for instructions, even if the child seems to be fine. Some poisons take time before they have an effect. Tell the poison control center the child's age, the name of the poison, how much poison he or she swallowed and when, whether he or she has vomited, and how long it will take to get to the nearest hospital emergency department. Before leaving, gather any items you find near the child—medications, empty containers or bottles, or plants—to give to the medical personnel to help them determine the right treatment. If your child is unconscious, drowsy, having convulsions, or having trouble breathing, call 911 (or your local emergency number).

Swallowed poisons

If your child has swallowed a poison, take the poison away and immediately call the poison control center for instructions. Do not give the child any fluids or try to induce vomiting unless you are told to do so because vomiting can worsen the problem with some poisons. Keep the child sitting up or lying facedown to prevent choking in case he or she vomits.

Exposure through the skin

If poisonous substances such as acids, lye, pesticides, or other chemicals come in contact with your child's skin, immediately brush off any material you can see and remove contaminated clothing. Wear rubber gloves if you have them. Wash the child's skin thoroughly with soap and water to remove as much of the poison as possible and call the poison control center for further instructions.

Inhaled poisons

If your child has inhaled smoke or poisonous gas or fumes, get him or her into the fresh air immediately and loosen tight clothing around the child's neck and waist. Call 911 (or your local emergency number) or the fire department immediately. If the child is not breathing, perform cardiopulmonary resuscitation (see page 668) until medical help arrives.

Shock

When bleeding drastically reduces blood flow to a child's organs and tissues, blood pressure drops dramatically, causing shock. Shock can also be caused by loss of fluids from vomiting or diarrhea, burns, infection, severe injuries, and failure of the heart to pump sufficient blood. A child needs immediate treatment after a serious injury to avoid going into shock. Signs of shock include:

- Confusion, restlessness, anxiety
- Pale or bluish, cool, clammy skin
- Widely dilated pupils
- Trembling or weakness in the arms and legs
- Very slow or rapid breathing or rapid pulse rate
- Extreme drowsiness
- Fainting

If you suspect that your child is in shock, call 911 (or your local emergency number) immediately and take the following steps while waiting for medical help to arrive:

1. Make sure the child is breathing. If not, perform cardiopulmonary resuscitation (CPR; see page 668). Treat whatever is causing the shock, such as severe bleeding (see page 674).
2. Keep the child lying down; don't move him or her unless it's necessary to get the child out of danger. Elevate his or her feet and legs above the level of the heart unless the child has a spinal, neck, or head injury. If the child has difficulty breathing, put him or her in a semireclining position. If the child vomits, place him or her on one side to prevent vomit from blocking the airway.
3. Loosen tight clothing and keep the child warm with a coat or blanket, but don't allow him or her to become overheated. Overheating could divert blood away from the child's vital organs. Do not offer anything to drink in case he or she needs surgery. Stay with the child, periodically checking to make sure he or she is still breathing and has a pulse.

Anaphylactic shock

Anaphylactic shock is a potentially life-threatening condition caused by an extreme allergic reaction to a medication, food, or insect bite or sting. Symptoms include coughing and wheezing; difficulty breathing; swelling, hives, or itching on many parts of the body; a flushed appearance; swollen lips, tongue, and ears; stomach cramps, nausea, and vomiting; severe swelling at the site of a bite or sting; dizziness; or unconsciousness. If your child has any of these symptoms, call your doctor immediately. Should your child have trouble breathing or pass out, call 911 (or your local emergency number) or take him or her to the nearest hospital emergency department. Lay the child down with his or her legs raised to improve circulation to the heart and brain while waiting for medical help to arrive. Some children with a known allergy to bee venom or a food or medication carry a prescribed premeasured dose of epinephrine (a form of adrenaline) to counteract anaphylactic shock. If your child's doctor has prescribed epinephrine for your child, give the child an injection of the medication at the first sign of anaphylactic shock.

Temperature extremes

Young children become affected by changes in temperature more quickly than do adults. Exposure to extreme hot or cold temperatures can damage the temperature-regulating mechanisms of a child's brain and be life threatening.

Heat exhaustion

Strenuous physical activity in hot weather can easily cause heat exhaustion, characterized by pale and clammy skin, dizziness, nausea, fatigue, and muscle cramps. If your child has any of these symptoms during hot weather, tell him or her to lie down and rest in the shade or in an air-conditioned room. Offer cool water and place a cool, wet cloth on his or her forehead. Untreated, heat exhaustion can lead to heatstroke (see below), which is more serious.

Heatstroke

Heatstroke, which often follows heat exhaustion, is a life-threatening condition that develops when the body cannot cool itself effectively during extremely hot weather. A child who has heatstroke does not sweat as much as usual, so body heat can't dissipate. The child's skin becomes flushed, hot, and often dry. Body temperature can rise to 104° to 106°F and the child can become confused or even lose consciousness. The primary goal in treating heatstroke is to lower the child's body temperature. Take the following steps right away if your child has heatstroke:

1. Call 911 (or your local emergency number).
2. Move the child into the shade or indoors and remove his or her clothing.
3. Place the child in a partially filled tub of cool (not cold) water or apply moist, cool towels or cold packs to his or her skin, putting a cloth between the cold pack and the skin. You could also spray cold water from a hose onto the child. Fan the child with a magazine or an electric fan.
4. Check the child's temperature frequently. Once the child's temperature has fallen to about 101°F, dry him

or her off to prevent the child from getting a chill. If his or her temperature begins to rise again, repeat the cooling process until medical help arrives.

Frostbite

Frostbite occurs when parts of a child's body are exposed to very cold temperatures and ice crystals form in the tissues, restricting blood flow. In the early stage, frostbitten skin is painful and red but the pain goes away as the child loses feeling in the area. The skin then turns white or grayish yellow and forms blisters. In severe cases, the skin may die and turn black. If your child has frostbite, take the following measures:

1. While outside, cover frostbitten skin with extra clothing or a blanket and bring the child indoors. Do not rub the frostbitten area.
2. Put the affected area of skin in warm water (about 100°F) or wrap it in blankets. Don't use a heating pad because it could burn frostbitten skin that has lost all sensation. Continue the warming until the skin turns pink or sensation returns.
3. Take your child to the doctor right away.

Preventing frostbite

Frostbite most often affects a child's fingers, nose, and ears. To prevent frostbite in cold weather, make sure your child wears warm mittens, a hat that covers the ears, and waterproof boots to protect the toes. Layer your child's clothing for maximum warmth.

Hypothermia

A fall in body temperature to 95°F or below is known as hypothermia, usually caused by immersion in frigid water, prolonged exposure to extremely cold weather, or wearing damp clothing in cold conditions. Hypothermia produces shivering, numbness, drowsiness, muscle weakness, and sometimes mental confusion. In severe cases, hypothermia can be life threatening. If you suspect that your child has hypothermia, call 911 (or your local emergency number) immediately and begin the following first-aid measures:

1. Maintain an open airway by laying the child on a flat surface and tilting his or her head back just until the child's ears are level with his or her shoulders. If your child has stopped breathing, perform cardiopulmonary resuscitation (see page 668).
2. Bring the child into a warm room as quickly as possible. Remove all wet clothing and wrap him or her in dry towels or blankets.
3. If the child is conscious, give him or her warm fluids, such as soup or broth, to drink. Never give alcoholic beverages to anyone with hypothermia because alcohol can cause the body to lose even more heat.
4. If the child cannot be moved indoors, cover him or her with a blanket or sleeping bag and lie close under the blanket to help warm him or her with your own body while you wait for medical help.

Glossary of common medical procedures and terms

amniocentesis A diagnostic test performed between the 14th and 18th weeks of pregnancy to detect abnormalities in the chromosomes or genes of the fetus. Using ultrasound imaging for guidance, a doctor inserts a thin, hollow needle through the woman's abdomen into the uterus and withdraws a small amount of the fluid that surrounds the fetus, which contains fetal cells. The sample is sent to a laboratory, where the cells are examined under a microscope. The sample may also be tested for elevated levels of a protein that could indicate the presence of a neural tube defect (see page 577). The test is offered to women who are at increased risk of having a baby with a genetic defect, including all women age 35 years and older.

angiogram An X-ray procedure used to diagnose and evaluate heart defects. The doctor threads a thin, flexible tube called a catheter through an artery in the upper arm or groin into a blood vessel or the heart and then injects a liquid dye. The dye allows the doctor to see the inside of the heart on an X-ray film. A child is sedated before the procedure so he or she does not feel discomfort and so that he or she will lie still during the angiogram. A local anesthetic is used at the insertion site. The procedure can take from a few minutes to 2 or 3 hours and may not require an overnight hospital stay.

antibody A protein produced by the immune system to fight a foreign substance in the body. Antibodies are formed in response to infectious organisms such as a bacterium or virus. The body also forms antibodies in response to some vaccinations, thereby acquiring lifelong or long-term protection against certain infections. Antibodies may also form in response to common substances, such as dust, producing an allergic response. The body can also form antibodies in response to transplanted tissue. Occasionally, the body mistakenly sees its own tissue as foreign and produces antibodies against it, resulting in an autoimmune disease, such as lupus (see page 556).

antitoxin A medication that is given, usually by injection, to neutralize the effects of a poison (toxin) produced by a particular bacterium, such as the one responsible for diphtheria, tetanus, or botulism. Because antitoxins don't kill the bacteria, antibiotics must also be given to eliminate the infection.

barium X-ray An imaging technique used to diagnose or monitor disorders of the digestive tract (the esophagus, stomach, and intestines) using liquid barium (a mineral that is visible on a video screen or on X-ray film) to highlight the area under examination. For a study of the esophagus, stomach, or upper part of the small intestine, the child may be asked to drink barium. For a study of the small intestine, the barium is either taken by mouth or introduced into the intestine through a thin, flexible tube called a catheter that is inserted into the mouth and threaded down the esophagus and stomach into the intestine. For a study of the colon and rectum, the barium is introduced through a catheter inserted into the rectum. The procedure is painless and does not require an overnight stay in the hospital.

biopsy A diagnostic test in which small samples of tissue or cells are removed from the body and examined under a microscope. Doctors use a biopsy to make or confirm a diagnosis of a disorder such as cancer or to evaluate or monitor an illness. Biopsies are done by cutting out a tiny piece of tissue or by withdrawing tissue or cells from the body through a hollow needle. For some biopsies, doctors obtain a tissue sample by inserting a flexible tube called an endoscope (which has a viewing lens and cutting instrument at the tip) into a natural body opening or incision.

cardiac catheterization A procedure in which a thin, flexible tube called a catheter is threaded through a blood vessel (usually in the upper arm or groin) and into the heart to monitor its functioning, to diagnose or evaluate heart defects, or to inject a liquid dye that can be seen on X-ray film. Although the procedure is painless, a young child may be given a sedative to make sure he or she lies still throughout the procedure, which can take from 1 to 3 hours.

catheter A thin, hollow, flexible tube made of plastic or rubber that is inserted into the body to drain or inject fluids, introduce medication, or help doctors evaluate disorders and perform medical procedures.

chemotherapy The use of powerful drugs to destroy cancer cells that are invading vital organs and can't be removed surgically, or that have spread from the original site to other parts of the body. Most chemotherapy drugs work by preventing cancer cells from dividing. Certain drugs may be used in combination and are either given by mouth or injected into the bloodstream or a muscle or directly into the abdomen or the fluid that surrounds the brain and spinal cord. The specific course of chemotherapy a child may undergo depends on the type of cancer, the degree of abnormal cell change, and the extent to which the cancer has spread. Chemotherapy can have side effects (see page 446).

chorionic villus sampling A diagnostic test that is performed between the 10th and 12th weeks of pregnancy to detect abnormalities of the chromosomes in the fetus. Using ultrasound imaging for guidance, the doctor inserts a thin, hollow needle through the woman's abdomen and uterus and withdraws a tiny sample of tissue from the chorionic villi, microscopic projections that form part of the placenta and contain the same genetic material as cells of the fetus. The sample can also be withdrawn through a thin, flexible tube called a catheter that is inserted through the woman's vagina into the cervix (the lower end of the uterus). The sample is then sent to a laboratory, where the cells are examined under a microscope for chromosomal abnormalities.

chromosomes Rod-shaped structures that package genes, the chemical units of heredity. Every person has 46 chromosomes (23 from each parent) inside each cell in his or her body. Because chromosomes contain so many genes, an irregularity in the number or structure of just one chromosome can interfere with the development and functioning of a fetus and have widespread effects, as in Down syndrome (see page 474).

complete blood cell count A test that measures the blood's major components, including red cells, white cells, and platelets. The test can provide much information about a child's health. For example, a low level of red blood cells indicates the presence of anemia (see page 412) and an elevated level of white blood cells indicates the presence of an infection.

computed tomography (CT) A diagnostic procedure that combines an X-ray machine with a computer to produce detailed, cross-sectional images of structures in the body. Doctors use CT scans to detect or evaluate abnormalities such as tumors, broken bones, or fluid buildup. During a CT scan, a child lies on a table that slides through a large, doughnut-shaped, rotating tube that takes a series of images. A computer transforms the images into a picture that a doctor (usually a radiologist) can interpret. The procedure is painless, takes about 30 minutes, and minimizes exposure to radiation. The confinement of being inside the tube can frighten a child, so he or she may be given a sedative so he or she will lie still during the procedure.

corticosteroids Synthetic hormones prescribed to reduce inflammation and suppress the activity of the immune system. Doctors also prescribe corticosteroids to replace the natural corticosteroids the body no longer can produce, as occurs in some disorders such as Addison's disease (see page 402). The drugs may be applied to the skin in creams, taken by mouth in pills, injected into an affected body part, transfused directly into the bloodstream, or inhaled into the airways.

culture A test used to diagnose infections by taking a sample of a disease-causing organism, such as a bacterium, from body tissue or fluid or from a wound and growing it in a nutrient-rich medium in the laboratory. Cultures help doctors identify specific infectious agents, decide whether or not to prescribe a medication, and choose what medication to prescribe.

cystogram X-ray examination of the bladder used to diagnose abnormalities of the bladder or urethra. Before the X-ray is taken, a dye that is visible on film is introduced into the bladder by way of a thin, hollow tube called a catheter. An X-ray or radionuclide scan is taken and the dye highlights the abnormality on film.

echocardiogram A test that can diagnose some heart defects using sound waves (ultrasound) to produce a picture of the structure of the heart. The image, displayed on a video monitor, shows the size, shape, and activity of the heart chambers and valves. Because the test cannot display the insides of blood vessels, a doctor may recommend another more definitive test called an angiogram to get more detailed information so he or she can make a diagnosis.

electrocardiogram (ECG or EKG) A painless test that records the flow of electricity through the heart to help doctors diagnose some heart abnormalities. Before the test, a nurse rubs a jellylike substance onto the child's chest and then places electrodes on the chest. The electrodes feed into a machine that records electrical waves from the heart's four chambers and prints out the recordings. A doctor reads the printout to determine if the heart rhythm is regular and the rhythm is coming from the proper location inside the heart.

intravenously Given through a vein. The term refers to the introduction of fluid or medication, or both, directly into a vein, usually using a needle or a thin, flexible tube called a catheter. When given intravenously, medications enter the general circulation faster than when they are taken by mouth.

lumbar puncture A procedure in which a doctor inserts a hollow needle between two bones (vertebrae) in the lower spine to remove a sample of cerebrospinal fluid (the fluid that surrounds and protects the brain and spinal cord). The sample is examined in a laboratory to help diagnose infection and evaluate the child for disorders of the brain and spinal cord. Occasionally, a lumbar puncture is also performed to inject drugs or other substances into the spinal canal. A local anesthetic is given to older children and adults before the procedure to numb the injection site. The procedure takes about 20 minutes.

magnetic resonance imaging (MRI) An imaging technique that links a powerful magnet with a computer to make detailed cross-sectional pictures of the body without X-rays or other radiation. MRIs provide sharper images than computed tomography scans and can detect less obvious injuries or abnormalities. During an MRI, a child lies on a table that slides through a large, rotating tube, which takes a series of images transformed by a computer into a picture that a doctor (usually a radiologist) can interpret. Because the confinement of being inside the tube can frighten a child, he or she may be given a sedative so he or she will lie still during the procedure, which takes about 30 minutes.

outpatient A patient who receives a test or procedure that is given in a doctor's office or clinic and does not require an overnight stay in the hospital. Increasing numbers of surgical procedures and diagnostic tests are done on an outpatient basis.

positron emission tomography (PET) A computerized imaging technique that produces two- or three-dimensional color-coded images that show the functioning of body organs or tissues. PET scans are usually used to diagnose disorders of the brain, heart, or blood vessels or to detect and evaluate cancerous tumors. The technique uses safe doses of very short-acting radioactive substances called radioisotopes that are injected or inhaled into the body. During a PET scan, a child lies on a table that slides into a doughnut-shaped scanning machine. The machine detects the radioisotopes as they are absorbed by the targeted organ or tissue and converts the information into a color image on a computer monitor that a doctor (usually a radiologist) can interpret. The test is painless and the amount of radiation exposure is minimal–roughly equal to that from two chest X-rays.

radiation The use of high-powered X-rays or radioactive implants to kill cancer cells at specific sites in the body. The radiation may be delivered by a machine that directs X-ray beams at the cancerous tissue. This kind of radiation therapy is usually done on an outpatient basis 5 days a week for several weeks. Radioactive implants can also be placed inside the body next to the cancerous tumor to provide a continuous, high dose of radiation designed to shrink the tumor. This type of radiation therapy usually requires a hospital stay. The radioactive material is left in place for 1 to 2 days and then removed. Both forms of radiation therapy have side effects.

radionuclide scan A painless diagnostic imaging technique that measures levels of radioactivity in targeted organs after a person has been given a mildly radioactive substance (radionuclide) by mouth or injection. A special device called a gamma camera detects the amount of radiation in the organ and a computer converts the information into an image that shows the functioning of the organ or tissue. Doctors use the technique to diagnose disorders such as infections and to detect and evaluate cancers. Because the amount of radiation in the substances is low, the procedure is harmless. A radionuclide scan can take from 1 to 5 hours.

toxins Poisonous substances produced by bacteria, insects, animals such as venomous snakes, and some plants. Exposure to a toxin can stimulate the immune system to produce antibodies to fight it. The effects of such exposure can vary from mild to life threatening.

ultrasound An imaging technique that uses high-frequency sound waves to create a picture of internal organs on a video screen. During an ultrasound, a child lies on an examining table and a doctor or ultrasound technician rubs a gel on the skin over the area of the body to be studied. The gel improves contact between the skin and the ultrasound transducer, a handheld wand that transmits sound waves as it is moved over the skin. The sound waves are converted into an image that the doctor (usually a radiologist) can interpret to diagnose, evaluate, or monitor an illness. Ultrasound scans do not use radiation and are very safe.

Index

A

D

E

F

G

H

I

J

K

L

M

N

O

P

R

S

T

U

V

W

Y